wk2

3 - 9, 18, 20
6 - 12
7 - 13, 17
8 - 5, 7, 8
9 - 21, 22

Handbook of
Evidence-Based
Therapies for Children
and Adolescents

Issues in Clinical Child Psychology

Series Editor: **Michael C. Roberts,** *University of Kansas—Lawrence, Kansas*

A continuation Order Plan is available for this series. A continuation order will bring delivery of each new volume immediately upon publication. Volumes are billed only upon actual shipment. For further information please contact the publisher.

Handbook of Evidence-Based Therapies for Children and Adolescents

Bridging Science and Practice

Edited by

Ric G. Steele
University of Kansas
Lawrence, Kansas

T. David Elkin
University of Mississippi
Jackson, Mississippi

Michael C. Roberts
University of Kansas
Lawrence, Kansas

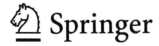 Springer

Ric G. Steele
Clinical Child Psychology Program
University of Kansas
Lawrence, KS 66045, USA
rsteele@ku.edu

T. David Elkin
Department of Psychiatry &
 Human Behavior
University of Mississippi
Jackson, MS, 39216, USA
delkin@psychiatry.umsmed.edu

Michael C. Roberts
Clinical Child Psychology Program
University of Kansas
Lawrence, KS 66045, USA
mroberts@ku.edu

ISBN: 978-0-387-73690-7   e-ISBN: 978-0-387-73691-4

Library of Congress Control Number: 2007934759

Printed on acid-free paper.

9 8 7 6 5 4 3 2 1

springer.com

RGS

To my parents, Ric and Sandra Steele, for their love and support.

TDE

To my parents, Mary and Tom Elkin, Ph.D. I told them I never wanted to be a psychologist. And to The Girls: Allie, Bailey Grace, Emma, Sarah, and Claire. SDG.

MCR

To my grandson, Caden, who rocks my world.

Contents

I

Establishing the Need and Criteria for Evidence-Based Therapies

1

Evidence-Based Therapies for Children and Adolescents: Problems and Prospects

RIC G. STEELE, MICHAEL C. ROBERTS, and T. DAVID ELKIN

In the last U.S. Surgeon General's report addressing the issue of children's mental health, David Satcher, M.D., Ph.D., estimated that approximately 20% of children and adolescents in the United States have mild to moderate symptoms of mental illness and that approximately 1 in 10 children has significant emotional health concerns that warrant professional intervention (U.S. Department of Health and Human Services, 1999). These figures are consistent with both earlier and subsequent estimates of mental health needs among school-aged children (e.g., Costello et al., 1996; Roberts et al., 1998; Sturm et al., 2003). More alarming, however, are reports indicating that between 65 and 80% of U.S. youth who need mental health services do not receive them (Kataoka et al., 2002; Sturm et al., 2003).

In a recent review and commentary addressing the disparity between mental health needs and services for youth, Knitzer and Cooper (2006) outlined several specific policy directives with the potential to expand and improve such services. Included in this list was the challenge of "overcoming obstacles to the adoption of evidence-based practices" (p. 674). In his response, Friedman (2006) noted some of the specifics of these obstacles, including the need for expanded evidence-based practices for use with various populations, improved access to information about evidence-based therapies (EBTs), and the identification and evaluation of

RIC G. STEELE, MICHAEL C. ROBERTS • University of Kansas and **T. DAVID ELKIN** • University of Mississippi Medical Center

innovative and promising interventions that are emerging from the literature. In many ways, these challenges are both the impetus and the outline for the current volume.

The primary purpose of the handbook is to provide a comprehensive review of evidence-based therapies across numerous disorders and conditions affecting children and adolescents. Consistent with the call for an expanded view of EBTs and with the need for identification of emerging and promising new therapies (Friedman, 2006), contributors to this volume were asked to include not just therapies with the highest levels of empirical support (i.e., "well-established" therapies; Chambless & Hollon, 1998), but also "possibly efficacious" and "promising" therapies. Recognizing that there are conditions for which there are no "well-established" therapies, our goal was to provide clinicians with the "best available evidence" (American Psychological Association, 2006, p. 278) for treatment options and, at the same time, alert clinical researchers to areas that are in need of further investigation and development.

We also approached this handbook with the goal of helping bridge the gap between clinical research and clinical practice. Evidence from a variety of sources suggests that practicing mental health professionals may not be utilizing EBTs to the extent that they could (e.g., Kazdin et al., 1990; Nelson et al., 2006; Sheehan et al., 2007). Supposing that this gap is due (in part) to a lack of information on EBTs among practicing mental health providers, the most recent APA criteria for accreditation in clinical, school, and counseling psychology specifically call for "training in empirically supported procedures" (APA, 2002). Despite this call, a recent APA resolution (2004) has noted a specific shortage in clinicians' access to appropriate evidence-based promotion, prevention, and treatment services for children and adolescents in particular.

We see this volume as having particular value in training programs, not just because of the coverage of the EBTs themselves, but also because of the focus that we placed on training issues. For example, Chapter 31 (Leffingwell & Collins) highlights promising approaches for teaching EBTs in graduate training programs. Beyond the chapter specifically on graduate training programs, however, this volume also addresses training issues by its inclusion of chapters on flexible implementation of EBTs (Chapter 25; Southam-Gerow et al.), the importance of therapist, client, and process variables (Chapter 26; Shirk & McMakin), key ethical issues that relate to the implementation of EBTs (Chapter 28; Rae & Fournier), and the importance of evidence-based assessment (Chapter 30; Phares & Curley).

In addition to graduate training programs, mental health service organizations and infrastructures also play a vital role in the dissemination of information regarding EBTs. Recent data indicate that prior training (e.g., taking a class in EBTs) and perceived institutional openness to EBTs accounted for approximately the same amount of variance in practitioners' self-reported EBT use (Nelson & Steele, 2007). Similarly, Sheehan and colleagues (2007) reported that agency-sponsored trainings were identified as the source of information about EBTs at approximately the same rate (on average) as respondents' graduate training programs. Such findings (as well as the shift toward economic policies that favor evidence-based practices; cf. Garber, 2001) underscore the need for mental health service administrators, directors, and training coordinators to be knowledgeable of current and emerging EBTs and to promote an institutional culture that is supportive of such therapies. In response to these needs, the current volume includes chapters designed to assist community mental health centers implement EBTs (Chapter 29; Smith-Boydston & Nelson) and to help individual therapists implement EBTs in "real-world" settings (Chapter 4; Higa & Chorpita) and within diverse populations (Chapter 27; Kotchick & Grover).

At its core, the EBT movement is concerned with ensuring that psychotherapies offered to individuals have adequate evidence for their effectiveness. Although this goal seems fairly straightforward, the movement is not without its critics. A number of authors have raised strong objections to an "overreliance" on the EBT or EST literature (Garfield, 1996; Levant, 2004; Persons & Silberschatz, 1998; Strupp, 2001). Authors have frequently raised concerns about the use of manualized treatments that may not be responsive to the session-to-session issues brought to therapy, a lack of attention to client-therapist relationships, and a failure to make "course alterations" when a given EBT is not producing results.

In our view, part of the controversy surrounding the implementation of EBTs can be attributed to a set of assumptions that may have been made by the APA Task Force on Promotion and Dissemination of Psychological Procedures (1995) and early proponents of empirically supported therapies (ESTs; Chambless et al., 1996). We liken these assumptions to those made by authors of cookbooks or textbooks on cooking. Although most would recognize the necessity of an oven and utensils to cook a chocolate soufflé, it would seem strange for such books to instruct the reader to "go to the kitchen" or to "remove the cooking utensils from the drawers." We take it for granted that someone cooking a soufflé would be in a kitchen with an oven and would possess the appropriate utensils.

Perhaps this is an oversimplification, but we believe the early writers on ESTs took it for granted that professional psychologists would (by virtue of their training as professional psychologists) be responsive to the idiosyncratic and dynamic needs of individual clients, practice the therapy in the context of a therapeutic relationship, and be sensitive to indications that a particular therapy might not be working well with a particular client. Indeed, Diane Chambless (2007), the chair of the original Division 12 Task Force, recognized that "ESTs are not a substitute for training in building a relationship with the client" and fully endorsed that therapeutic alliance and other process research is important to help ensure that students can form an effective working alliance with their clients. In retrospect, we wonder whether some of the controversy surrounding the identification and promotion of EBTs might have been alleviated if these assumptions had been more clearly articulated earlier in the discussion.

On the other hand, many important issues have been raised by opponents of the EBT movement. And, to some degree, the movement to the broader concept of evidence-based practice (APA, 2006) expands to explicitly include two additional elements of clinical expertise and patient characteristics—values and context—along with the best research evidence of ESTs. Granted, there is much less research into these additional elements. In our view, there is more scientific support currently for the evidence-based therapeutic approaches than for the other two EBT components, clinical expertise and client/patient values and preferences. These latter two components of the "three-legged stool" require much more empirical attention. Questions of how to inculcate expertise and competence, how to measure such competence, and how to maintain it over the therapist's career require considerably more scientific effort (Roberts et al., 2005). Questions of what are the relevant patient values, under what circumstances, for what problems, and how are they measured and integrated into professional practice are similarly less well developed but necessitate the attention of clinical researchers. Culture is one important "value" variable; treatment acceptability and therapeutic relationship are others. Throughout this book, we and the chapter authors have tried to make these issues more clearly linked—several chapters attempt to demonstrate the integral nature of these components. But we rely on the cliché that most clinical researchers and practitioners use at some point or another: *More research needs to be done.*

Rather than organizing the book into proponents versus opponents, we see a more valuable approach for the field is to advance the dialogue by demonstrating integration—forming into sides has fractionated professional psychology almost more than anything else has. Of course, the reaction and responses to each position have helped demonstrate points at which greater attention in research needs to be focused and where grater clarity in communication needs to be articulated. As in the case of negative reactions to manualized treatments, the objections helped advance the dialogue through responses such as by Kendall and Beidas (2007) calling for "flexibility within fidelity." If professionals are willing to listen with the same open ears they endeavor to use in therapy, they might not have as strong a reaction as they expressed toward the clinical researchers. If "opponents" of ESTs are not cast as "anti-science," and if the profession can lower the decibels so that communication can take place, then diplomacy might help the field become more amenable to advancement for the benefit of the profession and the clients we serve.

REFERENCES

American Psychological Association (2002). *Guidelines and Procedures for Accreditation of Programs in Professional Psychology.* Washington, DC.

American Psychological Association (2005). *Policy Statement on Evidence-Based Practice in Psychology.* Accessed on January 6, 2007, from http://www.apa.org/practice/ebpstatement.pdf.

American Psychological Association Presidential Task Force on Evidence-Based Practice (2006). Evidence-based practice in psychology. *American Psychologist, 61,* 271–285.

American Psychological Association (2004, February). *Resolution on Children's Mental Health approved by Council of Representatives.* Washington, DC.

Chambless, D. L. (2007). The role of empirically-supported treatments in teaching evidence-based practice. Paper presented at the annual meeting of the Council of University Directors of Clinical Psychology, Savannah, GA, January. PowerPoint slides retrieved February 10, 2007, from www.cudcp.org.

Chambless, D. L., & Hollon, S. D. (1998). Defining empirically supported therapies. *Journal of Consulting and Clinical Psychology, 66,* 7–18.

Chambless, D. L., Sanderson, W. C., Shaham, V., Bennett Johnson, S., Pope, K. S., Crits-Christoph, P., et al. (1996). An update on empirically validated therapies. *Clinical Psychologist, 49,* 5–18.

Costello, E. J., Angold, A., Burns, B. J., Erkanli, A., Stangl, D. K., & Tweed, D. L. (1996). The Great Smokey Mountains Study of Youth: Functional impairment and serious emotional disturbance. *Archives of General Psychiatry, 53,* 1137–1143.

Division 12 of the American Psychological Association Task Force on Promotion and Dissemination of Psychological Procedures. (1995). Training in and dissemination of empirically-validated psychological treatments: Report and recommendations. *The Clinical Psychologist, 48,* 3–23.

Friedman, R. M. (2006). Children's mental health: A discussion and elaboration on Knitzer and Cooper's article. *Data Trends, 137,* 1–7. Accessed on January 8, 2007, from http://datatrends.fmhi.usf.edu/summary_137.pdf.

Garber, A. M. (2001). Evidence-based coverage policy. *Health Affairs, 20,* 1–21. Accessed on February 12, 2007, from http://content.healthaffairs.org/cgi/reprint/20/5/62.pdf.

Garfield, S. L. (1996). Some problems associated with "validated" forms of psychotherapy. *Clinical Psychology: Science and Practice, 3,* 218–229.

Kataoka, S. H., Zhang, L., & Wells, K. B. (2002). Unmet need for mental health care among U.S. children: Variation by ethnicity and insurance status. *American Journal of Psychiatry, 159,* 1548–1555.

Kazdin, A. E., Siegel. T. C., & Bass, D. (1990). Drawing upon clinical practice to inform research on child and adolescent psychotherapy: A survey of practitioners. *Professional Psychology: Research and Practice, 21,* 189–198.

Kazdin, A. E., & Weisz, J. R. (1998). Identifying and developing empirically supported child and adolescent treatments. *Journal of Consulting and Clinical Psychology, 66,* 19–36.

Kendall, P. C., & Beidas, R. S. (2007). Smoothing the trail for dissemination of evidence-based practices for youth: Flexibility within fidelity. *Professional Psychology: Research and Practice, 38,* 13–20.

Knitzer, J., & Cooper, J. (2006). Beyond integration: Challenges for children's mental health. *Health Affairs, 25,* 670–679.

Levant, R. F. (2004). The empirically validated treatments movement: A practitioner/educator perspective. *Clinical Psychology: Science and Practice, 11,* 219–224.

Nelson, T. D., & Steele, R. G. (2007). Predictors of practitioner self-reported use of evidence-based practices: Practitioner training, clinical setting, and attitudes toward research. *Administration and Policy in Mental Health and Mental Health Services Research, 34,* 319–330.

Nelson, T. D., Steele, R. G., & Mize, J. (2006). Practitioner attitudes toward evidence-based practice: Themes and challenges. *Administration and Policy in Mental Health and Mental Health Services Research, 33 ,* 398–409.

Persons, J. B., & Silberschatz, G. (1998). Are results of randomized controlled trials useful to psychotherapists? *Journal of Consulting and Clinical Psychology, 66,* 126–135.

Roberts, M. C., Borden, K. A., Christiansen, M. D., & Lopez, S. J. (2005). Fostering a culture shift: Assessment of competence in the education and careers of professional psychologists. *Professional Psychology: Research and Practice, 36,* 355–361.

Roberts, R. E., Attkisson, C. C., & Rosenblatt, A. (1998). Prevalence of psychopathology among children and adolescents. *American Journal of Psychiatry, 155,* 715–725.

Sheehan, A. K., Walrath, C. M., & Holden, E. W. (2007). Evidence-based practice use, training, and implementation in the community-based service setting: A survey of children's mental health service providers. *Journal of Child and Family Studies, 16,* 169–182.

Strupp, H. H. (2001). Implications of the empirically supported treatment movement for psychoanalysis. *Psychoanalytic Dialogues, 11,* 615–619.

Sturm, R., Ringel, J. S., & Andreyeva, T. (2003). Geographic disparities in children's mental health care. *Pediatrics, 112,* e308–e315. Accessed on January 8, 2007, from http://www.pediatrics.org/cgi/content/full/112/4/e308.

U.S. Department of Health and Human Services (1999). *Mental health: A Report of the Surgeon General.* Rockville, MD: U.S. Department of Health and Human Services, Substance Abuse and Mental Health Services Administration, Center for Mental Health Services, National Institutes of Health, National Institute of Mental Health.

2

Empirically Supported Treatments and Evidence-Based Practice for Children and Adolescents

MICHAEL C. ROBERTS and ROCHELLE L. JAMES

A number of forces exert influence on professional psychology. Though these forces change over time, they continue to impact all aspects of the field. Psychologists recognized that the mental health professions had not yet developed an adequate scientific base for making treatment decisions and demonstrating the "worth" of psychological interventions. The rise of managed care concomitantly compelled many changes in the way psychologists provided treatment and were reimbursed (Roberts & Hurley, 1997). Increasing demands were made for evidence that psychological treatments would work if they were to be eligible for payment. As outlined by Steele and Roberts (2003), the movement toward empirically supported treatments (ESTs) and, correspondingly, evidence-based practice (EBP) came from

> (a) a strong desire on the part of psychologists oriented to the scientist-practitioner model to enhance the scientific base for clinical practice (Calhoun et al., 1998; Davison, 1998); (b) a focus on accountability in both practice and research (Weisz et al., 2000); and (c) the policies of managed care organizations, which increasingly provide financial reimbursements only to those therapies and interventions with established utility. (p. 308)

Although market forces might appear to be a driving force, initiatives internal to psychology motivated much of the effort, specifically; these

---

MICHAEL C. ROBERTS and ROCHELLE L. JAMES • University of Kansas, Clinical Child Psychology Program

included the scientist-practitioner model of integration in which science informs practice, which informs science in a reciprocating process.

The immense need for effective interventions has not abated over the decades of developments in mental health, especially for children and adolescents, who have been chronically underserved (Steele & Roberts, 2005). Although various efforts have been made over time to develop and evaluate effective treatments (e.g., Eysenck, 1952; Levitt, 1957, 1963), nothing seems to have catalyzed the profession to take action more than the efforts of the Task Force on Promotion and Dissemination of Psychological Procedures of the Division of Clinical Psychology of the American Psychological Association (APA). The task force established criteria that it used to identify and categorize effective treatments for specific disorders (Chambless et al., 1996, 1998). These designations were initially "empirically validated" with a later change in terminology to "empirically supported treatments," or ESTs. As will be examined later, reactions, both favorable and unfavorable, were swift and ongoing. Although the initial focus had been mostly on treatments for adults, the subsequent efforts, including ones by specialty practice divisions of the APA, extended the identification of ESTs to child/adolescent and pediatric psychology treatments (Kazdin & Weisz, 1998; Lonigan et al., 1998; Spirito, 1999).

EMPIRICALLY SUPPORTED TREATMENTS

In 1993, the APA Division of Clinical Psychology (Division 12) organized a Task Force on Promotion and Dissemination of Psychological Procedures, headed by Dianne Chambless. This task force examined and reported on the ways by which information about empirically validated treatments, later termed "empirically supported treatments," is disseminated to clinical psychology students, practicing clinical psychologists, third-party payers, and the general public. Subsequently, Division 12 approved the task force's report and published it in *The Clinical Psychologist* (Task Force, 1995). In this report, the task force delineated three categories and their criteria for classifying the treatments based on their level of empirical support. The criteria for well-established treatments required two studies using a between-group design from different researchers that demonstrate efficacy of treatment (demonstrating superiority to pill or psychological placebo or to another treatment and/or demonstrating equivalence to an established treatment) or a series of studies using a single-case design that demonstrated efficacy of treatment utilizing a rigorous experimental designs as well as a comparison of treatment intervention to another). In these criteria, the treatments must have manuals to guide implementation and permit replication. In all studies, the client characteristics must be detailed. To meet the criteria for the category of "probably efficacious," there needs to be two studies demonstrating treatment produced more effective outcomes than a control group, two studies from the same researchers meeting the well-established treatments criteria, or a small series of single-case design experiments. The third category, experimental treatments, refers to psychotherapies that do not meet the criteria for either of the two higher-level categories. The task force also listed 25 specific treatments that met its criteria for empirical support (Task Force, 1995).

As an additional component of its activities, the task force developed a list of treatments, including the 25 ESTs as well as other treatments, in which clinical psychology doctoral students and interns might obtain instruction or training. The task force surveyed clinical training directors and internship directors of APA-approved sites in regards to which of these treatments are included in the training of their students or interns. One in five APA-approved clinical programs failed to provide even minimal coverage of ESTs in their courses and practicum. In addition, most internships did not require competence in an EST. In light of these findings, the task force put forth several recommendations for training at the predoctoral, internship, and continuing education levels. A number of recommendations concerning the dissemination of information about ESTs to clinicians, third-party payers, and the public were also laid out in the task force's report (Task Force, 1995).

Following the 1995 Task Force report, Chambless and colleagues published updates on ESTs in both 1996 and 1998. The first update expanded the list of ESTs and attempted to clear up misconceptions about their use. The focus of this report lay in discussing the use of ESTs with ethnic minority individuals and the effects of the interplay of aptitude and treatment on treatment outcome (Chambless et al., 1996). The second update in 1998 reviewed the procedure for evaluating treatments according to the criteria as well as expanded the list of ESTs, particularly in the areas of couples and family therapies to treat psychological disorders, treatments for those with severe mental illness, and health psychology interventions (Chambless et al., 1998).

The discussion and evaluation of ESTs have rapidly increased since then as evidenced by several prominent journals dedicating special sections to the topic of ESTs. A special section of the *Journal of Consulting and Clinical Psychology* (1998) included articles evaluating specific areas of psychosocial interventions, such as child and adolescent treatments (Kazdin & Weisz, 1998), and articles commenting on issues related to ESTs (e.g., Calhoun et al., 1998). After the Chambless Task Force, another task force was formed to focus more specifically on empirically supported interventions for children and adolescents (Lonigan et al., 1998). The reports of this child-focused task force were published in a special issue of the *Journal of Clinical Child Psychology* (1998). This series of articles covered ESTs for children and adolescents with depression (Kaslow & Thompson, 1998), phobia and anxiety disorders (Ollendick & King, 1998), autism (Rogers, 1998), conduct disorder (Brestan & Eyberg, 1998), and attention deficit hyperactivity disorder (Pelham et al., 1998). The *Journal of Pediatric Psychology* also devoted several special sections (1999–2000) to ESTs for pediatric problems such as recurrent pediatric headache (Holden et al., 1999); recurrent abdominal pain (Janicke & Finney, 1999); procedure-related pain (Powers, 1999); disease-related pain (Walco et al., 1999); severe feeding problems (Kerwin, 1999); pediatric obesity (Jelalian &

Saelens, 1999); disease-related symptoms of asthma, diabetes, and cancer (McQuaid & Nassau, 1999); bedtime refusal and night waking (Mindell, 1999); nocturnal enuresis (Mellon & McGrath, 2000); and constipation and encopresis (McGrath et al., 2000).

In addition, several books provide detailed descriptions of treatments and their empirical support for each of a wide range of psychological problems. For example, *What Works for Whom?* by Roth and Fonagy (2005) provided evidence toward answering the question of which psychosocial treatments have been shown to be beneficial for which client populations. Books more specific to the psychological problems of childhood and adolescence include *What Works for Whom? A Critical Review of Treatments for Children and Adolescents* by Fonagy et al. (2002) and *Psychosocial Treatments for Child and Adolescent Disorders: Empirically Based Strategies for Clinical Practice* by Hibbs and Jensen (2005).

In the expanding discussions on ESTs, Chambless and Ollendick (2001) reviewed the criteria and treatments described by several task forces and other work groups and found that the various groups used slightly different criteria when classifying treatments. Nonetheless, different groups reviewing the same treatment generally came to compatible conclusions about that treatment's level of empirical support. Chambless and Ollendick integrated these various criteria into three general categories of empirical support and identified 108 adult and 37 child treatments as Category I or Category II ESTs. Thus, the number of treatments demonstrating substantial empirically support has multiplied well beyond the 25 ESTs listed by the original 1995 task force.

EVIDENCE-BASED PRACTICE

The concept and terminology of "evidence-based practice" (EBP) provide a more encompassing approach to applying research-based information to practice. Deriving from evidence-based movements in other countries and in American medicine, this concept has been embraced by most, if not all, health-care provider professions. In 2005, the Presidential Task Force on Evidence-Based Practice of the American Psychological Association (APA) was appointed to develop a position statement regarding the integration of science and practice for health services provided by professional psychologists. The work of the task force resulted in a policy statement approved as APA policy by the Council of Representatives (July 2005) and a full report published in the *American Psychologist* (APA Presidential Task Force on Evidence-Based Practice, 2006). While noting some of the controversy, the report provided the following definition: "Evidence-based practice in psychology (EBPP) is the integration of the best available research with clinical expertise in the context of patient characteristics, culture, and preferences" (APA Presidential Task Force on Evidence-Based Practice, 2006, p. 273). As the task force noted, the psychology position emphasized clinical expertise and gave broader attention to patient characteristics than the definition of EBP from the Institute of Medicine (IOM, 2001):

"Evidence-based practice is the integration of best research evidence with clinical expertise and patient values" (p. 147). Although the IOM definition moderated scientific evidence by clinical expertise and patient values, in effect, the psychology definition gave equal weight to science, clinician's expertise, and patient characteristics. Hence, the metaphor of a "three-legged stool" or "pyramid" has been used to describe equal footing, or balance, for the three components of EBP, at least for psychology.

The task force report on EBP described "best research evidence" as deriving from a variety of research strategies including clinical observations, qualitative research, systematic case studies, single-case designs, public health and ethnographic research, therapy process and outcome studies, randomized clinical trials (RCTs), and meta-analyses (p. 274). The report also defined clinical expertise as "competence attained by psychologists through education, training, and experience that results in effective practice" (p. 275) and outlined the components to include (1) case formulation and planned treatment based on assessment and diagnostic judgment, (2) skillful treatment provision and decision making with monitoring of progress, (3) interpersonal skills to develop a therapeutic relationship, (4) self-reflection and skill development, (5) consideration of research evidence, (6) awareness of influence from "individual, cultural, and contextual differences" (p. 277), (7) seeking other resources such as consultation and adjunctive services, and (8) having a "cogent rationale for clinical strategies" (p. 278). Patient characteristics include attention to the patient's belief systems and worldview, personal goals, perceptions of problems and treatment, personal situation, social and cultural characteristics (e.g., gender/ethnicity, race, and social class), developmental considerations, and variations in the way disorders are manifested. The report concluded that "the purpose of EBPP is to promote effective psychological practice and enhance public health by applying empirically supported principles of psychological assessment, case formulation, therapeutic relationship, and intervention" (p. 280).

Reactions to the EBP resolution and report (as well as to the drafts) included calls for changing the report, from those who wished to have greater emphasis on RCTs and those who wished to diminish any emphasis on them, from those who wanted ESTs to be recognized and those who wished to avoid "cookbook" psychotherapy viewed by them as promulgated by manualized treatments in RCTs, and from those who wanted less importance given to clinical expertise and those who wanted statements included such as "we [psychologists] are competent, we know what we're doing, and we do it well." The task force responded with the philosophy of balance—not privileging one component in the three parts of EBP: research base, clinical expertise, and patient characteristics. The EBP resolution was approved by the Council of Representatives with a strong endorsement, but many in the profession recognize it as a statement dominated by political realities within the organization. The EBP position statement does not endorse any particular treatment but points to a broader integration of all components. The EBP statement also does not establish any criteria by which to judge the applicability of interventions, approaches, or sets of information for the clinician to use. In 2006, another APA task force was formed to apply EBP principles to children, adolescents, and their families.

Other health-care professions have also adopted an orientation to evidence-based practice including various subfields of medicine, nursing, occupational therapy, physical therapy, public health, social work, rehabilitation, special education, speech/language/hearing specialists, and developmental disabilities (and even the nonhealth professions of librarian/information specialists). Additionally, other countries including Germany, the United Kingdom, Australia, and New Zealand have promoted EBP concepts. Canadian psychology, for example, through the Canadian Psychological Association (Section on Clinical Psychology) and the Canadian Register of Health Service Providers in Psychology, has taken initiatives to advance EBP through its policy and educational efforts.

Many aspects of EST can be incorporated into EBP, but they are not the same and will be treated distinctively. As perhaps a less rigorous approach, the EBP orientation may be less offensive to some in psychology who objected to what was perceived as an overreliance on empirically derived information of the EST movement and the neglect of the clinician's expertise and experience.

PROGRESS TOWARD DISSEMINATION AND ADOPTION OF ESTS FOR CHILDREN AND ADOLESCENTS

While clinical child psychology has made substantial progress in identifying and evaluating ESTs for children, the field has lagged behind adult-focused clinical psychology in the dissemination of its treatments during the years following the 1995 Task Force report. Herschell et al. (2004) conducted two reviews of publications from January 1995 through December 1999 that provided evidence to this effect. First, their PsycINFO search revealed that six of the seven empirical studies associated with EST dissemination focused on treatments for adults. Second, their survey of publications in the *Journal of Clinical Child Psychology* and the *Journal of Consulting and Clinical Psychology* found that, compared to child treatments, adult treatments were the focus of twice as many treatment evaluation and dissemination articles.

Several individual professionals, specialty workgroups, system reform projects, and national organizations have made substantial effort to close this gap between child and adult dissemination progress. For example, at the national level, the *Report of the Surgeon General's Conference on Children's Mental Health: A National Agenda* (U.S. Public Health Service, 2000) and the National Institute of Mental Health's (NIMH) *Blueprint for Change: Research on Child and Adolescent Mental Health* (2001) encouraged the development, implementation, and dissemination of ESTs as necessary for the progress of children's mental health. Yet, much improvement still needs to be done in the dissemination of child-focused ESTs.

Herschell et al. (2004) reviewed four methods that can be used to increase the dissemination of ESTs for children. First, treatment manuals give detailed descriptions of session activities, which facilitate standardizing treatment and maintaining treatment fidelity. Herschell et al. recommended that treatment manuals be more user-friendly for clinicians by including information on development, theory, therapeutic process factors, procedures for integrating various systems, and strategies for developing positive relationships with clients. For each session, treatment manuals should also contain integrity checklists and measures of therapist adherence and ability (Herschell et al., 2004).

Second, graduate education can serve an important role in disseminating ESTs to the future professionals of the field. Training in ESTs should begin early in students' graduate careers so that students may acquire an understanding of how flexibility and creativity play a part in the effective use of ESTs. Such training should consist of didactic classes covering a wide range of ESTs and supervised practicum experiences utilizing ESTs. It was even proposed that evidence of competency in a child EST be added to the graduation requirements (Herschell et al., 2004). In a survey of 172 doctoral students from 60 APA-accredited clinical, counseling, and school psychology programs, Karekla et al. (2004) found that early didactic and practicum training in ESTs and treatment manuals predicted a more positive attitude toward ESTs and manuals. In addition, those students who received early EST training were more likely to have plans to use ESTs and obtain additional training in ESTs in the future. In a 10-year follow-up to the 1995 Task Force survey, Woody et al. (2005) found that APA-accredited clinical psychology doctoral and predoctoral internship programs have increased EST dissemination through didactic training. However, supervised training in ESTs has decreased, with fewer than half of programs now providing it.

Third, continuing education (CE) can be used as a method of disseminating ESTs to clinical practitioners. Longer, more comprehensive CE formats that include follow-up components would provide additional opportunities for supervision to ensure that skills have been acquired and are being used properly. Advances in communication technology such as videoconferencing can also be utilized to provide CE to clinical practitioners in various locations and aid in making follow-up CE sessions possible (Herschell et al., 2004). Herschell et al. (2004) also suggested that APA provide more monitoring of CE and that states require clinicians who treat children to complete at least some of their CE credits in child ESTs. Focusing a series of CE workshops on a particular child EST would allow clinical practitioners the chance for more in-depth learning about an EST that they may wish to use with their clients.

Fourth, empirically supported training protocols can provide effective methods for using training as an EST dissemination tool (Herschell et al., 2004). Two types of research are needed in this area. Investigations of preexisting protocols' effectiveness need to be conducted. Analyses of training components are necessary to determine the critical components related to effectiveness, which would allow EST training protocols to be streamlined (Herschell et al., 2004).

In addition to improving these four dissemination strategies, there are several areas for future progress in dissemination of ESTs for children, including improvements in both research and theory; collaborations among researchers, clinicians, and policy makers; and the utilization of technology methods for dissemination. Herschell et al. (2004) called for more empirical examination of the processes by which ESTs for children can be disseminated, transported to community settings, and used effectively with those child populations that are underrepresented in the current research. Silverman et al. (2004) responded to this petition for more basic research with their own call for the development of more basic theory on effectiveness, transportability, and dissemination to explain the mechanisms by which they work and to direct research in these areas. Thus, clinical child psychology should build on its existing strengths such as its firm basis in highly developed theory as well as its focus on prevention programs and separate identity from downwardly extended adult treatments (Herschell et al., 2004).

Researchers, clinicians, and policy makers need to collaborate so that research is informed by practice, funding opportunities are available for research, and practice and public policy are grounded in empirical evidence. Practice research networks are models of such collaboration, such as outlined by Borkovec (2002, 2004). Similarly, Weisz and colleagues have proposed methods of collaboration between researchers and clinicians (Weisz & Addis, 2006; Weisz et al., 2004). Also, the utilization of technology methods such as audiotapes, videotapes, interactive CDs, the Internet, and telehealth will become increasingly useful in communicating information about ESTs in the future (Herschell et al., 2004). For example, Ollendick and Davis (2004) described a Web-based strategy that should facilitate clinical practitioners' ability to efficiently search through research literature and evaluate the evidence for particular treatments.

Weisz et al. (2004) also provided recommendations for future efforts in the dissemination of ESTs and EBP. Professionals in the field of psychology as well as across disciplines need to come to a consensus on the methods and criteria for identifying ESTs and the treatments classified as ESTs. Dissemination of ESTs must be accompanied by the dissemination of those empirically robust assessment and diagnosis procedures. Besides ESTs, EBP requires intermittent assessment to evaluate whether the treatment being employed is actually benefiting the client as well as modification of intervention strategies when indicated. Unfortunately, this process of "assess-treat-reassess-adjust treatment" has not yet become standard practice (Weisz et al., 2004, p. 303). This continual evaluation of outcomes should be conducted on all evidence-based practice. In contrast to the traditional medical-pharmaceutical model, Weisz et al. (2004) proposed a "deployment-focused model of intervention development and testing (p. 304)." In this model, constant collaboration between researchers and clinicians allows for the development of practice-ready treatments and the generation of empirical evidence in real-world settings for the effectiveness of the treatment as a whole as well as the individual components and mechanisms of change that contribute most to treatment gains. Consistent with Weisz et al.'s deployment-focused model, Shirk (2004) advocated for effectiveness trials as the next step in dissemination but cautioned researchers that they might have to challenge those beliefs of practitioners that pose a barrier to disseminating ESTs in clinic settings.

The actions the State of Hawaii took to comply with the Felix Consent Decree provide an example of large-scale efforts to address questions of treatment effectiveness and practitioner skepticism of outcome research. In 1994, the Felix Consent Decree outlined the settlement of a class action lawsuit brought against the State of Hawaii in federal court regarding the mental health services received by children with special needs in the state education system. This settlement mandated the State of Hawaii to establish a statewide system of care to provide children with all the mental health services they need to be able to benefit from their free public education (Chorpita et al., 2002). To develop a system of care, the state founded several local Family Guidance Centers (FGCS); contracted with private agencies to provide services; cultivated partnerships among the mental health system, the university, and the families of the children being served; and increased the quantity of services available to meet the rising need. Then, in October 1999, Hawaii's Child and Adolescent Mental Health Division (CAMHD) addressed the quality of services when it launched the Empirical Basis to Services (EBS) Task Force. The EBS Task Force employed a similar methodology as the national-level APA Division 12 task forces as well as extended their efforts by evaluating the effectiveness of treatments for children. In addition to publishing the findings, CAMHD took further steps to ensure the dissemination of ESTs to practitioners statewide by distributing easy-to-use practice guidelines, providing training and consultation in implementation of specific ESTs, and conducting quarterly assessments of treatment outcomes (Chorpita & Donkervoet, 2005; Chorpita et al., 2002). Thus, large-scale implementation of ESTs for children can be done.

CRITICISMS AND CHANGES OVER TIME

Many criticisms by virtually all sides have addressed the EST movement (and so far less so the more expansive EBP conceptualization). While proponents of EST applaud the increased focus on scientifically derived recommendations in the EST movement, opponents of EST point to an overreliance on the application of highly rigorous research methodology and a seemingly rigid set of criteria for inclusion of therapies on lists (McCrady, 2000).

The rigorous research methodology of randomized clinical trials (RCTs) has been challenged because it emphasizes internal validity to the neglect of external validity (i.e., neglect of "real-world" situations and diagnoses in the literature; Blatt, 2001; Goldfried & Wolfe, 1996). ESTs have been criticized for not attending to issues and types of problems and disorders exhibited by "real-world patients." Because results from RCTs are considered the highest level of scientific basis for therapy, RCTs have been criticized for overly restricting the diagnoses for inclusion of patients in the experimental trials. The restrictions on diagnoses limit generalizability of the treatment findings to a narrow category of presenting problems (Blatt, 2001; Goldfried & Wolfe, 1996; Havik & Vandenbos, 1996; Westen et al., 2004). This criticism results from the need to enhance internal validity while perhaps sacrificing external validity. Recently, RCT investigators have attempted to enhance the applicability of RCTs by lessening restrictiveness and by conducting effectiveness studies in community-based settings where, it is asserted, more complex cases are presented (cf., Doss & Weisz, 2006; Kazdin & Whitley, 2006).

Another criticism has been that some commentators consider ESTs to be too narrow as a conceptualization of psychotherapy and do not capture the essence of the process (Luborski, 2001; Strupp, 2001). For example, Jensen et al. (2005) found that most research does not attend to the nonspecific therapeutic variables such as therapeutic alliance, positive regard, therapist attention, positive expectations, and dose and intensity effects. In some ways, the clinical researchers working on ESTs appear to have assumed these elements to be important in psychotherapy but not the objects of concern when delineating the empirical base to psychological interventions. However, the EST advocates have noted the complexity of psychotherapy and the importance of variables that are categorized in patient values and clinical expertise in EBP (e.g., Chambless & Ollendick, 2001).

Because RCTs rely on treatment manuals to standardize therapy for scientific examination, derogation of EST also focused on manualized treatments as ill-equipped to handle what is perceived as a more complex therapeutic situation than a "cookbook" or manual can provide. Treatment manuals used in RCT research have raised concerns about applications to therapy outside the research lab setting because manualized treatments are thought to bind the therapist in a prescribed set of actions (Davison, 1998; Messer, 2004). Fonagy (2001), while noting some limitations, did suggest that manuals provide "a clear structured and coherent framework that guides the therapeutic process" (p. 647). Others have presented that rigidly following a therapy manual is not necessary for positive results, but the manual should be used to guide interventions (Abramowitz, 2006). Kendall and Beidas (2007, p. 16) call this "flexibility within fidelity" to the manual.

Other concerns about the EST lists revolve around the potential use to restrict payment to psychologists by managed care to only those treatments on the list; thus, some psychologists would not receive payment for therapies they currently do if the treatments are not on the EST list. The lists themselves imply approval for some therapeutic techniques and disapproval for others. Some have argued that therapies appear to be equally effective and that the implication of one treatment as better than another is detrimental to the profession (Slife et al., 2005).

Several surveys have established that ESTs are not widely utilized by practitioners (Mussell et al., 2000; Persons, 1995). Surveys of practitioners indicate many negative perceptions and lack of understanding about ESTs in particular (Addis & Krasnow, 2000; Aarons, 2004). This failure to implement may be due to a variety of barriers including inadequate training and dissemination of usable literature, therapists' resistance to change, misperceptions of treatment manuals, lack of economic incentives to adopt, difficulty in gaining skills, among others (e.g., Nelson et al., 2006). Several efforts are being made to increase dissemination and usefulness of information (e.g., Riley et al., 2007).

In contrast to the orientation to therapeutic techniques of the EST approach, others have called for a focus on therapeutic relationships (Wampold, 2001). The Division of Psychotherapy (Division 29 of APA) in its Task Force on Empirically Supported Therapy Relationships developed a list of empirically supported therapeutic relationships that resulted in a book, *Psychotherapy Relationships That Work* (Norcross, 2002). This task force presented evidence for such elements of relationships as therapeutic alliance, empathy, congruence, and positive regard. Norcross (2002) articulated the view that "concurrent use of empirically supported relationships and empirically supported treatments is likely to generate the best outcomes" (p. 442). In the child therapy area, Shirk and Karver (2003) found that relationship characteristics were related to therapeutic outcomes.

Instead of the EST approach, Beutler et al. (2002) have argued for a greater focus on empirically establishing principles of change rather than the prescriptive approach of therapies for specific disorders interpreted from the EST approach. In a later effort, Castonguay and Beutler (2006) presented the results of a task force of the Division of Clinical Psychology aimed at delineating empirically based principles of change in psychotherapy. In the same series of reports, Beutler et al. (2006) articulated a conceptualization of therapy that includes "aspects of the patient and therapist (participant factors), those relating to the development and role of the therapeutic relationship (relationship factors), and those that defined the application of formal interventions that are implemented by the therapist (techniques factors)" (p. 639). The techniques factors rely on ESTs.

While most of the criticisms of the EST philosophy and approach have been from those representing more traditional psychotherapy and those with less empirical support at this point, the criticisms of the EBP movement also have come from those with stronger scientific orientations. For example, concern was expressed that putting clinical expertise on a par with scientific evidence (in the three-legged-stool metaphor) implies that they are equally weighted and thus diminishes a reliance on empirically supported therapies. In contrast, in the more recent approach of the EST movement emphasizing flexibility in application of a treatment, the clinician's developed expertise determines how to adapt the scientifically based literature to the specific patient's needs. Additionally, EST proponents argue that knowing through scientific validation which therapies work with which types of clients under what conditions is an important and essential element of competent and ethical treatment of humans who are experiencing problems.

CONCLUDING REMARKS

The controversies surrounding ESTs and the recent emergence of EBP as overarching, even if imprecise, conceptualizations will likely continue. A growing and dynamic profession requires continual examination and reassessment of itself. The ESTs and EBP movement might have united some aspects of the field but to some degree appears also to have further divided the already noticeable gap between research and practice. Additionally, as noted, a critical consideration will be how information on effective practice is disseminated and successfully implemented. True to the model of integration of science-practice noted earlier, practitioners, clinical researchers, and policy makers will need to work together to create the next generation of treatments that rely on the science of behavior (Weisz et al., 2004).

A new research agenda needs development to innovate and evaluate education and training practices. Traditional modalities such as CE workshops and short courses may not be the most useful. Computer and Web-based information may seem more "cutting edge," but these resources have not been sufficiently evaluated (and indeed may suffer the same limitations of implementation following exposure in CE workshops). This dissemination and adoption research must parallel renewed efforts to empirically evaluate all of the components in EBP and their integration into successful conceptualizations. The children, adolescents, and their families treated by mental health providers deserve the most effective services possible. The profession and society can only hope that the current state of affairs is but a way-station on a journey to better practice in psychology.

REFERENCES

Aarons, G. A. (2004). Mental health provider attitudes toward adoption of evidence-based practice: The evidence-based practice attitude scale (EBPAS). *Mental Health Services Research, 6*, 61–74.

Addis, M. E., & Krasnow, A. D. (2000). A national survey of practicing psychologists' attitudes toward psychotherapy treatment manuals. *Journal of Consulting and Clinical Psychology, 68*, 331–339.

American Psychological Association Task Force on Evidence-Based Practice (2006). Evidence-based practice in psychology. *American Psychologist, 61*, 271–285.

Abramowitz, J. S. (2006). Toward a functional analytic approach to psychological complex patients: A comment on Ruscio and Holohan (2006). *Clinical Psychology: Science and Practice, 13*, 163–166.

Blatt, S. J. (2001). The effort to identify empirically supported psychological treatments and its implications for clinical research, practice, and training. *Psychoanalytic Dialogues, 11*, 633–644.

Beutler, L. E., Castonguay, L. G., & Follette, W. C. (2006). Therapeutic factors in dysphoric disorders. *Journal of Clinical Psychology, 62*, 639–647.

Beutler, L. E., Moleiro, C., & Talebi, H. (2002). How practitioners can systematically use empirical evidence in treatment selection. *Journal of Clinical Psychology, 58*, 1199–1212.

Borkovec, T. D. (2002).Training clinic research and the possibility of a National Training Clinics Practice Research Network. *Behavior Therapist, 25*, 98–103.

Borkovec, T. D. (2004). Research in training clinics and practice research networks: A route to the integration of science and practice. *Clinical Psychology: Science and Practice, 11,* 211–214.

Brestan, E. V., & Eyberg, S. M. (1998). Effective psychosocial treatments of conduct-disordered children and adolescents: 29 years, 82 studies, 5,272 kids. *Journal of Clinical Child Psychology, 27,* 180–189.

Calhoun, K. S., Moras, K., Pilkonis, P. A., & Rehm, L. P. (1998). Empirically supported treatments: Implications for training. *Journal of Consulting and Clinical Psychology, 66,* 151–162.

Castonguay, L. G., & Beutler, L. E. (2006). Principles of therapeutic change: A task force on participants, relationships, and techniques factors. *Journal of Clinical Psychology, 62,* 631–638.

Chambless, D. L., Baker, M. J., Baucom, D. H., Beutler, L. E., Calhoun, K. S., Crits-Christoph, P., et al. (1996). An update on empirically validated therapies. *Clinical Psychologist, 49,* 5–18.

Chambless, D. L., Baker, M. J., Baucom, D. H., Beutler, L. E., Calhoun, K. S., Crits-Chritoph, P., et al. (1998). Update on empirically validated therapies II. *The Clinical Psychologist, 51*(1), 3–16.

Chambless, D. L., & Ollendick, T. H. (2001). Empirically supported psychological interventions: Controversies and evidence. *Annual Review of Psychology, 52,* 685–716.

Chambless, D. L., Sanderson, W. C., Shoham, V., Johnson, S. B., Pope, K. S., Crits-Chritoph, P., et al. (1996). An update on empirically validated therapies. *The Clinical Psychologist, 49*(2), 5–18.

Chorpita, B. F., & Donkervoet, C. (2005). Implementation of the Felix Consent Decree in Hawaii: The impact of policy and practice development efforts on service delivery. In R. G. Steele & M. C. Roberts (Eds.), *Handbook of Mental Health Services for Children, Adolescents, and Families* (pp. 317–332). New York: Kluwer Academic/Plenum Publishers.

Chorpita, B. F., Yim, L. M., Donkervoet, J. C., Arensdorf, A., Amundsen, M. J., McGee, C., et al. (2002). Toward large-scale implementation of empirically supported treatments for children: A review and observations by the Hawaii Empirical Basis to Services Task Force. *Clinical Psychology: Science and Practice, 9,* 165–190.

Davison, G. C. (1998). Being bolder with the Boulder model: The challenge of education and training in empirically supported treatments. *Journal of Consulting and Clinical Psychology, 66,* 163–167.

Doss, A. J., & Weisz, J. R. (2006). Syndrome co-occurrence and treatment outcomes in youth mental health clinics. *Journal of Consulting and Clinical Psychology, 74,* 416–425.

Eysenck, H. J. (1952). The effects of psychotherapy: An evaluation. *Journal of Consulting Psychology, 16,* 319–324.

Fonagy, P. (2001). The talking cure in the cross fire of empiricism: The struggle for the hearts and minds of psychoanalytic clinicians: Commentary on paper by Lester Luborsky and Hans H. Strupp. *Psychoanalytic Dialogues, 11,* 647–658.

Fonagy, P., Target, M., Cottrell, D., Phillips, J., & Kurtz, Z. (2002). *What Works for Whom? A Critical Review of Treatments for Children and Adolescents.* New York: Guilford.

Goldfried, M. R., & Wolfe, B. E. (1996). Psychotherapy practice and research: Repairing a strained relationship. *American Psychologist, 51,* 1007–1016.

Havik, O. E., & Vandenbos, G. R. (1996). Limitations of manualized psychotherapy for everyday practice. *Clinical Psychology: Science and Practice, 3,* 264–267.

Herschell, A. D., McNeil, C. B., & McNeil, D. W. (2004). Clinical child psychology's progress in disseminating empirically supported treatments. *Clinical Psychology: Science and Practice, 11,* 267–288.

Hibbs, E. D., & Jensen, P. S. (Eds.) (2005). *Psychosocial Treatments for Child and Adolescent Disorders: Empirically Based Strategies for Clinical Practice,* 2nd ed. Washington, DC: American Psychological Association.

Holden, E. W., Deichmann, M. M., & Levy, J. D. (1999). Empirically supported treatments in pediatric psychology: Recurrent pediatric headache. *Journal of Pediatric Psychology, 24,* 91–109.

Institute of Medicine (2001). *Crossing the Quality Chasm: A New Health System for the 21st Century.* Washington, DC: National Academies Press.

Janicke, D. M., & Finney, J. W. (1999). Empirically supported treatments in pediatric psychology: Recurrent abdominal pain. *Journal of Pediatric Psychology, 24,* 115–128.

Jelalian, E., & Saelens, B. E. (1999). Empirically supported treatments in pediatric psychology: Pediatric obesity. *Journal of Pediatric Psychology, 24,* 223–248.

Jensen, P. S., Weersing, R., Hoagwood, K. E., & Goldman, E. (2005). What is the evidence for evidence-based treatments? A hard look at our soft underbelly. *Mental Health Services Research, 7,* 53–74.

Karekla, M., Lundgren, J. D., & Forsyth, J. P. (2004). A survey of graduate training in empirically supported and manualized treatments: A preliminary report. *Cognitive and Behavioral Practice, 11,* 230–242.

Kaslow, N. J., & Thompson, M. P. (1998). Applying the criteria for empirically supported treatments to studies of psychosocial interventions for child and adolescent depression. *Journal of Clinical Child Psychology, 27,* 146–155.

Kazdin, A. E., & Kendall, P. C. (1998). Current progress and future plans for developing effective treatments: Comments and perspectives. *Journal of Clinical Child Psychology, 27,* 217–226.

Kazdin, A. E., & Weisz, J. R. (1998). Identifying and developing empirically supported child and adolescent treatments. *Journal of Consulting and Clinical Psychology, 66,* 19–36.

Kazdin, A. E., & Whitley, M. K. (2006). Comorbidity, case complexity, and effects of evidence-based treatment for children referred for disruptive behavior. *Journal of Consulting and Clinical Psychology, 74,* 455–467.

Kendall, P., & Beidas, R. (2007). Smoothing the trail for dissemination of evidence-based practices for youth: Flexibility within fidelity. *Professional Psychology: Research and Practice, 38,* 13–20.

Kerwin, M. E. (1999). Empirically supported treatments in pediatric psychology: Severe feeding problems. *Journal of Pediatric Psychology, 24,* 193–214.

Levitt, E. E. (1957). The results of psychotherapy with children: An evaluation. *Journal of Consulting Psychology, 32,* 286–289.

Levitt, E. E. (1963). Psychotherapy with children: A further evaluation. *Behavior Research and Therapy, 60,* 326–329.

Lonigan, C. J., Elbert, J. C., & Johnson, S. B. (1998). Empirically supported psychosocial interventions for children: An overview. *Journal of Clinical Child Psychology, 27,* 138–145.

Luborski, L. (2001). The meaning of empirically supported treatment research for psychoanalytic and other long-term therapies. *Psychoanalytic Dialogues, 11,* 583–604.

McCrady, B. S. (2000). Alcohol use disorders and the Division 12 Task Force of the American Psychological Association. *Psychology of Addictive Behaviors, 14,* 267–276.

McGrath, M. L., Mellon, M. W., & Murphy, L. (2000). Empirically supported treatments in pediatric psychology: Constipation and encopresis. *Journal of Pediatric Psychology, 25,* 225–254.

McQuaid, E. L., & Nassau, J. H. (1999). Empirically supported treatments of disease-related symptoms in pediatric psychology: Asthma, diabetes, and cancer. *Journal of Pediatric Psychology, 24,* 305–328.

Mellon, M. W., & McGrath, M. L. (2000). Empirically supported treatments in pediatric psychology: Nocturnal enuresis. *Journal of Pediatric Psychology, 25,* 193–214.

Messer, S. B. (2004). Evidence-based practice: Beyond empirically supported treatments. *Professional Psychology: Research and Practice, 35,* 580–588.

Mindell, J. A. (1999). Empirically supported treatments in pediatric psychology: Bedtime refusal and night wakings in young children. *Journal of Pediatric Psychology, 24,* 465–481.

Mussell, M. P., Crosby, R. D., Crow, S. J., Knopke, A. J., Peterson, C. B., Wonderlich, S. A., & Mitchell, J. E. (2000). Utilization of empirically supported psychotherapy treatments for individuals with eating disorders: A survey of psychologists. *International Journal of Eating Disorders, 27,* 230–237.

National Institute of Mental Health (National Advisory Mental Health Workgroup on Child and Adolescent Mental Health Intervention Development and Deployment) (2001). *Blueprint for Change: Research on Child and Adolescent Mental Health.* Rockville, MD: National Institute of Mental Health.

Nelson, T. D., Steele, R. G., & Mize, J. (2006). Practitioner attitudes toward evidence-based practice: Themes and challenges. *Administration and Policy in Mental Health and Mental Health Services Research, 33,* 398–409.

Norcross, J. (2002). *Psychotherapy Relationships That Work: Therapist Contributions and Responsiveness to Patients.* New York: Oxford University Press.

Ollendick, T. H., & Davis, T. E. (2004). Empirically supported treatments for children and adolescents: Where to from here? *Clinical Psychology: Science and Practice, 11,* 289–294.

Ollendick, T. H., & King, N. J. (1998). Empirically supported treatments for children with phobia and anxiety disorders: Current status. *Journal of Clinical Child Psychology, 27,* 156–167.

Pelham, W. E., Wheeler, T., & Chronis, A. (1998). Empirically supported psychosocial treatments for attention deficit hyperactivity disorder. *Journal of Clinical Child Psychology, 27,* 190–205.

Persons, J. B. (1995). Why practicing psychologists are slow to adopt empirically-validated treatments. In S. C. Hayes, V. M. Follette, R. M. Dawes, & K. E. Grady (Eds.), *Scientific Standards of Psychological Practice: Issues and Recommendations* (pp. 141–157). Reno, NV: Context Press.

Powers, S. W. (1999). Empirically supported treatments in pediatric psychology: Procedure-related pain. *Journal of Pediatric Psychology, 24,* 131–146.

Riley, W. T., Schuman, M. F., Forman-Hoffman, V. L., Mihm, P., Applegate, B. W., & Asif, O. (2007). Responses of practicing psychologists to a website developed to promote empirically supported treatments. *Professional Psychology: Research and Practice, 38,* 44–53.

Roberts, M. C., & Hurley, L. K. (1997). *Managing Managed Care.* New York: Plenum.

Rogers, S. J. (1998). Empirically supported comprehensive treatments for young children with autism. *Journal of Clinical Child Psychology, 27,* 168–179.

Roth, A., & Fonagy, P. (2005). *What Works for Whom? A Critical Review of Psychotherapy Research,* 2nd ed. New York: Guilford.

Shirk, S. R. (2004). Dissemination of youth ESTs: Ready for prime time? *Clinical Psychology: Science and Practice, 11,* 308–312.

Shirk, S. R., & Karver, M. (2003). Prediction of treatment outcome from relationship variables in child and adolescent therapy: A meta-analytic review. *Journal of Consulting and Clinical Psychology, 71,* 452–464.

Silverman, W. K., Kurtines, W. K., & Hoagwood, K. (2004). Research progress on effectiveness, transportability, and dissemination of empirically supported treatments: Integrating theory and research. *Clinical Psychology: Science and Practice, 11,* 295–299.

Slife, B. D., Wiggins, B. J., & Graham, J. T. (2005). Avoiding an EST monopoly: Toward a pluralism of philosophies and methods. *Journal of Contemporary Psychotherapy, 35,* 83–97.

Spirito, A. (1999). Introduction: Special series on empirically supported treatments in pediatric psychology. *Journal of Pediatric Psychology, 24,* 97–90.

Steele, R. G., & Roberts, M. C. (2003). Therapy and interventions research with children and adolescents. In M. C. Roberts & S. S. Ilardi (Eds.), *Handbook of Research Methods in Clinical Psychology* (pp. 307–326). Malden, MA: Blackwell Publishing.

Steele, R. G., & Roberts, M. C. (2005). Mental health services for children: Adolescents, and families: Trends, models, and current status. In R. G. Steele & M. C. Roberts (Eds.), *Handbook of Mental Health Services for Children, Adolescents, and Families* (pp. 1–14). New York: Kluwer Academic/Plenum Publishers.

Strupp, H. H. (2001). Implications for the empirically supported treatment movement of psychoanalysis. *Psychoanalytic Dialogues, 11,* 605–619.

Task Force on Promotion and Dissemination of Psychological Procedures (1995). Training in and dissemination of empirically-validated psychological treatments. *The Clinical Psychologist, 48*(1), 3–23.

U.S. Public Health Service (2000). *Report of the Surgeon General's Conference on Children's Mental Health: A National Action Agenda.* Washington, DC: Department of Health and Human Services.

Walco, G. A., Sterling, C. N., Conte, P. M., & Engel, R. G. (1999). Empirically supported treatments in pediatric psychology: Disease-related pain. *Journal of Pediatric Psychology*, *24*, 155–167.

Wampold, B. E. (2001). *The Great Psychotherapy Debate: Model, Methods, and Findings.* Mahwah, NJ: Erlbaum.

Weisz, J. R., & Addis, M. E. (2006). The research-practice tango and other choreographic challenges: Using and testing evidence-based psychotherapies in clinical care settings. In C. D. Goodheart, A. E. Kazdin, & R. J. Sternberg (Eds.), *Evidence-Based Psychotherapy: Where Practice and Research Meet* (pp. 179–206). Washington, DC: American Psychological Association.

Weisz, J. R., Chu, B. C., & Polo, A. J. (2004). Treatment dissemination and evidence-based practice: Strengthening intervention through clinician-researcher collaboration. *Clinical Psychology: Science and Practice*, *11*, 300–307.

Weisz, J. R., & Hawley, K. M. (1998). Finding, evaluating, refining, and applying empirically supported treatments for children and adolescents. *Journal of Clinical Child Psychology*, *27*, 206–216.

Weisz, J. R., Hawley, K. M., Pilkonis, P. A., Woody, S. R., & Follette, W. C. (2000). Stressing the (other) three Rs in the search for empirically supported treatments: Review procedures, research quality, relevance to practice and the public interest. *Clinical Psychology: Science and Practice*, *7*, 243–258.

Westen, D., Novotny, C. M., & Thompson-Brenner, H. (2004). The empirical status of empirically supported psychotherapies: Assumptions, findings, and reporting in controlled clinical trials. *Psychological Bulletin*, *130*, 631–663.

Woody, S. R., Weisz, J., & McLean, C. (2005). Empirically supported treatments: 10 years later. *The Clinical Psychologist*, *58*(4), 5–11.

3

Methodological Issues in the Evaluation of Therapies

RIC G. STEELE, JENNIFER A. MIZE NELSON, and TIMOTHY D. NELSON

Implicit to the concept of "evidence-based therapy" (EBT) are the suppositions that mental health outcomes can be reliably measured, that changes in mental health outcomes can be attributed to the interventions delivered, and that results from outcome studies can be applied to individuals beyond the study sample. The first supposition, *that mental health outcomes can be reliably measured*, requires that assessment methods and processes (broadly defined) receive adequate empirical support to provide the "evidence" on which EBTs depend. A more complete evaluation and discussion of evidence-based assessment and its relationship to EBTs is taken up later in this volume (Phares & Curley, Chapter 30). The remaining assumptions (i.e., *that changes in mental health outcomes can be attributed to the interventions delivered* and *that results from outcome studies can be applied to individuals beyond the study sample*) form the substance of the present chapter.

Taking our lead from the National Institute of Mental Health (NIMH) Clinical Treatment and Services Research Workgroup (CTSRW, 1998), we propose that the needs of the mental health community follow a general developmental trajectory with regard to each particular intervention. Specifically, the CTSRW outlines a process of evaluating interventions that encompasses questions regarding efficacy and effectiveness, as well as questions regarding the larger ecologies within which interventions are provided, such as the degree to which interventions are used in practice settings (practice research) and the degree to which changes in policy or funding decisions influence quality of care (service systems research). In order to refine the active components of therapy, the needs of the field may alternate between studies that demonstrate that a therapy "can

RIC G. STEELE, JENNIFER A. MIZE NELSON, and TIMOTHY D. NELSON • University of Kansas, Clinical Child Psychology Program

work" (i.e., efficacy studies) and studies that demonstrate that a therapy "does work" in practice settings (effectiveness studies). Similarly, results of practice research (e.g., to what degree do clinicians use or adhere to treatment models?) may inform additional efficacy or effectiveness studies to improve upon the efficiency of therapy.

A number of authors have voiced concerns that therapies developed and tested in laboratory settings lack applicability in "real-world" settings (Persons & Silberschatz, 1998), and Shirk (2005) has noted several "polarity issues" that continue to divide clinical researchers from the potential consumers of that research. Perhaps contributing to these polarities, Simons and Wildes (2003) have noted that the frequent juxtaposition of internal validity (i.e., does the intervention produce results in the lab?) and external validity (i.e., do results generalize to actual clinical populations?) has solidified the perception of those two concepts existing on a linear continuum. While it is true that increases in internal reliability *may* have, or even *frequently have*, a deleterious effect on external validity, this association is not given and is not always necessary. Rather, Simons and Wildes suggested that internal and external validity exist as orthogonal dimensions and that studies may freely range within the four quadrants defined by those dimensions. The importance of this reconceptualization lies in the necessity of conducting research that has a high degree of internal validity, while at the same time being practical enough to allow generalization (or the eventual generalization) to clinical samples that do not meet the tightly controlled inclusion or exclusion criteria of many "efficacy" studies.

Consistent with Simons and Wildes' (2003) orthogonal view of internal and external validity, we now present a brief discussion of characteristics of efficacy/effectiveness research, practice research, and service systems research, with particular attention to aspects of the characteristics that facilitate translation of research findings into clinical practice. Rather than perpetuating the above-noted juxtaposition of efficacy and effectiveness research, the following section examines these two related research paradigms together, noting similarities and differences in the degree to which each strives to attain external and internal validity.

EFFICACY AND EFFECTIVENESS RESEARCH

The ultimate objective of *efficacy research* is to determine whether a treatment is capable of effecting positive therapeutic change, with the proximal goal of isolating treatment effects from all other sources of variance. Similarly, the ultimate objective of *effectiveness research* is to determine whether the treatment can produce positive therapeutic change as implemented under more externally valid (i.e., "real-world") conditions. The process of research design requires decisions regarding a number of issues that determine the degree to which experimental control is achieved.

As discussed below, efficacy and effectiveness studies may differ along a number of dimensions (e.g., inclusion/exclusion criteria), but both forms of research will demonstrate some degree of control over systematic variance. Uncontrolled systematic variance may come from a number of sources. Several sources of variance that pose threats to internal validity involve internal and external events separate from the components of treatment that can be responsible for change in participants' behavior from treatment inception to termination (i.e., threats of participants' maturation, developmental history, and measurement issues). Efficacy studies traditionally impose control of these threats by comparing participants receiving treatment to a control group of participants who do not receive the treatment in question but experience similar developmental and contextual events and complete the same assessment instruments at the same intervals. Such control groups may receive placebo or standard treatment or be waitlisted to receive the treatment of interest at a later time.

Additional threats to internal validity involve individual differences among participants (i.e., selection bias) as well as differential completion of efficacy or effectiveness trials (i.e., attrition). Attrition is an issue with regard to research conducted in both controlled and community settings; however, the structure of efficacy studies (Wierzbicki & Pekarik, 1993), as well as the use of the Consolidated Standards of Reporting Trials (CONSORT; Moher et al., 2001) and the Transparent Reporting of Evaluations with Nonrandomized Designs (TREND; Des Jarlais et al., 2004) recommendations, may allow for better tracking of the characteristics that lead to attrition. Furthermore, participants in efficacy studies often receive participation incentives that may counteract barriers to treatment adherence (e.g., offering treatment free of charge). To control for individual differences among participants, researchers use random assignment to determine whether participants will receive the treatment in question or be placed in the control group. This procedure assumes that each group will be made up of participants who share a similar range of variability in individual characteristics.

The combination of randomization and use of control groups has resulted in the traditional use of randomized controlled trials (RCTs) in efficacy research (see Chambless & Hollon, 1998, for proposed requirement of RCTs to establish an evidence base). As a result, RCTs have become the "gold standard" among researchers for evaluating the effects of psychological and psychiatric treatments (Wells, 1999). However, the characteristics of RCTs that were designed to maintain internal validity and ensure the isolation of treatment effects present challenges to generalizing results beyond the controlled setting. Below, we outline a number of issues that the clinical researcher, or the consumer of clinical research, might consider in the evaluation of efficacy or effectiveness designs.

Inclusion/Exclusion Criteria

Among the most noticeable differences between efficacy and effectiveness studies is the degree to which exclusion criteria are applied to study samples. Efficacy research is historically known for strict inclusion and exclusion criteria to guide the selection of participants. The primary issue regarding selection criteria involves whether children and adolescents presenting with comorbid conditions should be included; they have often been excluded to examine the effect of a treatment on symptom patterns exhibited by a single diagnosis. Critics of the EBT movement argue that children presenting with non-comorbidity are relatively rare in less controlled settings, suggesting that efficacy studies with homogenous samples are not useful (see Nelson et al., 2006, for discussion). Indeed, Southam-Gerow et al. (2003) reported that children presenting to community service clinics (for anxiety disorders) presented with more comorbidity than children presenting to a university-based research clinic; however, recent studies have suggested that comorbidity is not a significant predictor of treatment outcomes (e.g., Jensen-Doss & Weisz, 2006).

In contrast to efficacy studies, effectiveness research aims to capture the heterogeneity characteristic of applied settings in treatment studies. Despite the need to examine treatment outcomes among heterogeneous samples, this task is not easily accomplished, as evidenced by the reliance on nonreferred cases in the majority of therapy studies in the literature (Kazdin & Weisz, 1998). In response to this issue, some treatment researchers have begun to embrace less restrictive inclusion criteria in outcome studies. For example, Beidel et al. (2000) employed more relaxed inclusion criteria to combine a community sample with children seeking treatment, all of whom met diagnostic criteria for social phobia. Despite the relaxed criteria for admission, the results indicated that the treatment of interest (Social Effectiveness Therapy for Children) yielded decreased anxiety symptoms and improved social skills, as well as a clinically significant drop in the percentage of children meeting criteria for a diagnosis of social phobia, at posttreatment and follow-up compared to children receiving nonspecific control treatment (Beidel et al., 2000).

Jensen-Doss and Weisz (2006) offered a promising methodological technique for assessing the effect of comorbid diagnosis on treatment outcomes. Moving away from traditional, categorical conceptualization based on specific single versus comorbid diagnoses, they examined the effect of statistical interactions among multiple dimensions of psychopathology (i.e., different syndromes measured on the Child Behavior Checklist). This approach allowed them to demonstrate that "symptom co-occurrence" (e.g., high levels of two types of symptoms) was not generally a significant predictor of treatment outcome among a heterogeneous sample of children receiving outpatient community mental health services. Consistent with Weisz and colleagues' deployment-based model of treatment and development of interventions (Weisz et al., 2005), the above statistical technique allows for the examination of intervention efficacy in the context of the children with comorbid diagnoses who would eventually receive treatment in actual clinics. The results of the work of Jensen-Doss and Weisz (2006) also raised questions about the influence of comorbid conditions on the effectiveness of specific interventions.

Therapist Selection

In addition to the selection of participants, the selection of therapists to deliver treatments also constitutes an area of debate. To determine whether a treatment leads to therapeutic change across participants and over time, the content of the treatment must be well defined, and the treatment must be delivered in a standardized fashion across treatment providers. Otherwise, differences in treatment delivery would undermine the researchers' ability to isolate the unique effect of the treatment. These traditional requirements in efficacy research have led to detailed treatment manuals and the need for therapists who are well trained in the specifics of treatment delivery (e.g., often graduate students or staff working in a university setting for treatment developers).

The challenge arises when considering that practitioners struggle to find the time to become adequately trained to deliver emerging treatments with empirical support, which can lead to less fidelity to the treatments validated in efficacy studies and the subsequent difference in therapeutic effectiveness for clients in practice settings. Kazdin (2003a) raised this concern with respect to longstanding evaluations of problem-solving skills training (PSST) and parent management training (PMT) for children with conduct disorder. He noted the limitations of the extensive training that would be required for a practicing clinician to be competent in the delivery of these treatments, even though their efficacy has been demonstrated in multiple studies (e.g., Kazdin et al., 1992).

Unlike efficacy studies, in which university-based clinicians often have intensive training in a specific manualized protocol, clinicians in typical treatment settings often do not have extensive training with specific treatments. This lack of specialized training is likely the result of the diversity of client presentations typically seen in these settings, which require clinicians to deliver treatments for a wide range of problems. Because of the challenges of serving a diverse clientele, many clinicians rely more heavily on the therapeutic process, which is viewed as a mechanism of change for a broad range of clinical issues, rather than detailed, problem-specific manualized techniques (Nelson et al., 2006). In light of clinician use of more relational treatment strategies, some work has begun to emerge exploring the impact of therapeutic alliance on treatment outcomes (e.g., Shirk & McMakin, Chapter 26).

In the evaluation of specific treatments, differences between clinicians also pose a notable challenge for effectiveness research. The goal of providing evidence of treatment effectiveness in real settings can be difficult if the treatment of interest is not delivered to the same degree and in the same manner by different clinicians with different clients. However, because these differences are expected as a result of the nature of variability in practice, the inclusion of fidelity measures is considered an important part of conducting effectiveness research (Chambless & Hollon, 1998). For example, Borrelli and colleagues (2005) measured treatment fidelity over 10 years of published research and found that over half (54%) of the studies reviewed had not accounted for fidelity (i.e., no maintenance of therapist skills or use of a treatment manual, no checks of adherence to a specified treatment protocol).

Graczyk et al. (2003) conceptualized fidelity as a multifaceted construct that includes the degree to which (1) the proposed intervention structure is followed and (2) the timing of intervention delivery and dosage are consistent. Kållestad and Olweus (2003) were among the first to examine teacher- and school-level fidelity in the evaluation of school-based antibullying interventions (i.e., in their case, the Olweus Bullying Prevention Program). Teachers who perceived problematic levels of bullying in their schools and felt personally efficacious about affecting change were more likely to implement classroom-based intervention components. In turn, there was an observed effect of dosage whereby teachers who implemented essential intervention components (e.g., establishment of class bullying rules) had classrooms that reported more reduction in bullying problems, compared to classrooms where fewer intervention components were implemented (Olweus et al., 1999).

Outcome Measures

An additional issue to consider with respect to the generalizability of treatment findings involves the assessment and interpretation of treatment effects. There has been some criticism of the instruments typically used to evaluate change in both efficacy and effectiveness studies (see Kendall, 1999). Often, assessment instruments consist of measures of symptom levels or diagnostic criteria, with the expectation that clients will evidence symptom reduction or will meet fewer criteria for diagnosis after exposure to treatment (Kazdin & Weisz, 1998). However, some argue that symptom reduction at posttreatment may not necessarily mean that the treatment rendered longer-term change (see Kendall, 1999). For example, Kazdin (2006) suggested that rating scales may frequently fail to capture the degree of change that relates to components of everyday life and pointed to the value of gathering qualitative information about change to supplement more standard quantitative methods of assessing the clinical significance of treatment effects.

Similarly, Hoagwood and colleagues (1996) proposed a framework for more thoroughly evaluating treatment effects in multiple contexts. Specifically, they proposed a dynamic model for assessing not only individual symptoms but also functioning across different environments (e.g., home, school, community) and system-level changes (e.g., changes in the use of services or intensity of services) within a developmental framework. While these areas have not traditionally been the focus of outcomes evaluation (Jensen et al., 1996), studies employing broader measures of treatment outcomes have begun to emerge. Several research groups have examined long-term records of rearrest and incarceration as a functional outcome following juvenile boot camp and parole programming (Bottcher & Ezell, 2005) and multisystemic therapy (MST; Henggeler et al., 1997) among juvenile offenders.

Determination of Treatment Effects

Beyond the instrumentation used to determine treatment outcome, recent discussions of the statistical analyses and decision rules used to evaluate treatment responses may also enhance the clinical utility of efficacy and effectiveness trials (e.g., Kazdin, 2006; Kendall, 1999). Traditional mean-level comparison of the change in symptom levels between treatment and control groups has been criticized for not demarcating a degree of change that has clinical meaning. For example, some efficacy trials may have such large numbers of participants in each group that even the slightest change in overall symptom level is statistically significant. In response to this, the past decade has been marked by numerous calls for the inclusion of effect sizes, examinations of confidence intervals, and analyses of changes in functioning when presenting the results of treatment evaluations in order to determine the clinical significance of treatment effects (see Kendall, 1999).

Of particular promise is the use of the reliable change index (RCI) as a means of examining whether differences in pretreatment and posttreatment scores are due to measurement error or actual treatment effects (Jacobson & Truax, 1991; Ogles et al., 1996). In addition, normative comparison has also been identified as a more meaningful way to determine whether clients' functioning posttreatment can be justified as having reached a level where the treatment of interest made a meaningful difference (Achenbach, 2001). Sheldrick et al. (2001) demonstrated the use of both the RCI and normative comparisons in their summary of the body of research findings evaluating three treatments targeting conduct disorder among children and adolescents (i.e., video modeling parent-training, Problem Solving Skills Training, and Parent-Child Interaction Therapy). All three treatments were found to produce clinically significant changes of large magnitude across the majority of included studies (92% of studies, according to RCI analyses) and moderate changes in the percentage of samples that, on average, returned to within one standard deviation of the mean level of symptoms in the normative sample (40% of samples across included studies, according to normative comparison analyses).

Moderators of Treatment Outcome

For both efficacy and effectiveness studies, the examination of treatment moderators provides an additional avenue for making results more generalizable to specific populations (APA Presidential Task Force on Evidence-Based Practice, 2006; Kazdin, 1997; Paul, 1967). For example, the knowledge that participants with specific characteristics might not respond as well to a particular treatment would suggest the need to explore other treatment options and also highlights a potential area for further research. Responsiveness to recent calls to adequately describe the demographics of study samples has afforded the opportunity to examine gender, ethnic, socioeconomic, and diagnostic differences in treatment efficacy or effectiveness (Kazdin, 2003b; Kazdin et al., 1990).

Despite recognition of the importance of considering ethnicity as a moderator of treatment outcome (Kazdin et al., 1990), a recent review of psychotherapy outcomes for ethnic minority youth suggested that ethnicity was not a significant moderator of effectiveness in the studies reviewed (i.e., socioeconomic disadvantage accounted for the difference in one study where there were ethnic differences in outcome; Miranda et al., 2005). Therefore, the limited number of studies to date comparing treatment efficacy and effectiveness among ethnically diverse samples suggests that ethnic minorities share similar outcomes with nonminority populations. However, these null findings regarding ethnic differences should not serve to downplay the potential value of adapting empirically based treatments to be more culturally sensitive (e.g., Matos et al., 2006). Kotchick and Grover (Chapter 27) provide further discussion of the importance of examination of ethnicity vis-à-vis treatment outcomes.

With regard to diagnostic considerations, Birmaher and colleagues (2000) provided an example of the importance of examining treatment moderators in a clinical trial comparing the efficacy of cognitive behavioral therapy, systematic behavioral family therapy, and nondirective supportive therapy in the treatment of adolescent depression. Depression severity at intake and chronic parent-child conflict both served as treatment moderators, weakening treatment effects and predicting recurrent depressive symptoms at follow-up. These results suggested that further development of effective treatments for adolescent depression may do well to consider longer and more intensive intervention for adolescents with more severe presentation at intake (e.g., combining medication with psychotherapy), as well as including family conflict reduction strategies for adolescents who present with this risk for recurrence (Birmaher et al., 2000).

Evidence of Consumer and Provider Satisfaction

Beyond the evaluation of treatment outcomes, several additional issues are important when researching the effectiveness and feasibility of new and emerging treatments (Nelson & Steele, 2006). Unlike their counterparts receiving treatment in efficacy trials, individuals seeking treatment in typical clinical settings have input into the types of treatment provided. Thus, client satisfaction is an important construct to measure as part of the overall evaluation of new treatments. Even if a treatment demonstrates a measurable impact, clients who are dissatisfied with its components (e.g., length, techniques employed) may not choose that treatment or be invested enough for the technique to yield benefits in applied settings. Indeed, Hawley and Weisz (2005) noted that youth- and parent-reported therapeutic alliance were each related to consumer satisfaction and that youth alliance was related to youth- and parent-reported symptom improvement in a community-based outpatient mental health services clinic.

In response to the growing awareness of consumer issues in treatment development, a number of consumer satisfaction measures have been recently developed. For example, Attkisson and colleagues (Attkisson

& Greenfield, 1999, 2004; Greenfield & Attkisson, 2004), Varni and colleagues (2004), and others (Center for Mental Health Services, 1997) have developed measures of client satisfaction for adults as well as for parents and children receiving mental health and/or medical services. Although informal means of assessing consumer satisfaction have been successfully employed (e.g., Huebner et al., 2004), the use of standardized measures may allow for greater comparisons across treatments, sites, or modes of therapy.

Practicing clinicians also have a choice in the treatments they utilize in their work with clients. Given the resistance to using manualized treatments in applied settings, the assessment of clinician satisfaction is an important issue during the development and initial evaluation of a treatment. Huebner and colleagues (2004) included a formal evaluation of provider satisfaction within the context of a large program evaluation for the Healthy Steps for Young Children Program. In this evaluation, health-care providers using the program completed a brief survey specifically designed to evaluate the perceived usefulness of the program to providers. Although more general standardized measures for provider evaluations are not yet widely available, more general clinician attitude surveys might serve as useful models in evaluating clinicians' satisfaction (Aarons, 2005; Addis & Krasnow, 2000).

Single-Subject Design

While RCTs may remain the standard for demonstrating efficacy and effectiveness in treating many disorders, such methods may not be feasible for conditions with very low incidence rates or in relatively small clinical settings. Accordingly, Chambless and Hollon (1998) suggested guidelines for the recognition of effective therapies that are based on studies using single-subject or "small-n" designs. Such designs have been thought of as the one methodology most viable for bridging the research and practice gap (Persons & Silberschatz, 1998). Despite the need for smaller numbers of participants, the *sine qua non* of such studies remains the demonstration of experimental control. This occurs primarily via two methods, the ABAB and the multiple-baseline designs (see Anderson & Kim, 2003, for a full description of these methods).

Using an ABAB experimental design in a nonacademic clinical setting, Moore et al. (1995) examined the effectiveness of a cognitive-behavioral intervention designed to reduce anticipatory anxiety and delay preceding daily insulin injections in a 14-year-old girl with diabetes. Results indicated decreased anxiety and reduced treatment time under the CBT condition, relative to baseline and return-to-baseline conditions. Moore and colleagues' methodology serves as an excellent model of how the ABAB design can be employed in a nonacademic clinical setting.

Similar to the reversal (ABAB) design, the multiple-baseline approach allows causal inferences to be made about the efficacy of treatment by demonstrating specific treatment effects across different conditions (e.g., vocal tics, motor tics) within the same individual, across different individuals presenting with the same problem condition, or within the same individual with a single problem occurring across multiple settings (see also Anderson & Kim, 2003). Using this approach, Plumer and Stoner (2005) investigated the effects of two classroom-based interventions (classroom-wide peer tutoring and peer coaching) to improve the social behaviors of children with ADHD. Three children with ADHD were observed during the baseline condition, after which a classroom-wide peer tutoring condition was implemented. This resulted in changes in social behavior during structured classroom time, but not during unstructured social settings. When peer coaching was added during the final phase of the study, children's social behaviors in unstructured social settings improved as well.

Although the use of small-n and single-subject designs has been remarkably useful in the development and evaluation of interventions, the interpretation of the results of such studies has historically been based on visual inspection of the data. Chambless and Hollon (1998) noted that comparison of two active treatments might be more challenging and that reliance on visual inspection to determine significance sometimes results in disagreements across reporters. To address these concerns, Crosbie (1993) provided a more quantitative approach, the interrupted time series analysis (ITSA), to determine the statistical significance of differences across conditions in single-subject or small-n designs. Slifer et al. (2002) used this approach in their examination of the use of differential reinforcement and contingency management on procedural distress in a 7-year-old girl who received regular subcutaneous injections. In this case, visual inspection of the pre- and posttreatment distress data was complicated by a reasonably high degree of variability. ITSA allowed a more quantitative evaluation of change in terms of mean level of distress, as well as change in slope of the pattern of distress (i.e., greater decreases in distress with more counter-conditioning trials).

PRACTICE RESEARCH

At a different level of abstraction, practice research is concerned with studying clinical services as they are actually delivered in the field. This area of research can be conceptualized as investigating two fundamental and related issues. First, practice research describes the nature of mental health services that are provided in applied settings. Questions of what treatments are being used, who is providing services, and the quality and cost of services are particularly relevant issues for understanding the realities of current practice. Second, practice research explores how treatments with research support are disseminated into widespread clinical practice. In this area, treatment transportability, factors influencing provider treatment decisions, and institutional obstacles to adopting new evidence-based approaches are some of the important topics of investigation.

Describing Treatment in Practice

Despite the general consensus that treatments with rigorous research support are not widely used in practice (Connor-Smith & Weisz, 2003; Kazdin et al., 1990), relatively little research has detailed exactly what treatments are being used in applied settings. Such work will be vital in identifying the most common treatment approaches and understanding the degree of the gap between the treatment literature and typical clinical care. A related issue in describing treatment services is *where* mental health services for children and adolescents are being provided. Understanding patterns of service delivery across different types of clinical settings (e.g., Community Mental Health Centers, private practice, hospitals, schools) will be important in efficiently targeting EBT dissemination and training efforts. Likewise, studying *who* is providing mental health services is an emerging issue in practice research. Research describing who is providing treatment and the relative effectiveness of different treatment providers is needed in order to better understand the nature of typical mental health service delivery.

Quality of Care

Another major issue in the area of practice research is the quality of clinical care provided in applied settings. The degree to which the most appropriate treatments are implemented by competent professionals with positive outcomes is an important indicator of quality of care; however, such information is still rare in the treatment literature. Research describing the quality of care in clinical settings and examining quality assurance mechanisms can also be useful in evaluating systems of care for children and adolescents (see below). Bridging practice research and service system research, future quality-of-care studies might investigate the effects of fragmented services, financial considerations, or therapist adherence to treatment protocols on treatment outcomes (see Schoenwald et al., 2004, for an innovative example of research addressing quality of care).

Cost-Effectiveness of Treatment

In light of the growing influence of economic factors on service delivery, the examination of the cost-effectiveness of treatment has emerged as an important area for study. Although numerous methods of measuring costs and cost-effectiveness have been proposed, Yates (2003) described a framework that incorporates both direct and indirect costs associated with an intervention. While the direct costs of an intervention (i.e., labor, materials) must be considered, it is also important to include indirect costs (i.e., training, supervision, preparation) in calculating the cost-effectiveness of a treatment. The amount of therapist and client time and money necessary to effect a meaningful change can be calculated and evaluated within this framework.

Treatment Transportability

Another emerging focus of practice research is concerned with the ability of treatments with research support to move from research settings to widespread clinical practice. Nelson and Steele (2006) argued that the ability of a given treatment to successfully move into clinical settings is related to the treatment's validation on several dimensions. Beyond evidence for efficacy and effectiveness, they suggested that treatments that are demonstrated to be appealing to service providers and potential clients are more likely to be adopted and successfully implemented in applied settings. Likewise, the cost-effectiveness of a treatment can impact the likelihood of its implementation in practice (Chambless & Hollon, 1998). More generally, research on the process of disseminating treatments into clinical settings has been identified as an important area for investigation, with a specific emphasis on the social processes involved in this endeavor (Stirman et al., 2004). By better understanding the process of dissemination, EBTs can be more efficiently transported from research to clinical practice.

Factors Influencing Provider Decisions

In addition to studying the transportability of particular treatments, research investigating the various influences on provider treatment decisions is an emerging area of practice research. Recently, some work has described clinician preferences and attitudes toward EBTs in general (Aarons, 2005; Nelson et al., 2006) as well as specific components of EBTs (Addis & Krasnow, 2000). Research investigating the relative influences of treatment research, colleagues and supervisor opinions, clinical training, clinical judgment, and provider characteristics would be helpful in better understanding the factors associated with provider treatment decisions. As an example of this kind of research, Henderson et al. (2006) examined the adoption and implementation of the TAPP-C program in community settings and found that, although the majority (82%) of health professionals in the study indicated adoption of the TAPP-C program, only 29% indicated routine implementation of the program. Further, results suggested that different factors (e.g., perceived self-efficacy, perceived innovation characteristics) predict adoption and implementation at various stages of diffusion. As noted by Henderson et al. (2006) and Nelson and Steele (2006), inclusion of "front-line" providers (and their reactions to treatment characteristics) in the initial development of new EBTs is likely to positively impact the eventual utilization of the final product.

Institutional Obstacles and Opportunities

Research focusing on institutional influences on services is an important component of practice research. Recognizing that different clinical settings may provide unique challenges to implementing EBTs (e.g., Smith-Boydston & Nelson, Chapter 29), research identifying potential institutional obstacles to adopting EBTs would be valuable. Perhaps most helpful would be research on the effects of economic and policy restrictions within clinical settings on quality of care and client outcomes. Conversely, research exploring institutional opportunities for group training and supervision might help to maximize institutional capacity for widespread adoption of EBTs.

Overall, practice research is still a developing area of study within the EBT literature. More work is needed to describe clinical services as they are typically delivered in the field. Likewise, more research on the dissemination of treatments with research support is needed. As studies describing clinical practice and dissemination processes become more widely available, this body of research will likely assist in efforts to facilitate the use of EBTs in a variety of settings.

SERVICE SYSTEMS RESEARCH

In contrast to efficacy and effectiveness studies, which focus on individual or group responses to particular interventions, *service systems research* examines the large-scale organizational, financial, and policy decisions and characteristics that affect service delivery (CTSRW, 1998). As such, the results of such research have the potential to broadly impact how and what services are delivered and may be particularly important when considering the transportation of evidence-based services into community settings (see Schiffman et al., 2006).

As described in more detail elsewhere (Chorpita & Donkervoet, 2005; Chorpita et al., 2002), the overhaul of mental health services provided to children and youth in Hawaii serves as an excellent example of the impact of service system evaluation and of the dissemination of evidence-based services on a large-scale basis. A review of the history of the implementation of the Felix Decree (i.e., a court mandate to establish a statewide system of care for children and youth in need of psychological or psychoeducational services; Chorpita & Donkervoet, 2005) reveals large-scale system evaluation at a variety of levels, including the number of children served, the types of services rendered, the "match" between youth need and services rendered, the outcomes of services provided, and annual costs of services.

As part of this ongoing systems research effort, Schiffman and colleagues (2006) examined the diagnostic characteristics of, and the services identified for, children and adolescents registered for services with the Child and Adolescent Mental Health Division (CAMHD) of the Hawaii Department of Health. Results indicated that the majority of youth (90%) presenting to the CAMHD did so with problem areas for which evidence-based services had been targeted by the Evidence-Based Services (EBS) committee. Schiffman and colleagues noted that these results speak to the strength of the evidence-based services literature as well as to the responsiveness of the CAMHD to the dissemination of evidence-based services. However, a large number of children presenting with at least one problem area not specifically addressed by an evidence-based intervention speaks to the need for continued efforts in terms of intervention development.

The Fort Bragg (Bickman et al., 1995) and the Stark County Evaluation studies (Bickman et al., 1999) serve as additional examples of large-scale service system research projects, designed to examine the type of services provided, the cost-efficacy of those services, and the clinical outcomes rendered in large service systems. In the Fort Bragg demonstration project, a quasi-experimental design was used to examine service and outcome variables across two types of mental health service systems (see Bickman & Mulvaney, 2005). The Stark County evaluation project examined similar outcomes and processes but employed a randomized experimental design. Both studies allowed a comprehensive examination of system-level variables (e.g., access to services, total costs) as well as some sense of system-level effects on individual outcomes (e.g., percentage of consumers evidencing clinical improvement).

Similarly, the national evaluation of the *Comprehensive Community Mental Health Services for Children and Their Families* program has provided a wealth of information regarding the impact of systems-of-care in mental health services (Holden et al., 2005). Across a number of individual studies, the evaluation program has examined the populations served by the system-of-care communities, the evolution of systems-of-care services over time, the relative improvement of youth served in systems-of-care, the costs associated with implementation, and consumer satisfaction with services (Holden & Brennan, 2002; Holden et al., 2002, 2005). Consistent with the recommendations of the American Psychological Association Presidential Task Force on Evidence-Based Practice (2006), more recent investigations in the national evaluation program have examined differential response to treatment patterns across individual pre-referral consumer characteristics (e.g., ethnicity, history of substance abuse, history of out-of-home placements; Walrath et al., 2006).

On a smaller scale, Huebner and colleagues (2004) examined a number of systemic variables in a quasi-experimental evaluation of a support and educational program implemented within a health maintenance organization. Variables assessed included some program evaluation (outcomes and satisfaction) components but also included service system variables including number and variability of services provided, impact on standard of care, and service utilization. Similarly, Olson and Netherton (1996) reported on systems-relevant variables affected by the Pediatric Consultation Liaison Service at the University of Oklahoma Health Science Center. Again, while some practice or outcome variables were examined (e.g., provider or patient satisfaction), measured constructs included a number of service system variables such as service utilization patterns. As noted above, and consistent with the CTSRW model (1998), some "blurring" of the lines between genres of research (practice/service systems) may translate into greater clinical utility and provide important cross-fertilization for further research endeavors.

These examples highlight a number of important methodological issues when considering service system research. First, regardless of the size of the system under investigation (e.g., local, regional, state, or national), randomized experimental designs may not be possible. To the extent that randomization increases the strength of inferences that can be reached from investigations, randomization is preferred. However, other research designs can and will add value to the service system research literature. Regardless of the research design employed, careful consideration of comparison samples and statistical controls is necessary (Bickman & Mulvaney, 2005).

For a number of the studies noted above, multiple sites were required to adequately examine the impact of policy or organizational changes on systems. As Chorpita and Donkervoet (2005) noted, the use of multiple clinical sites introduces the possibility of nonequivalent treatment, treatment adherence, or measurement across sites. Careful attention must be provided to nullify these potential sources of uncontrolled variance.

On a related note, because service system research is usually conducted in "real-world" settings with consumers who are in need of the services being evaluated, care should be given to include multiple stakeholders in the design and evaluation of the system (Hernandez et al., 1998). Stakeholders may include the families of children being served, providers, administrators, members of community-based organizations that provide ancillary services to the consumers, and members of child-services agencies from outside the mental health system. Members of these diverse groups will necessarily have different metrics for evaluating the system in question. Such diversity of metrics can bring additional richness to the methodologies employed in the evaluation (Kazdin, 2001, 2006).

CONCLUSIONS

The movement toward adoption of EBTs in clinical settings has spurred considerable discussion regarding the most appropriate methods for treatment evaluation research. Consistent with the recommendations from the NIMH Clinical Treatment and Services Research Workgroup (CTSRW, 1998) and numerous authors, we argue for an expansion of the topics and methods of inquiry used in the EBT literature. In addition to continued adaptations of more traditional methods of investigation (e.g., efficacy and effectiveness studies), we highlight the importance of several emerging issues to be addressed in future research. For example, the integration of cost analyses into ongoing treatment evaluation research will be essential in demonstrating not only that treatments are effective but also that they are cost-effective. Similarly, obtaining multiple perspectives on emerging and established treatments (e.g., consumer satisfaction, provider acceptability) will be crucial in developing and disseminating protocols that are well received and successfully implemented. Another major issue to be addressed in the EBT literature will be the moderators and mediators of treatment effectiveness (e.g., issues related to comorbidity, gender, and ethnicity) and the continued explication of the conditions under which treatments are effective. Research demonstrating that EBTs can be extended to diverse populations and are consistent with community values will be crucial in validating the usefulness of EBTs in affecting positive mental health outcomes for children and adolescents. Finally, the growing EBT literature will need to more clearly demonstrate the applicability of evidence-based protocols to community practice. Such research will necessarily include efficacy/effectiveness studies as well as practice and service system research to determine the degree to which EBTs are being implemented in practice settings and the impact of such therapies on service delivery.

REFERENCES

Aarons, G. A. (2005). Measuring provider attitudes toward evidence-based practice: Considerations of organizational context and individual differences. *Child and Adolescent Psychiatric Clinics of North America, 14,* 255–271.

Achenbach, T. M. (2001). What are norms and why do we need valid ones? *Clinical Psychology: Science and Practice, 8,* 446–450.

Addis, M. E., & Krasnow, A. D. (2000). A national survey of practicing psychologists' attitudes toward psychotherapy treatment manuals. *Journal of Consulting and Clinical Psychology, 68,* 331–339.

American Psychological Association Presidential Task Force on Evidence-Based Practice (2006). Evidence-based practice in psychology. *American Psychologist, 61,* 271–285.

Anderson, C. M., & Kim, C. (2003). Evaluating treatment efficacy with single-case designs. In M. C. Roberts & S. S. Ilardi (Eds.), *Handbook of Research Methods in Clinical Psychology* (pp. 73–91). Malden, MA: Blackwell Publishing.

Attkisson, C. C., & Greenfield, T. K. (1999). The UCSF Client Satisfaction Scales: I. The Client Satisfaction Questionnaire-8. In M. E. Maruish (Ed.), *The Use of Psychological Testing for Treatment Planning and Outcomes Assessment,* 2nd ed. (pp. 1333–1346). Mahwah, NJ: Lawrence Erlbaum Associates.

Attkisson, C. C., & Greenfield, T. K. (2004). The UCSF Client Satisfaction Scales: I. The Client Satisfaction Questionnaire-8. In M. E. Maruish (Ed.), *The Use of Psychological Testing for Treatment Planning and Outcomes Assessment: Volume 3: Instruments for Adults,* 3rd ed. (pp. 799–811). Mahwah, NJ: Lawrence Erlbaum Associates.

Beidel, D. C., Turner, S. M., & Morris, T. L. (2000). Behavioral treatment of childhood social phobia. *Journal of Consulting and Clinical Psychology, 68,* 1072–1080.

Bickman, L., Guthrie, P. R., Foster, E. M., Lambert, E. W., Summerfelt, W. T., Breda, C. S., et al. (1995). *Evaluating Managed Mental Health Services: The Fort Bragg Experiment.* New York: Plenum.

Bickman, L., & Mulvaney, S. (2005). Large-scale evaluations of children's mental health services: The Ft. Bragg and Stark County studies. In R. G. Steele & M. C. Roberts (Eds.), *Handbook of Mental Health Services for Children, Adolescents, and Families* (pp. 371–386). New York: Kluwer.

Bickman, L., Noser, K., & Summerfelt, W. T. (1999). Long-term effects of a system of care on children and adolescents. *The Journal of Behavioral Health Services and Research, 26,* 185–202.

Birmaher, B., Brent, D. A., Kolko, D., Baugher, M., Bridge, J., Holder, D., et al. (2000). Clinical outcome after short-term psychotherapy for adolescents with major depressive disorder. *Archives of General Psychiatry, 57,* 29–35.

Borrelli, B., Sepinwall, D., Ernst, D., Bellg, A. J., Czajkowski, S., Breger, R., et al. (2005). A new tool to assess treatment fidelity and evaluation of treatment fidelity across 10 years of health behavior research. *Journal of Consulting and Clinical Psychology, 73,* 852–860.

Bottcher, J., & Ezell, M. E. (2005). Examining the effectiveness of boot camps: A randomized experiment with a long-term follow-up. *Journal of Research in Crime and Delinquency, 42,* 309–332.

Center for Mental Health Services (1997). *The Family Satisfaction Questionnaire—Abbreviated Version (FSQ-A).* Unpublished manuscript.

Chambless, D. L., & Hollon, S. D. (1998). Defining empirically supported therapies. *Journal of Consulting and Clinical Psychology, 66,* 7–18.

Chorpita, B. F., & Donkervoet, C. (2005). Implementation of the Felix Consent Decree in Hawaii: The impact of policy and practice development efforts on service delivery. In R. G. Steele & M. C. Roberts (Eds.), *Handbook of Mental Health Services for Children, Adolescents, and Families* (pp. 317–332). New York: Kluwer.

Chorpita, B. F., Yim, L. M., Donkervoet, J. C., Arensdorf, A., Amundsen, M. J., McGee, C., et al. (2002). Toward large-scale implementation of empirically supported treatments for children: A review and observations by the Hawaii Empirical Basis to Services Task Force. *Clinical Psychology: Science and Practice, 9,* 165–190.

Clinical Treatment and Services Research Workgroup (CTSRW) (1998). *Bridging Science and Service: A Report by the National Advisory Mental Health Council's Clinical Treatment and Services Research Workgroup.* Bethesda, MD: National Institutes of Health, National Institute of Mental Health. Retrieved May 19, 2006, from http://www.nimh.nih.gov/publicat/nimhbridge.pdf.

Connor-Smith, J. K., & Weisz, J. R. (2003). Applying treatment outcome research in clinical practice: Techniques for adapting interventions to the real world. *Child and Adolescent Mental Health, 8,* 3–10.

Crosbie, J. (1993). Interrupted time-series analyses with brief single-subject data. *Journal of Consulting and Clinical Psychology, 61,* 966–974.

Des Jarlais, D. C., Lyles, C., Crepaz, N., & the TREND Group (2004). Improving the reporting quality of nonrandomized evaluations of behavioral and public health interventions: The TREND statement. *American Journal of Public Health, 94,* 361–366.

Graczyk, P. A., Domitrovich, C. E., & Zins, J. E. (2003). Facilitating the implementation of evidence-based prevention and mental health promotion efforts in schools. In M. D. Weist, S. W. Evans, & N. A. Lever (Eds.), *Handbook of School Mental Health: Advancing Practice and Research* (pp. 301–318). New York: Kluwer Academic/Plenum Publishers.

Greenfield, T. K., & Attkisson, C. C. (2004). The UCSF Client Satisfaction Scales: II. The Service Satisfaction Scale-30. In M.E. Maruish (Ed.), *The Use of Psychological Testing for Treatment Planning and Outcomes Assessment: Volume 3: Instruments for Adults,* 3rd ed. (pp. 813–837). Mahwah, NJ: Lawrence Erlbaum Associates.

Hawley, K. M., & Weisz, J. R. (2005). Youth versus parent working alliance in usual clinical care: Distinctive associations with retention, satisfaction, and treatment outcome. *Journal of Clinical Child and Adolescent Psychology, 34,* 117–128.

Henderson, J. L., MacKay, S., & Peterson-Badali, M. (2006). Closing the research-practice gap: Factors affecting adoption and implementation of a children's mental health program. *Journal of Clinical Child and Adolescent Psychology, 35,* 2–12.

Henggeler, S. W., Melton, G. B., Brondino, M. J., Scherer, D. G., & Hanley, J. H. (1997). Multisystemic therapy with violent and chronic juvenile offenders and their families: The role of treatment fidelity in successful dissemination. *Journal of Consulting and Clinical Psychology, 65,* 821–833.

Hernandez, M., Hodges, S., & Cascardi, M. (1998). The ecology of outcomes: System accountability in children's mental health. *The Journal of Behavioral Health Services & Research, 25,* 136–150.

Hoagwood, K., Jensen, P. S., Petti, T., & Burns, B. J. (1996). Outcomes of mental health care for children and adolescents: I. A comprehensive conceptual model. *Journal of the American Academy of Child and Adolescent Psychiatry, 35,* 1055–1063.

Holden, E. W., & Brennan, A. M. (Eds.) (2002). Special issue: Evaluating systems of care: The National Evaluation of the Comprehensive Community Mental Health Services for Children and Their Families Program. *Children's Services: Social Policy, Research, and Practice, 5,* 1–74.

Holden, E. W., De Carolis, G., & Huff, B. (2002). Policy implications of the National Evaluation of the Comprehensive Community Mental Health Services for Children and Their Families Program. *Children's Services: Social Policy, Research, and Practice, 5,* 57–66.

Holden, E. W., Stephens, R. L., & Santiago, R. L. (2005). Methodological challenges in the national evaluation of the Comprehensive Community Mental Health Services for Children and Their Families program. In R. G. Steele & M. C. Roberts (Eds.), *Handbook of Mental Health Services for Children, Adolescents, and Families* (pp. 387–401). New York: Kluwer.

Huebner, C. E., Barlow, W. E., Tyll, L. T., Johnston, B. D., & Thompson, R. S. (2004). Expanding developmental and behavioral services for newborns in primary care: Program design, delivery, and evaluation framework. *American Journal of Preventive Medicine, 26,* 344–355.

Jacobson, N. S., & Truax, P. (1991). Clinical significance: A statistical approach to defining meaningful change in psychotherapy research. *Journal of Consulting and Clinical Psychology, 59,* 12–19.

Jensen, P. S., Hoagwood, K., & Petti, T. (1996). Outcomes of mental health care for children and adolescents: II. Literature review and application of a comprehensive model. *Journal of the American Academy of Child and Adolescent Psychiatry, 35,* 1064–1077.

Jensen-Doss, A., & Weisz, J. R. (2006). Syndrome co-occurrence and treatment outcomes in youth mental health clinics. *Journal of Consulting and Clinical Psychology, 74,* 416–425.

Kallestad, J. H., & Olweus, D. (2003). Predicting teachers' and schools' implementation of the Olweus Bullying Prevention Program: A multilevel study. *Prevention and Treatment, 6.*

Kazdin, A. E. (1997). A model for developing effective treatments: Progression and interplay of theory, research, and practice. *Journal of Clinical Child Psychology, 26,* 114–129.

Kazdin, A. E. (2001). Almost clinically significant ($p < .10$): Current measures may only approach clinical significance. *Clinical Psychology: Science and Practice, 8,* 455–462.

Kazdin, A. E. (2003a). Problem-solving skills training and parent management training for conduct disorder. In A. E. Kazdin & J. R Weisz (Eds.), *Evidence-Based Psychotherapies for Children and Adolescents* (pp. 241–262). New York: Guilford.

Kazdin, A. E. (2003b). Psychotherapy for children and adolescents. *Annual Review of Psychology, 54,* 253–276.

Kazdin, A. E. (2006). Arbitrary metrics: Implications for identifying evidence-based treatments. *American Psychologist, 61,* 42–49.

Kazdin, A. E., Siegel, T., & Bass, D. (1990). Drawing on clinical practice to inform research on child and adolescent psychotherapy: Survey of practitioners. *Professional Psychology: Research and Practice, 21,* 189–198.

Kazdin, A. E., Siegel, T., & Bass, D. (1992). Cognitive problem-solving skills training and parent management training in the treatment of antisocial behavior in children. *Journal of Consulting and Clinical Psychology, 60,* 733–747.

Kazdin, A. E., & Weisz, J. R. (1998). Identifying and developing empirically supported child and adolescent treatments. *Journal of Consulting and Clinical Psychology, 66,* 19–36.

Kendall, P. C. (Ed.) (1999). Special section: Clinical significance. *Journal of Consulting and Clinical Psychology, 67,* 283–339.

Matos, M., Torres, R., Santiago, R., Jurado, M., & Rodriguez, I. (2006). Adaptation of parent-child interaction therapy for Puerto Rican families: A preliminary study. *Family Process, 45,* 205–222.

Miranda, J., Guillermo, B., Lau, A., Kohn, L., Hwang, W., & LaFromboise, T. (2005). State of the science on psychosocial interventions for ethnic minorities. *Annual Review of Clinical Psychology, 1,* 113–142.

Moher, D., Schulz, K. F., & Altman, D. (2001). The CONSORT statement: Revised recommendations for improving the quality of reports of parallel-group randomized trials. *Journal of the American Medical Association, 285,* 1987–1991.

Moore, K. E., Geffken, G. R., & Royal, G. P. (1995). Behavioral intervention to reduce child distress during self-injection. *Clinical Pediatrics, 34,* 530–534.

Nelson, T. D., & Steele, R. G. (2006). Beyond efficacy and effectiveness: A multifaceted approach to treatment evaluation. *Professional Psychology: Research and Practice, 37,* 389–397.

Nelson, T. D., Steele, R. G., & Mize, J. A. (2006). Practitioner attitudes toward evidence-based practice. *Administrative Policy in Mental Health and Mental Health Services Research, 33,* 398–409.

Ogles, B. M., Lambert, M. J., & Masters, K. S. (1996). *Assessing Outcome in Clinical Practice.* Boston: Allyn & Bacon.

Olson, R., & Netherton, S. D. (1996). Consultation and liaison in a children's hospital. In M. C. Roberts (Ed.), *Model Programs in Child and Family Mental Health* (pp. 249–264). Mahwah: NJ: Lawrence Erlbaum Associates.

Olweus, D., Limber, S., & Mihalic, S. F. (1999). *Blueprints for Violence Prevention, Book Nine: Bullying Prevention Program*. Boulder, CO: Center for the Study and Prevention of Violence.

Paul, G. L. (1967). Outcome research in psychotherapy. *Journal of Consulting Psychology, 31*, 109–118.

Persons, J. B., & Silberschatz, G. (1998). Are results of randomized controlled trials useful to psychotherapists? *Journal of Consulting and Clinical Psychology, 66*, 126–135.

Plumer, P. J., & Stoner, G. (2005). The relative effects of classwide peer tutoring and peer coaching on the positive social behaviors of children with ADHD. *Journal of Attention Disorders, 9*, 290–300.

Schiffman, J., Becker, K. D., & Daleiden, E. L. (2006). Evidence-based services in a statewide public mental health system: Do the services fit the problems? *Journal of Clinical Child and Adolescent Psychology, 35*, 13–19.

Schoenwald, S. K., Sheidow, A. J., & Letourneau, E. J. (2004). Toward effective quality assurance in evidence-based practice: Links between expert consultation, therapist fidelity, and child outcomes. *Journal of Clinical Child and Adolescent Psychology, 33*, 94–104.

Sheldrick, R. C., Kendall, P. C., & Heimberg, R. G. (2001). The clinical significance of treatments: A comparison of three treatments for conduct disordered children. *Clinical Psychology: Science and Practice, 8*, 418–430.

Shirk, S. R. (2005). President's message: Dialogue and persistent polarities between research and practice. *In Balance: Society of Clinical Child and Adolescent Psychology Newsletter, 20*(3), 1–2.

Simons, A. D., & Wildes, J. E. (2003). Therapy and interventions research with adults. In M. C. Roberts & S. S. Ilardi (Eds.), *Handbook of Research Methods in Clinical Psychology* (pp. 329–351). Malden, MA: Blackwell Publishing.

Slifer, K. J., Eischen, S. E., & Busby, S. (2002). Using counterconditioning to treat behavioural distress during subcutaneous injections in a paediatric rehabilitation patient. *Brain Injury, 16*, 901–916.

Southam-Gerow, M. A., Weisz, J. R., & Kendall, P. C. (2003). Youth with anxiety disorders in research and service clinics: Examining client differences and similarities. *Journal of Clinical Child and Adolescent Psychology, 32*, 375–385.

Stirman, S. W., Crits-Christoph, P., & DeRubeis, R. J. (2004). Achieving successful dissemination of empirically supported psychotherapies: A synthesis of dissemination theory. *Clinical Psychology: Science and Practice, 11*, 343–359.

Varni, J. W., Burwinkle, T. M., Dickinson, P., Sherman, S. A., Dixon, P., Ervice, J. A., et al. (2004). Evaluation of the built environment at a children's convalescent hospital: Development of the Pediatric Quality of Life Inventory^{TM} parent and staff satisfaction measures for pediatric health care facilities. *Journal of Developmental and Behavioral Pediatrics, 25*, 10–20.

Walrath, C. M., Ybarra, M. L., & Holden, E. W. (2006). Understanding the pre-referral factors associated with differential 6-month outcomes among children receiving system-of-care services. *Psychological Services, 3*, 35–50.

Weisz, J. R., Jensen, A. L., & McLeod, B. D. (2005). Development and dissemination of child and adolescent psychotherapies: Milestones, methods, and a new deployment-focused model. In E. D. Hibbs & P. S. Jensen (Eds.), *Psychosocial Treatments for Child and Adolescent Disorders: Empirically Based Strategies for Clinical Practice*, 2nd ed. (pp. 9–39). Washington, DC: American Psychological Association.

Wells, K. B. (1999). Treatment research at the crossroads: The scientific interface of clinical trials and effectiveness research. *American Journal of Psychiatry, 156*, 5–10.

Wierzbicki, M., & Pekarik, G. (1993). A meta-analysis of psychotherapy dropout. *Professional Psychology: Research and Practice, 24*, 190–195.

Yates, B. T. (2003). Toward the incorporation of costs, cost-effectiveness analysis, and cost-benefit analysis into clinical research. In A. E. Kazdin (Ed.), *Methodological Issues and Strategies in Clinical Research*, 3rd ed. (pp. 711–727). Washington, DC: American Psychological Association.

4

Evidence-Based Therapies: Translating Research into Practice

CHARMAINE K. HIGA and BRUCE F. CHORPITA

A plethora of evidence exists supporting the use of certain clinical practices for children and adolescents over others (e.g., Kazdin et al., 1990; Weiss & Weisz, 1995; Weisz et al., 1995), yet current research shows that practitioners rarely use these interventions in their own practice (e.g., Weersing et al., 2002) and that therapy conducted in community settings is not as effective as therapy conducted in research settings (e.g., Weiss et al., 1995, 1999). Thus, practices with evidence of being helpful are not available to most children and adolescents who seek treatment. An even greater challenge involves recent evidence suggesting that the relative advantages of evidence-based practices documented in the laboratory may not hold up in real-world settings (e.g., Barrington et al., 2005). Thus, at least two related problems appear to face the field: (1) Despite years of documentation of the promising effects of evidence-based practices, their penetration into practice settings is extremely limited; and (2) the quality and relevance of laboratory findings on treatment may not universally apply to real-world applied settings. However, despite leading researchers' having emphasized moving treatment research into practice settings for over a decade (e.g., Kazdin et al., 1990; Weisz et al., 1995) and policy makers and funding sources encouraging the rapid development of dissemination research (e.g., Chambers et al., 2005; National Advisory Mental Health Council Workgroup on Child and Adolescent Mental Health Intervention Development and Deployment, 2001; National Institutes of Health, 2002; Norquist et al., 1999), only a handful of evidence-based practices have been examined in "real-world" settings in the youth mental health literature to date (Barrington et al., 2005; Henggeler et al., 1992; Mufson et al., 2004). To address these matters, this chapter begins with a discussion

---

CHARMAINE K. HIGA and BRUCE F. CHORPITA • University of Hawai'i at Mānoa

of the possible reasons for the relatively slow translation of research to practice, follows with a brief review of current models of dissemination, and finishes with a summary of an alternative perspective to addressing not only problems with dissemination but also problems with the relevance and generalizability of intervention research.

BARRIERS TO DISSEMINATION

There are a multitude of obstacles to the much-sought-after connection between science and practice. One way to organize these stumbling blocks is by putting them into a larger framework for understanding human behavior. For decades, researchers in a number of different fields have theorized that human change behavior is related to (1) *knowledge* about the targeted concept and (2) *attitude* toward this concept. For example, researchers have used this knowledge-attitude-practice framework to examine family planning and contraception use in underdeveloped countries (e.g., Rehan, 1984), recycling behavior (e.g., Arbuthnot, 1974), and tobacco use among college students (e.g., Torabi et al., 2002). This framework could be used to help better understand the obstacles the field is currently facing with regard to the adoption of evidence-based practices.

Knowledge Barriers

Knowledge of evidence-based practices has many facets, from awareness of the concept to the more technical, "how-to" aspects of applying specific evidence-based interventions. As such, there are a number of knowledge-related barriers to translating research into practice.

Defining Evidence

First, one would assume that with the growing interest in and attention to this area over the last decade, as well as the many task forces and workgroups developed to address this concern specifically [e.g., Task Force on Psychological Intervention Guidelines of the American Psychological Association, 1995; Task Force on Promotion and Dissemination of Psychological Procedures, Division of Clinical Psychology, APA, 1995; APA Division 12, Section 1 Task Force on Empirically Supported Psychosocial Interventions for Children (Lonigan et al., 1998)], there would be at least some consensus on the definition of evidence. For instance, the Division 12 Task Force (Lonigan et al., 1995) differentiated *efficacy*, the scientific or internal validity of the outcome research, from *effectiveness*, the external validity or generalizability of the treatment in real-world settings. ESTs were categorized into two levels: *probably efficacious* and *well-established* (Chambless et al., 1998; Chambless & Hollon, 1998). In contrast, the Substance Abuse and Mental Health Services Administration (SAMHSA) separates evidence-based programs into three different categories: *promising*, *effective*, and *model*. *Promising programs* have been evaluated and implemented and are considered "scientifically defensible" but have not yet yielded consistently positive outcomes required for effective program status. *Effective programs* are well implemented and evaluated and produce a consistent positive pattern of results. The only difference between *effective programs* and *model programs* is that developers of *model programs* have agreed to work with SAMHSA/CSAP to provide materials, training, and technical assistance for nationwide implementation (U.S. Department of Health and Human Services, SAMHSA, n.d.). The inconsistency and complexity of the evidence-based taxonomies are clearly obstacles to the therapist seeking to select and implement the most effective therapeutic strategies.

Restrictive and Uninformative Definitions of Evidence

Another knowledge-related barrier to bridging the science-practice gap is that as a result of the highly restrictive definitions used to identify empirically supported treatments, for some treatment targets, there are no treatments that meet the strict criteria. For example, although numerous treatment programs are reported in the literature for autism, based on previous definitions, none meets the criteria for well-established or probably efficacious status (Chorpita et al., 2002; Rogers, 1998). This is highly problematic for those involved in the provision of services for youth afflicted with problems in such areas where there is no one treatment deemed "evidence-based." As such, some researchers have proposed a third *possibly efficacious* level that does not require that the treatment programs used manuals (Chorpita et al., 2002). Broadening the definition of evidence-based treatments in this manner shows us that in fact, for autism, not all treatments have won and not all must have prizes (cf. Luborsky et al., 1975).

A related definitional problem is that the current evidence base does not communicate information regarding client and context characteristics associated with each treatment. In other words, if one wanted to know more than simply if a treatment is evidence-based or not, such as for whom did the treatment work and in what context, one could not easily draw inferences from the existing lists of evidence-based treatments (Chambless et al., 1998; Lonigan et al., 1998; SAMHSA, 2006). As one attempt to address this issue, Chorpita and colleagues (2005a) proposed a Distillation and Matching Model (DMM). *Distillation* is described as the view that individual techniques (e.g., exposure, time out, etc.) can be gleaned from larger treatment packages (e.g., parent management training), and using statistical *matching* procedures akin to data mining, study or patient characteristics that are most important in the selection of evidence-based treatments (e.g., age, gender, setting, etc.) can be identified via the literature (Chorpita et al., 2005a).

Too Many and Too Few Evidence-Based Treatments

The DMM may also prove fruitful in addressing two other separate but related barriers to practitioner awareness of evidence-based practices. If a practitioner decided to treat a depressed child using cognitive-behavioral therapy (CBT), he or she might find it frustrating that there are at least 13 different treatment manuals to choose from that were used in RCTs. The lack of a tool to help select among multiple evidence-based treatments is one problem that the DMM could potentially address, either by bypassing the need to choose among complete treatment packages and yielding an aggregate summary of the techniques consistent across the manuals (Chorpita et al., 2005a) or by suggesting the most appropriate manual in terms of similarity to that aggregate summary. In other words, instead of trying to choose one of the 13 depression treatment manuals, a practitioner might decide to use the five most common techniques across all of the evidence-based protocols for depression (e.g., cognitive coping, activity selection, psychoeducation, problem solving, and relaxation; Chorpita et al., 2005a).

Having too many manuals to choose from is problematic, but it is definitely preferable over having none to choose from. Too often the field has heard complaints from community clinicians, clinic directors, and even graduate students that the manuals described in RCTs are difficult to find. Furthermore, given that most protocols undergo numerous revisions, the original protocol tested in a trial is often times no longer available (e.g., Anastopoulos et al., 1993; Barrett, 1998; Weisz et al., 1997).

Awareness Knowledge Barrier

Selecting and finding evidence-based treatment manuals may be challenging, but this assumes that practitioners can get past the first step of becoming aware of and identifying these treatments. In a study of youth mental health providers' attitudes toward evidence-based practices, program managers (many of whom were supervisors of the direct care staff) reported very little familiarity with the terms "evidence-based practice" and "empirically supported treatment" (Aarons, 2004). It seems that an even bigger and initial problem to address is the lack of a simple communication tool for practitioners to access the research. Given that the main vehicle researchers have relied on for decades to communicate their findings is through scientific journals, without a more user-friendly "dissemination engine," practitioners in the field have little chance of gaining awareness of these practices supported by the evidence.

How-to-Knowledge Barrier

Finally, the largest and, some might argue, the most challenging knowledge-related barrier to dissemination is that the training and supervision requirements to learn evidence-based practices are substantial (e.g., Connor-Smith & Weisz, 2003). If a practitioner could find an evidence-based protocol for childhood depression, there is little, if any, research demonstrating that CBT implemented without substantial training, supervision, and quality control would do better than the interventions the practitioner is already implementing. Attention to these issues of training and dissemination will likely dominate the research agenda for the foreseeable future (e.g., Weingardt, 2004).

Attitude Barriers

A practitioner may be aware of evidence-based practices and may have even been trained in an evidence-based procedure, but these together may not predict whether or not he or she will decide to use this intervention in his or her own practice. This is because it is believed that a provider's attitude toward evidence-based practices together with how knowledgeable he or she is about the procedure will predict the likelihood that he or she will adopt it into practice (e.g., Rogers, 2003).

Individual Differences

In an effort to examine practitioners' attitudes toward evidence-based practice, Addis and Krasnow (2000) surveyed practicing psychologists about manual-based psychotherapy. Although predictions that fewer number of years in practice (more recently educated) would be related to more positive attitudes were only weakly supported, results clearly supported hypotheses that theoretical orientation and practice setting are related to attitudes toward manual-based treatment (i.e., cognitive-behavioral orientation and academic setting predicted more positive attitudes; Addis & Krasnow, 2000).

In contrast to findings reported by Addis and Krasnow (2000), Aarons (2004) found that the strongest individual difference variable that predicted positive attitudes toward evidence-based practice was internship status in providers of youth mental health. Interns reported higher levels of openness to change and found evidence-based practices more appealing than staff providers, suggesting that professional internships may be an opportune time to expose developing practitioners to evidence-based practices (Aarons, 2004). More studies are needed to better understand individual difference variables related to practitioner attitudes toward evidence-based practices.

Specific Practitioner Attitudes

There are a number of different reasons why a practitioner might have a negative attitude toward evidence-based practices. Addis et al. (1999) described six thematic concerns commonly voiced by practitioners about manual-based psychotherapies: (1) unmet client needs, (2) restriction of clinical innovation, (3) feasibility of manual-based treatments, (4) effects on the therapeutic relationship, (5) treatment credibility, and (6) competence and job satisfaction. Some of the most commonly cited concerns by practitioners about manualized psychotherapy are related to beliefs that manuals do not allow clinicians to address individual client needs, do not work with "real" patients with multiple problems, and restrict practitioner creativity (Addis et al., 1999). The common theme is that the traditional "cookie cutter," "lock-step," session-by-session manual-driven approach is practically cumbersome and clinically unappealing.

One proposed method of addressing these concerns and at the same time remaining evidence-based is via the use of modular protocols (e.g., Carroll, 1998; Clarke et al., 1990; Curry et al., 2000). Chorpita and colleagues (2005b) described modularity as "breaking complex [therapeutic] activities into simpler parts that may function independently" and modules as "self-contained functional units that connect with other units but do not rely on those other units for their own stable operations" (p. 142). In other words, most cognitive-behavioral therapy for child anxiety includes the following: exposure, modeling, cognitive coping, relaxation, and psychoeducation. By breaking down CBT for child anxiety into modules, practitioners can choose to employ only the most appropriate therapeutic activities for each of their cases. For example, treatment for a young, anxious child who presents with a specific phobia might focus on modeling and exposure, whereas treatment for an adolescent with more generalized symptoms of anxiety might focus on cognitive coping and relaxation. Modularity also allows practitioners the flexibility to incorporate other evidence-based modules into treatment when treatment progress is hindered due to another interfering problem. For instance, during the course of treatment for separation anxiety, a clinician might choose to implement a tangible rewards module if he or she finds that the child's motivation to complete homework exposure tasks is interfering with treatment progress or an active ignoring module if the child tantrums to avoid or escape a fearful situation. Thus, modular protocols can allow practitioners to tailor their evidence-based interventions to fit the individual needs of their clients (Chorpita et al., 2004, 2005b; Chorpita & Weisz, 2005). Modular designs can also address practitioner feasibility concerns related to training and implementation. For example, because a number of protocols have overlapping modules (e.g., rewards), practitioner training is potentially less burdensome and comprehensibility is more parsimonious (Chorpita et al., 2005b; Chorpita & Weisz, 2005). The promise of such an approach has preliminary support but would benefit from further empirical testing. Some additional ways that clinical researchers can address attitude-related barriers will be discussed below.

Practice (Contextual) Barriers

The knowledge-attitude-practice framework is useful in understanding which individual factors are related to the eventual adoption of certain behaviors. However, given that most providers of youth mental health services work in settings with other people as part of a system, the context in which the individual is embedded is also very important to consider.

Few Incentives to Change

In many cases, there are countless motivating reasons to choose not to adopt evidence-based practices and to continue doing things the way they have been, with few incentives to adopt a completely new way of doing treatment. For instance, unlike with medicine or other professions, federal authorities do not regulate mental health services. Whereas a new medication must receive FDA approval before it can be prescribed (and not be considered an off-label prescription), mental health treatments are not required to undergo extensive evaluation before their use. And although governing bodies have taken more of an interest in regulation of the practices clinicians provide, these at least initially have been motivated by cost-containment motives, such that brevity is emphasized over specific content of the intervention (Hayes et al., 1999). Given that licensing in most states requires continuing education, some clinicians might be motivated to learn evidence-based procedures in their practice. However, in our work on the Child STEPs Clinic Treatment Project (CTP), we found that a majority of practitioners in community outpatient clinics do not hold a state license (Nakamura et al., 2005), and so this motivating factor may be less powerful. Furthermore, as staff turnover rates are high in the mental health field (e.g., Torrey et al., 2001), agencies are much less motivated to invest in training practitioners who may not be with the agency for very long.

Many Costs to Change

In addition to having few reasons to adopt evidence-based practices, there are considerable costs associated with training in most manualized treatments, including materials and trainer costs as well as costs to the agency in lost productivity time due to practitioner participation in training and, in some cases, continuing education via booster sessions, supervision time, etc. (e.g., Strosahl, 1998; Torrey et al., 2001). As such, learning how to use new treatment procedures is timely and costly, and for many practitioners, new learning must occur outside their normal work hours or they experience a loss in wages as a result of not meeting productivity benchmarks placed on them by clinic administration (e.g., Hatgis et al., 2001). In the Child STEPs CTP, one challenge being faced is that many of the clinicians participating in the study are on a fee-for-service pay schedule with their agency, so any time they spend working outside direct clinical contact (e.g., training and consultation with manual experts), they are not earning a paycheck; therefore, finding time to meet with them can sometimes be very challenging (Ho et al., 2007). These costs, coupled with the fact that there are few incentives to investing personal time into learning new treatment procedures, make the slow adoption of evidence-based practices less surprising.

MODELS OF DISSEMINATION

In order to address these numerous barriers, differing models of dissemination have developed and evolved. We will briefly describe two models of dissemination in the context of moving treatment outcomes research into practice settings (for a more thorough review of dissemination models, see Southam-Gerow et al., in press). Before moving to a summary of these models, we want to comment briefly on terminology. The focus here is on how researchers translate or decode information from research to practitioners, implying a unidirectional or hierarchical relationship. The term *translational research* grew out of a U.S. Food and Drug Administration philosophy and, accordingly, has been termed the "medical-pharmaceutical" model by some authors (Weisz et al., 2005). The concept proposes that treatments initially be developed via wisdom from basic laboratory research and then tested first in lab-based efficacy experiments. Only after extensive efficacy research is an intervention then brought into the community setting to measure the public health impact (e.g., Greenwald & Cullen, 1984; Norquist et al., 1999). In an ideal world, the lab setting would be a close approximation to the real world so that findings from lab-based efficacy trials could easily be generalized to practice settings. Unfortunately, the targets of impact in efficacy trials often differ widely from those in real-world settings (see Schoenwald & Hoagwood, 2001; Southam-Gerow et al., in press). Research on programs that were widely disseminated before they were examined for effectiveness has indicated that identifying whether practices shown to be efficacious in a highly controlled setting might be transportable to another setting is an important missing link in much of the previous dissemination research. For example, the Home-Builders Model of Family Preservation Services and the Healthy Families America program were both widely disseminated before they were examined in the settings to which they were disseminated, and subsequent studies found that they were not effective at preventing foster care placement (Heneghan et al., 1996) or child abuse and neglect (Duggan et al., 1999; Olds et al., 2002), respectively. As such, leading researchers in the field have argued for the importance of studying interventions that have demonstrated efficacy in research settings in the community settings they are to be disseminated to before widespread diffusion takes place (e.g., Schoenwald & Hoagwood, 2001; Weisz, 2004).

Deployment-Focused Model

Weisz (2004) described a deployment-focused model of dissemination that addresses the missing link between efficacy and dissemination by breaking the traditional stage III research (NIH, 2003) into three separate steps and adding a final step for a total of 6 steps: (1) construction, refinement, and manualizing of the intervention protocol; (2) initial efficacy trial under controlled conditions to establish evidence of benefit; (3) single-case applications in practice settings, with progressive adaptations to the protocol; (4) partial effectiveness tests of one or more practice setting targets (referred youth, community setting, community practitioners, etc.); (5) full tests of effectiveness and dissemination; and (6) tests of sustainability in practice contexts. He further argued that other foci of interest that have typically been examined in research settings must also be first examined in community settings before assumptions can be made about their generalizability. Some of these include the (1) necessary and sufficient components of treatment packages, (2) moderators of outcome that set boundaries around treatment impact, (3) hypothesized mediators of outcome, (4) treatment costs relative to benefits, (5) organizational factors in the systems and settings where the treatments are being used related to effectiveness of use, and (6) variations in treatment procedures, packaging, training, and delivery designed to improve fit between treatment and various settings of deployment. Using the NIH model, even research that examines the adaptation of a therapy for use in a community setting is defined as Stage I (NIH, 2003). This strict definition and requirement that any changes to protocols be "run through the gauntlet" of stages of research could potentially impede the deployment of evidence-based procedures to children and families who might benefit from them, and Weisz's (2004) model attempts to address this problem.

Multilevel Contextual Model

Schoenwald and Hoagwood (2001) described similar procedures for researching the transportability of efficacious interventions to usual care settings. They argued for a model of dissemination research that is a cross between efficacy and effectiveness and that emphasizes multilevel factors, including organizational and system factors as well as other factors traditionally emphasized in child intervention research. Federal and foundation-sponsored initiatives have also incorporated such multilevel thinking into strategies to disseminate evidence-based practices for adults with serious mental illnesses (Torrey et al., 2001). Multilevel contextual models such as these reflect the "emerging concept that broad-based implementation has a systemic nature and underpinnings, with facilitators and barriers at the level of policy and regulations, the level of the organization, the level at which service provision or treatment occurs, and the levels of the consumer and family member" (Stuart et al., 2002, p. 328). Youth receiving mental health care are nested within a mental health system (providers and agencies) that is influenced by policy and funding mechanisms, and each level influences and interacts with all other levels. Consistent with this model, recent findings show that in multisystemic therapy, therapist adherence, organizational climate, and organizational structure all have direct effects on posttreatment child outcomes (Schoenwald et al., 2003).

FROM TRANSLATION TO DISSEMINATION TO DIFFUSION

Recently, mental health researchers have found the cross-fertilization of ideas from public health, sociology, anthropology, and even marketing helpful in reconceptualizing the psychological services approach. Rogers' (2003) classic model of diffusion of innovation is especially useful. The utility of that model here is that it may reveal the relative strengths and weaknesses of current models as well as point to gaps in thinking about these issues as they have been developed within the EBT context. Rogers (2003) describes diffusion as "the process by which (1) an *innovation* (2) is *communicated* through certain *channels* (3) over *time* (4) among the members of a *social system*" (p. 11).

Innovation

The perceived attributes of an innovation or technology determine how quickly or slowly it will be adopted. If evidence-based practices are perceived as having (1) *relative advantage* (better than the practices they supercede), (2) *compatibility* (consistent with values, experiences, and needs of potential adopters), (3) minimal *complexity* (not difficult to understand and use), (4) *trialability* (free to try before completely adopting it), and (5) *observability* (results are visible to others), they will be adopted more quickly. Although evidence-based practices appear to provide relative advantage over current practices, in many cases they are not compatible with the interventions practitioners currently use, and learning to use them proficiently is not an easy task. Moreover, practitioners may not feel they have trialability if their clinics invest in materials and training in a new intervention. Given that much of the research on youth mental health has been conducted in lab-based settings, a common argument about evidence-based practices is that clinicians have not truly observed positive results of these practices with the kinds of youth they treat (e.g., Weisz et al., 2005).

In an effort to increase the staying power of an innovation, Rogers (2003) suggested that adopters who actively participate in customizing an innovation to fit their unique situation will be more likely to sustain their use of the innovation (Rogers, 2003). This concept supports the use of a deployment-focused model of dissemination where the study design calls for reinventions and examination of these reinventions (Weisz, 2004).

Communication

The characteristics of the communication channel—or how information about the innovation is transmitted—also affect the adoption rate of an innovation. Although mass media channels are a rapid and efficient way to build awareness knowledge about an innovation, interpersonal channels are generally more effective in persuading an adopter to implement an innovation, especially if the two people communicating about an innovation share similar attributes (i.e., beliefs, educational level, SES, etc.; Rogers, 2003). Rogers called this "homophily" and contrasts it with the term "heterophily," which is defined as "the degree to which two or more individuals who interact are different in certain attributes" (p. 19). He argued that heterophilious interpersonal communication channels slow the rate of innovation adoption. This has especially problematic implications for dissemination of evidence-based interventions given that it is almost always the case where researchers are seen as quite different from those practicing in the community. Rogers (2003) suggested that the more attributes on which people are different (e.g., educational level, field of training, theoretical orientation, age, etc.), the less likely adoption of an innovation is to occur. This means that researchers and innovators of evidence-based treatments must find unique ways to promote change by selecting key people who are homophilious with the adoptee majority yet are also able to advance the innovation. One way to accomplish this could include hiring staff that are similar to the targeted group. Another way is by training community partners to work with the dissemination team (e.g., Hardy et al., 2004). Related to this, diffusion research shows that most people do not evaluate an innovation on the basis of scientific studies of its consequences, but rather on more subjective evaluation of information conveyed to them from other adopters. In other words, when arguing for the importance of using evidence-based treatments to practitioners, it is more important that leaders in the field focus on enhancing subjective evaluation via people who are most like the potential adopters. Potential avenues to explore further include the use of testimonials by homophilious practitioners who have experienced success with the evidence-based procedure as well as clinical vignettes with practitioners and clients that are as similar to the potential adoptee as possible.

Time

In addition to factors associated with the innovation itself as well as how information about the innovation is communicated to potential adopters, there appears to be a common temporal pattern in the diffusion process. Rogers (2003) called this the innovation-decision process and described a progression that all individuals go through at varying speeds from first knowing about an innovation, to the formation of an attitude about the innovation, to a decision to adopt or reject the innovation, to implementation of the innovation, and finally to confirmation of this decision. Individual differences shape how innovative a person is, which determines the speed at which the person will move through the innovation-decision process. Individuals who are more innovative or move more quickly through the process tend to be more educated, are more able to cope with ambiguity, and have a greater exposure to mass media (Rogers, 2003). Rogers identified several adopter categories that describe how quickly or slowly a person moves through the innovation-decision process and collectively, the number of people adopting an innovation progresses over time to form an S-shaped curve such that only a few individuals rapidly adopt a given innovation at first (*Innovators*). The *Early Adopters* (13.5%) then communicate with the *Early Majority* (34%) about their experiences with the innovation. Only after observing the consequences of adoption via interpersonal communication channels does the *Late Majority* (34%) make decisions regarding adoption or rejection of the innovation. People in this adoption category tend to be of lower socioeconomic status and make little use of mass media channels (Rogers, 2003). After the majority of individuals have adopted an innovation, the rate of adoption slows until the *Laggards* (16%) decide to either adopt or reject the innovation. Future dissemination research should focus on individual practitioner variables that moderate adoption of evidence-based practices and whether focusing dissemination efforts on early adopters is a cost-effective and feasible approach to translating research into practice.

Social System

The rate of adoption and the shape of the S-curve are dependent on the characteristics of the social system in which they are embedded. The structure of social systems and, specifically, the way decisions are made in social structures determine the rate and staying power of innovations. If one individual with authority decides for the group that an innovation will be adopted (e.g., clinical supervisor), the rate of adoption is quick, but the staying power will not be as strong as it would be if each individual were allowed to make this decision on his own. On the other end of the spectrum, if the entire social system must make a collective decision about the adoption of an innovation, the slope of the S-curve is much more gradual. However, according to Rogers (2003), if *change agents* or individuals who influence clients' innovation-decisions in a desirable direction utilize *opinion leaders*, individuals within the social system who informally influence the attitudes and adoption behavior of others in the system, the number of adopters per unit of time increases exponentially. Opinion leaders are individuals within the social system to whom other people look to help them make decisions about adoption of innovations (Rogers, 2003). Investing resources in change agents who actively work to identify and support well-established opinion leaders in community agencies would be one way to enhance the diffusion of evidence-based treatments in practice settings. For example, Glisson and Schoenwald (2005) described an organizational and community intervention strategy that specifically targeted the mismatch between the innovation and the social context to which it was to be disseminated. Their Availability, Responsiveness, and Continuity (ARC) intervention strategy used change agents (i.e., doctoral- and masters-level practitioners in clinical psychology, social work, industrial organizational psychology, and counseling) who worked to bridge the technical-social or research-practice gap in a sequence of phases: (1) identifying and forming personal relationships with community opinion leaders, organizations, and key stakeholders, and collecting data about the problem and its effect on the community; (2) working with service providers, opinion leaders, etc. on coming to a collective understanding of how the community can begin to better understand and address the targeted problem; (3) ensuring that agreements are followed through; and (4) promoting self-regulation of the system after the intervention has terminated (Glisson & Schoenwald, 2005). Although there is no clear evidence yet whether this model or some other approach will work best, it is clear that the prevailing model of dissemination (which is to publish a lot, train a little, supervise less, and address organizations not at all) is in need of repair.

CONCLUSION

Taken together, it appears that the translation of research into practice depends on an awareness of the synergistic relationship between the innovation and the social context it is to be disseminated to. In other words, in order to accomplish diffusion of evidence-based practices, attention needs to be paid to both the social aspects of the adoption of evidence-based practices in youth mental health systems as well as the design of the technology itself. In the state of Hawaii, a quality improvement and clinical decision-making model serves as one example of this type of endeavor. Daleiden and Chorpita (2005) described a systemwide implementation of an evidence-based clinical decision-making model adopted by the Hawai'i Child and Adolescent Mental Health Division. This model was intended to incorporate aspects of the innovation—evidence-based practices—into the existing clinical decision-making processes.

Social context was also addressed through the facilitation of a culture of investigation, learning, and testing of claims. Thus, the foundation of the model drew from the traditional individualized case conceptualization model, in which individual cases are evaluated for their progress. Rather than mandating evidence-based practices, then, the model suggested an order to the decision-making structure, such that practice strategies be reviewed mainly in the absence of clinical progress. Thus, individual case results served as the primary evidence base, after which the larger evidence base of the scientific literature was consulted. This framework helped to establish commitment to the notion of accountability and verifiable results as a first step. Evidence-based practices were then seen as one set of tools to assist practitioners in their efforts to demonstrate success. To that end, extensive work was done to reanalyze the literature and organize it in a way that both optimized and simplified informed decision making about clinical practice (see Chorpita et al., 2002).

One additional innovation that was developed to facilitate this decision-making framework was a clinical reporting system using "clinical dashboards" that communicated important quantitative and qualitative case information (Daleiden & Chorpita, 2005). Dashboards included ratings on specific targets of intervention (e.g., specific phobia) plotted over time so that practitioners could observe case progress at a glance (see Figure 1). Specific therapeutic practices (e.g., practice or exposure, cognitive restructuring, rewards, etc.) that the practitioner had implemented were also plotted over time so that the relationship between case progress and therapeutic activities could easily be observed. Thus, only when case progress ratings suggested non-improvement or problem worsening were practitioners encouraged to examine their current practices against the summary of suggested evidence-based practices. In this way, the clinical dashboard helped to foster a culture of accountability, openness, and results and became a part of routine business procedures that incorporated and encouraged the use of evidence-based practices when clinical conditions warranted.

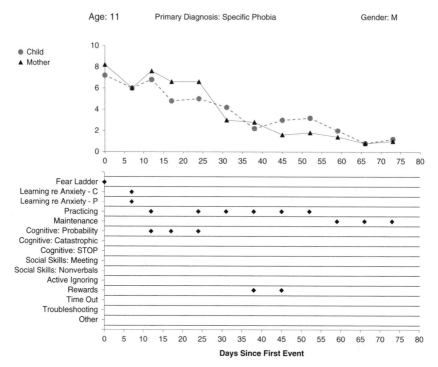

Figure 1. Example of a clinical dashboard for an 11-year-old boy receiving cognitive behavioral treatment for specific phobia.

Models such as these that focus on and appreciate the symbiotic nature of the relationship between the practice innovation (evidence-based practices) and the social context (youth mental health systems) in which it is embedded will be important to test in the future as psychological interventions move out of the laboratory and into the "real world." Our hope is that other models continue to emerge that fuse organizational intervention with the technology of evidence-based practices and that the profession can continue to learn better ways to allow research findings to inform and improve clinical practice.

REFERENCES

Aarons, G. A. (2004). Mental health provider attitudes toward adoption of evidence-based practice: The evidence-based practice attitude scale (EBPAS). *Mental Health Services Research, 6* , 61–74.

Addis, M. E., & Krasnow, A. D. (2000). A national survey of practicing psychologists' attitudes toward psychotherapy treatment manuals. *Journal of Consulting & Clinical Psychology, 68*, 331–339.

Addis, M. E., Wade, W. A., & Hatgis, C. (1999). Barriers to dissemination of evidence-based practices: Addressing practitioners' concerns about manual-based psychotherapies. *Clinical Psychology: Science and Practice, 6*, 430–441.

Anastopoulos, A. D., Shelton, T. L., DuPaul, G. J., & Guevremont, D. C. (1993). Parent training for attention-deficit hyperactivity disorder: Its impact on parent functioning. *Journal of Abnormal Child Psychology, 21*, 581–596.

Arbuthnot, J. (1974). Environmental knowledge and recycling behavior as a function of attitudes and personality characteristics. *Personality and Social Psychology Bulletin, 1* , 119–121.

Barrett, P. M. (1998). Evaluation of cognitive-behavioral group treatments for childhood anxiety disorders. *Journal of Clinical Child Psychology, 27*, 459–468.

Barrington, J., Prior, M., Richardson, M., & Allen, K. (2005). Effectiveness of CBT versus standard treatment for childhood anxiety disorders in a community clinic setting. *Behaviour Change, 22*, 29–43.

Carroll, K. M. (1998). *A Cognitive Behavioral Approach: Treating Cocaine Addiction* (Therapy Manual for Drug Addiction NIH Publication Number 98-4308). Rockville, MD: U.S. Department of Health and Human Services, National Institutes of Health.

Chambers, D. A., Ringeisen, H., & Hickman, E. E. (2005). Federal, state, and foundation initiatives around evidence-based practices child and adolescent mental health. *Child and Adolescent Psychiatric Clinics of North America, 14* , 307–327.

Chambless, D. L., Baker, M. J., Baucom, D. H., Beutler, L. E., Calhoun, K. S., Crits-Christoph, P., et al. (1998). Update on empirically validated therapies II. *The Clinical Psychologist, 51*, 3–16.

Chambless, D. L., & Hollon, S. D. (1998). Defining empirically supported therapies. *Journal of Consulting and Clinical Psychology, 66*, 7–18.

Chorpita, B. F., Daleiden, E. L., & Weisz, J. R. (2005a). Identifying and selecting the common elements of evidence-based interventions: A distillation and matching model. *Mental Health Services Research, 7*, 5–20.

Chorpita, B. F., Daleiden, E. L., & Weisz, J. R. (2005b). Modularity in the design and application of therapeutic interventions. *Applied and Preventive Psychology, 11*, 141–156.

Chorpita, B. F., Taylor, A. A., Francis, S. E., Moffitt, C., & Austin, A. A. (2004). Efficacy of modular cognitive behavior therapy for childhood anxiety disorders. *Behavior Therapy, 35*, 263–287.

Chorpita, B. F., & Weisz, J. R. (2005). *MATCH-ADC: A Modular Approach to Treatment for Children with Anxiety, Depression, or Conduct Problems.* Unpublished treatment manual.

Chorpita, B. F., Yim, L. M., Donkervoet, J. C., Arensdorf, A., Amundsen, M. J., McGee, C., et al. (2002). Toward large-scale implementation of empirically supported treatments for children: A review and observations by the Hawaii Empirical Basis to Services Task Force. *Clinical Psychology: Science & Practice, 9*, 165–190.

Clarke, G., Lewinsohn, P., & Hops, H. (1990). *Leader's Manual for Adolescent Groups: Adolescent Coping with Depression Course.* Portland, OR: Kaiser Permanente Center for Health Research.

Connor-Smith, J. K., & Weisz, J. R. (2003). Applying treatment outcome research in clinical practice: Techniques for adapting interventions to the real world. *Child and Adolescent Mental Health, 8* , 3–10.

Curry, J. F., Wells, K. C., Brent, D. A., Clarke, G. N., Rohde, P., Albano, A. M., et al. (2000). *Treatment for Adolescents with Depression Study Cognitive Behavior Therapy Manual: Introduction, Rationale, and Adolescent Sessions.* Unpublished manuscript, Duke University Medical Center.

Daleiden, E. L., & Chorpita, B. F. (2005). From data to wisdom: Quality improvement strategies supporting large-scale implementation of evidence-based services. *Child and Adolescent Psychiatric Clinics of North America, 14*, 329–349.

Duggan, A., McFarlane, E., Windham, A. M., Rohde, C., Salkever, D. S., Fuddy, L., et al. (1999). Evaluation of Hawaii's Healthy Start program. *The Future of Children, 9*, 66–90.

Glisson, C., & Schoenwald, S. K. (2005). The ARC organizational and community intervention strategy for implementing evidence-based children's mental health treatments. *Mental Health Services Research, 7*, 243–259.

Greenwald, P., & Cullen, J. W. (1984). The scientific approach to cancer control. *CA: A Cancer Journal for Clinicians, 34*, 328–332.

Hardy, C. M., Wynn, T. A., Huckaby, F., Lisovicz, N., & White-Johnson, F. (2004). African American community health advisors trained as research partners. *Family & Community Health, 28,* 28–40.

Hatgis, C., Addis, M. E., Krasnow, A. D., Khazan, I. Z., Jacob, K L., Chiancola, S., et al. (2001). Cross-fertilization versus transmission: Recommendations for developing a bi-directional approach to psychotherapy dissemination research. *Applied & Preventive Psychology, 10,* 37–49.

Hayes, S. C., Barlow, D. H., & Nelson-Gray, R. O. (1999). *The Scientist Practitioner: Research and Accountability in the Age of Managed Care,* 2nd ed. Needham Heights, MA: Allyn & Bacon.

Heneghan, A. M., Horwitz, S. M., & Leventhal, J. M. (1996). Evaluating intensive family preservation programs: A methodological review. *Pediatrics, 97,* 535–542.

Henggeler, S. W., Melton, G. B., & Smith, L. A. (1992). Family preservation using multisystemic therapy: An effective alternative to incarcerating serious juvenile offenders. *Journal of Consulting and Clinical Psychology, 60,* 953–961.

Ho, A.C., Weisz, J.R., Austin, A.A., Chorpita, B.F., Wells, K.C., Southam-Gerow, M.A., & the Research Network on Youth Mental Health. (2007). Bridging science and community practice: Clinician and organization engagement in community clinics in the Clinic Treatment Project. *Emotional and Behavioral Disorders in Youth, 7,* 13–16.

Kazdin, A. E., Bass, D., Ayers, W. A., & Rodgers, A. (1990). Empirical and clinical focus of child and adolescent psychotherapy research. *Journal of Consulting and Clinical Psychology, 58,* 729–740.

Lonigan, C. J., Elbert, J. C., & Bennett Johnson, S. (1998). Empirically supported psychosocial interventions for children: An overview. *Journal of Clinical Child Psychology, 27,* 138–145.

Luborsky, L., Singer, B., & Luborsky, L. (1975). Comparative studies of psychotherapies: Is it true that "everyone has won and all must have prizes"? *Archives of General Psychiatry, 32,* 995–1008.

Mufson, L., Dorta, K. P., Wickramaratne, P., Nomura, Y., Olfson, M., & Myrna, M. W. (2004). A randomized effectiveness trial of interpersonal psychotherapy for depressed adolescents. *Archives of General Psychiatry, 61 ,* 577–584.

Nakamura, B. J., Smith, R. L., & Chorpita, B. F. (2005). Child STEPs Clinic Treatment Project: Therapist diversity and comparisons with existing randomized trials. In B. F. Chorpita & J. R. Weisz (Chairs), *Bridging Science and Community Practice: An Overview of the Child STEPs Clinic Treatment Project.* Symposium presented at the annual convention of the Association of Behavioral and Cognitive Therapies, Washington, DC.

National Advisory Mental Health Council Workgroup on Child and Adolescent Mental Health Intervention Development and Deployment (2001). *Blueprint for Change: Research on Child and Adolescent Mental health.* Washington, DC.

National Institutes of Health (2002). *State Implementation of Evidence-Based Practices: Bridging Science and Service* (NIMH and SAMHSA RFA MH-03-007). Retrieved September 13, 2006, from http://grants1.nih.gov/grants/guide/rfa-files/RFA-MH-03-007.html.

National Institutes of Health (2003). *Behavioral Therapies Development Program* (NIDA and NIAA PA-03-126). Retrieved September 13, 2006, from http://grants.nih.gov/grants/guide/pa-files/PA-03-126.html.

Norquist, G., Lebowitz, B., & Hyman, S. (1999). Expanding the frontier of treatment research. *Prevention & Treatment, 2 ,* np. Retrieved September 13, 2006, from the PsycARTICLES database.

Olds, D. L., Robinson, J., O'Brien, R., Luckey, D. W., Pettitt, L. M., Henderson, C. R., et al. (2002). Home visiting by paraprofessionals and by nurses: A randomized, controlled study. *Pediatrics, 110,* 486–496.

Rehan, N. (1984). Knowledge, attitude and practice of family planning in Hausa women. *Social Science & Medicine, 18 ,* 839–844.

Rogers, E. M. (2003). *Diffusion of Innovations,* 5th ed. New York: The Free Press.

Rogers, S. (1998). Empirically supported comprehensive treatments for young children with autism. *Journal of Clinical Child Psychology, 27,* 168–179.

Schoenwald, S. K., & Hoagwood, K. (2001). Effectiveness, transportability, and dissemination of interventions: What matters when? *Psychiatric Services, 52,* 1190–1197.

Schoenwald, S. K., Sheidow, A. J., Letourneau, E. J., & Liao, J. G. (2003). Transportability of multisystemic therapy: Evidence for multilevel influences. *Mental Health Services Research, 5* , 223–239.

Southam-Gerow, M. A., Austin, A. A., & Marder, A. M. (in press). Transportability and dissemination of psychological treatments: Research models and methods. In D. McKay (Ed.), *Handbook of Research Methods in Abnormal and Clinical Psychology.* Newbury Park, CA: Sage.

Strosahl, K. (1998). The dissemination of manual-based psychotherapies in managed care: Promises, problems, and prospects. *Clinical Psychology: Science and Practice, 5* , 382–386.

Stuart, G. W., Burland, J., Ganju, V., Levounis, P., & Kiosk, S. (2002). Educational best practices. *Administration and Policy in Mental Health, 29* , 325–333.

Task Force on Promotion and Dissemination of Psychological Procedures, Division of Clinical Psychology, American Psychological Association (1995). Training in and dissemination of empirically-validated psychological treatments: Report and recommendations. *The Clinical Psychologist, 48,* 3–23.

Task Force on Psychological Intervention Guidelines of the American Psychological Association (1995). *Template for Developing Guidelines: Interventions for Mental Disorders and Psychosocial Aspects of Physical Disorders.* Washington, DC: American Psychological Association.

Torabi, M. R., Yang, J., & Li, J. (2002). Comparison of tobacco use knowledge, attitude and practice among college students in china and the United States. *Health Promotion International, 17* , 247–253.

Torrey, W. C., Drake, R. E., Dixon, L., Burns, B. J., Flynn, L., Rush, A. J., et al. (2001). Implementing evidence-based practices for persons with severe mental illnesses. *Psychiatric Services, 52* , 45–50.

U.S. Department of Health and Human Services, Substance Abuse and Mental Health Services Administration (n.d.). *National Registry of Evidence-Based Programs and Practices: Model Programs.* Retrieved September 13, 2006, from http://modelprograms.samhsa.gov/template_cf.cfm?page=model_list.

Weersing, V. R., Weisz, J. R., & Donenberg, G. R. (2002). Development of the Therapy Procedures Checklist: A therapist-report measure of technique use in child and adolescent treatment. *Journal of Clinical Child Psychology, 31,* 168–180.

Weingardt, K. R. (2004). The role of instructional design and technology in the dissemination of empirically supported, manual-based therapies. *Clinical Psychology: Science and Practice, 11,* 313–331.

Weiss, B., Catron, T., Harris, V., & Phung, T. M. (1999). The effectiveness of traditional child psychotherapy. *Journal of Consulting and Clinical Psychology, 67* , 82–94.

Weiss, B., & Weisz, J. R. (1995). Relative effectiveness of behavioral and nonbehavioral child psychotherapy. *Journal of Consulting and Clinical Psychology, 63,* 317–320.

Weisz, J. R. (2004). *Psychotherapy for Children and Adolescents: Evidence-Based Treatments and Case Examples.* Cambridge: Cambridge University Press.

Weisz, J. R., Donenberg, G. R., Han, S. S., & Weiss, B. (1995). Bridging the gap between laboratory and clinic in child and adolescent psychotherapy. *Journal of Consulting and Clinical Psychology, 63* , 688–701.

Weisz, J. R., Jensen, A. L., & McLeod, B. D. (2005). Development and dissemination of child and adolescent psychotherapies: Milestones, methods, and a new deployment-focused model. In E. D. Hibbs & P. S. Jensen (Eds.), *Psychosocial Treatments for Child and Adolescent Disorders: Empirically Based Strategies for Clinical Practice,* 2nd ed. (pp. 9–39). Washington, DC: American Psychological Association.

Weisz, J. R., Thurber, C. A., Sweeney, L., Proffitt, V. D., & LeGagnoux, G. L. (1997). Brief treatment of mild-to-moderate child depression using primary and secondary control enhancement training. *Journal of Consulting and Clinical Psychology, 65,* 703–707.

Weisz, J. R., Weiss, B., Han, S. S., Granger, D. A., & Morton, T. (1995). Effects of psychotherapy with children and adolescents revisited: A meta-analysis of treatment outcome studies. *Psychological Bulletin, 117,* 450–468.

II

Evidence-Based Therapies for Specific Disorders or Conditions

Anxiety Disorders

5

Psychosocial Treatments for Phobic and Anxiety Disorders in Youth

WENDY K. SILVERMAN and ARMANDO A. PINA

Over the past decade, the field has made significant strides in developing and testing psychosocial treatments for phobic and anxiety disorders in children and adolescents. However, treatments vary in the amount of research evidence accumulated supporting their efficacy. The purpose of the present chapter is to report on the evidence-based status of these treatments with the hope of providing a guide for clinical and school psychologists, practitioners, educators, and public mental health system administrators as they make determinations concerning the adoption of treatments for phobic and anxiety disorders in youth.

For this chapter, psychosocial treatments for phobic and anxiety disorders in youth were identified by searching the research literature using PsycINFO and MEDLINE. Selection of treatment studies was narrowed by focusing on psychosocial treatments targeting the most prevalent phobic and anxiety disorders classified in the *Diagnostic and Statistical Manual of Mental Disorders* (American Psychiatric Association, 1987, 1994) (i.e., DSM-III-R or IV; APA, 1987, 1994), namely, separation anxiety disorder (SAD), social phobia (SOP), generalized anxiety disorder (GAD), and specific phobia (SP). The search and selection led to 30 studies and most used multisource assessments, state-of-the-art diagnostic methods, randomization to conditions, manualized treatment protocols, treatment fidelity checks, reliable and valid outcome assessment measures, and follow-ups. To report on the evidence-based status of the

Support for this chapter comes in part from NIMH Grant 63997 awarded Wendy Silverman and IMHR Grant 2006PA 139 awarded to Armando Pina.

WENDY K. SILVERMAN • Florida International University and **ARMANDO A. PINA** • Arizona State University

psychosocial treatments evaluated in the 30 studies selected, we relied on the criteria of Chambless and Hollon (1998) (described in Chapter 2). Thus, the label names used to classify the psychosocial treatments were *efficacious, efficacious and specific,* and *probably efficacious.*

The chapter begins by reporting on the evidence-based status of psychosocial treatments evaluated in the 30 selected studies. Then the chapter briefly describes psychosocial treatments evaluated for youth diagnosed with either SAD, SOP, or GAD as their primary diagnosis. Treatments evaluated in samples of youth with SOP as their primary diagnosis are described next, followed by treatments evaluated in samples of youth with school phobia or school refusal behavior, and then treatments for SP. Our grouping of treatments by these diagnoses is a reflection of the research literature. For each grouping there is a table showing basic details about each study. We conclude the chapter with recommendations and a case example of a child who presented to our clinic due to difficulties with excessive fear and anxiety.

EVIDENCE-BASED STATUS OF PSYCHOSOCIAL TREATMENTS FOR PHOBIC AND ANXIETY DISORDERS IN YOUTH

The criteria of Chambless and Hollon (1998) were used to classify psychosocial treatments evaluated in the 30 identified studies. As shown in Table 1, individual cognitive-behavioral therapy (ICBT), group cognitive-behavioral therapy (GCBT), and two variants of GCBT met Chambless and Hollon's (1998) *efficacious* criteria because at least two experiments showed each of these treatments to be statistically significantly superior to no treatment (waitlist). The remaining psychosocial treatments met criteria for *possibly efficacious,* and no treatment met criteria for *efficacious and specific.* As Table 1 also shows, most *possibly efficacious* treatments received supportive evidence from one study. However, ICBT with parents, ICBT for school refusal behavior, and ICBT for school refusal behavior with parent/teacher training each received supportive evidence from two studies. In the absence of one good experiment per treatment demonstrating its efficacy relative to no treatment, psychological pill placebo, or alternative treatment, each of these treatments was labeled *possibly efficacious.* School-based GCBT also received supportive evidence from two studies, but these studies had significant limitations (e.g., lacked power, used nonequivalent attention controls, reported equivocal findings). Consequently, we believe the efficacy of school-based GCBT necessitates replication. Lastly, as shown in Table 1, two studies are listed with the label name "family cognitive-behavioral therapy" (Bögels & Siqueland, 2006; Wood et al., 2006). Unlike the other paired citations corresponding to the remaining treatments listed in Table 1, these two studies report on two different types of treatment procedures despite both using labels that refer to "family." We thus classified these two variants of family cognitive-behavioral therapy as *possibly efficacious* pending replication (Chambless & Hollon, 1998).

Table 1. Evidence-Based Status of Psychosocial Treatments for Phobic and Anxiety Disorders in Youth

Psychological Treatment	Citation for Efficacy Evidence
Efficacious Treatments	
Individual cognitive-behavioral therapy	Kendall (1994); Kendall et al. (1997); Barrett et al. (1996); Flannery-Schroeder & Kendall (2000)
Group cognitive-behavioral therapy	Barrett (1998); Flannery-Schroeder & Kendall (2000); Mendlowitz et al. (1999)
Group cognitive-behavioral therapy with parents	Barrett (1998); Silverman et al. (1999b); Spence et al. (2006)
Group cognitive-behavioral therapy for social phobia	Spence et al. (2000); Hayward et al. (2000); Gallagher et al. (2004)
Possibly Efficacious Treatments	
Individual cognitive-behavioral therapy with parents	Barrett et al. (1996); Manassis et al. (2002)
Emotive imagery for darkness phobia	Cornwall et al. (1996)
Individual cognitive-behavioral therapy for school refusal behavior with Parent/Teacher Training	King et al. (1998); Heyne et al. (2002)
Individual cognitive-behavioral therapy for school refusal behavior	Last et al. (1998); Heyne et al. (2002)
Group cognitive-behavioral therapy with Parental Anxiety Management for anxious parents	Cobham et al. (1998)
In vivo behavioral exposures for spider phobia	Muris et al. (1998)
Exposures coupled with contingency management for specific phobia	Silverman et al. (1999a)
Exposures coupled with self-control for specific phobia	Silverman et al. (1999a)
Social effectiveness training for children for social phobia	Beidel et al. (2000)
FRIENDS	Shortt et al. (2001)
One-session exposure treatment for specific phobia	Öst et al. (2001)
School-based group cognitive-behavioral therapy for social phobia	Masia et al. (2001)
School-based group cognitive-behavioral therapy	Ginsburg and Drake (2002); Muris et al. (2002)
Parent/Teacher Training for school refusal behavior	Heyne et al. (2002)
Individual cognitive-behavioral therapy with Cognitive Therapy for parents	Nauta et al. (2003)
School-based social effectiveness training for children with social phobia	Baer & Garland (2005)
Parent group cognitive-behavioral therapy	Thienemann et al. (2006)
Family cognitive-behavioral therapy	Bögels & Siqueland (2006); Wood et al. (2006)
Group cognitive-behavioral therapy with parents (face-to-face and Internet delivery)	Spence et al. (2006)

Psychosocial Treatment of Anxiety Disorders

Seventeen studies were identified as reporting on the efficacy of treatment packages for youth with a primary or principal diagnosis of SAD, SOP, or GAD; treatment efficacy was ascertained. Table 2 presents the main characteristics of these 17 treatment studies and key findings. Based on our review of these 17 studies, we found that for youth who present with SAD, SOP, or GAD, ICBT, GBCT, and GCBT with parents are *efficacious* treatments (below we describe the main aspects of the efficacious treatments). *Possibly efficacious* treatments also were identified; namely, ICBT with parents, GCBT with parental anxiety management for anxious parents, FRIENDS, school-based GCBT, ICBT with cognitive therapy for parents, parent-group CBT, and the two variants of family CBT.

The efficacy of the main ICBT program, the Coping Cat (Kendall, 2000), was first examined in Kendall (1994). The Coping Cat program prescribes four key cognitive components: (1) identifying cognitive and somatic-physiological reactions to anxiety; (2) clarifying thoughts in anxiety-provoking situations (e.g., unrealistic, threatening, negative attributions or expectations); (3) developing plans to cope with anxiety-provoking situations (e.g., changing anxious self-statements); and (4) self-evaluation and reward. Additionally, behavioral strategies are used including *in vivo* or imaginary exposures and relaxation. The Coping Cat (Kendall, 2000) has served as a prototype for subsequent treatments.

The publication of Kendall (1994) spurred a number of subsequent trials examining ICBT (Coping Cat) variants (e.g., Barrett et al., 1996; Barrett, 1998). For example, Barrett (1998) in Australia reported on the efficacy of a modified version of the Coping Cat program, the "Coping Koala." Barrett (1998) adapted Kendall's procedures for use in a group format, namely, GCBT as well as GCBT with parents. In Barrett's study, GCBT was delivered by two therapists and involved training youth in cognitive and behavioral strategies as outlined in the Coping Cat/Koala manuals. GCBT with parents involved the same procedures, as well as a Family Anxiety Management (FAM) module. The FAM aspect of the treatment focused on training parents in managing their child's emotional upsets and in communication and problem-solving. Barrett (1998) found both GCBTs to be efficacious, as detailed in Table 2.

The positive findings reported by Barrett (1998) have been replicated by other investigators (e.g., Flannery-Schroeder & Kendall, 2000; Manassis et al., 2002; Mendlowitz et al., 1999), including the efficacy of GCBT with parents (e.g., Mendlowitz et al., 1999; Silverman et al., 1999b). Recently, Spence et al. (2006) demonstrated delivery of GCBT with parents using a combined face-to-face and Internet format. In Spence et al. (2006), youth were seen in 10 group treatment sessions, but half of the sessions did not involve face-to-face therapist and group meetings but involved using the Internet to obtain psychoeducational information. Half of the parent sessions in the combined face-to-face and Internet treatment were face to face with a therapist and in group meetings and the other half were done over the Internet at home, including a three-month booster session. Youth Internet sessions focused on identifying physiological symptoms

Table 2. Psychosocial Treatments for Heterogeneous Anxiety Disorders in Children and Adolescents

Study	Sample Characteristics	Treatment	Pre- to Posttreatment Gains (% recovered, rating scales) and Maintenance over Time
Kendall (1994)	N = 47, ages 9 to 13 years (19 girls)	ICBT 16 to 20/16 to 20 sessions/weeks	ICBT = 64% improved on youth and parent scales. Teacher ratings did not show improvements. At 1-year follow-up, gains were maintained.
Barrett et al. (1996)	N = 70, ages 7 to 14 years (34 girls)	ICBT, ICBT + FAM 12/- sessions/weeks	ICBT = 57.1%, ICBT + FAM = 84%. Both ICBTs improved on youth and parent scales. At 1-year follow-up, gains were maintained.
Kendall et al. (1997)	N = 94, ages 9 to 13 years (25 girls)	ICBT 16 to 20/16 to 20 sessions/weeks	ICBT = 71% ICBT improved on youth and parent scales. A father measure of child anxiety/depression did not show improvements. At 1-year follow-up, gains were maintained.
Barrett (1998)	N = 50, ages 7 to 14 years (28 girls)	GCBT, GCBT + FAM 12/12 sessions/weeks	GCBT = 55.9%, GCBT + FAM = 70.7%. Both GCBTs improved on youth and parent scales. GCBT + FAM improved more than GCBT on clinician-rated child functioning and on youth fear ratings. At 1-year follow-up, gains were maintained.
Cobham et al. (1998)	N = 61, ages 7 to 14 years (33 girls)	GCBT, GCBT + PAM 10/14 sessions/weeks	For youth whose parents were "nonanxious," GCBT = 82%, GCBT + PAM = 80%. For youth whose parents were "anxious," GCBT = 39%, GCBT+PAM = 77%. Both GCBTs improved on youth scales. At 6- and 12-month follow-up, gains were maintained.
Silverman et al. (1999b)	N = 41, ages 6 to 16 years (22 girls)	GCBT 10/10 sessions/weeks	GCBT = 64%. GCBT improved on youth and parent scales. At 3-, 6-, and 12-month follow-up, gains were maintained.
Mendlowitz et al. (1999)	N = 62, ages 7 to 12 years (39 girls)	GCBT, GCBT + parent, GCBT parent only 12/12 - sessions/weeks	Diagnostic recovery was not reported. Both GCBTs improved on youth and parent scales. Girls improved more than boys on anxiety and social support ratings. GCBT + parent improved more on active coping ratings. No follow-up.
Flannery-Schroeder & Kendall (2000)	N = 37, ages 8 to 14 years (18 girls)	ICBT, GCBT -/12 sessions/weeks	ICBT = 73%, GCBT = 50%. Both CBTs improved on youth and parent scales. No improvements were found on social activities or teacher ratings. Only ICBT improved on child-rated state-anxiety. At 3-month follow-up, gains were maintained.

(Continued)

Table 2. *(Continued)*

Study	Sample Characteristics	Treatment	Pre- to Posttreatment Gains (% recovered, rating scales) and Maintenance over Time
Shortt et al. (2001)	$N = 64$, ages 6 to 10 years (42 girls)	FRIENDS 10/10 sessions/weeks	FRIENDS = 69%. FRIENDS improved on youth and mother scales. Fathers' ratings did not show improvements. At 1-year follow-up, gains were maintained.
Manassis et al. (2002)	$N = 78$, ages 8 to 12 years (36 girls)	ICBT, GCBT (both with parent present) 12/12 sessions/weeks	Diagnostic recovery was not reported. Both CBTs improved on anxiety and depression, but ICBT showed greater improvement. No follow-up.
Muris et al. (2002)	$N = 20$, ages 9 to 12 (20 girls)	GCBT 12/ sessions/weeks	Diagnostic recovery not reported. GCBT improved on youth-rated anxiety. No follow-up.
Ginsburg & Drake (2002)	$N = 12$, ages 14 to 17 years (10 girls)	GCBT 10/10 sessions/weeks	GCBT = 75%. GCBT improved on clinician ratings and youth-rated anxiety. No follow-up.
Nauta et al. (2003)	$N = 76$, ages 7 to 18 years (40 girls)	ICBT, ICBT + CT 12/12 sessions/weeks	ICBT = 68%, ICBT + CT = 69%. Both ICBTs improved on youth and parent ratings. At 3-month follow-up, gains were maintained.
Thienemann et al. (2006)	$N = 24$, ages 7 to 16 years (7 girls)	Parent GCBT 8/8 sessions/weeks	Parent GCBT = 25%. Parent GCBT improved on mother's ratings about the child's anxiety, attitudes toward the child, and clinician's ratings of child functioning. No follow-up.
Bögels & Siqueland (2006)	$N = 17$, ages 8 to 17 years (8 girls)	Family CBT –/– sessions/weeks	Family CBT = 46%. Family CBT improved on youth-rated anxiety and parent ratings. At 3- and 12-month follow-up, gains were maintained.
Wood et al. (2006)	$N = 38$, ages 6 to 13 years (14 girls)	Family CBT, ICBT 12 to 16 sessions/weeks	Family CBT = 78.9%, ICBT = 52.6%. Family CBT and ICBT improved on youth- and parent-rated anxiety. Family CBT improved more than ICBT on parent-rated anxiety. No follow-up.
Spence et al. (2006)	$N = 65$, ages 7 to 14 years (30 girls)	GCBT with parents (face-to-face), GCBT with parents (face-to-face and Internet) 10/10 sessions/weeks	GCBT with parents (face-to-face) = 65%, GCBT with parents (face-to-face and Internet) = 56%. Both GCBTs improved on child and parent ratings. At 6-month follow-up, gains were maintained.

– designates "not reported." N = number of completers. CBT = cognitive-behavioral treatment, FAM = family anxiety management, GCBT = group cognitive-behavioral treatment, ICBT = individual cognitive-behavioral treatment, PAM = parental anxiety management.
CT = cognitive therapy for parents. All parent and clinician's ratings are about the child. A table with details about specific improvements on rating scales is available from the second author.

of anxiety, learning about relaxation, problem-solving, self-reinforcement, and the importance of practice. Youth face-to-face group sessions focused on cognitive restructuring, graded exposures, and relapse prevention. Table 2 presents the key findings from Spence et al. (2006).

Psychosocial Treatment of Social Phobia (or Social Anxiety Disorder)

Six studies were identified reporting on the efficacy of treatment packages targeting SOP. Table 3 presents the main characteristics of these six studies and their key findings.

We found that when SOP is the primary or principal diagnosis, GBCT for SOP is an *efficacious* treatment. There also are *possibly efficacious*

Table 3. Psychosocial Treatments for Social Phobia in Children and Adolescents

Study	Sample Characteristics	Treatment	Pre- to Posttreatment Gains (% recovered, rating scales) and Maintenance over Time
Beidel et al. (2000)	N = 50, ages 8 to 12 years (30 girls)	SET-C 25/12 sessions/ weeks	SET-C = 67%. SET-C improved on youth and parent scales. At 6-month follow-up, gains were maintained and recovery rose to 85%.
Spence et al. (2000)	N = 50, ages 7 to 14 years (19 girls)	GCBT, GCBT + Parent Involvement 12/12 sessions/ weeks	GCBT = 58%, GCBT + parent involvement = 87.5%. Both GCBTs improved on youth and parent ratings. At 6- and 12-month follow-up, gains were maintained.
Hayward et al. (2000)	N = 35, mean age = 15.8 (35 girls)	GCBT 16/16 sessions/ weeks	GCBT = 45%. GCBT improved on youth and parent ratings. At the 1-year follow-up, gains were generally maintained in terms of diagnoses but not on youth social anxiety symptom ratings.
Masia et al. (2001)	N = 6, ages 14 to 17 years (3 girls)	Modified SET-C 14/14 sessions/ weeks	Modified SET-C = 50%. Modified SET-C improved on youth and clinician ratings. No follow-up.
Gallagher et al. (2003)	N = 23, ages 8 to 11 years (12 girls)	GCBT 3/3 sessions/ weeks	No improvements after treatment. At three-month follow-up, GCBT improved on youth, parent, and clinician ratings.
Baer & Garland (2005)	N = 11, ages 13 to 18 years (7 girls)	Modified SET-C 12/sessions/ weeks	Modified SET-C = 36%. Modified SET-C improved on clinician ratings of child functioning and youth depression ratings. No follow-up.

– designates "not reported." *N* = number of completers. GCBT = group cognitive-behavioral treatment, SET-C = social effectiveness training for children. All parent and clinician's ratings are about the child. A table with details about specific improvements on rating scales is available from the second author.

treatments: namely, social effectiveness training for children (SET-C), school-based GCBT, and school-based modified SET-C.

GCBT for SOP consists of key CBT components (i.e., cognitive challenging and graded exposures, relaxation), but emphasis is placed on social skills training, including handling socially challenging situations. SET-C (Beidel et al., 2000) targets social anxiety and fear as well as interpersonal skills and includes child and parent education, social skills training, in vivo exposures, and peer generalization experiences. Social skills training and peer generalizations are conducted in small-group sessions, and in vivo exposures are conducted in individual sessions.

Since the publication of Beidel et al. (2000), SET-C variants have been evaluated in a small number of studies (see Table 3). Baer and Garland (2005), for example, modified SET-C by excluding Beidel et al.s peer generalization sessions and contingent reinforcement procedures, resulting in less positive findings than Beidel et al. (2000). See Table 3 for a summary of the key findings of these studies.

Psychosocial Treatment of School Phobia or School Refusal Behavior

Three studies were identified as reporting on the efficacy of treatment packages targeting school phobia or school refusal behavior. Table 4 presents the main characteristics of these three studies and their key findings.

Based on our review of these three studies, we found that for youth who present with school phobia or school refusal behavior as the primary principal problem, no treatment met the *efficacious* criteria. However, three treatments did meet the *possibly efficacious* criteria: namely, ICBT for school refusal behavior or school phobia, ICBT for school refusal behavior with Parent and Teacher Training, and Parent and Teacher Training.

In Last et al. (1998), ICBT for school refusal behavior or school phobia consisted of graduated in vivo exposure and coping self-statements training. With the graduated in vivo exposures, the focus was on returning the child to school. Coping self-statements training focused on identifying maladaptive thoughts when anticipating and confronting anxiety-provoking situations and replacing those thoughts with more adaptive coping self-statements.

In King et al. (1998), youth received ICBT with parent/teacher training (referred by authors as "CBT"). In the ICBT with parent/teacher training, a modified version of the Coping Cat was administered. Specifically, youth were trained to use relaxation and recognize and assess self-talk during anxiety-provoking situations, particularly anxiety-producing and anxiety-reducing self-talk. Youth were then required to apply these skills during imaginary or in vivo or exposures along with self-evaluation and reward. The treated youth received ICBT; parents (in five sessions) and teachers (in one session) were trained to use child behavior management strategies such as establishing routines, ignoring somatic complaints, and delivering reinforcement to increase school attendance.

In Heyne et al. (2002), youth with school refusal behavior received ICBT, ICBT with parent and teacher training (ICBT plus PTT), or parent and teacher training (PTT). Heyne et al. described the ICBT condition as incorporating relaxation training, social skills training, cognitive therapy, and desensitization (emotive imagery and *in vivo* exposures). In ICBT plus PTT and PTT, parents received cognitive therapy to highlight their role in influencing child change. Parents and teachers received training in behavior management strategies (e.g., reinforcement). See Table 4 for a summary of the key findings of these studies.

Psychosocial Treatment of Specific Phobias

Four studies were identified as reporting on the efficacy of treatment packages or procedures targeting specific phobia or simple phobia. Table 5 presents the main characteristics of these four studies and their key findings. Based on our review of these four studies, we found that for youth who present with specific phobia or simple phobia as the primary or principal diagnosis, no psychosocial treatment met the *efficacious* criteria, but emotive imagery for darkness phobia, *in vivo* exposures for spider phobia, exposures with contingency management or self-control, and a one-session *in vivo* exposure (and with parent) did meet criteria for *possibly efficacious*. Because each study involved the use of graded behavioral exposures in various formats/approaches, each is briefly described below.

Table 4. Psychosocial Treatments for School Phobia or School Refusal Behavior in Children and Adolescents

Study	Sample Characteristics	Treatment	Pre- to Posttreatment Gains (% recovered, rating scales) and Maintenance over Time
Last et al. (1998)	*N* = 41, ages 6 to 17 years (28 girls)	ICBT 12/12 sessions/ weeks	ICBT = 65%. ICBT improved on mean percentage of hours spent in the classroom and on youth-rated anxiety and depression. At 4-week follow-up, gains were maintained.
King et al. (1998)	*N* = 34, ages 5 to 15 years (16 girls)	ICBT + PTT 6/4 sessions/ weeks	Diagnostic recovery not reported. ICBT + PTT improved on number of full days present at school and on youth, parent, and teacher ratings. At 3-month follow-up, gains were maintained.
Heyne et al. (2002)	*N* = 61, ages 7 to 14 years (28 girls)	ICBT, ICBT + PTT, PTT 8/16 session/ weeks	Diagnostic recovery not reported. All treatments improved on number of full days present at school and on youth ratings. At 2-week follow-up, gains were maintained.

N = number of completers. ICBT = individual cognitive-behavioral treatment, PTT = parent and teacher training. All parent and teacher's ratings are about the child. A table with details about specific improvements on rating scales is available from the second author.

Table 5. Psychosocial Treatments for Fears and Specific Phobias in Children and Adolescents

Study	Sample Characteristics	Type of Fear/Phobia(s)	Treatment	Pre- to Posttreatment Gains (% recovered, rating scales) and Maintenance over time
Cornwall et al. (1996)	$N = 24$, ages 7 to 10 years (number of girls not reported)	Darkness	EI 6/6 sessions/weeks	Diagnostic recovery not reported. EI improved on youth and observer ratings. At 3-month follow-up, gains were maintained.
Muris et al. (1998)	$N = 26$, ages 8 to 17 years (26 girls)	Spiders	EMDR, *in vivo* exposures, CE. All followed by *in vivo* exposures. 1/1 session/week	Diagnostic recovery not reported. EMDR improved on state anxiety. *In vivo* exposures improved on state anxiety, youth-rated fear, and observer ratings. CE did not improve. After these treatments were followed by *in vivo* exposures, there were improvements on youth and observer ratings. No follow-up.
Silverman et al. (1999a)	$N = 81$, ages 6 to 16 years (50 girls)	Nighttime fears, small animals, school, thunder/lightening, doctors, blood/injections, planes, camera flashes, loud noises, swimming/water, costumed characters	Exposures with self-control (SC), exposures with contingency management (CM) 10/10 sessions/weeks	SC = 88%, CM = 56%. SC and CM improved on youth, parent, and clinician ratings. At 3-, 6-, and 12-month follow-up, gains were maintained.
Öst et al. (2001)	$N = 60$, ages 7 to 17 years (37 girls)	Small animals, blood injections, enclosed spaces, thunderstorms, deep water, loud noise, mummies, yogurt	One-session behavioral exposure treatment, one-session behavioral exposure treatment with parent 1/1 session/week	Diagnostic recovery not reported. Both treatments improved on youth and clinician ratings. At one-year follow-up, gains were maintained.

N = number of completers. EI = emotive imagery. EMDR = eye movement desensitization and reprocessing. CE = computerized exposures. All parent and teacher ratings are about the child. A table with details about specific improvements on rating scales is available from the second author.

Emotive imagery prescribes the child to think of situations that evoke positive imagery while engaging in graded exposures to fear-provoking stimuli (e.g., darkness in the study of Cornwall et al., 1996). In Muris et al. (1998), youth with a specific phobia of spiders were assigned to one of three 2.5-hour conditions: eye movement desensitization and reprocessing (EMDR; Shapiro, 1995), *in vivo* exposures, or computerized exposures. *In vivo* exposures consisted of graded confrontations with the phobic stimulus (e.g., looking at a spider from a distance, letting the spider walk on one's arm). Computerized exposures consisted of graded confrontations with the phobic stimulus on a computer screen (e.g., looking at a static cartoon spider and then a moving tarantula). After completing one of these conditions, youth participated in *in vivo* exposures lasting 1.5 hours.

Silverman et al. (1999a) also investigated the efficacy of exposure for the treatment of phobias. Youth with various phobias received one of two exposure treatments (administered *in vivo* or in imagination depending on the type of phobia). In one condition, exposures were coupled with cognitive therapy, referred to as "self-control" (SC), and in the other condition exposures were coupled with behavior therapy, referred to as "contingency management" (CM). Youth also were randomized to an active credible psychological control condition, education support (ES).

Lastly, Öst et al. (2001) reported on a single-session exposure treatment for phobias. Specifically, youth received one-session behavioral exposure treatment (child-alone) or one-session behavioral exposure treatment with parent participation (parent-present). In child-alone, graded *in vivo* exposures were conducted. In parent-present, in addition to graded *in vivo* exposures, the parent observed the child conducting exposures, modeled handling the phobic stimulus/event, and provided comfort to the child when experiencing high anxiety. See Table 5 for a summary of the key findings of these studies.

RECOMMENDATIONS AND CASE EXAMPLE

Based on the 30 studies selected for review, we recommend clinical and school psychologists, practitioners, educators, and public mental health system administrators consider using treatments found to be *efficacious* based on Chambless and Hollon's (1998) criteria: namely, ICBT, GCBT, GCBT with parents, and GCBT for SOP. Service providers interested in delivering these CBTs should engage in similar therapist training procedures used in the trials evaluating these psychosocial treatments. For instance, in some trials, therapist training consisted of 5 to 12 hours of didactic instruction using CBT manuals, weekly case supervision, or both (see Bögels & Siqueland, 2006; King et al., 1998; Muris et al., 1998; Nauta et al., 2003; Silverman et al., 1999b; Wood et al., 2006). To illustrate how we have used some of these CBT procedures, we describe a case example of a 9-year-old boy who presented with his mother to our clinic.

Case Example

On the basis of child and parent interview data (i.e., Anxiety Disorders Interview Schedule for DSM-IV—Child and Parent versions, Silverman & Albano, 1996; Silverman et al., 2001), a 9-year-old European-American boy was found to meet DSM-IV criteria for SAD. The problem began when the boy was 5 years old, in kindergarten, when his mother did not pick him up from school on time. He described the situation in which he ran out of the class, his mother was not there to pick him up, and he was asked to wait at the school's main office. While he waited for his mother, the school's assistant principal tried to reach his mother over the telephone. The assistant principal was unable to reach the boy's mother. The boy described the experience of waiting for his mother as distressful, and since then both the boy and his mother have reported that his avoidance of being alone continually increased. At first, his avoidance of being alone did not present many difficulties, but as time progressed, it became more difficult for him to be separated from his mother. This led to several areas of interference for the boy and his family, such as difficulties attending or staying in school, and difficulties concentrating in school due to excessive preoccupation with not being picked up. Outside school, he avoided taking showers and using the bathroom alone and had difficulties sleeping alone and attending sleepovers. When the boy and his mother presented to the clinic, the duration of the separation anxiety problems was four years.

The child was treated with an exposure-based treatment involving cognitive and behavioral procedures. Table 6 shows a session-by-session description of the exposure-based CBT program. Treatment sessions lasted about 45 minutes with the boy and 15 minutes with the mother. Table 7 shows the fear hierarchy devised in sessions 2 and 3 along with the boy's subjective ratings of distress (on a 9-point scale) using the Feelings Thermometer (Silverman & Albano, 1996). The treatment involved first using a contingency management plan in which positive reinforcement was provided contingent on the child's successful completion of gradual exposures to being alone. The most difficult situation was not being picked up from school on time, which he rated 8. By the end of session 6, the boy successfully completed *in vivo* exposure tasks 1 to 5 listed on Table 7, and his subjective ratings of distress had decreased to 0 by the end of the exposures. Figure 1 shows an example of a contingency management contract used to facilitate implementation of one of his exposures.

Sessions 7 to 10 involved exploring with the boy the various things about being alone that he found scary (e.g., "when I am home with a sitter and mom is late arriving from work, I worry that she is badly hurt from being in a car accident") and using specific self-control/cognitive strategies (e.g., a four-step coping plan). For example, he was prompted to imagine Mom was late and to elaborate on how this situation made him feel. Then he was prompted to come up with alternative outcomes to his mother being late ("other things that might be happening") and alternative solutions (e.g., "things I can do while I wait for Mom to get home"). Figure 2 shows

Table 6. Cognitive and Behavioral Treatment of Phobic and Anxiety Disorders

Session-by-Session Description

1. Begin building rapport, discussion of presenting problem, emphasize importance of skills training, behavioral and cognitive strategies, and the idea of using a hierarchy. Explain out-of- session activities and the importance of practice (STIC jobs; Kendall, 2000; STIC = Show That I Can).
2. Review treatment rationale and goals using a fear/anxiety hierarchy and rewards.
3. Finalize hierarchy and specific rewards with the child. Explain home-based contingency contracting program (e.g., contingency management, CM). Devise first contract; assign first STIC (starting with low anxiety-provoking situation).
4. Review STIC. Conduct in-session exposure and provide feedback, modeling, and reinforcement for exposure. For STIC, devise contract for child exposure.
5. Review STIC. Conduct in-session exposure and provide feedback. For STIC, devise contract for child exposure.
6. Review STIC. Devise contract for child exposure.
7. Review STIC. Introduce cognitive component of program (e.g., self-control, SC). Specifically, teach the identification of faulty cognitions, generation of incompatible self-statements, explore alternatives, etc. For STIC, devise contract for child exposure.
8. Review STIC; continue SC. Conduct in-session exposure. Explain fading of rewards (to begin next session). For STIC, devise final contract
9. Review STIC. Present four-step coping plan ("STOP"). S = Scared?, T = Thoughts, O = Other[*thoughts*], P = Praise. For STIC, use the four-step plan for next exposure.
10. Review STIC. Conduct in-session exposure using coping plan. For STIC, use four-step plan for next exposure.
11. Review STIC and progress. Continue to practice four-step plan. Discuss relapse prevention strategies. For STIC, use four-step plan for next exposure.
12. Review STIC, progress, and relapse prevention.

Table adapted from Silverman et al. (1999b).

Table 7. Fear Hierarchy with Child's Ratings of Distress

Situation	Distress Ratings (0–8)
1. Playing video games while being alone in his bedroom	2
2. Watching TV while being alone in his bedroom	3
3. Playing with his toys while being alone in a room of the house	3
4. Using the toilet while being alone in the bathroom	4
5. Taking showers while being alone in the bathroom	5
6. Mom being late from work while he is home with sitter	6
7. Sleeping over at other kids' houses	7
8. Being alone in a room (e.g., at home or our clinic)	7
9. Sleeping alone in his bedroom	8
10. Not being picked up from school on time	8

Date __August 11, 2006__   Contract Number __5__
                                                  Session Number __6__

Child-Parent Contract

Let it be known that on this ___Friday___ day, the ___11___ of
                            (day of week)   (date)

___August___ in the year ___2006___, a contract between
(month)

_____John_____ and the parents ___Ms. Smith___
(Child's name)   (Parents' names)

concerning the child's anxiety about ___taking shower alone___ was signed, witnessed

by ___Dr. Silverman___.
   (therapist's name)

The above parents and child hereby agree that if ___John___
                                               (Child's name)

successfully _Goes into the bathroom at 5:00pm, with his towel and clean clothes,_

then takes a shower that lasts at least 15 minutes, without calling on mom (or anybody else),

ends his shower after a timer goes off (set at 15 minutes), and gests dressed in the bathroom

then _Mom will take John to buy a basketball trading card of no more than $5.00_ .
     (reward child will receive)

This task is to be done by the child _Saturday, 12_ , and the parents are
                                       (when)

to give child the above mentioned reward _Saturday, 12_ .
                                            (when)

Child's signature _____John Smith_____

Parents' signatures _____Ms. J. Smith_____

Therapist's signature _____Dr. Silverman_____

Figure 1. Example of a contract for conducting an *in vivo* exposure and administering a reward.

an example of the four-step coping plan used to implement the cognitive strategy. By the end of the fear-related imagery exposure and use of the four-step coping plan shown in Figure 2, the child had successfully reduced his subjective ratings of distress. That is, the boy's rating (on the 9-point scale) decreased from 6 (initial rating of distress) to 4 (midway through the procedure) to 1 (after the procedure). This cognitive strategy was used in treatment (and prescribed for use out of treatment) for the remaining sessions, coupled with *in vivo* behavioral exposures. At the posttreatment and 12-month follow-up assessment sessions, the ADIS-C/P was readministered. At both assessment points, the boy reported minimal distress about

S = Scared?

   Situation: ___Mom is late from work while I am home with a sitter.___

   _____

T = Thoughts

   What are your thoughts?___Mom was in a car accident and she is badly hurt.___

   _____

O = Other (*thoughts*)

   What can happen instead?___If there would have been an accident someone would___

   had called. Mom is stuck in traffic, stopped to buy food for dinner, or at the food market.

P = Praise (*yourself*)

   What can you tell yourself? ___I did a good job at changing my thoughts.___

   I am proud of myself. I am able to stop myself from panicking when mom is late.

Figure 2. Example of the four-step coping plan.

being separated from his mother (or being alone); he no longer met DSM-IV criteria for SAD; and both the boy and his mother reported improved functioning. He now stayed in school with no difficulties, had no difficulties concentrating in school, took showers/used the bathroom alone, and attended sleepovers and even summer camp, on a regular basis.

SUMMARY AND CONCLUSIONS

This chapter provided a review of the current status of evidence-based psychosocial treatments. Our hope is that this review will serve as a useful guide for practitioners and program administrators in making determinations about the adoption of treatments for phobic and anxiety disorders in youth. Our search of the treatment research literature led to 30 studies that met the criteria for robustness suggested by the American Psychological Association's Task Force on Promotion and Dissemination of Psychological Procedures (1995, 2000). Specifically, we found that ICBT, GCBT, GCBT with parents, and GCBT for SOP met the *efficacious* treatment criteria of Chambless and Hollon (1998). The remaining treatments met the *possibly efficacious* criteria; and no treatment met the *efficacious and specific* criteria. Based on this review, practitioners should consider training and then delivering the CBT programs labeled *efficacious* to children and adolescents who present to their clinics. We concluded the chapter with a case example to illustrate how we have used CBT to reduce SAD in a 9-year-old boy who presented with his mother to our clinic.

REFERENCES

Achenbach, T. M. (1991). *Manual for the Child Behavior Checklist/4-18.* Burlington, VT: University of Vermont, Department of Psychiatry.

Achenbach T. M., & Edelbrock, C. (1986). *Manual for the Teacher Report Form.* Burlington, VT: University of Vermont, Department of Psychiatry.

American Psychiatric Association (1987). *Diagnostic and Statistical Manual of Mental Disorders,* 3rd ed., rev. Washington, DC.

American Psychiatric Association (1994). *Diagnostic and Statistical Manual of Mental Disorders,* 4th ed. Washington, DC.

Baer, S., & Garland, J. (2005). Pilot study of community-based cognitive behavioral group therapy for adolescents with social phobia. *Journal of the American Academy of Child and Adolescent Psychiatry, 44,* 258–264.

Barrett, P. M. (1998). Evaluation of cognitive-behavioral group treatments for childhood anxiety disorders. *Journal of Clinical Child Psychology, 27,* 459–468.

Barrett, P. M., Dadds, M. R., & Rapee, R. M. (1996). Family treatment of childhood anxiety: A controlled trial. *Journal of Consulting and Clinical Psychology, 64,* 333–342.

Barlow D. H., Craske, M. G., Cerny, G., & Klosko, J. S. (1989). Behavioral treatment of panic disorder. *Behavior Therapy, 20,* 261–282.

Barlow D. H., Rapee R. M., & Brown T. A. (1992). Behavioral treatment for generalized anxiety disorder. *Behavior Therapy, 23,* 551–570.

Beidel, D. C., Turner, S. M., & Morris, T. L. (1995). A new inventory to assess childhood social anxiety and phobia: The Social Phobia and Anxiety Inventory for Children. *Psychosocial Assessment, 7,* 73–79.

Beidel, D. C., Turner, S. M., & Morris, T. L. (2000). Behavioral treatment of childhood social phobia. *Journal of Consulting and Clinical Psychology, 68,* 1072–1080.

Beidel, D. C., Turner, S. M., Young, B., & Paulson, A. (2005). Social effectiveness training for children: Three-year follow-up. *Journal of Consulting and Clinical Psychology, 73,* 721–725.

Borkovec, T. D., & Costello, E. (1993). Efficacy of applied relaxation and cognitive-behavioral therapy in the treatment of generalized anxiety disorder. *Journal of Consulting and Clinical Psychology, 61,* 611–619.

Bögels, S. M., & Siqueland, L. (2006). Family cognitive behavioral therapy for children and adolescents with clinical anxiety disorders. *Journal of the American Academy of Child and Adolescent Psychiatry, 45,* 134–141.

Chambless, D. L., & Hollon, S. D. (1998). Defining empirically supported therapies. *Journal of Consulting and Clinical Psychology, 66,* 7–18.

Chambless, D. L., & Ollendick, T. H. (2001). Empirically supported psychosocial interventions: Controversies and evidence. *Annual Review of Psychology, 52,* 685–716.

Chambless, D. L., Sanderson, W. C., Shoham, V., Johnson, S. B., Pope, K. S., Crits-Christoph, P., et al. (1996). An update on empirically validated therapies. *The Clinical Psychologist, 49,* 5–18.

Cobham, V. E., Dadds, M. R., & Spence, S. H. (1998). The role of parental anxiety in the treatment of childhood anxiety. *Journal of Consulting and Clinical Psychology, 66,* 893–905.

Cornwall, E., Spence, S. H., & Schotte, D. (1996). The effectiveness of emotive imagery in the treatment of darkness phobia in children. *Behaviour Change, 13,* 223–229.

Flannery-Schroeder, E. C., & Kendall, P. C. (2000). Group and individual cognitive-behavioral treatments for youth with anxiety disorders: A randomized clinical trial. *Cognitive Therapy and Research, 24,* 251–278.

Gallagher, H. M., Rabian, B. A., & McCloskey, M. S. (2003). A brief group cognitive behavioral intervention for social phobia in childhood. *Journal of Anxiety Disorders, 18,* 459–479.

Ginsburg, G. S., & Drake, K. (2002). School-based treatment for anxious African-American adolescents: A controlled pilot study. *Journal of the American Academy of Child and Adolescent Psychiatry, 41,* 768–775.

Hayward, C., Varady, S., Albano, A. M., Thienemann, M., Henderson, L., & Schatzberg, A. F. (2000). Cognitive-behavioral group therapy for social phobia in female adolescents:

Results of a pilot study. *Journal of the American Academy of Child and Adolescent Psychiatry, 39,* 721–726.

Heimberg, R. G., Becker, R. E., Goldfinger, K., & Vermilyea, J. A. (1985). Treatment of social phobia by exposure, cognitive restructuring and homework assignments. *Journal of Nervous and Mental Disease, 173,* 236–245.

Heyne, D., King, N., Tonge, B., Rollings, S., Young, D., Pritchard, M., et al. (2002). Evaluation of child therapy and caregiver training in the treatment of school refusal. *Journal of the American Academy of Child and Adolescent Psychiatry, 41 ,* 687–695.

Howard, B. L., & Kendall, P. C. (1996). Cognitive-behavioral family therapy for anxiety-disordered children: A multiple-baseline evaluation. *Cognitive Therapy and Research, 20,* 423–443.

Kendall, P. C. (1994). Treating anxiety disorders in children: Results of a randomized clinical trial. *Journal of Consulting and Clinical Psychology, 62,* 200–210.

Kendall, P. C., Flannery-Schroeder, E., Panichelli-Mindel, S. M., Southam-Gerow, M., Henin, A., & Warman, M. (1997). Therapy for youth with anxiety disorders: A second randomized clinical trial. *Journal of Consulting and Clinical Psychology, 65,* 366–380.

Kendall, P.C., Safford, S., Flannery-Schroeder, E., & Webb, A. (2004). Child anxiety treatment: Outcomes in adolescence and impact on substance use and depression at 7.4-year follow-up. *Journal of Consulting and Clinical Psychology, 72,* 276–287.

Kendall, P. C., & Southam-Gerow, M. A. (1996). Long-term follow-up of a cognitive-behavioral therapy for anxiety-disordered youth. *Journal of Consulting and Clinical Psychology, 64,* 724–730.

King, N. J., Tonge, B. J., Heyne, D., Pritchard, M., Rollings, S., Young, D., et al. (1998). Cognitive-behavioral treatment of school-refusing children: A controlled evaluation. *Journal of the American Academy of Child and Adolescent Psychiatry, 37,* 395–403.

Kovacs, M. (1992). *Children's Depression Inventory Manual.* North Tonawanda, NY: Multi-Health Systems, Inc.

Last, C. G., Hansen, C., & Franco, N. (1998). Cognitive-behavioral treatment of school phobia. *Journal of the American Academy of Child and Adolescent Psychiatry, 37 ,* 404–411.

Masia, C. L., Klein, R. G., Storch, E. A., & Corda, B. (2001). School-based behavioral treatment for social anxiety disorder in adolescents: Results of a pilot study. *Journal of the American Academy of Child and Adolescent Psychiatry, 40 ,* 780–786.

Manassis, K., Mendlowitz, S. L., Scapillato, D., Avery, D., Fiksenbaum, L., Freire, M., et al. (2002). Group and individual cognitive behavioral therapy for childhood anxiety disorders: A randomized trail. *Journal of the American Academy of Child and Adolescent Psychiatry, 41,* 1423–1430.

Mendlowitz, S. L., Manassis, K., Bradley, S., Scapillato, D., Miezitis, S., & Shaw, B. F. (1999). Cognitive-behavioral group treatments in childhood anxiety disorders: The role of parental involvement. *Journal of the American Academy of Child and Adolescent Psychiatry, 38,* 1223–1229.

Muris, P., Meesters, C., & Gobel, M. (2002a). Cognitive coping versus emotional disclosure in the treatment of anxious children: A pilot-study. *Cognitive Behaviour Therapy, 31 ,* 59–67.

Muris, P., Meesters, C., & Melick, M. (2002b). Treatment of childhood anxiety disorders: A preliminary comparison between cognitive-behavioral group therapy and a psychosocial placebo intervention. *Journal of Behavior Therapy and Experimental Psychiatry, 33,* 143–158.

Muris, P., Merckelbach, H., Holdrinet, I., & Sijsenaar, M. (1998). Treating phobic children: Effects of EMDR versus exposure. *Journal of Consulting and Clinical Psychology, 66 ,* 193–198.

Nathan, P. E., & Gorman, J. M. (2002). *A Guide to Treatments That Work,* 2nd ed. London: Oxford University Press.

Nauta, M. H., Schooling, A., Emmelkamp, P. M. G., & Minderaa, R. B. (2003). Cognitive- behavioral theory for children with anxiety disorders in a clinical setting: No additional effect of a cognitive parent training. *Journal of the American Academy of Child and Adolescent Psychiatry, 42,* 1270–1278.

Ollendick, T. H. (1983). Reliability and validity of the revised Fear Survey Schedule for Children (FSSC-R). *Behaviour Research and Therapy, 21,* 685–692.

Öst, L., Svensson, L., Hellström, K., & Lindwall, R. (2001). One-session treatment of specific phobia in youth: A randomized clinical trial. *Journal of Consulting and Clinical Psychology*, *69*, 814–824.

Rapee, R. M. (1997). Potential role of childrearing practices in the development of anxiety and depression. *Clinical Psychology Review*, *17*, 47–67.

Reynolds, C. R., & Richmond, B. O. (1978). What I think and feel: A revised measure of children's manifest anxiety. *Journal of Abnormal Child Psychology*, *6*, 271–280.

Ronan, K. R., Kendall, P. C., & Rowe, M. (1994). Negative affectivity in children: Development and validation of a self-assessment questionnaire. *Cognitive Therapy and Research*, *18*, 509–528.

Roth, A., & Fonagy, P. (1996). *What Works for Whom? A Critical Review of Psychotherapy*. New York: Guilford Press.

Shapiro, F. (1995). *Eye Movement Desensitization and Reprocessing: Basic Principles, Protocol and Procedures*. New York: Guildford Press.

Shortt, A. L., Barrett, P. M., & Fox, T. L. (2001). Evaluating the FRIENDS program: A cognitive-behavioral group treatment for anxious children and their parents. *Journal of Clinical Child and Adolescent Psychology*, *30*, 525–535.

Silverman W. K., & Albano, A. M. (1996). *Anxiety Disorders Interview Schedule for DSM-IV: Child and Parent Versions*. New York: Oxford University Press.

Silverman, W. K., Kurtines, W. M., Ginsburg, G. S., Weems, C. F., Rabian, B., & Serafini, L. T. (1999a). Contingency management, self-control, and education support in the treatment of childhood phobic disorders: A randomized clinical trial. *Journal of Consulting and Clinical Psychology*, *67*, 675–687.

Silverman, W. K., Kurtines, W. M., Ginsburg, G. S., Weems, C. F., Lumpkin, P. W., & Carmichael, D. H. (1999b). Treating anxiety disorders in children with group cognitive-behavioral therapy: A randomized clinical trial. *Journal of Consulting and Clinical Psychology*, *67*, 995–1003.

Silverman, W. K., & Nelles, W. B. (1988). The Anxiety Disorders Interview Schedule for Children. *Journal of the American Academy of Child and Adolescent Psychiatry*, *27*, 772–778.

Southam-Gerow, M. A., Flannery-Schroeder, E. C., & Kendall, P. C. (2003a). A psychometric evaluation of the parent report form of the State-Trait Anxiety Inventory for Children—Trait Version. *Journal of Anxiety Disorders*, *17*, 427–446.

Southam-Gerow, M. A., Weisz, J. R., & Kendall, P. C. (2003b). Youth with anxiety disorders in research and service clinics: Examining client differences and similarities. *Journal of Clinical Child and Adolescent Psychology*, *32*, 375–385.

Spence, S. H. (1995). *Social Skills Training: Enhancing Social Competence with Children and Adolescents*. Windsor, UK: NFER-Nelson.

Spence, S. H., Donovan, C., & Brechman-Toussaint, M. (2000). The treatment of childhood social phobia: The effectiveness of a social skills training-based, cognitive-behavioral intervention, with and without parental involvement. *Journal of Child Psychology and Psychiatry*, *41*, 713–726.

Spielberger, C. D. (1973). *Preliminary Test Manual for the State-Trait Anxiety Inventory for Children*. Palo Alto, CA: Consulting Psychologists Press.

Spielberger, C. D., Gorsuch, R. L., & Lushene, R. E. (1970). *Manual for the State-Trait Anxiety Inventory*. Palo Alto, CA: Consulting Psychologists Press.

Spirito, A. (1999). Introduction to the special series on empirically supported treatments in pediatric psychology. *Journal of Pediatric Psychology*, *24*, 87–90.

Thienemann, M., Moore, P., & Tompkins, K. (2006). A parent only group intervention for children with anxiety disorders: Pilot study. *Journal of the American Academy of Child and Adolescent Psychiatry*, *45*, 37–46.

Wood, J. J., Piacentini, J. C., Southam-Gerow, M. A., Chu, B., & Sigman, M. (2006). Family cognitive behavioral therapy for child anxiety disorders. *Journal of the American Academy of Child and Adolescent Psychiatry*, *45*, 314–321.

6

Panic Disorder in Adolescents

THOMAS H. OLLENDICK and DONNA PINCUS

The prevalence of child and adolescent psychiatric disorders has been estimated to be about 15% (Kazdin, 2000; Ollendick & Hersen, 1998). Anxiety disorders are among the most common of these psychiatric disorders. As defined by DSM-IV (*Diagnostic and Statistical Manual*, 4th edition, American Psychiatric Association, 1994), ICD-10 (International Classification of Diseases Manual; World Health Organization, 1992), and their earlier variants, anxiety disorders comprise about 20% of these psychiatric disorders. Although generalized anxiety disorder, separation anxiety disorder, social phobia, and specific phobia are among the most common anxiety disorders in childhood and adolescence, panic disorder (PD) occurs in a significant minority of these youths. For example, in child and adolescent community samples, PD has been reported to range between 0.5% and 5.0% (e.g., Essau et al., 1999; Hayward et al., 1997, 2000; Moreau & Follet, 1993) and in outpatient psychiatric clinics from 0.2% to 10% (Biederman et al., 1997; Kearney et al., 1997; Last & Strauss, 1989). Although most cases of PD occur in adolescent females, they also occur in children and adolescents of both sexes (Ollendick et al., 1994, 2004). Moreover, up to 40% of adults with PD report that their disorders began in their teenage years (Moreau & Follet, 1993). The peak onset of PD in these studies has been reported to be between 15–19 years of age; however, about 15% report their first panic attack (PA) occurred before they were 10 years of age (Thyer et al., 1985). These prevalence rates, along with emerging evidence that the onset of PD may be even younger in successive generations (Battaglia et al., 1998), indicate the pressing need to study the symptom picture, developmental course, etiology, and treatment of PD in children and adolescents.

THOMAS H. OLLENDICK • Child Study Center, Department of Psychology, Virginia Polytechnic Institute and State University and **DONNA PINCUS** • Center for Anxiety and Related Disorders, Department of Psychology, Boston University

PD is a disabling condition accompanied by psychosocial, family, peer, and academic difficulties (Birmaher & Ollendick, 2004; Moreau & Weissman, 1992; Ollendick et al., 2004). In addition, PD is associated with increased risk for a host of adult disorders including other anxiety disorders, major depressive disorder (MDD), and substance abuse (Birmaher & Ollendick, 2004; Strauss et al., 2000). Moreover, such adverse outcomes are most prevalent in adults whose PD started early in life (before 17 years of age; see Weissman et al., 1997). Despite this, it takes about 12 years from the onset of reported symptoms for adults to initiate and seek treatment (Moreau & Follet, 1993), and it appears that very few youngsters with PD seek help at all (Essau et al., 1999, 2000; King et al., 1993; Ollendick, 1995, 1998).

In this chapter, we review the current literature on the symptom picture, developmental course, etiology, and treatment of PD in children and adolescents. In addition, we present a case study and offer directions for future research and clinical practice.

SYMPTOM PICTURE

In order to meet diagnostic criteria for PD, the child or adolescent must experience recurrent panic attacks (PAs). Therefore, we will first describe the symptom picture of PAs and then the picture of PD in children and adolescents.

Panic Attacks (PAs)

A PA is an acute anxiety episode in which a set of emotional, cognitive, and somatic symptoms are experienced in the absence of real danger. The episode is typically intense and is accompanied by at least 4 of 13 symptoms, as described in DSM-IV (APA, 1994): emotional symptoms (e.g., feelings of unreality or being detached from oneself, feelings of choking), somatic symptoms (e.g., palpitations, chest pain, tingling sensations, chills or hot flushes, dizziness, nausea, sweating, trembling or shaking), and cognitive symptoms (e.g., fear of losing control or going crazy, fear of dying). The PA typically reaches its peak in intensity within a few minutes (i.e., 5 to 10 minutes) before gradually subsiding (i.e., 15 to 30 minutes later). Typically, individuals report that something is wrong or that something bad is going to happen but that they do not know exactly *what* is going to happen, *when* it will happen, *where* it will happen, and, perhaps most important of all, *why* it will happen. As a consequence, the young person might believe that he or she is going to go crazy, lose control, faint, develop a severe illness, or even die. The above-noted symptoms by themselves can increase the youngster's level of anxiety and create a vicious circle, which serves to worsen and maintain PA frequency, intensity, and duration (APA, 1998).

Three types of PA have been described: (1) uncued, (2) situationally bound, and (3) situationally predisposed (APA, 1994). Uncued PAs are unexpected, spontaneous, and seemingly "out of the blue." Situationally bound PAs almost always occur immediately upon exposure to, or in anticipation of, a specific event (e.g., the presence of a phobic object, separation from a caregiver). Situationally predisposed PAs, while also triggered by certain situations (e.g., a threatening or embarrassing situation), do not always occur immediately after exposure to the external trigger (APA, 1998). It is important to note that PAs may initially be uncued but, over time, become paired with or associated with specific stimuli (e.g., elevator, shopping center, being in a crowed place) and subsequently result in situationally bound or situationally predisposed attacks. Frequently, regardless of the type of PA, avoidance behaviors ensue.

Community studies using structured psychiatric interviews have found that 2% to 18% of adolescents between 12 and 18 years of age have experienced at least one four-symptom PA during their lives (Essau et al., 1999; Hayward et al., 1997, 2000). Studies using self-report questionnaires have yielded considerably higher prevalence rates, reaching between 43% and 60% (King et al., 1993, 1997); however, reliance on self-report questionnaires tends to produce increased rates of false-positive cases, and many of these cases turn out not to be true cases of PA when followed up with structured psychiatric interviews. PAs tend to be equally prevalent in males and females (Essau et al., 1999; Hayward et al., 2000; King et al., 1993) but tend to be more severe in females (Hayward et al., 1989, 2000; King et al., 1997). PAs can occur in children but are much less prevalent than in adolescents (Ollendick, 1998). Ten to 30% of youngsters with PA develop moderate to severe avoidance behaviors (e.g., agoraphobia) of specific situations (e.g., school, restaurants, malls, crowds) for fear they might experience another attack (Essau et al., 1999; Hayward et al., 2000; King et al., 1993).

Panic Disorder (PD)

PD is characterized primarily by recurrent, unexpected, or uncued PAs. In addition, it is characterized by at least one month of persistent concern about having another PA (anticipatory anxiety), worry about the implications and consequences of the PA, and/or significant impairment in functioning (APA, 1994, 1998). In addition, to diagnose PD, the PA should not be accounted for primarily by other physical or psychiatric illnesses. The ICD-10 (World Health Organization, 1992) includes similar diagnostic criteria.

Clinical studies (Alessi & Magen, 1988; Biederman et al., 1997; Kearney et al., 1997; Last & Strauss, 1989; Moreau & Follet, 1993; Ollendick, 1995) have shown that older adolescents who are Caucasian, female, and of middle class are more likely to present to outpatient clinics for treatment of PD. Similar to the adult literature, more than half of these adolescents report palpitations, tremor, dizziness, shortness of breath, faintness, sweating, chest pressure/pain, and fear of dying. Although PD in children has been reported in the clinical literature, it appears that this disorder is less frequent and perhaps less severe in youngsters (Mattis & Ollendick, 1997a; Nelles & Barlow, 1988).

Diagnosis

Up to 90% of children and adolescents with PD are comorbid with other anxiety and/or depressive disorders (Alessi & Magen, 1988; Biederman et al., 1997; Essau et al., 2000). PD has also been shown to be comorbid with other psychiatric disorders in children and adolescents, including attention deficit hyperactive disorder, oppositional defiant disorder, and bipolar disorder (Biederman et al., 1997; Last & Strauss, 1989; Ollendick et al., 2004).

Differential diagnosis is important in children and adolescents who present primarily with other disorders. For example, youngsters with primary mood disorders and other anxiety disorders can experience PAs (APA, 1994, 1998). In such instances, a differential diagnosis is imperative and the secondary diagnosis of PD would be made only if the PA is not explained by the other psychiatric disorder. For example, if socially anxious or separation-anxious youths experience PAs, but *only* when they are exposed to potentially embarrassing or evaluative situations or situations in which they might be separated from their parent(s), respectively, the diagnosis of PD would not be made.

Children and adolescents with certain medical conditions (e.g., hyperthyroidism, diabetes, asthma) may also experience anxiety symptoms secondary to their medical condition that resemble PAs, and, as result, they can be misdiagnosed with PD. On the other hand, inasmuch as PD is frequently accompanied by a number of somatic symptoms, youths with PD can be and frequently are misdiagnosed with a spate of medical conditions including pulmonary (e.g., asthma), cardiovascular (e.g., angina, arrhythmias, myocardial infarction), neurological (e.g., seizures, vestibular dysfunctions, syncope), and gastrointestinal illnesses (e.g., irritable bowel syndrome) (APA, 1998). Therefore, clinicians need to be aware of these conditions and to show good clinical judgment when these medical illnesses need to be ruled out (Birmaher & Ollendick, 2004; Ollendick et al., 2004).

Substances, including street drugs (e.g., cocaine, caffeine), over-the-counter medications, and acute withdrawal from prescribed medications and other substances (e.g., benzodiazepines, alcohol) can also induce PAs. In these instances, PD would be diagnosed only if the PAs have occurred before or lasted long enough after the substance has been discontinued (APA, 1994). Finally, a child can be experiencing anxiety symptoms and PAs due to exposure to real current or past threatening situations such as exposure to violence or sexual or physical abuse. Such possibilities should be routinely explored in the clinical interview prior to commencement of psychosocial or pharmacological treatment (Birmaher & Ollendick, 2004).

DEVELOPMENTAL COURSE

No longitudinal studies of children and adolescents with PD have been published, and so the developmental course of this disorder is unknown. In adults, however, PD has been reported to wax and wane. In longitudinal studies of adults, approximately one-third show improvement, one-third remain subsyndromal, and one-third continue to fulfill criteria for PD even years after their diagnosis.

Although the developmental course of PAs and PD has not yet been tracked with children and adolescents, female sex, puberty, negative affectivity (NA: an increased sensitivity to negative stimuli with resulting distress and fearfulness), anxiety sensitivity (AS: an increased tendency to respond fearfully to anxiety symptoms), internal attributions of responsibility in response to negative events, and the presence of MDD have been associated with the onset of full-blown PAs in youths (Hayward et al., 1997, 2000; Kearney et al., 1997; Lau et al., 1996; Mattis & Ollendick, 1997a). Although the findings are less robust, family conflict and stress have also been shown to be predictive of PAs in adolescents (King et al., 1997; Macauly & Kleinknecht, 1989).

Female sex, MDD, high AS, and family history of MDD and PD have been associated with higher rates of PD in youth as well (e.g., Biederman et al., 2001; Kearney et al., 1997). Earlier studies suggested that childhood separation anxiety disorder might herald the development of PD during late adolescence and adulthood (see reviews by Ollendick & Huntzinger, 1990, and Silove et al., 1996). However, more recent studies have failed to affirm this intuitive relationship (Essau et al., 1999; Hayward et al., 2000).

ETIOLOGY

There are several groups of children and adolescents who are at risk to develop anxiety disorders including PD. These children include offspring of anxious and/or depressed parents, so-called behaviorally inhibited children (Kagan et al., 1988; Muris & Ollendick, 2005), and, more controversially, children with psychological characteristics such as anxiety sensitivity and insecure attachment that portend anxiety outcomes (Mattis & Ollendick, 1997a; Ollendick et al., 2004). Although space in this chapter does not permit an explication of these etiologic pathways to the onset of PAs and PD, it appears reasonable to conclude that multiple pathways exist, including those associated with genetic, temperamental, cognitive, familial, and environmental risk factors. Moreover, it appears that any one pathway, including those associated with any one of these risk factors, does not necessarily result in PD. Such a conclusion is consistent with the tenets of developmental psychopathology: namely, that multiple pathways can lead to any one disorder (the principle of equifinality) and that any one pathway can result in a diversity of outcomes, only one of which is PD (the principle of multifinality) (Ollendick & Hirshfeld-Becker, 2002; Toth & Cicchetti, 1999).

TREATMENT

This section reviews the psychosocial treatments for PD and briefly comments upon pharmacological treatments. As we shall see, there is considerably less support for pharmacological treatments of PD in children and adolescents but emerging evidentiary support for psychosocial treatments, at least for the cognitive-behavioral treatments. Moreover, all of the available studies with children and adolescents address the acute treatment of PD. Studies evaluating the effects of continuation (to avoid relapses) and maintenance (to avoid recurrences) of treatment are nonexistent in the child and adolescent literature, and rare in the adult literature. Such studies are sorely needed, not only for PD but for other childhood psychiatric disorders as well (March & Ollendick, 2004).

Psychoeducation

For both psychosocial and pharmacological treatments, education about PAs and PD is important. Children and their parents should be educated about the symptom picture, developmental course, etiology (if known), and the assessment and treatment of the disorder. Psychoeducation can increase compliance with treatment, reduce anxiety, and improve the child's self-esteem (e.g., the child can come to see that having PAs is not a sign of personal weakness) and overall family relationships (e.g., parents can come to see that child is not pretending or exaggerating his or her symptoms, and that they are not to blame for their child's symptoms). Although no studies have been published on the effects of psychoeducation alone for children and adolescents with PD, for other disorders including depression, anxiety, bipolar, and even schizophrenia, psychoeducation in combination with active treatments has been found to be helpful (e.g., Brent et al., 1993). The American Psychiatric Association's (1998) Practice Guidelines for the Treatment of Patients with Panic Disorder also stress the importance of psychoeducation whether psychosocial or pharmacological interventions are implemented subsequently.

Psychosocial Interventions

Evidence-based psychosocial treatments for the treatment of PD have been based largely on cognitive and cognitive-behavioral theories (Chambless & Ollendick, 2001). The primary proponents of the cognitive model have been Beck and Clark (Beck & Emery, 1985; Clark et al., 1985). In its simplest form, this model suggests that the insidious spiral into panic is due to catastrophic misinterpretations of otherwise normally occurring bodily sensations. Implicit in this theory is the notion that nothing particularly unique is occurring in the individual from a neurobiological perspective; rather, it is primarily a "psychological" account of the development and maintenance of panic. Mild chest pain experienced after exercise, for example, might be interpreted in an at-risk or psychologically vulnerable youngster as an impending heart attack in which the young person believes he or she might actually die. Individual differences in the tendency to misinterpret somatic events would differentiate the child or adolescent who develops PAs and the one who does not. Youngsters high in AS (i.e., anxiety sensitivity), for example, might more likely be vulnerable to the onset of PAs and the development of PD (Ollendick, 1998). Treatment, according to this theory, consists largely of a mixture of cognitive techniques and behavioral experiments designed to modify the faulty misinterpretations of bodily sensations and the processes that serve to maintain them. Considerable support for this model has been garnered in recent years for the treatment of PAs and PD in adults (cf., Clark, 1996; Clark et al., 1999). However, to our knowledge, the cognitive approach has not been used nor evaluated with children and adolescents at this time.

The primary proponent of the cognitive-behavioral model has been Barlow (1988), and the treatment evolving from this perspective has come to be called *Panic Control Treatment*. According to Barlow, several risk factors are required in order for PAs and PD to develop. First, a person must have the tendency to be neurobiologically overreactive to stress. In particular, some individuals seem to react to the stress of negative life events with considerable apprehension, believing that some drastic or terrible thing will happen to them. Such apprehension leads to a fight-or-flight response that is, in all likelihood, triggered prematurely and unnecessarily. That is, the response exceeds the demands of the stimulus event. Barlow refers to this premature, unnecessary, and extreme response as a "false alarm." Over time, through a process of conditioning, false alarms become associated with bodily sensations (e.g., rapid heartbeat, difficulty breathing) and PAs follow. After repeated conditioning trials, the person becomes extremely sensitive to the physical sensations so that even slight bodily changes associated with exercise or fatigue, for example, trigger an alarm reaction and a resultant PA. Subsequently, the individual develops anxious apprehension over the possibility that future alarms or PAs will occur. This tendency to develop anxious apprehension is viewed as a psychological vulnerability that arises from developmental experiences in which predictability and control are largely absent. Finally, avoidance behavior may develop depending on the person's coping skills and perceptions of safety.

Treatment from this model is comprised of three primary components: relaxation training and breathing retraining to address neurobiological sensitivities to stress, interoceptive exposure to address heightened somatic symptoms, and cognitive restructuring to address faulty misinterpretations associated with the somatic symptoms. In effect, this model consists of cognitive therapy (similar to that espoused by Beck and Clark) as well as behavioral therapy (relaxation training, breathing retraining, interoceptive exposure). Considerable support for this cognitive-behavioral model has been garnered in recent years in the treatment of PAs and PD in adults (Barlow et al., 2000).

Mattis and Ollendick (1997b) adapted Barlow's model of panic to children and suggested a pathway through which stressful separation experiences, in combination with individual differences in temperament characteristics and attachment styles, result in development of panic. They proposed that children respond to stressful separation experiences differently depending on their temperament (in particular, behavioral inhibition) and the nature of their attachment relationships with significant adults (in particular, insecure-ambivalent/resistant relationships). According to this

model, children who are characterized by this constellation of variables
and events are at high risk for the development of PAs and eventual PD.
Inasmuch as these children have difficulty being soothed and comforted
by their caregivers in times of stress (e.g., separations), they experience
intense alarm reactions and have little sense of predictability or control over
these events. These "at-risk" children learn to associate distress in these
situations with physical or somatic symptoms (e.g., pounding heart, shaky
hands), resulting in a cascade of false alarms. Next, as suggested by Mattis
and Ollendick, the child begins to display anxious apprehension over the
possibility of future alarms or panic attacks. Anxious apprehension is
viewed as a psychological vulnerability, encapsulated in the notion of AS
(anxiety sensitivity). PA symptoms are likely to occur when these at-risk
children perceive little control over what will happen to them and/or little
ability to predict what will happen to them in the future. Agoraphobic
avoidance develops when the children begin to withdraw from unfamiliar
people and situations as a way of coping with and reducing their distress
(see Mattis & Ollendick, 2002).

Treatment studies based on Barlow's model and Mattis and Ollendick's
adaptation of it have shown promising outcomes with adolescents. Two
controlled single-case studies lend initial support to its use, as does a
randomized, controlled clinical trial. In addition, one intensive clinical
trial, based on an extension of this model, is currently underway. In the
first single-case study, Barlow and Seidner (1983) treated three adolescent
agoraphobic youths with an early rendition of Panic Control Treatment.
The adolescents were treated in a 10-session group-therapy format and
were accompanied by their mothers, who were enlisted to facilitate and
reward behavior change. Treatment consisted of panic management procedures, cognitive restructuring, and instructions to engage in structured
homework sessions, which involved graduated exposure to feared situations. Parents were educated on the nature of panic disorder and agoraphobia and were taught procedures for dealing with anxiety that were
neither reinforcing of anxiety-related behaviors nor punishing to the
adolescent. Parents encouraged and supported their teens to practice
between sessions and practiced with them at least once a week. Following
treatment, two of the three adolescents showed marked improvement
in their symptoms; however, the other adolescent did not show significant change. In fact, treatment resulted in a slight increment in phobic
avoidance for this adolescent. Barlow and Seidner (1983) suggested that
treatment outcome was related to the extent of parent-adolescent conflict in
the families; that is, for the two families in which a reasonably good parent-
adolescent relationship was evident, treatment was successful, while for
the remaining family, the presence of parent-adolescent conflict seemingly
interfered with treatment outcome. Although only two of the three adolescents responded positively, the treatment appeared promising.

Based on this early study, Ollendick (1995) used a controlled multiple-
baseline design to illustrate the controlling effects of the adapted version
of Panic Control Treatment in the treatment of four adolescents who
presented with PD with agoraphobia. The adolescents ranged in age from

13 to 17 years; however, their PAs began when they were between 9 and 13 years of age—nearly four years, on average, prior to the beginning of treatment. Adolescents were treated individually and alone, but, as in Barlow and Seidner (1983), their mothers were enlisted to facilitate behavior change. Treatment consisted of information about panic (i.e., psychoeducation), relaxation training and breathing retraining, cognitive restructuring, interoceptive exposure, participant modeling (e.g., therapist and then parent demonstrating approach behavior in agoraphobic situations), *in vivo* exposure, and profuse praise and social reinforcement. Treatment was individualized and varied in duration, lasting between 10 and 12 sessions. Treatment was effective for all four adolescents in eliminating panic attacks, reducing agoraphobic avoidance, decreasing accompanying negative mood states, and increasing self-efficacy for coping with previously avoided situations and panic attacks should they occur in the future. Follow-up over a six-month interval affirmed the lasting effects of the treatment.

Mattis and her colleagues recently completed the first randomized controlled trial of a developmental adaptation of Panic Control Treatment (PCT-A) and a self-monitoring control condition in the treatment of PD in adolescents (Mattis et al., in preparation). Three aspects of PD were addressed in this 11-week intervention: (1) the cognitive aspect of PD or the tendency to misinterpret physical sensations as catastrophic; (2) the tendency to hyperventilate, thus creating and/or intensifying physical sensations of panic; and (3) conditioned fear reactions to the physical sensations. Key components of treatment included correcting misinformation about panic, breathing retraining, cognitive restructuring, and interoceptive and *in vivo* exposure. In the interoceptive exposure component of treatment, the adolescents were taught to face their primary fear: namely, the physical sensations of panic. Exercises such as shaking their head from side to side for 30 seconds, running in place for 1 minute, holding their breath for 30 seconds, rotating in a chair for 1 minute, hyperventilating for 1 minute, and breathing through a thin straw for 2 minutes were used to facilitate exposure to the interoceptive physical sensations. Adolescents were informed that they would be learning different "tools" or strategies to address their panic and to control the resultant anxiety they experienced. Specifically, "Changing My Breathing" was described as a tool for reducing the frequency and intensity of unwanted or undesired physical sensations; "Being a Detective" was introduced as the process of evaluating and changing anxious, worrisome, catastrophic, and nonproductive thoughts; and "Facing My Fears" was the strategy for reducing avoidance through interoceptive and graduated *in vivo* exposure exercises. Adolescents were further informed that the goal of using these tools was to break the cycle of panic by reducing physical panic sensations, anxious thoughts, and avoidance while also altering the relations among the components. For example, changing anxious thoughts about a situation also reduced physical sensations the adolescent experienced; in turn, the reduced physical sensations led to decreased avoidance of that situation. Eleven sessions, all manualized, were delivered by trained doctoral-level staff and graduate students.

Twenty-five adolescents (19 females, 6 males), aged 14–17 years, participated in this trial. A total of 13 adolescents received the PCT-A treatment, and 12 received a self-monitoring control condition in which they waited 8 weeks and then were offered PCT-A treatment. All adolescents received a principal diagnosis of panic disorder with or without agoraphobia. A multimodal assessment was utilized, including self-report measures of anxiety, depression, anxiety sensitivity, and panic frequency and intensity; a diagnostic interview [Anxiety Disorder Interview Schedule for Children/Parents (ADIS-C/P)] and a behavioral measure (Behavioral Approach Task) during which physiological monitoring (heart rate) were obtained. All adolescents were assessed at pretreatment, posttreatment, and at 3-, 6-, and 12-month follow-up, to track the maintenance of change.

Results of the study showed a significant reduction in the severity and frequency of PAs as well as significant decreases in AS in those adolescents receiving PCT-A relative to those in the monitoring control condition (Mattis et al., in preparation). In addition, findings showed that the PCT-A group evidenced a greater reduction in clinician-rated severity ratings of PD than those in the control group. Almost all adolescents in the PCT-A group showed reductions in PD to the nonclinical level, whereas those adolescents in the control group maintained clinical levels of PD. Additionally, only the PCT-A group showed significant reductions on self-report measures of anxiety and depression. These findings, along with the two single-case studies, provide considerable support for the preliminary efficacy of this innovative developmental adaptation of Panic Control Treatment.

Interestingly, the most common reason for treatment refusal in the above clinical trial was the length and timing of the treatment. The 11 weekly one-hour sessions were distributed over a three-month period. In addition, the treatment did not include therapist-assisted *in vivo* exposure, as was evident in the Ollendick (1995) study. Some families contacted the clinic expressing a desire for more immediate relief of their adolescent's symptoms, including extreme anxiety, school refusal, and avoidance of normal teenage activities. Some of them inquired whether a more "intensive" form of treatment was possible so as to facilitate more rapidly their child's school reentry and involvement in daily activities.

These issues prompted a pilot study and a randomized clinical trial that is currently investigating the efficacy of an eight-day intensive format of treatment for adolescents with PD with agoraphobia. It was reasoned that such intensive intervention would be particularly useful for those adolescents who were not attending school and who were suffering academically and socially due to their agoraphobic avoidance. Further, a briefer form of PCT could also be helpful for those adolescents who have limited access to appropriate forms of therapy and need to travel to a distant location to receive psychological treatment, or for those who have not succeeded with other more traditional "weekly" therapies. In addition, for those adolescents with more severe agoraphobia, it was hypothesized that therapist-assisted *in vivo* exposure would be extremely helpful in motivating and rewarding adolescents to enter these fear-producing situations.

In response to these needs, in an open clinical trial, Pincus et al. (2004) recently examined the efficacy of this eight-day intensive treatment, called Adolescent Intensive Panic Control Treatment with Situational Exposure (APE). Modeled after a similar program for adults developed by Spiegel and Barlow (2000), APE extends PCT-A in several ways. First, APE is conducted over eight consecutive days, whereas PCT-A is conducted over a three-month period of time. Second, the session structure of APE is different from PCT-A in that each session is extended in duration, rather than the 50-minute sessions used in PCT-A. In sessions 1–3 of APE, for example, adolescents meet with the therapist for approximately 2–3 hours each session and receive education about the nature of anxiety and panic, the physiology of anxiety, and the cognitive component of panic attacks. They are also taught skills such as cognitive restructuring and hypothesis testing. Adolescents also learn how to create a personalized "Fear and Avoidance Hierarchy" and are taught the concepts of interoceptive exposure, situational exposure, and habituation. Adolescents and their parents are given an educational workbook and are instructed to complete specific chapter readings and exercises in the evenings between sessions. During sessions 4–7, therapists assist the adolescent in conducting *in vivo* situational and interoceptive exposure exercises, so that the adolescent can begin to enter previously avoided situations and confront panic symptomatology. These four sessions last approximately 5–7 hours per session, and the focus is on helping the adolescent enter situations listed on his or her "Fear and Avoidance Hierarchy."

Third, APE differs from PCT-A in the level of parent involvement. In PCT-A, parents were provided a brief handout educating them about their teenager's panic disorder. However, their participation in therapy sessions was minimal. In APE, parents were more heavily involved in treatment sessions. Parents joined treatment sessions for at least 30 minutes per session and were asked to learn similar skills as their adolescent. Therapists modeled for parents how to conduct situational exposures. They were asked to conduct interoceptive exercises with their children in session with therapist guidance and were educated about issues such as the importance of eliminating "safety" behaviors at home. Parents learned how to take on the important role of "coach" in encouraging adolescents not to avoid feared situations. Thus, parental involvement in APE was more extensive than in PCT-A.

Results of this open clinical trial indicated that the clinical severity ratings of panic disorder significantly decreased from pre-to posttreatment, with 14 of 18 adolescents displaying nonclinical levels of panic disorder by posttreatment. At one-month posttreatment, 17 of 18 adolescents showed nonclinical levels of PD with agoraphobia and reported that panic was no longer significantly interfering with their lives. The frequency of panic attacks also decreased substantially; at 1 month following treatment, adolescents reported a mean of 2.2 panic attacks per week (as compared to 11.4 per week at pretreatment), and at 3 months following treatment, the number of reported panic attacks was further decreased to an average of 1.5 per week. Adolescents' anxiety sensitivity also decreased from pre- to posttreatment and was maintained at follow-up points. Numerous collateral changes were also reported by families, including improved academic performance, improved social functioning, and improved family functioning. Adolescents reported decreased depression and decreased avoidance of situations due to panic. Parents reported feeling more knowledgeable about the factors that cause and maintain panic and reported feeling more confident in their ability to effectively deal with adolescents during a panic attack. They also reported improved family interactions, as they utilized skills learned in therapy to positively encourage adolescents' nonavoidance of previously avoided situations. In sum, this open trial showed initial support for an intensive treatment format for adolescent panic disorder.

Based on these promising findings, a randomized control clinical trial is currently underway to evaluate the efficacy and acceptability of this brief intensive treatment, relative to a no-treatment control; the study is also designed to investigate the relative advantage of involving parents in the treatment. Ninety adolescents are being randomly assigned to one of three treatment conditions: (1) intensive treatment with parent involvement, (2) intensive treatment without parent involvement, and (3) a waitlist control condition. An additional purpose of the study is to explore mechanisms of action of treatment. Currently, we have limited knowledge about the possible mechanisms of therapeutic action in interventions for youth, with or without parental involvement (Prins & Ollendick, 2003), and thus, the investigation of this issue is an important one. Long-term follow-up of treatment gains is also lacking to date; as a result, maintenance of adolescents' improvements will be tracked for one year posttreatment in this study.

At this point in time, it is obvious that psychosocial treatments based on cognitive-behavioral principles appear highly promising with adolescents. However, it is evident that these interventions have not yet been examined with children who present with PD. The reasons for this state of affairs is not at all clear, especially since very similar procedures have been used effectively with children who present with other forms of phobic and anxiety disorders (see Ollendick & King, 1998, 2000, and Ollendick et al., 2006, for reviews). Many of these cognitive-behavioral treatments enjoy empirically validated status. It is perhaps even more alarming that no other psychosocial treatments (i.e., interpersonal psychotherapy, psychodynamic therapy, family therapy) have been evaluated with children and adolescents who present with PAs or PD. Clearly, the development and evaluation of other psychosocial treatments for PAs and PD in children and adolescents are in an embryonic stage and are in need of systematic inquiry. Still, cognitive-behavioral evidence-based treatments do exist and enjoy considerable evidentiary support.

Phamacological Interventions: A Brief Note

No randomized controlled trials (RCTs) for the pharmacological treatment of PD in children and adolescents have yet been completed

(Birmaher & Ollendick, 2004). In adults, RCTs comparing the following classes of medications with placebo have been shown to be effective in the treatment of PD: the selective serotonin reuptake inhibitors (SSRIs) (60–80% vs. 36–60%), the tricyclic antidepressants (TCAs) (45–70% vs. 15–50%), and the high-potency benzodiazepines (55–75% vs. 15–50%). The SSRIs have been the first choice due to their ease of administration and the minimal side-effects profile, and they are thought to be less dangerous in case of an overdose. Although the monoamine oxidase inhibitors (MAOIs) are also effective in the treatment of PD in adults (APA, 1998), they are used primarily for those patients who have not responded well to other treatments; however, they also carry the risk of hypertensive crisis and require dietary restrictions.

In children and adolescents, anecdotal case reports have shown that benzodiazepines (e.g., Biederman, 1987; Simeon et al., 1992) and the SSRIs (e.g., Fairbanks et al., 1997; Renaud et al., 1999) may be effective treatments for PD. For example, in a prospective open trial, Renaud and colleagues (1999) treated 12 children and adolescents with PD with SSRIs for a period of 6–8 weeks. The youths were followed for six months and evaluated periodically with clinician-based and self-report rating scales for anxiety and depression, global functioning, and side effects. Nearly 75% of the youths showed improvement without experiencing significant side effects. At the end of the trial, 8 (67%) no longer fulfilled criteria for PD, whereas 4 (33%) continued to have significant and persisting residual symptoms.

On the basis of the adult literature, open clinical trials, and the fact that SSRIs have been effective in the treatment of children and adolescents with other anxiety and major depressive disorders (e.g., Emslie et al., 1997), Birmaher and Ollendick (2004) suggested that the SSRIs are a promising treatment for children and adolescents with PD as well. However, it is also evident that RCTs evaluating the effects of SSRI in youth with PD are sorely needed at this time.

CASE EXAMPLE

Presenting Information

"Kathleen K" is a 16-year-old female with panic disorder and agoraphobia whose parents called the Center for Anxiety and Related Disorders at Boston University stating that they were extremely worried about their daughter, who was having "out-of-the-blue" panic attacks several times every day and was having difficulty attending school. Mr. and Mrs. K stated that they were frustrated with their inability to help their daughter. Despite their attempts to help her relax, they described Kathleen as "inconsolable" during her panic episodes and reported that she would frequently cry and beg them to help her. Mr. and Mrs. K stated that Kathleen's panic attacks were "ruling" the family, and, without help, they feared that Kathleen would stop going to school altogether and would miss out on other developmentally appropriate activities such as dances, parties, and other social functions.

When Kathleen was initially assessed, she reported having 3 to 4 panic attacks per day (approximately 15–20 per week), which she stated "overwhelmed" her to the point where she had to leave the classroom or activity in which she was engaged. Kathleen stated that during a panic attack, her heart raced, she felt short of breath, and she became extremely nauseous. Kathleen indicated that her typical coping strategy for dealing with her panic attacks was to use her cell phone at school and to call her mother every time she had a panic attack in order to have her mother "talk her through it." Kathleen stated that she also carried a water bottle around everywhere, because water tended to "calm her down." She did not know why this was the case but that it simply seemed to "work." Kathleen's mother stated that she never knew what to say to help Kathleen, and although she tried to encourage her to cope on her own, she often wound up feeling badly for her and would "give in" and pick her up from school. Mrs. K stated that she arranged for special accommodations for Kathleen at school so that Kathleen would be permitted to leave the classroom at any moment if she felt a panic attack coming on.

Kathleen's mother further stated that she and Kathleen fought a lot at home, largely because she was unsure how hard to "push" her to continue to participate in activities. Kathleen's mother became tearful as she disclosed her own fears about whether she was being a "bad" mother when she felt it necessary to push her to stay in an activity rather than pick her up and drive her home. She also stated that she sometimes thought she should feel grateful that her 16- year-old daughter wanted to spend so much time with her, even though she secretly feared that panic disorder was the "glue" that was keeping her feeling emotionally close to her daughter.

Kathleen's mother and father reported that Kathleen's panic disorder has wreaked havoc on the entire family. Each morning began with a fight regarding whether or not Kathleen was "really sick" or whether her stomachaches and related physical symptoms before school were due to anxiety. Although Kathleen expressed a desire to spend time with friends outside school, she also indicated that she feared she would have a panic attack in those situations also and there would be no one there to help her who "really understands." As a result, Kathleen avoided many activities with her friends and typically made excuses for why she could not attend various functions. Kathleen reported that due to panic she avoided getting a part-time job during the summer months, which was another source of conflict in the family. Kathleen stated that she feared she would not be able to keep steady hours at a job because she might have a panic attack and have to leave. Mrs. K stated that she had started to push Kathleen to do more without her but that this caused constant fighting in their home.

Kathleen was an "A" student, was an accomplished athlete, and had many friends. In fact, her father reported that she was actually in the "popular" crowd at school and was always being invited to go out to parties, dances, and ski trips (but rarely went). She played on the school soccer and track teams and spent a lot of free time e-mailing her friends from her home computer. However, Kathleen stated that she had only one close friend who knew about her panic attacks and that she tried to hide her panic and her frustration from her other friends.

Case Formulation

Kathleen's case presentation and the pattern of family interactions that have developed in response to her panic attacks are quite representative of adolescents presenting for treatment for panic disorder and agoraphobia. Kathleen experienced frequent out-of-the-blue panic attacks, and she was constantly worried about the onset of another attack. As a result of her panic, she began avoiding developmentally appropriate activities, such as dances, parties, outings with friends, and school. Although her parents desperately wanted to see her have fun and to be a "normal teenager," Kathleen was torn between wanting the developmentally appropriate level of independence that most 16-year-olds desire and feeling she needed to be close to her mother or father in case a panic attack occurred. Thus, Kathleen's panic was interfering in her healthy adolescent development. As is commonly seen in families with a teenager with panic disorder, Kathleen's parents desperately wanted to help her but were unsure of what to do or how to help her. From a cognitive-behavioral perspective, Kathleen's thoughts about panic, "I am definitely going to have a panic attack," were triggering unwanted physical sensations (e.g., heart racing, nausea) and in turn her physical sensations retriggered or instigated such thoughts. A vicious cycle was evident. Kathleen's primary behavioral reaction to these physical sensations was to avoid situations in which these feelings were present. As a result, her negative thoughts about panic were being maintained and it was becoming more and more difficult for her to enter new situations in which she expected to have a panic attack.

Treatment

Kathleen and her parents were treated in the intensive eight-day program in order to more quickly facilitate her return to school and her involvement in developmentally appropriate activities. During sessions 1–3 of treatment, Kathleen was taught the cycle of panic and anxiety, the physiology of anxiety and panic, and how to become aware of the "triggers" of panic attacks. She was also taught how to restructure maladaptive thoughts that might trigger her panic attacks. Interoceptive exposure exercises, such as spinning in a chair, running in place, and breathing through a thin straw, were also used. Kathleen stated that these exercises triggered physical sensations that were similar to her naturally occurring panic attacks, and she was amazed to see that her physical sensations could be resolved after only a few minutes. Kathleen stated that although she thought her panic attacks were "out of the blue," it was very helpful for her to understand that her panic attacks were actually triggered by select thoughts, physical feelings, or behaviors. Kathleen was seen for 2 hours for each of these first three sessions, and her parents were invited to join in during the last 30 minutes of each session. When her parents joined each session, Kathleen taught her parents each of the skills she had learned. Kathleen stated that she most enjoyed teaching her parents the intero-ceptive exposure exercises as she felt this helped them relate to the physical sensations she experienced on a regular basis during her panic attacks. Kathleen and her parents were quite cooperative and participated in each session, and they completed homework and readings each evening prior to the next day's session.

During days 4–7 of treatment, Kathleen was accompanied by a doctoral-level therapist to "face her fears" and "ride the wave" of anxiety during *in vivo* exposure exercises derived from her Fear and Avoidance Hierarchy. During each exposure practice, Kathleen understood that the most important thing was to stay in the situation until her anxiety had abated. She began her exposure practices by drinking caffeine to heighten her physical sensations. Over the course of four days, Kathleen conducted exposures in classroom settings, in restaurants, on the subway, at a crowded concert, and at the movies. Kathleen was asked to enter these situations without her "safety behaviors," such as her cell phone or water bottle. On the final exposure day, Kathleen was able to perform interoceptive exercises prior to conducting the exposure practice to make it "harder." Kathleen expressed that she could feel her confidence grow as she started entering situations that she had previously avoided.

Kathleen's parents also received instruction in how to conduct a successful exposure practice with Kathleen. They stated that they felt a huge burden lifted off them when they were taught that anxiety and panic would not hurt Kathleen and that the most appropriate way to help Kathleen was to help her not to avoid things and to encourage her to use her newly learned coping skills to enter developmentally appropriate activities. Kathleen's mother and father were taught to praise Kathleen when she was successful in entering previously avoided activities, even if they began with praising smaller steps toward the activity. Mr. and Mrs. K were also instructed to begin having quality time with Kathleen that was entirely separate from dealing with panic disorder; for example, Kathleen stated that she would enjoy things like going to the mall with her mother or having dinner out with her father. Thus, Mr. and Mrs. K learned the importance of quality time with Kathleen to help their relationship remain emotionally close, even though they no longer had such a prominent role in helping Kathleen with her panic attacks. The final session (session 8) was conducted for two hours and was spent making a plan for continued exposure practice and to discuss relapse prevention strategies.

Outcome

When assessed at one month posttreatment, Kathleen and her parents reported significant reductions in the frequency and severity of Kathleen's panic attacks. Kathleen reported that she was only having 2 to 3 panic attacks per week (down from 15–20 per week at pretreatment). Furthermore, she reported that even these panic attacks no longer caused her as much distress, as she understood that the anxiety would not cause her any real harm and would dissipate after a few minutes if she did not continue to think the "worry thoughts" that triggered her attacks. In fact, Kathleen had become very skilled at restructuring her maladaptive thoughts about her panic attacks, and by the posttreatment assessment, Kathleen proudly stated that she was able to restructure worry thoughts "in her head" without having to write them down on paper. Kathleen's family stated that Kathleen's improvements had positive effects on the entire family. They reported that Kathleen was no longer calling her parents from school, had returned to school full-time, and had begun to enjoy developmentally appropriate activities with her friends, including going to football games, playing sports, and going to concerts. In fact, Mr. and Mrs. K stated that Kathleen even went on an overnight ski trip over three hours away from their home with friends, which was a huge accomplishment for Kathleen and the first time she had done so. Mr. and Mrs. K stated that they were thrilled no longer to have the role of staying on the phone for hours during the day to help Kathleen with her panic attacks, as this never really worked for Kathleen anyway. Instead, they ended treatment stating that the new skills Kathleen learned helped her to regain a healthy level of teenage independence. The regularly scheduled "quality time" was reportedly working to help Kathleen and her parents remain emotionally close.

CONCLUSIONS

Although significant advances have been made, the study of PAs and PD in children and adolescents is truly in its own stage of early development (Birmaher & Ollendick, 2004; Mattis & Ollendick, 2002). Moreover, although it was initially thought that children could not develop PAs and PD due to cognitive limitations, it now seems clear that children (and adolescents) can and do develop these disorders. Moreover, as with adults, these disorders are frequently comorbid with other anxiety and affective disorders and, albeit less frequently, comorbid with externalizing disorders such as substance abuse and conduct disturbance. The effects of these disorders on the developing child are considerable; many of these children experience academic, behavioral, emotional, and social difficulties. The evidence base for psychosocial treatments, especially so for cognitive-behavioral treatments, is very promising; however, it is also apparent that the evidentiary base for other psychosocial interventions is nonexistent and that the support for pharmacological interventions is truly in a nascent stage. Thus, although much has been discovered about PAs and PD in children and adolescents in recent years, much, much more remains to be learned.

REFERENCES

Alessi, N. E., & Magen, J. (1988). Panic disorders in psychiatrically hospitalized children. *American Journal of Psychiatry, 145,* 1450–1452.

American Psychiatric Association (1994). *Diagnostic and Statistical Manual of Mental Disorders,* 4th ed. Washington, DC.

American Psychiatric Association (1998). Practice guidelines for the treatment of patients with panic disorder. *American Journal of Psychiatry, 155,* 1–34.

Barlow, D. H. (1988). *Anxiety and Its Disorders: The Nature and Treatment of Anxiety and Panic.* New York: Guilford Press.

Barlow, D. H., Gorman, J. M., Shear, M. K., & Woods, S. W. (2000). Cognitive-behavioral therapy, imipramine, or their combination for panic disorder: A randomized controlled trial. *Journal of the American Medical Association, 283*(19), 2529–2536.

Barlow, D. H., & Seidner, A. L. (1983). Treatment of adolescent agoraphobics: Effects on parent-adolescent relations. *Behaviour Research and Therapy, 21,* 519–526.

Battaglia, M., Bertella, S., Bajo, S., Binaghi, F., & Bellodi, L. (1998). Anticipation of age at onset in panic disorder. *American Journal of Psychiatry, 155,* 590–595.

Beck, A. T., & Emery, G. (1985). *Anxiety Disorders and Phobias: A Cognitive Perspective.* Philadelphia: Center for Cognitive Therapy.

Biederman, J. (1987). Clonazepam in the treatment of prepubertal children with panic-like symptoms. *Journal of Clinical Psychiatry, 48* (Suppl), 38–41.

Biederman, J., Faraone, S. V., Hirshfeld-Becker, D. R., Friedman, D., Robin, J. A., & Rosenbaum, J. F. (2001). Patterns of psychopathology and dysfunction in high-risk children of parents with panic disorder and major depression. *American Journal of Psychiatry, 158*(1), 49–57.

Biederman, J., Faraone, S. V., Marrs, A., Moore, P., Garcia, J., Ablon, S., et al. (1997). Panic disorder and agoraphobia in consecutively referred children and adolescents. *Journal of the American Academy of Child and Adolescent Psychiatry, 36,* 214–223.

Birmaher, B., & Ollendick, T. H. (2004). Childhood onset panic disorder. In T. H. Ollendick & J. S. March (Eds.), *Phobic and Anxiety Disorders in Children and Adolescents: A Clinician's Guide to Effective Psychosocial and Pharmacological Interventions.* New York: Oxford University Press.

Birmaher, B., Waterman, G. S., Ryan, N. D., Cully, M., Balach, L., Ingram, J., et al. (1994). Fluoxetine for childhood anxiety disorders. *Journal of the American Academy of Child and Adolescent Psychiatry, 33,* 993–999.

Brent, D. A., Holder, D., Kolko, D., Birmaher, B., Baugher, M., Roth, C., et al. (1997). A clinical psychotherapy trial for adolescent depression comparing cognitive, family, and supportive therapy. *Archives of General Psychiatry, 54,* 877–885.

Brent, D. A., Poling, K., McKain, B., & Baugher, M. (1993). A psychoeducational program for families of affectively ill children and adolescents. *Journal of the American Academy of Child & Adolescent Psychiatry, 32,* 770–774.

Chambless, D. L., & Ollendick, T. H. (2001). Empirically supported psychological interventions: Controversies and evidence. *Annual Review of Psychology, 52,* 685–716.

Clark, D. M. (1996). Panic disorder: From theory to therapy. In P. M. Salkovskis (Ed.), *Frontiers of Cognitive Therapy* (pp. 318–344). New York: Guilford Press.

Clark, D. M., Salkovskis, P. M., & Chalkley, A. J. (1985). Respiratory control as a treatment for panic attacks. *Journal of Behavior Therapy and Experimental Psychiatry, 16,* 23–30.

Clark, D. M., Salkovskis, P. M., Hackmann, A., Wells, A., Ludgate, J., & Gelder, M. (1999). Brief cognitive therapy for panic disorder: A randomized controlled trial. *Journal of Consulting and Clinical Psychology, 67,* 583–589.

Emslie, G. J., Rush, A. J., Weinberg, W. A., Kowatch, R. A., Hughes, C. W., Carmody, T., et al. (1997). A double-blind, randomized, placebo-controlled trial of fluoxetine in children and adolescents with depression. *Archives of General Psychiatry, 54,* 1031–1037.

Essau, C. A., Conradt, J., & Petermann, F. (1999). Frequency of panic attacks and panic disorder in adolescents. *Depression & Anxiety, 9,* 19–26.

Essau, C. A., Conradt, J., & Petermann, F. (2000). Frequency, comorbidity, and psychosocial impairment of anxiety disorders in German adolescents. *Journal of Anxiety Disorders, 14,* 263–279.

Fairbanks, J. M., Pine, D. S., Tancer, N. K., Dummit III, E. S., Kentgen, L. M., Asche, B. K., et al. (1997). Open fluoxetine treatment of mixed anxiety disorders in children and adolescents. *Journal of the American Academy of Child and Adolescent Psychiatry, 7*, 17–29.

Ginsburg, G. S., & Drake, K. L. (in press). Anxiety sensitivity and panic attack symptomatology among low-income African-American adolescents. *Journal of Anxiety Disorders*.

Hayward, C., Killen, J. D., Kraemer, H. C., & Barr Taylor, C. (2000). Predictors of panic attacks in adolescents. *Journal of the American Academy of Child and Adolescent Psychiatry, 39*, 207–214.

Hayward, C., Killen, J. D., Kraemer, H. C., Blair-Greiner, A., Strachowski, D., Cunning, D., et al. (1997). Assessment and phenomenology of nonclinical panic attacks in adolescent girls. *Journal of Anxiety Disorders, 11*, 17–32.

Hayward, C., Killen, J. D., & Taylor, C. B. (1989). Panic attacks in young adolescents. *American Journal of Psychiatry, 146*, 1061–1062.

Kagan, J., Reznick, J. S., & Snidman, N. (1988). Biological bases of childhood shyness. *Science, 240*, 167–171.

Kazdin, A. E. (2000). *Psychotherapy for Children and Adolescents: Directions for Research and Practice*. New York: Oxford University Press.

Kearney, C. A., Albano, A. M., Eisen, A. R., Allan, W. D., & Barlow, D. H. (1997). The phenomenology of panic disorder in youngsters: An empirical study of a clinical sample. *Journal of Anxiety Disorders, 11*, 49–62.

Kendall, P. C., Flannery-Schroeder, E., Panichelli-Mindel, S., Southam-Gerow, M., Henin, A., & Warman, M. (1997). Therapy for youth with anxiety disorders: A second randomized clinical trial. *Journal of Consulting and Clinical Psychology, 65*, 366–380.

King, N. J., Gullone, E., Tonge, B. J., & Ollendick, T. H. (1993). Self-reports of panic attacks and manifest anxiety in adolescents. *Behaviour Research and Therapy, 31*, 111–116.

King, N. J., Ollendick, T. H., Mattis, S. G., Yang, B., & Tonge, B. (1997). Nonclinical panic attacks in adolescents: Prevalence, symptomatology and associated features. *Behaviour Change, 13*, 171–183.

Last, C. G., & Strauss, C. C. (1989). Panic disorder in children and adolescents. *Journal of Anxiety Disorders, 3*, 87–95.

Macaulay, J. L., & Kleinknecht, R. A. (1989). Panic and Panic attacks in adolescents. *Journal of Anxiety Disorders, 23*, 349–358.

March, J. S., & Ollendick, T. H. (2004). Integrated psychosocial and pharmacological treatments. In T. H. Ollendick & J. S. March (Eds.). *Phobic and Anxiety Disorders in Children and Adolescents: A Clinician's Guide to Effective Psychosocial and Pharmacological Interventions*. New York: Oxford University Press.

Mattis, S. G. (2002). Personal communication. Boston University.

Mattis, S. G., & Ollendick, T. H. (1997a). Children's cognitive responses to the somatic symptoms of panic. *Journal of Abnormal Child Psychology, 25*, 47–57.

Mattis, S. G., & Ollendick, T. H. (1997b). Panic in children and adolescents: A developmental analysis. In T. H. Ollendick & R. J. Prinz (Eds.), *Advances in Clinical Child Psychology*, Vol. 19 (pp. 27–74). New York: Plenum Press.

Mattis, S. G., & Ollendick, T. H. (2002). *Panic Disorder and Anxiety in Adolescents*. London: British Psychological Society.

Mattis, S. G., Pincus, D. B., Ehrenreich, J. T., & Barlow, D. H. (manuscript in preparation). Cognitive behavioral treatment of panic disorder in adolescence.

Moreau, D. L., & Follet, C. (1993). Panic disorder in children and adolescents. *Child and Adolescent Psychiatric Clinics North America, 2*, 581–602.

Moreau, D. L., & Weissman, M. M. (1992). Panic disorder in children and adolescents: A review. *American Journal of Psychiatry, 149*, 1306–1314.

Muris, P., & Ollendick, T. H. (2005). The role of temperament in the etiology of child psychopathology. *Clinical Child and Family Psychology Review, 8*, 271–289.

Nelles, W. B., & Barlow, D. H. (1988). Do children panic? *Clinical Psychology Review, 8*, 359–372.

Ollendick, T. H. (1995). Cognitive-behavioral treatment of panic disorder with agoraphobia in adolescents: A multiple baseline design analysis. *Behavior Therapy, 26*, 517–531.

Ollendick, T. H. (1998). Panic disorder in children and adolescents: New developments, new directions. *Journal of Clinical Child Psychology, 27*, 234–245.

Ollendick, T. H., & Hersen, M. (Eds.) (1998). *Handbook of Child Psychopathology*, 3rd ed. New York: Plenum Press.

Ollendick, T. H., & Hirshfeld-Becker, D. R. (2002). The developmental psychopathology of social anxiety disorder. *Biological Psychiatry, 51*, 44–58.

Ollendick, T. H. & Huntzinger, R. M. (1990). Separation anxiety disorders in children. In M. Hersen & C. G. Last (Eds.), *Handbook of Child and Adult Psychopathology: A Longitudinal Perspective* (pp. 133–149). New York: Pergamon Press.

Ollendick, T. H., & King, N. J. (1998). Empirically supported treatments for children with phobic and anxiety disorders: Current status. *Journal of Clinical Child Psychology, 27*, 156–167.

Ollendick, T. H., & King, N. J. (2000). Empirically supported treatments for children and adolescents. In P. C. Kendall (Ed.), *Child and Adolescent Therapy: Cognitive-Behavioral Procedures*, 2nd ed. (pp. 386–425). New York: Guilford Press.

Ollendick, T. H., King, N. J., & Chorpita, B. (2006). Empirically supported treatments for children and adolescents. In P. C. Kendall (Ed.), *Child and Adolescent Therapy*, 3rd ed. (pp. 492–520). New York: Guilford Press.

Ollendick, T. H., Mattis, S. G., & Birmaher, B. (2004). Panic disorder. In T. L. Morris & J. S. March (Eds.), *Anxiety Disorders in Children and Adolescents*, 2nd ed. (pp. 189–211). New York: Guilford Press.

Ollendick, T. H., Mattis, S. G., & King, N. J. (1994). Panic in children and adolescents: A review. *Journal of Child Psychology and Psychiatry, 35*, 113–134.

Pincus, D. B., Barlow, D. H., & Spiegel, D. (2004). *Eight-Day Intensive Treatment for Panic Disorder and Agoraphobia in Adolescents.* Paper presented in the Symposium, Intensive Treatments for Child and Adolescent Anxiety: New Findings (D. Pincus, Chairperson) at the Annual Meeting of the American Psychological Association, Honolulu, HI, August.

Prins, P. M. J., & Ollendick, T. H. (2003). Cognitive change and enhanced coping: Missing mediational links in cognitive behavior therapy with anxiety-disordered children. *Clinical Child and Family Psychology Review, 6*, 87–105.

Renaud, J., Birmaher, B., Wassick, S. C., & Bridge, J. (1999). Use of selective serotonin reuptake inhibitors for the treatment of childhood panic disorder: A pilot study. *Journal of Child and Adolescent Psychopharmacology, 9*, 73–83.

Research Units of Pediatric Psychopharmacology (RUPP) Anxiety Group (in press). Flovoxamine for anxiety in children. *New England Journal of Medicine.*

Silove, D., Manicavasagar, V., Curtis, J., & Blaszczynski, A. (1996). Is early separation anxiety a risk factor for adult panic disorder?: A critical review. *Comprehensive Psychiatry, 37*, 167–179.

Simeon, J., Ferguson, B., Knott, V., Roberts, N., Gauthier, B., Dubois, C., & Wiggins, D. (1992). Clinical, cognitive and neurophysiological effects of alprazolam in children with overanxious and avoidant disorders. *Journal of the American Academy of Child and Adolescent Psychiatry, 31*, 29–33.

Spiegel, D. A., & Barlow, D. H. (2000). *Eight-day treatment of panic disorder with moderate to severe agoraphobia: Preliminary outcome data.* Poster presented at the 34th Meeting of the Association for Advancement of Behavior Therapy, New Orleans, LA.

Strauss, J., Birmaher, B., Bridge, J., Axelson, D., Chiappetta, L., Brent, D., & Ryan, N. (2000). Anxiety disorders in suicidal youth. *Canadian Journal of Psychiatry—Revue Canadienne de Psychiatrie, 45*(8),739–745.

Thyer, B. A., Parrish, R. T., Curtis, G. C., Nesse, R. M., & Cameron, O. G. (1985). Ages of onset of DSM-III anxiety disorders. *Comprehensive Psychiatry, 26*, 113–122.

Toth, S. L., & Cicchetti, D. (1999). Developmental psychopathology and child psychotherapy. In S. W. Russ & T. H. Ollendick (Eds.), *Handbook of Psychotherapies with Children and Families*. New York: Kluwer Academic/Plenum Publishers.

Weissman, M. M., Bland, R. C., Canino, G. J., Faravelli, C., Greenwald, S., Hwu, H., et al. (1997). The Cross-National Epidemiology of Panic Disorder Study. *Archives of General Psychiatry, 54*, 305–309.

World Health Organization (1992). *International Statistical Classification of Diseases and Related Health Problems (ICD-10).*

7

Evidence-Based Treatment of Pediatric Obsessive-Compulsive Disorder

ERIC A. STORCH, MICHAEL LARSON, JENNIFER ADKINS, GARY R. GEFFKEN, TANYA K. MURPHY, and WAYNE K. GOODMAN

Previously thought to be rare, recent research has identified pediatric obsessive-compulsive disorder (OCD) as one of the most common childhood psychiatric illnesses, with a point-prevalence rate between 1 and 4% (Douglass et al., 1995; Rapoport et al., 2000). Symptoms frequently begin in childhood (DeVaugh-Geiss et al., 1992), with insidious onset, and pursue a protracted yet fluctuating course (Murphy et al., 2004). Not surprisingly, pediatric OCD is related to significant functional impairment within academic, family, and social domains largely due to distress and frequency of ritual engagement (Piacentini et al., 2003).

Advances in psychological and pharmacological interventions strongly suggest that early detection and treatment can improve prognosis [Leonard et al., 1993; Pediatric OCD Treatment Study Team (POTS), 2004]. Unfortunately, dissemination of efficacious psychological treatment has significantly lagged behind that of medications, making successful treatment difficult to obtain (Larson et al., 2005; Lewin et al., 2005). For example, the Obsessive-Compulsive Foundation estimates that approximately 5 million Americans with OCD lack access to evidence-based psychological treatment (Obsessive-Compulsive Foundation, 2004). With this issue in

ERIC A. STORCH, JENNIFER ADKINS, GARY R. GEFFKEN, TANYA K. MURPHY, WAYNE K. GOODMAN, • Department of Psychiatry, University of Florida, ERIC A. STORCH, GARY R. GEFFKEN • Department of Pediatrics, University of Florida and MICHAEL LARSON, GARY R. GEFFKEN • Department of Clinical and Health Psychology, University of Florida

mind, this chapter reviews empirically supported treatments for pediatric OCD highlighting theory, application, and extant outcome data.

ETIOLOGY

Although the cause of OCD remains unknown, there are multiple biobehavioral etiological theories. In all likelihood, the cause of OCD is multidetermined and includes cognitive-behavioral and biological factors (Storch, 2005). For example, cognitive-behavioral theory indicates that a neutral stimulus (or event) becomes conditioned to elicit distress due to its association with another feared situation. Subsequent to the acquisition of the conditioned fear, compulsive behaviors develop to reduce or avoid distress because they temporarily ameliorate the distress associated with obsessions through operant mechanisms (negative reinforcement). Cognitively, individuals with OCD frequently misattribute the meaning of intrusive thoughts. For example, intrusive thoughts might be interpreted such that an individual perceives responsibility for causing or failing to prevent harm, leading to obsessional patterns to reduce associated distress. Attempts to neutralize intrusive thoughts (obsessions) via rituals or avoidance prevent the disconfirmation of the patient's fears and maintain the reinforcement cycle.

A more biological model hypothesizes that abnormal serotonin metabolism is implicated in the expression of obsessive and compulsive symptoms. This hypothesis is supported by data from successful treatment-outcome studies with serotonin-enhancing agents [i.e., serotonin reuptake inhibitors (SRIs); Geller et al., 2003]. Evidence from genetic, neuroimaging, and neuroendocrine studies also provide support for the neurochemical etiological model of pediatric OCD (see Lewin et al., 2005, for a review). For example, positron emission tomography studies suggest that abnormal metabolism in the globus pallidus, orbitofrontal cortex, neostriatum, and thalamus may be linked to OCD symptoms (McGuire et al., 1994), whereas imaging studies have identified hyperactivity in the anterior cingulate cortex (Ursu et al., 2003). Together, these data suggest that a functional disturbance in the frontal-limbic-basal ganglia system may mediate OCD symptoms in children.

EVIDENCE-BASED PEDIATRIC OCD THERAPIES

Cognitive-behavioral therapy (CBT) with exposure and response prevention (E/RP) and pharmacotherapy, particularly selective serotonin reuptake inhibitors (SSRIs), are empirically supported treatment modalities for OCD in the pediatric population (Abramowitz, 1997). Yet implementation of such treatments in the clinical setting has lagged behind the supporting empirical literature. The recent emphasis on utilization of empirically supported treatments in mental health professions (Task Force on Promotion and Dissemination of Psychological Procedures, 1995) and

high levels of treatment success emphasize the importance of understanding the effectiveness/efficacy, advantages, challenges, and proper
utilization of these treatment modalities.

Cognitive-Behavioral Therapy

The efficacy of CBT in children has been demonstrated in several controlled
trials (Barrett et al., 2004; de Hann et al., 1998; Foa et al., 2005; Pediatric
OCD Treatment Study Team, 2004; Storch et al., 2007) and numerous
open trials (Benazon et al., 2002; Fischer et al., 1998; Franklin et al., 1998;
March et al., 1994; Piacentini et al., 1994, 2002; Thienemann et al., 2001;
Waters et al., 2001; Wever & Rey, 1997). The general findings of these
studies are presented below. An in-depth summary, including tables with
most study findings, can be found in Barrett et al. (2004).

In the first controlled trial of CBT for pediatric OCD, de Haan
and colleagues (1998) compared E/RP and clomipramine treatments
over 12 weeks. As measured by the Children's Yale-Brown Obsessive-
Compulsive Scale (CY-BOCS; Scahill et al., 1997), a nearly 60% reduction
in OCD symptoms was demonstrated in children treated with E/RP, while
patients treated with clomipramine demonstrated a 33% reduction in
OCD symptoms. Children treated with E/RP exhibited a faster rate of
improvement relative to those treated with clomipramine.

The recent Pediatric OCD Treatment Study (POTS, 2004) randomized
controlled trial found that CBT alone, sertraline alone, or a combination
of the treatments was more effective than placebo. On the CY-BOCS,
combined treatment was superior to CBT, sertraline, and placebo. CBT
alone did not differ from sertraline; both treatments were superior
to placebo. Approximately 54% of patients in the combined treatment
condition experienced symptom remission as defined by the DSM-IV-TR,
compared to 39% for CBT alone and 21% for sertraline alone, leading to
the conclusion that children and adolescents diagnosed with OCD should
be treated with a combination of CBT plus SSRI or with CBT alone.

Most recently, Barrett et al. (2004) randomized 77 youth to individual
family CBT (CBFT), group CBFT, or a 4–6-week waitlist. A 65% and 61%
reduction in CY-BOCS scores at posttreatment for individual and group
CBFT were found. At six-month follow-up, 65% of individual CBFT and
87% of group CBFT participants were OCD diagnosis-free. Improvements
were maintained at 18-month follow-up, with 70% of individual CBFT and
84% of group CBFT participants remaining OCD diagnosis-free (Barrett
et al., 2005).

Finally, the first author of this chapter is completing a randomized
controlled trial of weekly or intensive (daily psychotherapy sessions) family-
based CBT ($n = 40$; Storch et al., 2007). Assessments were conducted
at three time points: pretreatment, posttreatment, and three-month
follow-up. Intensive CBT was as effective as weekly treatment with some
advantages present immediately after treatment. No group differences were
found at follow-up, with gains being largely maintained over time. At
posttreatment, 75% (15/20) of the children in the intensive group and 50%

(10/20) in the weekly group met remission status criteria. Ninety percent (18/20) of the children in the intensive group and 65% (13/20) in the weekly group were considered treatment responders.

Importantly, these trials suggest that CBT alone or with concurrent pharmacotherapy is the front-line treatment for OCD. These results stand in contrast with play-based, supportive, insight-oriented, psychoanalytic, and psychodynamic therapies, which lack evidence showing effectiveness in the treatment of pediatric OCD (Lewin et al., 2005).

Group Treatment

In addition to individual approaches, CBT for pediatric OCD has also been demonstrated effective in the group setting. A controlled trial of CBT that utilized an active family component and group setting found consistent short- and long-term reductions in OCD symptoms in both individual and group CBFT treatment groups compared to waitlist controls (Barrett et al., 2004, 2005). Specific findings of this research are reviewed above. Other open trials that employed group CBT with adolescents demonstrated significant improvements in OCD symptomatology (Fischer et al., 1998; Thienemann et al., 2001). Overall, improvements in adolescents enrolled in the group setting have been slightly less robust than for those who participated in individual CBT, suggesting that, when possible, individual treatment is the preferred modality.

Intensive CBT

Despite the high rates of treatment success, not all patients respond to traditional therapeutic approaches. An alternative for such cases of intractable OCD or for those who do not have access to local CBT providers is to refer the youth to an intensive CBT program (Franklin et al., 1998; Lewin et al., 2005; Storch & Geffken, 2004). There are several such intensive treatment programs geared toward youth, including the University of Florida's OCD Program, Rogers Memorial Hospital, University of Pennsylvania Center for the Treatment and Study of Anxiety, and Saint Louis Behavioral Medicine Institute (Obsessive-Compulsive Foundation, 2005). Intensive CBT generally involves 90-minute therapy sessions held daily for approximately two to four weeks. Treatment incorporates identical principles to standard weekly CBT; however, children undergo a concentrated course of therapy characterized by an aggressive targeting of symptoms. Preliminary results of studies in difficult-to-treat pediatric OCD patients support its use and should stimulate future research and trials among refractory cases (Franklin et al., 1998; Storch et al., 2004, 2007).

Other Psychosocial Therapies

Whereas CBT has a strong evidence base, play-based, supportive, and psychoanalytic therapies have not been demonstrated as effective for OCD treatment. At best, any supporting evidence for each modality derives from case reports or anecdotal clinical accounts (e.g., Gold-Steinberg & Logan, 1999). Unfortunately, many children remain untreated or treated via nonevidence-based therapies, highlighting the need for parity in training among mental health professionals (Storch, 2005). Also problematic is that many clinicians who state that they practice CBT for OCD are, in fact, not employing exposure-based strategies in their treatment plan (Gallant et al., 2005). For example, a recent survey of 227 school psychologists found that 82.4% stated that they use CBT as their primary psychological approach to treating pediatric OCD. Yet only 7.1% reported that they incorporated exposure-based components within their treatment plan (Gallant et al., 2005). This juxtaposition between what is being implemented in clinical practice and what is shown as effective in research highlights the need for greater dissemination of knowledge about empirically supported methods for the treatment of OCD and increased education of practitioners about the benefits of CBT in an effort to bridge the gap between research and practice (POTS, 2004; Storch & Merlo, 2006).

Pharmacotherapy

As stated previously, pharmacological treatments are effective and commonly used in the treatment of pediatric OCD (Geller et al., 2003). Randomized, placebo-controlled trials of serotonin-enhancing medications, including clomipramine (DeVeaugh-Geiss et al., 1992; Flament et al., 1985), sertraline (Cook et al., 2001; March et al., 1998), fluoxetine (Geller et al., 2001; Liebowitz et al., 2002; Riddle et al., 1992), and fluvoxamine (Riddle et al., 2001), demonstrate clinically significant reductions in OCD symptoms among pediatric patients. For example, Liebowitz et al. (2002) found a 16-week course of fluoxetine treatment to be superior to placebo, with fluoxetine-treated children exhibiting significantly lower CY-BOCS scores and a higher percentage of patients rated as "much" or "very much" improved on the CGI-I. Similarly, Geller et al. (2001) showed that 13 weeks of fluoxetine treatment was associated with significantly greater improvement in OCD symptoms as measured by the CY-BOCS compared to placebo control. March et al. (1998) demonstrated that patients treated with sertraline show significantly greater improvements than placebo-controlled patients on the CY-BOCS and the NIMH-GOCS. Forty-two percent of sertraline-treated patients and 26% of placebo-treated patients showed "much" or "much much" improvement on the CGI-I after treatment. Cook et al. (2001) found that 72% of children and 61% of adolescents demonstrated at least a 25% reduction in OCD symptoms as measured by the CY-BOCS. This large body of evidence for the effectiveness of pharmacotherapy in the treatment of pediatric OCD has led to Food and Drug Administration (FDA) approval for the use of fluoxetine, sertraline, and fluvoxamine in clinical treatment (Center for Drug Evaluation and Research, 2005).

Pharmacological treatment of OCD emerged from the hypothesis that disruption in the serotonin neurotransmitter system contributes to OCD symptoms (Ellingrod, 1998; Thoren et al., 1980; Zak et al., 1988). The afore-mentioned controlled trials focused on SSRIs as the front-line treatment in adjusting serotonin levels; however, a meta-analysis of pharmacotherapy trials in children identified clomipramine [a tricyclic antidepressant (TCA)] to be significantly superior over SSRIs in reducing OCD symptoms (Geller et al., 2003). However, due to the risk profile, adverse effects, and required EKG and blood-level monitoring associated with TCAs (e.g., antiadren-ergic, anticholinergic, and antihistaminergic adverse effects), SSRIs (with a relatively minimal side-effect profile) remain the consensus first-line medication for pediatric OCD (Cook et al., 2001; Geller et al., 2001, 2003; Riddle et al., 2001).

SSRIs tend to work relatively slowly. It is therefore important not to discontinue medication if immediate improvement in OCD symptoms is not demonstrated. Current recommendations indicate that patients continue to take SSRIs for at least 12 weeks, giving slow responders a chance for improvement (Thomsen, 1998); however, some studies did not demonstrate significant reduction compared to placebo until 16 weeks of treatment (Liebowitz et al., 2002). In addition, poor clinical response to one SSRI is not necessarily predictive of failure with other SSRIs, suggesting adequate trials of multiple SSRIs may be necessary before changing medications (Practice Parameters, 1998). It is important to reiterate, however, that medication alone is not as effective as medication combined with CBT or CBT alone (Thomsen, 1998).

In some cases, children are unresponsive to both CBT and trials with multiple SSRIs. In these situations, second-line pharmacological treat-ments often involve augmentation with medications such as clomipramine (Dougherty et al., 2002; Grados & Riddle, 2001), with preliminary results suggesting significant improvement in OCD symptomatology (Figueroa et al., 1998; Simeon et al., 1990). This combination of medications requires vigilant monitoring of blood work, EKGs, and potential side effects.

An important consideration regarding pharmacological treatment of pediatric OCD is the recent literature indicating potentially increased suicidal ideation in children and adolescents treated with SSRIs. As noted above, fluoxetine, sertraline, and fluvoxamine are Food and Drug Admin-istration (FDA)–approved for the treatment of pediatric OCD (Center for Drug Evaluation and Research, 2005). While research into the safety of SSRI use in depressed children is burgeoning out of necessity, no trials to date have examined the risk of suicidality and SSRI intake in pediatric OCD. Given the link between SSRI use and increased suicidality, clinicians should adhere to current findings and warnings associated with SSRI use in depressed children (Center for Drug Evaluation and Research, 2005; Committee on Safety of Medicines, 2004).

COGNITIVE-BEHAVIORAL TREATMENT FOR PEDIATRIC
OCD: PRACTICAL APPLICATION

Cognitive-behavioral therapists combine techniques based on the cognitive and behavioral conceptualizations of OCD. To address the classical and operant conditioning mechanisms that theoretically establish and maintain OCD behaviors, CBT therapists engage their patients in E/RP exercises. To address cognitive distortions that are common in OCD, E/RP is combined with cognitive restructuring techniques.

To successfully implement E/RP exercises, it is essential to choose an exposure exercise that is anxiety-provoking, yet not so much so that the patient is unable to refrain from compulsive behavior. Thus, a ritual hierarchy, or list of anxiety-provoking situations that motivate rituals that is rank-ordered from least to most distressing, is developed early in the therapy process. Exposure exercises typically begin with tasks that are minimally or moderately anxiety-provoking (i.e., lower on the hierarchy). For example, a child who exhibits obsessions regarding contamination and responds with excessive hand washing would be exposed to situations that provoke the contamination obsession (e.g., placing bare hands on a dirty floor). Thereafter, the patient would stay in that situation without washing his or her hands until the anxious arousal decreases significantly [based on subjective ratings of distress (SUDS) and behavioral observations]. By completing this exercise without washing hands, the patient is accomplishing two behavioral goals. First, from an operant conditioning perspective, by refraining from washing hands during the exposure, the compulsive behavior was not negatively reinforced, thus weakening the association between hand washing and distress reduction. Second, from a classical conditioning perspective, the exposure sets up a situation where the conditioned stimulus (obsessions about exposure to potential contaminants) is presented in absence of the unconditioned stimulus (e.g., getting violently ill). Thus, with subsequent exposures, the conditioned response (anxious arousal) will be weaker. With a decrease in the anxious arousal, it becomes easier to refrain from compulsive behavior.

Although data regarding the role of cognitions in symptom presentation for children with OCD are inconclusive, cognitive restructuring techniques are often utilized in the treatment of pediatric OCD (Storch, 2005; March et al., 2001; Piacentini & Langley, 2004; Larson et al., 2005). Children are taught to recognize cognitive distortions (e.g., I will get sick if I don't go to the bathroom before meals) as "just my OCD," to identify types of cognitive distortions, and to use specific strategies to address particular types of distortions (Lewin et al., 2005; March & Mulle, 1998). For example, if a child is exaggerating the likelihood or magnitude of a particular feared event, then the child may be coached to use reminders about the realistic likelihood and severity of that negative outcome (e.g., "It probably will not happen and it wouldn't be that bad if it did"). Another treatment strategy to help children better conceptualize and implement the cognitive aspects of treatment is "bossing back" the OCD (March & Mulle, 1998). When "bossing" their OCD, children verbalize the irrational or unlikely nature of their obsessions and provide an opposite to the thought by "telling the OCD" that they are going to do something different and that it cannot hurt them. In addition, giving the OCD an undesirable nickname, visualizing it as something the child has control over, and portraying treatment as a "fight" against the nasty OCD can help children better conceptualize treatment and become more engaged (i.e., making treatment more fun).

Developmental Adaptations

As with any pediatric psychosocial intervention, a variety of developmental issues must be considered. From the onset of therapy, accurate assessment is a challenge with children, as they may have difficulty recognizing/reporting obsessions and the relationship between obsessions and compulsive behavior. To address this issue, CBT therapists may use treatment exercises as an opportunity to gain further information and to teach the child about obsessions. Specifically, a therapist may get a child started with an exposure exercise and then ask the child during a state of clear distress, "What are you thinking?" The therapist can use this information to gain a better understanding of the nature of the child's presentation and coach the child in use of cognitive restructuring techniques. In children who do not acknowledge the presence of specific cognitive components, therapists can defer to a sense of discomfort as the trigger for ritual engagement. Additionally, psychoeducation and metaphors used in therapy must be adjusted to meet the cognitive development of the child, while adequately conveying the conceptual basis of the therapy. Finally, younger children tend to focus on the present. Thus, the temporary distress associated with E/RP may have a stronger effect on their motivation to engage in therapy than the abstract future positive gains. This is particularly difficult in children who do not find their obsessions or ritual engagement distressing. To address this, many CBT therapists use contingency management techniques involving positive consequences for completion of therapy exercises and negative consequences for refusal to attempt therapy exercises.

Caregiver Involvement

The importance of family involvement in treatment of pediatric OCD is generally accepted in the research and clinical fields (Barrett et al., 2004; Piacentini & Langley, 2004). Of particular importance is assessing accommodating behaviors that are assisting in the maintenance of the child's OCD. Systematically identifying and reducing family accommodation can make it difficult for a child to engage in these behaviors and, thus, increases the likelihood that a child will make efforts to engage in alternate behaviors when faced with distressing obsessions. Family members, typically parents, are also trained to lead the child through exposure exercises. Thus, steps on the hierarchy can be targeted outside therapy sessions, thereby increasing the speed of treatment progress and enhancing generalization of skills. Additionally, family members and other caregivers can act as accountability agents and may be actively involved in contingency management of therapy compliance.

Therapy Intensity

Traditionally, CBT for pediatric OCD takes place in the context of a 1- to 1.5-hour in-office therapy session on a weekly basis; however, a variety of factors can change to increase the intensity of the therapy as needed for the child. For example, exposure sessions can be moved outside the therapy office into more relevant environments (e.g., public bathrooms, school, home, public places). The duration of the sessions may also be increased to accommodate for multiple in-session exposure exercises, or the frequency of the sessions may be increased to multiple times per week. Although the comparative efficacy of these methods of intervention has not been well established, some data suggest increased frequency of sessions may increase the effectiveness for children who do not respond to once-weekly sessions (Storch et al., 2007).

Prognostic Indicators

As concluded by the POTS (2004) trial, CBT should be considered for most children (and adults) with OCD, given its strong empirical support. However, variables that may impact response remain unclear and, again, the literature lags behind that of adults. Given this, we briefly review treatment response predictors in the adult and child literatures, at times making downward extensions to children.

OCD Severity

Among adults, some have found illness severity to be negatively related to outcome (de Haan et al., 1997; Keijsers et al., 1994), whereas others have not (Cottraux et al., 1993; Steketee & Shapiro, 1995). We typically recommend CBT for most cases, although more severe cases likely require additional care (e.g., pharmacological, intensive CBT).

Symptom Typology

Although CBT appears effective for a wide range of OCD symptoms (e.g., washing, checking, repeating, etc.), adults with compulsive hoarding symptoms often show poor response to CBT (Abramowitz et al., 2003; Black et al., 1998). Similarly, those with mental rituals or purely obsessions seem to have a worse prognosis (Mataix-Cols et al., 2002). Current theories suggest that the poor prognosis associated with hoarding and mental rituals is due to limited motivation to change, increased dropout rates in treatment, poor insight, less habituation to distress, magical ideas, and perfectionistic tendencies that are seen as beneficial and frequently reinforced by society (e.g., a child who is compulsively perfectionistic is praised by his or her teacher for neat work; see Steketee & Frost, 2003). In addition, mental rituals are more difficult to treat because they are not always recognized, are not overt (i.e., can be used to mitigate heightened anxiety without the knowledge of parents or clinicians), and are difficult to prevent. To date, no known research has investigated CBT for youth with purely compulsive hoarding or mental rituals, leaving questions about the efficacy of CBT and reasons for potential treatment resistance in youth with these presentations.

Psychiatric Comorbidity

Comorbid psychiatric conditions can have a significant impact on treatment. Generally, OCD-specific CBT should not be initiated when OCD is not the primary diagnosis (Treadwell & Tolin, in press). Although the presence of comorbidity might predict poor outcome for children undertaking CBT, there is currently little empirical literature as to moderators of treatment response for pediatric OCD. Among adults, severe depression has been linked to less favorable treatment gains, although patients still experience significant clinical improvement (Abramowitz et al., 2000). Attention deficit hyperactivity disorder (ADHD) should be managed via medication to maximize attention and participation. Disruptive behavior and oppositionality have also been linked to poor medication response (Geller et al., 2003); our clinical experience suggests that this relationship generalizes to the CBT model. Impaired intellectual or developmental functioning that interferes with the youth's ability to be a collaborative partner in the therapeutic process and/or the ability to voluntarily refrain from rituals often negatively impact treatment. In such cases, behavioral parent training and medication may be appropriate adjunctive treatments.

Family Factors

Family factors, such as accommodation, expressed emotion (e.g., critical, hostile, or emotionally charged patterns of interaction), and general chaos appear to predict poor response and relapse among adults (Chambless & Steketee, 1999; Leonard et al., 1993). Our clinical experiences have suggested similar relations among children.

Motivational Problems

Not surprisingly, low motivation among adult OCD patients has been associated with attenuated outcome (de Haan et al., 1997; Keijsers et al., 1994), most likely due to poor treatment adherence (Araujo et al., 1996). Although little empirical data exists for children, our clinical experiences suggest that such findings hold true across the age span. Assessment of motivation in-session includes primarily looking at the level of engagement in exposure/homework exercises as well as directly asking the child about his OCD experience, how she would benefit from changing her OCD behaviors, and how important it is for him to alter OCD behaviors. Providing immediate contingencies for treatment engagement is also helpful in maintaining increased motivation levels.

CASE EXAMPLE

Presenting Information

Amanda is an 8-year-old female with OCD who presented with a variety of compulsive behaviors including reassurance seeking (e.g., "Are you sure I got that question right on my homework?"), questioning (e.g., "What did you say?"), repetition (e.g., restating herself to her parents to ensure they understand exactly what she said), excessive revising (e.g., spending hours on a homework due to starting over repeatedly until she gets it perfect), excessive toileting (e.g., going to the bathroom frequently, especially before leaving the house, or having to sit down to meals), and ritualized dressing (e.g., wiping off feet before putting on socks, tying and retying shoes until they "feel right"). Although Amanda could not express her obsessions, it appeared that most of her thoughts centered on exactness, perfectionism, and personal comfort. Amanda did not report personal distress regarding her OCD symptoms and would become oppositional and aggressive when she was prevented from engaging in compulsive behaviors.

Amanda was an only child and reported positive relationships with her parents; however, it was evident that Amanda's compulsive behaviors placed significant strain on their relationship. Both parents reported difficulty contending with Amanda's aggressive behavior and had not placed limits on her compulsive behavior to avoid her angry outbursts, which included verbal and physical aggression. Further, Amanda's parents engaged in a variety of accommodating behaviors such as answering questions, delaying departure times from home, and helping Amanda complete her homework assignments.

Academically, Amanda was an A student. Due to compulsive exactness, she took longer than other students to complete tasks. Therefore, her teacher allowed her to shorten assignments or complete in-school assignments at home. Amanda was described by her teacher as a "joy" in school, she had many friends, and she was especially helpful with children who had special needs. Amanda's only behavioral problems in the classroom were repeated questioning of the teacher regarding classroom instructions and reporting other students' behavioral problems to the teacher.

Amanda and her parents were administered the Children's Yale-Brown Obsessive Compulsive Scale (CY-BOCS; Scahill et al., 1997; Goodman et al., 1989), a measure of OCD severity where a symptom rating score of 0–8 = not clinically significant, 8–15 = mild, 16–23 = moderate, 24–31 = severe, and 32–40 = extreme. Amanda's total score was a 32 (Compulsion and Obsession Scale scores of 16 each), falling in the extreme range.

Case Formulation

Although pediatric OCD is largely idiosyncratic, Amanda's behavioral presentation is fairly representative of children presenting for treatment of OCD. She exhibited obsessions about exactness and personal comfort. When placed in situations that elicited these obsessions, she became anxious and engaged in a variety of compulsive behaviors to reduce her anxiety. From an operant conditioning perspective, Amanda's ritual engagement was negatively reinforced via anxiety reduction, thus increasing the likelihood of engaging in rituals upon future exposures to anxiety-provoking stimuli. From a cognitive perspective, her constant engagement in rituals prevented Amanda from discovering that the feared outcomes (e.g., making a poor grade) would not occur if she refrained from ritual engagement.

Treatment

Amanda and her parents presented for 14 75-minute CBT sessions over a 16-week period generally following the treatment guidelines put forth by March & Mulle (1998; readers interested in learning more about the clinical implementation of E/RP principles are referred to this manual as a frequently used guide for the treatment of pediatric OCD). Each family member participated actively in treatment. Due to her parents' opposition to psychotropic medication, Amanda's sole treatment for her OCD and oppositional behavior was CBT with parent training.

Amanda's treatment began with psychoeducation for her and her parents. The behavioral aspects of OCD were emphasized, as these were more concrete and understandable to an 8-year-old. Developmentally appropriate metaphors were used to explain the process by which engagement in rituals may make you "feel better fast" with the cost of making you feel worse the next time. E/RP was explained as a treatment that can reverse this process. Amanda was told that her body needed to spend a little more time feeling uncomfortable so she could learn that nothing bad would happen. It was also explained that each time she did this it would get easier. Visual graphs of subjective distress over time were used to further explain this process to Amanda and her parents. Finally, the concept of labeling her subjective distress was explained to Amanda as a way for her to communicate her anxiety to her parents and therapist.

The psychoeducation and treatment explanation were used as a basis for building an exposure hierarchy. Due to a combination of shyness and oppositionality, Amanda had difficulty generating potential exposure exercises. To address this, Amanda's therapist and her parents generated a list of exposure exercises that would cause moderate to severe distress. Amanda was then asked to verbally rate her distress for each of these situations on a scale of 1 to 10. She had difficulty doing this, so she was given a slide algometer and asked to slide the ruler, revealing the red color underneath it, to show how anxiety-provoking each event would be. After some initial resistance, Amanda successfully used this tool to generate distress ratings.

Following generation of the exposure hierarchy, Amanda began E/RP exercises in session. During these exposures, three key points or rules were given: (1) You must put yourself in a situation that makes you uncomfortable; (2) you cannot do any tricks or rituals to make you feel better quick; and (3) you have to stay in that situation until you feel comfortable. Amanda's initial exposures included putting her shoes on without checking to make sure her feet were clean, drawing an imperfect picture, eating dinner without first going to the bathroom, and only rinsing twice after brushing her teeth. Following success with these exercises as discrete activities, the behavior became a standard to which Amanda would be held throughout the day and all parental accommodations regarding that behavior were removed. For example, after Amanda conducted repeated successful exposures to putting on her shoes without first checking her feet, she was expected to do so throughout the day and her father no longer helped her put on her shoes before school. Rituals were systematically targeted at a rate of one to two behaviors per week, and assignments were given to engage in extensions of exposures performed each week in session. Some examples of Amanda's homework include completing schoolwork in an allotted amount of time, walking around the house with her shoes untied or barefoot, and not brushing her teeth at night.

Given her modest difficulty identifying cognitive aspects of her OCD, the cognitive therapy components of CBT were initially left out; however, after a few weeks of in-session and at-home E/RP exercises, Amanda was again asked to identify her thoughts. The most effective way to generate cognitive distortions with Amanda was to ask her, "What are you thinking?" when she was engaged in an exposure exercise. After generating a list of cognitive distortions, Amanda was asked to come up with arguments. For the anxious thought "I'll feel bad if I don't use the bathroom before eating," Amanda responded, "If I have to go to the bathroom at dinner, I can go then." For the anxious thought "My feet might itch if I don't check before putting my shoes on," she replied, "They hardly ever itch," and "This is my OCD talking." To further illustrate the effect of thoughts on emotions, vignettes involving children Amanda's age were presented and she was asked to identify how the children's thoughts made them feel. Amanda was coached to use cognitive restructuring during E/RP exercises and throughout the day when she had a thought that made her worry. Her parents were asked to model or prompt cognitive restructuring during E/RP exercises.

Outcome

At the end of treatment, Amanda and her parents reported significant reductions in obsessive and compulsive behavior. Although she continued to exhibit a mild level of compulsive behavior, both Amanda and her parents reported that her symptoms no longer interfered with her daily functioning. Their report is consistent with Amanda's score on the CY-BOCS, which dropped from a pretreatment total score of 32 (severe) to a posttreatment total score of 8 (mild). Three months after Amanda completed treatment, she and her parents reported that Amanda was currently exhibiting "no OCD." Her total score on the CY-BOCS at this point was 4 (not clinically significant).

Amanda's case is typical of the course of E/RP in youth. Symptoms gradually decreased as previously conditioned associations were extinguished and she learned that she could function well without her ritual engagement. Her parent's involvement in decreasing accommodating behaviors, facilitating rewarding experiences for exposure exercises, and ensuring treatment was consistent and monitored played a large role in her treatment success. The additional reinforcement of being able to play with friends and engage in more social activities because she was not obsessing about homework or other difficulties provided added incentive for recovery.

CONCLUSION

Over the last decade, the empirical basis for the treatment of OCD in children and adults has expanded substantially, with considerable evidence for CBT and pharmacotherapy. At the same time, important gaps in professional knowledge remain, with clinical practice lagging behind research findings. One of the primary issues centers on dissemination of CBT, as many pediatric (and adult) patients with OCD continue to receive nonevidence-based psychological therapies. A second major issue concerns effective augmentation for nonresponders. It will be important for future efforts to comprehensively examine such factors to promote effective treatment for youth with OCD.

REFERENCES

Abramowitz, J. S. (1997). Effectiveness of psychological and pharmacological treatments for obsessive-compulsive disorder: A quantitative review. *Journal of Consulting and Clinical Psychology, 65,* 44–52.

Abramowitz, J. S., Franklin, M. E., Schwartz, S. A., & Furr, J. M. (2003). Symptom presentation and outcome of cognitive-behavioral therapy for obsessive-compulsive disorder. *Journal of Consulting and Clinical Psychology, 71,* 1049–1057.

Abramowitz, J. S., Franklin, M. E., Street, G. P., Kozak, M. J., & Foa, E. B. (2000). Effects of comorbid depression on response to treatment for obsessive-compulsive disorder. *Behavior Therapy, 31,* 517–528.

Araujo, L. A., Ito, L. M., & Marks, I. (1996). Early compliance and other factors predicting outcome of exposure for obsessive-compulsive disorder. *British Journal of Psychiatry, 169,* 747–752.

Barrett, P., Farrell, L., Dadds, M., & Boulter, N. (2005). Cognitive-behavioral family treatment of childhood obsessive-compulsive disorder: Long-term follow-up and predictors of outcome. *Journal of the American Academy of Child and Adolescent Psychiatry, 44,* 1005–1014.

Barrett, P., Healy-Farrell, L., & March, J. S. (2004). Cognitive-behavioral family treatment of childhood obsessive-compulsive disorder: A controlled trial. *Journal of the American Academy of Child and Adolescent Psychiatry, 43,* 46–62.

Benazon, N. R., Ager, J., & Rosenberg, D. R. (2002). Cognitive behavior therapy in treatment-naive children and adolescents with obsessive-compulsive disorder: An open trial. *Behavior Research and Therapy, 40,* 529–539.

Black, D. W., Monahan, P., Gable, J., Blum, N., Clancy, G., & Baker, P. (1998). Hoarding and treatment response in 38 nondepressed subjects with obsessive-compulsive disorder. *Journal of Clinical Psychiatry, 59,* 420–425.

Center for Drug Evaluation and Research (2005). *Worsening depression and suicidality in patients being treated with antidepressant medications.* Retrieved April 10, 2005, from www.fda.gov/cder/drug/antidepressants/AntidepressanstPHA.htm.

Chambless, D. L., & Steketee, G. (1999). Expressed emotion and behavior therapy outcome: A prospective study with obsessive compulsive and agoraphobic outpatients. *Journal of Consulting and Clinical Psychology, 67,* 658–665.

Committee on Safety of Medicines. (2004). Use of selective serotonin reuptake inhibitors (SSRIs) in children and adolescents with major depressive disorder (MDD)—Only fluoxetine (Prozac) shown to have a favourable balance of risks and benefits for the treatment of MDD in the under 18s. Retrieved April 20, 2005, from http://medicines.mhra.gov.uk/ourwork/monitorsafequalmed/safetymessages/ssris_spc_061204.pdf.

Cook, E. H., Wagner, K. D., March, J. S., Biederman, J., Landau, P., Wolkow, R., et al. (2001). Long-term sertraline treatment of children and adolescents with obsessive-compulsive disorder. *Journal of the American Academy of Child and Adolescent Psychiatry, 40,* 1175–1181.

Cottraux, J., Messy, P., Marks, I. M., Mollard, E., & Bouvard, M. (1993). Predictive factors in the treatment of obsessive-compulsive disorders with fluvoxamine and/or behavior therapy. *Behavioural Psychotherapy, 21,* 45–50.

de Hann, E., Hoogduin, K. A. L., Buitelaar, J. K., & Keijesers, G. P. J. (1998). Behavior therapy versus clomipramine for the treatment of obsessive-compulsive disorder in children and adolescents. *Journal of the American Academy of Child and Adolescent Psychiatry, 37,* 1022–1029.

de Haan, E., van Oppen, P., van Balkom, A. J., Spinhoven, P., Hoogduin, K. A., & Van Dyck, R. (1997). Prediction of outcome and early vs. late improvement in OCD patients treated with cognitive behaviour therapy and pharmacotherapy. *Acta Psychiatrica Scandinavica, 96,* 354–361.

DeVeaugh-Geiss, J., Moroz, G., Biederman, J. B., Cantwell, D., Fontaine, R., Greist, J. H., et al. (1992). Clomipramine hydrochloride in childhood and adolescent obsessive-compulsive disorder: A multicenter trial. *Journal of the American Academy of Child and Adolescent Psychiatry, 31,* 45–49.

Dougherty, D. D., Rauch, S. L., & Jenike, M. A. (2002). Pharmacological treatments for obsessive compulsive disorder. In *A Guide to Treatments That Work,* 2nd ed. (pp. 387–410). New York: Oxford University Press.

Douglass, H. M., Moffitt, T. E., Dar, R., McGee, R., & Silva, P. (1995). Obsessive-compulsive disorder in a birth cohort of 18-year-olds: Prevalence and predictors. *Journal of the American Academy of Child and Adolescent Psychiatry, 34,* 1424–1431.

Ellingrod, V. L. (1998). Pharmacotherapy of primary obsessive-compulsive disorder: Review of the literature. *Pharmacotherapy, 18,* 936–960.

Figueroa, Y., Rosenberg, D. R., Birmaher, B., & Keshavan, M. S. (1998). Combination treatment with clomipramine and selective serotonin reuptake inhibitors for obsessive-compulsive disorder in children and adolescents. *Journal of Child and Adolescent Psychopharmacology, 8,* 61–67.

Fischer, D., Himle, J. A., & Hanna, G. L. (1998). Group behavioral therapy for adolescents with obsessive-compulsive disorder: Preliminary outcomes. *Research in Social Work, 8,* 629–636.

Flament, M. F., Rapoport, J. L., Berg, C. J., Sceery, W., Kilts, C., Mellstrom, B., et al. (1985). Clomipramine treatment of childhood obsessive-compulsive disorder: A double-blind controlled study. *Archives of General Psychiatry, 46,* 1088–1092.

Foa, E. B., Liebowitz, M. R., Kozak, M. J., Davies, S., Campeas, R., Franklin, M. E., et al. (2005). Randomized, placebo-controlled trial of exposure and ritual prevention, clomipramine, and their combination in the treatment of obsessive-compulsive disorder. *American Journal of Psychiatry, 162,* 151–161.

Franklin, M. E., Kozak, M. J., Cashman, L. A., Coles, M. E., Rheingold, A. A., & Foa, E. (1998). Cognitive-behavioral treatment of pediatric obsessive-compulsive disorder: An open clinical trial. *Journal of the American Academy of Child and Adolescent Psychiatry*, *37*, 412–419.

Gallant, J., Storch, E. A., Valderhaug, R., & Geffken, G. R. (2005). *School Psychologists' Views and Management of Obsessive-Compulsive Disorder in Children and Adolescents*. Unpublished manuscript.

Geller, D. A., Biederman, J., Stewart, S. E., Mullin, B., Farrell, C., Wagner, K. D., et al. (2003a). Impact of comorbidity on treatment response to paroxetine in pediatric obsessive-compulsive disorder: Is the use of exclusion criteria empirically supported in randomized clinical trials? *Journal of Child and Adolescent Psychchopharmacology*, *13*S, S19–29.

Geller, D. A., Biederman, J., Stewart, S. E., Mullin, B., Martin, A., Spencer, T., et al. (2003b). Which SSRI? A meta-analysis of pharmacotherapy trials in pediatric obsessive-compulsive disorder. *American Journal of Psychiatry*, *160*, 1919–1928.

Geller, D. A., Hoog, S. L., Heiligenstein, J. H., Ricardi, R. K., Tamura, R., Kluszynski, S., et al. (2001). Fluoxetine treatment for obsessive-compulsive disorder in children and adolescents: A placebo-controlled clinical trial. *Journal of the American Academy of Child and Adolescent Psychiatry*, *40*, 773–779.

Gold-Steinberg, S., & Logan, D. (1999). Integrating play therapy in the treatment of children with obsessive-compulsive disorder. *American Journal of Orthopsychiatry*, *69*, 495–503.

Goodman, W.K., Price, L.H., Rasmussen, S.A., Mazure, C., Fleischman, R.L., Hill, C.L., et al. (1989). The Yale-Brown Obsessive Compulsive Scale: I. Development, use, and reliability. *Archives of General Psychiatry*, *46*, 1006–1011.

Grados, M. A., & Riddle, M. A. (2001). Pharmacological treatment of childhood obsessive-compulsive disorder: From theory to practice. *Journal of Clinical Child Psychology*, *30*, 67–79.

Keijsers, G. P., Hoogduin, C. A., & Schaap, C. P. (1994). Predictors of treatment outcome in the behavioural treatment of obsessive-compulsive disorder. *British Journal of Psychiatry*, *165*, 781–786.

Larson, M. J., Storch, E. A., Lewin, A. B., Geffken, G. R., Murphy, T. K., & Goodman, W. K. (2005). Update on the treatment of pediatric obsessive-compulsive disorder. *Current Psychiatry Reviews*, *1*, 281–291.

Leonard, H. L., Swedo, S. E., Lenane, M. C., Rettew, D. C., Hamburger, S. D., Bartko, J. J., et al. (1993). A 2- to 7-year follow-up study of 54 obsessive-compulsive children and adolescents. *Archives of General Psychiatry*, *50*, 429–439.

Lewin, A. B., Storch, E. A., Adkins, J. W., Murphy, T. K., & Geffken, G. R. (2005). Current directions in pediatric obsessive-compulsive disorder. *Pediatric Annals*, *34*, 128–134.

Lewin, A. B., Storch, E. A., Merlo, L. J., Adkins, J. W., Murphy, T. K., & Geffken, G. R. (in press). Intensive cognitive-behavioral therapy for pediatric obsessive-compulsive disorder: A treatment protocol for mental health providers. *Psychological Services*.

Liebowitz, M. R., Turner, S. M., Piacentini, J., Beidel, D. C., Clarvit, S. R., Davies, S. O., et al. (2002). Fluoxetine in children and adolescents with OCDL: A placebo-controlled trial. *Journal of the American Academy of Child and Adolescent Psychiatry*, *41*, 1431–1438.

March, J. S., Biederman, J., Wolkow, R., Safferman, A., Mardekian, J., Cook, E. H., et al. (1998). Sertraline in children and adolescents with obsessive-compulsive disorder: A multicenter randomized control trial. *Journal of the American Medical Association*, *280*, 1752–1756.

March, J. S., Franklin, M. E., Nelson, A., & Foa, E. (2001). Cognitive-behavioral psychotherapy for pediatric obsessive-compulsive disorder. *Journal of Clinical Child Psychology*, *30*, 8–18.

March, J. S., & Mulle, K. (1998). *OCD in Children and Adolescents: A Cognitive Behavioral Treatment Manual*. New York: Guilford Press.

March, J. S., Mulle, K., & Herbel, B. (1994). Behavioral psychotherapy for children and adolescents with obsessive-compulsive disorder: An open trial of a new protocol-driven treatment package. *Journal of the American Academy of Child and Adolescent Psychiatry*, *33*, 333–341.

Mataix-Cols, D., Marks, I. M., Greist, J. H., Kobak, K. A., & Baer, L. (2002). Obsessive-compulsive symptom dimensions as predictors of compliance with and response to behaviour therapy: Results from a controlled trial. *Psychotherapy and Psychosomatics*, *71*, 255–262.

McGuire, P. K., Bench, C. J., Frith, C. D., Marks, I. M., Frackowiak, R. S., & Dolan, R. J. (1994). Functional anatomy of obsessive-compulsive phenomena. *British Journal of Psychiatry, 164,* 459–468.

Murphy, T. K., Sajid, M., Soto, O., Shapira, N., Edge, P., Yang, M., et al. (2004). Detecting pediatric autoimmune neuropsychiatric disorders associated with streptococcus in children with obsessive-compulsive disorder and tics. *Biological Psychiatry, 55,* 61–68.

Obsessive-Compulsive Foundation. http://www.ocfoundation.org/ocf1130d.htm; accessed on December 18, 2004.

Obsessive-Compulsive Foundation. http://www.ocfoundation.org/1003/index.html; accessed on October 19, 2005.

Pediatric OCD Treatment Study Team (2004). Cognitive-behavior therapy, sertraline, and their combination for children and adolescents with obsessive-compulsive disorder. *Journal of the American Medical Association, 292,* 1969–1976.

Piacentini, J., Bergman, R. L., Jacobs, C., McCracken, J., & Kretchman, J. (2002). Open trial of cognitive-behavioral therapy for childhood obsessive-compulsive disorder. *Journal of Anxiety Disorders, 16,* 207–219.

Piacentini, J., Bergman, R. L., Keller, M., & McCracken, J. (2003). Functional impairment in children and adolescents with obsessive-compulsive disorder. *Journal of Child and Adolescent Psychopharmacology, 13S-1,* S61–S69.

Piacentini, J., Gitow, A., Jaffer, M., Graae, F., & Whitaker, A. (1994). Outpatient behavioral treatment of child and adolescent obsessive-compulsive disorder. *Journal of Anxiety Disorders, 8,* 277–289.

Piacentini, J., & Langley, A. K. (2004). Cognitive-behavioral therapy for children who have obsessive-compulsive disorder. *Journal of Clinical Psychology, 60,* 1181–1194.

Practice Parameters (1998). Practice parameters for the assessment and treatment of children and adolescents with obsessive-compulsive disorder. *Journal of the American Academy of Child and Adolescent Psychiatry, 37S,* 27S–45S.

Rapoport, J. L., Inoff-Germain, G., Weissman, M. M., Greenwald, S., & Narrow, W. E. (2000). Childhood obsessive-compulsive disorder in the NIMH MECA study: Parent versus child identification of cases. Methods for the Epidemiology of Child and Adolescent Mental Disorders. *Journal of Anxiety Disorders, 14,* 535–548.

Riddle, M. A., Reeve, E. A., Yaryura-Tobias, J. A., Yang, H. M., Claghorn, J. L., Gaffney, G., et al. (2001). Fluvoxamine for children and adolescents with obsessive-compulsive disorder: A randomized, controlled, multicenter trial. *Journal of the American Academy of Child and Adolescent Psychiatry, 40,* 222–229.

Riddle, M. A., Scahill, L., King, R., Harding, M., Anderson, G., Ort, S. I., et al. (1992). Double-blind, crossover trial of fluoxetine and placebo in children and adolescents with obsessive-compulsive disorder. *Journal of the American Academy of Child and Adolescent Psychiatry, 31,* 1062–1069.

Scahill, L., Riddle, M. A., McSwiggin-Hardin, M., Ort, S. I., King, R. A., Goodman, W. K., et al. (1997). Children's Yale-Brown Obsessive Compulsive Scale: Reliability and validity. *Journal of the American Academy of Child and Adolescent Psychiatry, 36,* 844–852.

Simeon, J. G., Thatte, S., & Wiggins, D. (1990). Treatment of adolescent obsessive-compulsive disorder with clomipramine-fluoxetine combination. *Psychopharmacological Bulletin, 26,* 285–290.

Steketee, G., & Frost, R. (2003). Compulsive hoarding: Current status of the research. *Clinical Psychology Review, 23,* 905–927.

Steketee, G., & Shapiro, L. J. (1995). Predicting behavioral treatment outcome for agoraphobia and obsessive-compulsive disorder. *Clinical Psychology Review, 15,* 315–346.

Storch, E. A. (2005a). But is it OCD? A guide to detection and effective treatment. *Contemporary Pediatrics, 22*(11), 58–70.

Storch, E. A. (2005b). Update on childhood anxiety. *Pediatric Annals, 34,* 78–81.

Storch, E. A., & Geffken, G. R. (2004). *Intensive Cognitive Behavior Therapy for Pediatric Obsessive-Compulsive Disorder.* Paper presented at the Anxiety Disorders Association of America, Miami, FL.

Storch, E. A., Geffken, G. R., Merlo, L. J., Mann, G., Duke, D., Munson, M., Adkins, J., Grabill, K., Murphy, T. K., & Goodmann, W. K., (2007). Cognitive-Behavioral Therapy for Pediatric Obsessive-Compulsive Disorder: Comparison of Intensive and Weekly

Approaches. *Journal of the American Academy of Child and Adolescent Psychiatry, 46,* 469–478.

Storch, E. A., Gerdes, A., Atkins, J., Geffken, G. R., Star, J., & Murphy, T. (2004). Behavioral treatment of child with pediatric autoimmune neuropsychiatric disorder associated with group A streptococcal infection. *Journal of the American Academy of Child and Adolescent Psychiatry, 43,* 510–511.

Storch, E. A., & Merlo, L. J. (2006). Evaluation and treatment of the patient with obsessive-compulsive disorder. *Journal of Family Practice, 55,* 329–333.

Task Force on Promotion and Dissemination of Psychological Procedures (1995). Training in and dissemination of empirically-valid psychological treatments: Report and recommendations. *Clinical Psychologist, 48,* 3–23.

Thienemann, M., Martin, J., Cregger, B., Thompson, H. B., & Dyer-Friedman, J. (2001). Manual-driven group cognitive-behavioral therapy of adolescents with obsessive-compulsive disorder: A pilot study. *Journal of the American Academy of Child and Adolescent Psychiatry, 40,* 1254–1260.

Thomsen, P. H. (1998). Obsessive-compulsive disorder in children and adolescents. Clinical guidelines. *European Journal of Child & Adolescent Psychiatry, 7,* 1–11.

Thoren, P., Asberg, M., & Cronholm, B. (1980). Clomipramine treatment of obsessive compulsive disorder: A controlled clinical trial. *Archives of General Psychiatry, 37,* 1281–1285.

Treadwell, K., & Tolin, D. (2007). Clinical challenges in the treatment of pediatric OCD. In E. A. Storch, G. Geffken, & T. Murphy (Eds.), *Handbook of Child and Adolescent Obsessive-Compulsive Disorder.* Mahwah, NJ: Lawrence Erlbaum, 273–294.

Ursu, S., Stenger, V. A., Shear, M. K., Jones, M. R., & Carter, C. S. (2003). Overactive action monitoring in obsessive-compulsive disorder: Evidence from functional magnetic resonance imaging. *Psychological Science, 14,* 347–353.

Waters, T., Barrett, P., & March, J. S. (2001). Cognitive-behavioral family treatment of childhood obsessive-compulsive disorder: An open clinical trial. *American Journal of Psychotherapy, 55,* 105–113.

Wever, C., & Rey, J. (1997). Juvenile obsessive-compulsive disorder. *Australia New Zealand Journal of Psychiatry, 31,* 105–113.

Zak, J. P., Miller, J. A., Jr., Sheehan, D. V., & Fanous, B. S. (1988). The potential role of serotonin reuptake inhibitors in the treatment of obsessive compulsive disorder. *Journal of Clinical Psychiatry, 49S,* 23–29.

8

Interventions for Posttraumatic Stress in Children and Adolescents Following Natural Disasters and Acts of Terrorism

ANNETTE M. LA GRECA

In recent years, devastating natural disasters (e.g., hurricanes, earthquakes, floods, tsunamis) and acts of violence (e.g., school shootings, terrorist attacks) have focused tremendous attention on how such events affect children and adolescents. Ample evidence suggests that exposure to such events may cause children and adolescents significant distress and psychological impairment (Gurwitch et al., 2002; La Greca et al., 2002; Silverman & La Greca, 2002).

In terms of natural disasters, Hurricane Katrina, one of the worst natural disasters in U.S. history, struck Louisiana and the U.S. Gulf Coast in August 2005 and inflicted catastrophic devastation and mass casualties in New Orleans and along the Gulf Coast. In fact, as of this writing, more than a year later, many of the affected areas are enduring a very slow and painful recovery. Hurricane Rita struck Louisiana only a month after Katrina and also brought flooding and destruction to coastal areas. Moreover, between 2004 and 2005, seven hurricanes struck the state of Florida, causing widespread destruction and numerous casualties.

In addition to these and other natural disasters in the United States, catastrophic natural disasters affect many parts of the world. Major earthquakes in Turkey (1999) and Pakistan (2005) brought about tremendous destruction and mass casualties. Similarly, in December 2004, the Indian

ANNETTE M. LA GRECA • University of Miami

Ocean earthquake and tsunami devastated parts of Asia, killing about 200,000 people.

Acts of terrorism have also resulted in substantial trauma and loss of life both in the United States and abroad. For example, the terrorist attacks of September 11, 2001, on the World Trade Center and Pentagon, produced substantial loss of life and led to heightened concerns within the United States and abroad about the occurrence of future attacks and how to deal with mental health issues among survivors and those directly affected.

In the aftermath of destructive disasters and shocking acts of terrorism, empirical reports have revealed severe and persistent stress reactions among children and adolescents[1] exposed to such events (Gurwitch et al., 2002; La Greca & Prinstein, 2002; Silverman & La Greca, 2002). For example, in the wake of the terrorist attacks on the World Trade Center, it was estimated that 75,000 youth in the New York City schools were experiencing posttraumatic stress disorder (PTSD) (Hoven et al., 2005), thereby representing a tremendous public mental health concern.

In the context of these recent and recurring events, it is critical to understand how disasters and terrorist attacks affect children and how they cope with and recover from such events. Developing interventions for children's reactions to natural disasters and acts of terrorism and preventing serious, persistent adjustment problems in their aftermath have become challenging and important mental health concerns (Vernberg, 2002). The goal of this chapter is to review evidence-based approaches to treating children following these kinds of traumatic events.

To set the stage for this review, the first chapter section describes the symptoms and prevalence of PTSD in children following disasters and acts of terrorism as well as other trauma-related reactions. The second section briefly describes risk factors for posttraumatic stress reactions. The third section reviews the current state of intervention research. The chapter ends with a summary of best practices for delivering interventions in the aftermath of disasters/terrorism.

POSTTRAUMATIC STRESS REACTIONS FOLLOWING DISASTERS AND ACTS OF TERRORISM

Natural disasters and acts of terrorism represent traumatic events for children and adolescents that can result in acute stress, posttraumatic stress (PTS) symptoms, and posttraumatic stress disorder (PTSD) (Gurwitch et al., 2002; Silverman & La Greca, 2002; Yule et al., 2002). Immediately after a disaster or terrorist attack, there may be a brief period of "shock" or numbing, or even elation and relief at being alive (Vogel & Vernberg, 1993). Beyond these initial reactions, however, children

---

[1] To simplify the text, the term "children" or "youth" will be used throughout the chapter to refer to children *and* adolescents, unless otherwise specified.

commonly report symptoms of acute stress as well as PTS within the first few weeks or months after the events (Silverman & La Greca, 2002). Moreover, these stress reactions can be severe and persistent (e.g., La Greca & Prinstein, 2002; Yule et al., 2002).

Posttraumatic Stress

PTSD refers to a set of symptoms that develop following exposure to an unusually severe stressor or event that causes or is capable of causing death, injury, or threat to the physical integrity of oneself or another person (American Psychiatric Association, 1994). For a diagnosis of PTSD, a child's reaction to the traumatic event must include intense fear, helplessness, or disorganized behavior, and specific criteria must be met for three symptom clusters: reexperiencing, avoidance/numbing, and hyperarousal (American Psychiatric Association, 1994). These symptoms must be manifest for at least one month (acute PTSD) and be accompanied by significant impairment in the functioning (problems in school, social, or family relations); the diagnosis is chronic PTSD if symptoms persist for more than three months.

Reexperiencing symptoms include recurrent or intrusive thoughts or dreams about the event and intense distress at cues or reminders of the event. Young children may display repetitive play with traumatic themes or a reenactment of traumatic events in play, drawings, or verbalizations. Following acts of violence, children have described a specific vivid image or sound that disturbed them or reported traumatic dreams with a strong feeling of life threat (Nader & Mello, 2002). Reexperiencing symptoms are extremely common in youth following traumatic events, such as natural disasters and terrorist attacks. For example, 3 months after Hurricane Andrew, a Category 5 hurricane with sustained winds above 150 miles per hour, almost 90% of children with high levels of exposure to the hurricane reported reexperiencing symptoms (Vernberg et al., 1996), and 78% reported such symptoms 10 months after the disaster (La Greca et al., 1996).

Avoidance or numbing symptoms include avoiding thoughts, feelings, or conversations about the event; avoiding reminders of the event; having diminished interest in normal activities; and feeling detached or removed from other people. Children may report lessened interest in play or usual activities and also feeling distant from parents and friends. Avoidance and numbing are the least commonly reported symptoms of PTSD (e.g., Vernberg et al., 1996) and thus may represent good markers for the presence of a PTSD diagnosis (Lonigan et al., 1998).

Hyperarousal symptoms include difficulty sleeping or concentrating, irritability, angry outbursts, hypervigilance, and an exaggerated startle response. The symptoms must be newly occurring since the trauma event. Startle reactions are very common after exposure to unexpected, violent events, like shootings (Nader & Mello, 2002) or bombings (Gurwitch et al., 2002).

The *prevalence of PTSD* in children and adolescents following disasters and acts of terrorism is difficult to estimate because studies have been extremely diverse with respect to the type of trauma evaluated, the sampling procedures and assessment methods used, and the length of time since the traumatic event. However, rates of PTS symptoms and PTSD diagnoses are often high.

In community studies, approximately 24% to 39% of children and adolescents exposed to destructive natural disasters have been found to meet criteria for a PTSD diagnosis in the first few weeks or months following the event (American Academy of Child and Adolescent Psychiatry, 1998). Subclinical levels of PTS are substantially higher, with more than 50% of the children in large community samples reporting at least moderate levels of PTS during the first two to four months following an event (e.g., Vernberg et al., 1996).

Youth who witness death and physical injury in conjunction with acts of violence, or who are exposed to disasters that are associated with mass casualties, may display even higher rates of PTSD and PTS symptoms. Gurwitch et al. (2002) estimate that rates of PTSD vary from 28% to 50% among children exposed to terrorist events (e.g., kidnapping, hostage situations). Following an earthquake in Armenia that killed over 25,000 people, Goenjian and colleagues (1995, 1997) found that rates of "likely PTSD" in adolescents exceeded 50% a year or more after the disaster.

Although little is known about the *developmental course of PTS*, such symptoms emerge in the days or weeks following a trauma event and can take months or years to dissipate (Gurwitch et al., 2002; La Greca et al., 1996; Yule et al., 2000, 2002). However, the typical developmental course of symptoms appears to be one of lessening frequency and intensity over time. For example, among British adolescents who survived the sinking of the cruise ship *Jupiter* in 1988, 51.5% were estimated to develop PTSD at some time point after the disaster (compared with 3.4% of the matched controls); the duration of PTSD was less than a year for 30% of the survivors, with additional youth "remitting" each subsequent year (Yule et al., 2000, 2002).

Although findings suggest a steady reduction in PTS symptoms and diagnoses of PTSD over time, a significant minority of youth do not "recover," and continue to report difficulties years later. For example, Yule and colleagues (2000, 2002) studied adolescent survivors of the *Jupiter* sinking, finding that PTSD was present in 17.5% of the adolescents who were reevaluated 5 to 8 years' postdisaster (or 34% of the initial cases of PTSD). Youngsters who display persistent and elevated symptoms of PTS following disasters are important to target for interventions.

Other Disaster Reactions and Issues of Comorbidity

In addition to PTSD, other trauma reactions have been identified (Vogel & Vernberg, 1993). Moreover, rates of comorbidity are extremely high among youth who display PTSD (American Academy of Child and Adolescent Psychiatry, 1998). Evaluating and understanding these other trauma reactions can aid mental health providers in delivering more effective interventions.

Regardless of whether PTSD symptoms are present, exposure to disasters and acts of terrorism is associated with high levels of anxiety in youth (e.g., Lonigan et al., 1991; Yule et al., 2002). Five to eight years after the *Jupiter* sinking, adolescent survivors displayed high rates of anxiety disorders compared to matched controls, including specific phobia (23.6% vs. 9.2%), panic disorder (12.0% vs. 2.3%), separation anxiety (6.8% vs. 0%), and "any" anxiety disorder (40.7% vs. 18.4%) (Bolton et al., 2000; Yule et al., 2002). Similarly, a survey of children in the New York City public schools conducted six months after September 11, 2001, revealed elevations in agoraphobia (15%), separation anxiety (12.3%), and panic (9%) relative to community rates prior to the attacks (Hoven et al., 2005).

Symptoms of *depression* have also been reported following natural disasters and acts of terrorism (Goenjian et al., 1997; Gurwitch et al., 2002; Nolen-Hoeksema & Morrow, 1991) and are common after disasters that involve loss of loved ones (Goenjian et al., 1995, 1997; Gurwitch et al., 2002; Yule et al., 2002). For example, in the long-term follow-up of survivors of the *Jupiter* sinking (Bolton et al., 2000; Yule et al., 2002), 61 youth developed both major depression and PTSD; in 93% of these cases, depression developed at the same time or after PTSD.

Safety and security concerns also are common reactions to disasters (Silverman & La Greca, 2002). Following the 1995 bombing of the Federal Building in Oklahoma City, Gurwitch and colleagues (2002) observed high levels of children's separation fears (e.g., clinging to parents); in addition, children had a heightened sense of vigilance and a decreased sense of safety and security. With "unpredictable" acts of violence, fears of reoccurrence, ongoing security concerns, and preoccupation with revenge may be evident (Gurwitch et al., 2002; Nader & Mello, 2002).

Many children and adolescents evidence increased *fears* following a disaster that are often linked to the traumatic event that was experienced. For example, fears of water, thunder, and rainstorms have been reported following hurricanes (Vogel & Vernberg, 1993).

In summary, PTSD, anxiety disorders, and depressive disorders are the most common clinical problems documented in youth following disasters; anxiety and depression also may be comorbid with PTSD. Consequently, it is desirable to obtain a comprehensive assessment of youngsters' psychological functioning following disasters and to consider using treatment procedures for addressing comorbid symptoms of anxiety, depression, and/or fears—or other behavior problems.

UNDERSTANDING FACTORS THAT CONTRIBUTE TO CHILDREN'S PTS REACTIONS

Understanding the risk and resilience factors that play a role in development or maintenance of children's disaster reactions is important for the development of evidence-based interventions and for identifying youth, early on, who may need psychological services. Specifically, across a wide range of disasters, the development of PTS symptoms in youth has been associated with the following: (1) traumatic exposure, (2) preexisting characteristics of the child, (3) characteristics of the postdisaster recovery environment, and (4) the child's psychological resources.

Aspects of Traumatic Exposure

First and foremost, the *presence or perception of life threat* is critical for the emergence of children's disaster reactions (Green et al., 1991). The more children perceive that their lives or the lives of loved ones are threatened, the higher their reports of PTS symptoms (e.g., La Greca et al., 1996; Lonigan et al., 1991). In fact, disasters that lead to the *death of a loved one* (parent, friend), especially a violent death, are strongly linked to the development of PTSD symptoms (Gurwitch et al., 2002; see Gibson, 2006a). The terms "complicated grief" and "traumatic grief" have been used to describe these losses, as they are complicated by feelings of grief and guilt.

Loss of possessions and disruption of everyday life also contribute to PTS symptoms following disasters (La Greca et al., 1996; Vernberg et al., 1996). Many youngsters are faced with a cascading series of life stressors that are set into motion by the disaster, such as the loss of one's home and possessions, a change of schools, shifts in parental employment and finances, friends moving away, altered leisure activities, and so on. These stressors challenge children's adaptation.

Duration and intensity of life-threatening events are also associated with PTS symptom severity (Nader & Mello, 2002; Vernberg, 2002). Disaster reactions are further influenced by exposure to either *single or multiple incidents*, with greater distress often following multiple exposures (Robin et al., 1997).

Preexisting Characteristics of the Child

Demographic characteristics may be viewed as markers for other variables that play a more direct role in the development of children's PTS reactions. However, demographic characteristics may be useful for identifying youth who are at high risk for adverse postdisaster reactions.

With respect to *age*, few studies have had sufficiently large samples of youth to adequately evaluate developmental differences in children's disaster reactions. Understanding developmental aspects of children's reactions is also hampered by the fact that diverse manifestations of PTSD exist at different ages (American Academy of Child and Adolescent Psychiatry, 1998).

Regarding *gender*, girls often report more PTSD symptoms than boys following disasters (Gurwitch et al., 2002; Yule et al., 2002). A recent meta-analysis (Tolin & Foa, 2006) found that girls and women were more likely to meet diagnostic criteria for PTSD than boys and men and that these gender effects were stronger for disaster victims than for victims of terrorism. It is not clear to what extent these gender differences are also a manifestation of different base rates of psychopathology, with girls and women reporting higher levels of anxiety, depression, and other internalizing problems than boys or men (Tolin & Foa, 2006).

Community studies following natural disasters generally show that *minority youth* report higher levels of PTS symptoms and have more difficulty recovering from such events than nonminority youth (e.g., La Greca et al., 1996, 1998; Lonigan et al., 1994; Rabalais et al., 2002). Following destructive disasters, youth from minority and/or low-income backgrounds may have less financial resources to deal with the rebuilding process, which could prolong the life disruption that ensues after disasters. Minority youth also may have had other predisaster trauma exposure, which could sensitize them to the effects of disasters (Berton & Stabb, 1996).

Children's *prior psychosocial functioning* also is a factor. In particular, preexisting *anxiety* is a significant risk factor for postdisaster PTSD symptoms (e.g., La Greca et al., 1998; Lonigan et al., 1994). Other findings point to predisaster *depression, stress,* and *ruminative coping styles* as risk factors for postdisaster stress reactions (Nolen-Hoeksema & Morrow, 1991).

Aspects of the Recovery Environment

Several aspects of the recovery environment may affect children's disaster reactions. Specifically, *social support from significant others* has been found to mitigate the impact of disasters on youth (e.g., La Greca & Prinstein, 2002).

Parents' psychosocial functioning, including their levels of psychopathology and their own reactions to the disaster, also affects children's postdisaster functioning (e.g., Swenson et al., 1996). For example, Green et al. (1991) found that parental psychopathology predicted higher levels of PTSD symptoms in children and adolescents following the Buffalo Creek dam collapse.

Major life events (e.g., death of a family member; parental divorce or separation) occurring in the months following a disaster also impede disaster recovery and are associated with greater persistence of PTS symptoms in children (La Greca et al., 1996). Youngsters who encounter major life stressors following a disaster represent a high-risk group for severe and persistent PTS.

Children's Psychological Resources

Finally, children's psychological resources (e.g., coping skills, intelligence) play a role in their disaster reactions. Children with more negative *coping strategies* (e.g., anger, blaming others) report higher levels and greater persistence of PTS after disasters (e.g., La Greca et al., 1996). Efforts to promote adaptive coping may be useful for postdisaster interventions with children.

EVIDENCE-BASED INTERVENTIONS FOR POSTTRAUMATIC STRESS

Unfortunately, there is a dearth of outcome studies on postdisaster interventions for children (Vernberg, 2002). The few well-controlled studies have focused on children with persistent PTSD, occurring a year or more after the disaster/event. Considerably less is known about interventions designed for the immediate aftermath of disaster or during the short-term recovery phase.

This gap in our understanding of how to intervene with children and adolescents is related to the tremendous challenges to conducting research, especially controlled-outcome studies, in the aftermath of disasters and acts of terrorism. Difficulties in securing funding for research, in obtaining IRB approval in a timely manner, and in working with individuals and communities that are undergoing substantial stress, disorganization, and chaos add to the normal challenges of conducting treatment outcome research (see La Greca, 2006, for further details).

Intervention goals differ substantially based on the postdisaster timeframe and the context in which they are delivered. A useful way to conceptualize postdisaster interventions is whether they pertain to the immediate aftermath of the event, the short-term recovery and rebuilding phase, or the long-term recovery phase. Below, the review of interventions follows this framework.

Postimpact Phase

The postimpact phase focuses on the actual disaster event and its immediate aftermath, typically the first few weeks' postdisaster (Vernberg, 2002). After a devastating natural disaster or act of terrorism, most or all children and adolescents directly exposed to the event will display some degree of stress reactions. In particular, children and their families will be concerned with personal safety and security issues. Concerns about food, shelter, and basic physical needs may also require attention, especially in destructive natural disasters. Psychological interventions provided during this time period are designed to be *brief and present-focused;* their main goal is to *reduce or prevent long-term psychological difficulties.* The main interventions used in this period are Critical Incident Stress Debriefing, Psychological First Aid, and psychoeducational materials.

Critical Incident Stress Debriefing (CISD), also referred to as "debriefing," is a crisis intervention designed to relieve and prevent trauma-related distress in normal individuals who are experiencing abnormally stressful events (e.g., Chemtob et al., 1997). CISD provides opportunities for children and adolescents to express feelings, normalize their responses to the disaster, and learn about common reactions to the disaster in the context of a supportive setting (Chemtob et al., 1997). CISD is delivered to groups or individuals, usually by mental health workers or disaster responders working in the field (e.g., community shelters for disaster survivors; schools in affected areas). Despite its appeal, there is no empirical support for its effectiveness (Rose et al., 2003), although research is limited by small samples, lack of adequate control groups, and limited follow-up evaluations. In fact, there is only one well-controlled study of the use of CISD with a large sample of children (n = 158) that employed adequate controls and included an 8-month follow-up (Stallard et al., 2006), although it focused on child survivors (7–18 years) of motor vehicle accidents. The findings revealed that levels of PTSD improved significantly for all youth at follow-up and did not differ for those who received CISD and those who did not.

Concerns regarding the use of CISD with children and adolescents include that the intervention may "retraumatize" children and that these brief interventions may be insufficient to address the multiple, complex, and cascading stressors that result from disasters and acts of terrorism, which may last for months or years (Brymer et al., in press; Ruzek et al., in press). Moreover, the provision of CISD may reduce the likelihood of further help seeking, as individuals may believe that they have received sufficient mental health care (Brymer et al., in press; Ruzek et al., in press).

Psychological First Aid (PFA) is another intervention used in the immediate aftermath of disasters that can be implemented in field settings, such as schools or community crisis centers (Amaya-Jackson & March, 1995; Brymer et al., in press). PFA was developed by disaster mental health experts from the National Child Traumatic Stress Network (www.nctsn.org), in response to concerns about the effectiveness of "debriefing." PFA is an "evidence-informed" approach that also is culturally informed, appropriate for developmental levels across lifespan, and designed to be delivered in flexible manner (Brymer et al., in press; Ruzek et al., in press). According to Brymer et al. (in press), the main elements of PFA include promoting (1) a sense of safety, (2) "calming," (3) self- and community efficacy, (4) connectedness, and (5) hope. PFA provides children with an opportunity to express their feelings, clarify any areas of confusion, and identify areas of need. (See the Field Operating Guide for PFA that is posted on the NCTSN Web site.) PFA also allows disaster responders to identify children who are having severe postdisaster reactions, so that they may receive more intensive psychological assistance.

PFA appears promising as part of a comprehensive, postdisaster intervention strategy. To date, however, there are no controlled evaluations of PFA (Brymer et al., in press; Ruzek et al., in press), in large part due to the challenges of conducting postdisaster research. Potential concerns with PFA are that the intervention is complex and requires trained personnel to administer; that few individuals have been trained to administer PFA, although there are ongoing efforts to train paraprofessionals; and that many children and youth who are affected by disasters and acts of terrorism may not be present in the field settings where the intervention is typically delivered.

Finally, several relief organizations and mental health associations have developed *psychoeducational materials*, such as brochures, pamphlets, and fact sheets (often available via the Internet) (see Table 1). The materials provide advice on how to help children cope with disasters and/or terrorist events. Generally, these materials suggest that adults encourage children to express feelings in developmentally appropriate ways (through discussion, drawings, journal writing, or storytelling); address fears, worries, or security concerns children may have; and help children return to normal roles and routines.

The appeal of psychoeducational materials is their relative ease of distribution in the postdisaster environment; however, no evidence is available on their effectiveness. Moreover, the information contained in some brochures and pamphlets may not be evidence-informed. Other issues include that dissemination depends on computer and Internet connections, which may not be available in the aftermath of a disaster. In addition, some sophistication may be needed to adapt the materials to the current disaster/event or age of the child/adolescent, although the information may be useful to mental health professionals who are working with disaster survivors.

In summary, at this point in time, there is no evidence that psychological interventions delivered in the immediate aftermath of disasters and other traumatic events are effective for reducing short- or long-term distress (Gibson, 2006b), although PFA and psychoeducation appear promising. Efforts to conduct controlled field studies of early interventions are very much needed.

Table 1. *Summary of Interventions for Children and Youth*

Immediate Impact Phase
   Critical Incident Stress Debriefing (Chemtob et al., 1997)
   Psychological First Aid (Brymer et al., in press; see www.nctsn.org for manual)
   Fact sheets, brochures, and Web sites (selected)
      National Child Traumatic Stress Network (www.nctsn.org)
      National Center for Posttraumatic Stress Disorder (www.ncptsd.va.gov)
      National Institute of Mental Health (www.nimh.nih.gov/publicat/violence.cfm)
      American Psychological Association (www.apa.org, www.apa.org/practice/kids.html)
      American Academy of Child and Adolescent Psychiatry (www.aacap.org)
      FEMA (www.fema.gov/kids)
      American Red Cross (www.redcross.org/disaster/safety/guide.html)
      American Academy of Child and Adolescent Psychiatry (www.aacap.org)

Short-Term Recovery Phase
   School-based cognitive-behavior therapy (Wolmer et al., 2005)
   Community-based "stress and coping" interventions (selected)
      After the Storm (La Greca et al., 2005)
      The Bushfire and Me (Storm et al., 1994)
      Helping Children Prepare for and Cope with Natural Disasters (La Greca et al., 1994)
      Healing After Trauma (Gurwitch & Messenbaugh, 1998)
      Helping America Cope (La Greca et al., 2001)

Long-Term Recovery Phase
   Multi-Modality Trauma Treatment (March et al., 1998)
   Brief trauma/grief-focused psychotherapy (Goenjian et al., 1997)
   School-based psychosocial intervention (Chemtob et al., 2002)
   EMDR (Chemtob et al., 2002)

Short-Term Recovery and Reconstruction Phase

This phase begins the first few weeks after the disaster and continues for several months to a year postdisaster. During this period, children's persistent and chronic stress reactions begin to emerge. In addition, youth with high levels of exposure to the disaster are likely to experience major life stressors (e.g., relocation, disruption of routines and social ties) that interfere with their recovery. As a result, the primary goals of psychological interventions for this recovery phase are to reduce or prevent persistent psychological difficulties from developing and to improve youngsters' adaptive functioning. Because some children will begin to "recover," interventions typically focus on "high-risk" youth, or youth who have already demonstrated high levels of PTS.

Unfortunately, no controlled-outcome studies are available for the interventions developed for this short-term recovery phase. Although cognitive-behavioral therapy (CBT) approaches, such as anxiety management and guided exposure, have been used effectively with traumatic events that affect *individual* children and adolescents (e.g., motor vehicle accidents), these treatments are difficult or impractical to implement with large numbers of disaster-affected youth who are also undergoing significant postdisaster life stressors (e.g., relocation, loss of family member; see Ruzek et al., in press). The interventions delivered in the short-term recovery phase include detailed psychoeducational materials (see Table 1), sometimes used in combination with CBT.

Wolmer and colleagues (2005) recently reported on the long-term follow-up of a classroom-based "School Reactivation Program" that was delivered 4 to 5 months after a major earthquake in Turkey in 1999; this devastating natural disaster led to 18,000 deaths and destroyed nearly 150,000 homes. The intervention was described as a combination of psychoeducation and CBT and was led by teachers over a 4-week period, in eight 2-hour meetings. At enrollment there were 202 participants, aged 9–17 years (*M* age = 11.5 years). Rates of PTSD were reduced from 32% (pretreatment) to 17% among treated children, and the posttreatment levels were similar to those of comparison children who were in areas unaffected by the earthquake. At the three-year follow-up, 67 (33%) of the treated children were evaluated and compared to 220 untreated control youth who had similar levels of PTS symptoms and disaster exposure. The results revealed significant decreases in symptoms of PTS, grief, and dissociation for both treated children and control youth. However, a large proportion of youth in both groups reported moderate (30–33%) to severe (17–18%) levels of PTS symptoms. On the positive side, teacher ratings for academics, social behavior, and general conduct were higher for treated versus untreated youth, suggesting that a positive effect on adaptive functioning may have been associated with this intervention.

Other community- or school-based interventions using psychoeducational materials and/or CBT strategies have been developed for the short-term recovery phase (see Table 1). Although they have not been evaluated empirically, many are "empirically informed" and appear promising.

Specifically, several disaster researchers have developed manuals for use in schools or group settings to help youngsters cope with large-scale disasters (see Table 1). Manuals focusing on natural disasters include *The Bushfire and Me: A Story of What Happened to Me and My Family* (Storm et al., 1994), *After the Storm* (La Greca et al., 2005), and *Helping Children Prepare for and Cope with Natural Disasters* (La Greca et al., 1994); manuals focusing on coping with terrorism include *Healing After Trauma Skills* (Gurwitch & Messenbaugh, 1998) and *Helping America Cope: A Guide to Help Parents and Children Cope with the September 11th Terrorist Attacks* (La Greca et al., 2001). *After the Storm* and *Helping America Cope* were designed for a parent or caring adult to use with children, although they have been adapted for use in school and community settings.

These manuals are intended to reduce or prevent long-term stress reactions and to identify children with severe reactions who may need more intensive assistance. The manuals typically cover strategies for helping children to "process" the traumatic events in a supportive manner, develop effective coping strategies for dealing with ongoing stressors that result from the trauma, maintain regular routines, increase social support, and prepare for future events. These manuals contain "lessons" that teachers, parents, or mental health providers could use with children in disaster-affected areas, and they review "risk factors" to help adults identify children with stress reactions.

For example, both *Helping American Cope* (La Greca et al., 2001) and *After the Storm* (La Greca et al., 2005) were developed for school-aged children. Over 1.5 million copies of *Helping American Cope* were distributed (by the BellSouth Foundation and the United Way) to families in the Northeast U.S. the year following the terrorist attacks on the Pentagon and World Trade Center. *After the Storm* was used extensively in Louisiana after Hurricanes Katrina and Rita. Both manuals share key elements: providing information about the disaster; providing information about children's stress reactions and how to identify them; enhancing children's social support; and enhancing children's coping skills. The lessons are presented in an interesting and interactive format and cover strategies that might help most children cope with disaster, such as using positive (and avoiding negative) coping to deal with stressors, maintaining normal roles and routines, keeping healthy and fit (including ways to encourage nighttime sleeping), and limiting media exposure to disaster-related images. Other lessons promote children's coping with "change," fears and worries, intrusive thoughts and dreams, anger, sadness, and future events.

Although promising, none of the intervention materials available for this phase of disaster recovery has been evaluated. Potential limitations of these materials are that they require Internet connections (for downloads) or substantial funding to print the number of copies needed after large-scale disasters. The manuals typically require an 8th-grade reading level and may need some adaptation to fit the particular circumstances of a new disaster or to be used effectively by different professionals (e.g., parent versus teacher versus school or mental health counselor).

Other ideas for helping children cope with disasters and terrorist events include having public ceremonies, memorials, or other disaster-related rituals that provide an opportunity for survivors to remember the event and place it in context (Vernberg & Vogel, 1993). Rituals may serve several important psychological functions, including public expression of shared grief and support, reassurance that victims are remembered, review and reinterpretation of disaster experiences, and obtaining a sense of closure on a difficult life event (Vernberg & Vogel, 1993).

Long-Term Recovery Phase

A year or more after destructive disasters and major terrorist events, many children will have recovered; however, a significant minority will experience persistent, chronic stress reactions that may be complicated by secondary stressors (e.g., relocation, loss of family member). Interventions conducted a year or more after a traumatic event typically target individuals or small groups of youngsters with persistent or chronic PTSD. A few evidence-based interventions are available.

Cognitive-Behavioral Treatments

Interventions for adults experiencing PTSD following a wide range of traumatic events suggest that exposure-based cognitive-behavioral treatment (CBT) is effective (Foa et al., 1999, 2005). Based on emotional processing theory, exposure-based CBT targets pathological elements of the individual's fear structure (an aspect of PTSD), as well as dysfunctional beliefs, by having the individual systematically carry out therapist-prescribed exposures—either imaginal or *in vivo*—to provide information that is incompatible with the pathological elements that underlie the fear structure (Foa & Rothbaum, 1998). Exposure to memories of the traumatic event is thought to promote habituation by targeting stimulus-response associations and correcting distorted cognitions. Foa and colleagues (2005) have reported that prolonged exposure alone is also effective for the treatment of PTSD among adult rape victims. Prolonged exposure involves psychoeducation, breathing retraining, imaginal exposure to the trauma memory, and *in vivo* exposure to trauma reminders. Among children and youth, several well-controlled studies of CBT with sexual abuse victims provide a moderate level of evidence for its effectiveness (e.g., Cohen et al., 2005; Deblinger et al., 2006).

Despite the promising findings, *no* well-controlled studies, using random assignment to treatment, have focused on adults or children exposed to disasters or terrorist attacks (Gibson, 2006b). The studies of children and youth reviewed below contain treatment elements that are similar to (or based on) CBT, often with elements of exposure.

Multi-Modality Trauma Treatment

March and colleagues (1998) evaluated an exposure-based CBT intervention, Multi-Modality Trauma Treatment (MMTT), with 17 children and adolescents (*M* age = 12.1 years; range = 10 to 15) who displayed PTSD after a single-stressor traumatic incident (e.g., car accidents, shootings, accidental injuries), including disaster-related incidents (severe storms, fires). The participants' average duration of PTSD ranged from 1.5 to 2.5 years.

Based on emotional processing theory, MMTT was designed as a group-administered CBT that focused on (1) habituating conditioned anxiety through narrative exposures, (2) modifying maladaptive trauma-related cognitions through positive self-talk and cognitive restructuring, (3) teaching adaptive coping strategies for disturbing feelings and physiological reactions, and (4) reducing co-occurring symptoms such as anxiety, anger, depression, grief, and disruptive behaviors through problem-solving and self-management strategies. Imaginal exposures were used during certain treatment sessions, and *in vivo* exposures were to be completed as homework. This 18-week intervention was evaluated using a single-case multiple-baseline design, with controls for time, location, and school type (elementary versus junior high). Results revealed significant improvement on clinician-reported PTSD outcome measures from pre- to posttreatment that were maintained at six-month follow-up. Improvements also were observed for child ratings of depression, anxiety, and anger; only teacher ratings of child externalizing problems did not show significant improvement. Of the 14 treatment completers, 8 (57%) no longer met criteria for PTSD at posttreatment and 12 (86%) no longer met criteria at six months' follow-up.

These findings represent important, initial evidence for the efficacy of exposure-based CBT for youth with PTSD. Further research is necessary to determine whether similar effects would be obtained in a randomized controlled trial with a larger sample of disaster-exposed children.

Brief Trauma/Grief-Focused Psychotherapy

Goenjian and colleagues (1997) evaluated a school-based brief trauma/grief-focused intervention that contains components similar to those found in exposure-based CBT, with 64 adolescents (*M* age = 13.2 years) from four schools who had experienced a devastating earthquake in Armenia and who displayed high levels of PTS and depressive reactions 1.5 years later. All participants had been exposed to life threat, mutilating injuries, or horrific deaths during the earthquake and continued to live in the area where the earthquake occurred. Because study personnel were limited, schools and students were not randomly assigned. Students from the schools closest to the authors' clinics participated in the treatment (*n* = 35); students from the schools farthest from the clinic were not treated (*n* = 29).

The intervention included two individual and four classroom sessions over three weeks. It addressed several areas, including reconstructing and reprocessing traumatic experiences and associated thoughts and feelings; identifying reminders and cues to past traumatic events and improving tolerance for and reactivity to the cues/reminders; enhancing social support-seeking behaviors; enhancing coping strategies for accepting and adapting to changes and loss; dealing with grief and bereavement by reconstituting a nontraumatic mental representation of any deceased persons; and identifying missed developmental opportunities and promoting positive development.

Adolescents' PTS and depressive reactions were evaluated prior to the intervention and 18 months' postintervention (i.e., 3 years' postdisaster). The treated adolescents reported significantly lower PTS reactions than the untreated adolescents at 18 months' posttreatment. Estimated rates of depression did not change from pretreatment to follow-up for the treated adolescents (46% at each time point) but increased significantly for the untreated adolescents (from 35% to 75%).

Goenjian et al. (2005) reported a second follow-up, five years after the disaster (two years after the above study). Among treated adolescents, improvements in PTS symptoms were three times greater than for adolescents in the untreated comparison group. Treated adolescents also tended to improve in depressive symptoms, in contrast to untreated adolescents, who showed increases.

Although this was a nonrandomized trial, the findings suggest that youth with persistent, significant disaster reactions who do not receive any intervention are not likely to recover but are likely to show persistent, deleterious effects. The findings highlight the importance of developing and evaluating randomized clinical trials for child disaster victims.

School-Based Psychosocial Intervention

Chemtob et al. (2002) have reported the largest and most well-controlled study to evaluate the efficacy of a manualized, school-based, psychosocial intervention to treat children with persistent disaster-related trauma symptoms. Children (grades 2–6; $n = 3,864$) enrolled in all 10 public elementary schools on the Hawaiian island of Kauai, which was struck by Hurricane Iniki in September 1992, were screened for high levels of PTSD symptoms 2 years' postdisaster; 248 children who were exposed to Iniki and who had PTSD symptom scores above the 94th percentile were identified as having severe trauma symptoms. The children were randomly assigned to one of three consecutively treated cohorts, with the children awaiting treatment serving as waitlist controls. Within each cohort, children were randomly assigned to individual or group treatment, to compare the two treatment modalities.

The manualized treatment consisted of four weekly sessions that focused on helping children master disaster-related psychological challenges; the sessions were (1) restoring a sense of safety, (2) grieving losses and renewing attachments, (3) adaptively expressing disaster-related anger, and (4) achieving closure about the disaster to move forward.

The intervention provided a context for children to review their disaster-related experiences in a structured, supportive way. For example, in Session 2 ("Loss"), children were engaged in play, art, and talk aimed at helping them identify any losses, express feelings about the losses, and identify forward-looking ways of integrating the loss into the present (which could be construed as an exposure-based procedure). Similar activities were used in the individual and group treatment approaches, with the group approach involving cooperative play and discussion.

Children reported significant reductions in PTS symptoms that were maintained at 12-month follow-up. For a subset of the youth with clinician-ratings of PTSD symptoms ($n = 37$), treated children had fewer trauma symptoms (11.65) compared with untreated children (20.32). Although the group and individual treatment approaches did not differ, more children completed the group treatment (95%) than the individual treatment (85%). This study is important because it demonstrates the feasibility of screening a large population of disaster-affected children two years' postdisaster and the feasibility and efficacy of a brief school-based psychosocial intervention.

Eye Movement Desensitization Processing (EMDR)

Chemtob et al. (2002) reported the results of another treatment—EMDR—for school-aged children with disaster-related PTS symptoms. The participants were 32 children ($M = 8.4$ years) who were treatment nonresponders at one-year follow-up of a prior intervention for disaster-related symptoms (presumably the intervention described above) and who met criteria for disaster-related PTSD.

EMDR was used, in part, because efficacy data using EMDR with single-event trauma appeared promising. The study evaluated two groups in an ABA design plus follow-up. Group 1 was assessed at pretreatment, provided treatment (three weekly sessions), and reassessed at posttreatment. Group 2 consisted of waitlisted children who were assessed at baseline, and then, following treatment for Group 1, were reassessed at pretreatment, provided treatment, and assessed at posttreatment. Both groups were administered six-month follow-up assessments.

The elements of EMDR included (1) identifying a distressing memory and related imagery and sensations, and assessing its subjective distress, (2) identifying trauma-related negative self-cognitions and positive self-cognitions, (3) inducing sets of eye movements by asking the child to track the back-and-forth movements of the therapist's hand while concentrating on memory-related images, thoughts, and sensations, and (4) in the "reprocessing" stage, the child is asked to focus on positive cognitions regarding the memory during further sets of eye movements.

On child-reported symptoms of PTS, anxiety, and depression, both the "immediate" and "delayed" treatment groups showed significant declines from pre- to posttreatment that were maintained at six-month follow-up. Despite encouraging findings, inferences cannot be drawn about the efficacy of EMDR, because the study was not designed as a comparative evaluation. The components of EMDR are similar to components of exposure-based CBT, including imaginal exposure, rehearsal of the trauma-related experience, and support by a trained clinician, which might also account for the positive treatment results.

SUMMARY OF PSYCHOSOCIAL INTERVENTIONS AND CHAPTER CONCLUSIONS

It is clear from the above review that, despite the high degree of need, there is a paucity of evidence-based procedures for intervening with children and adolescents in the immediate, short-term, and long-term aftermaths of disasters and acts of terrorism. The very limited evidence that is available is restricted to the treatment of children and adolescents with persistent PTSD a year or more after the traumatic event; this evidence suggests that cognitive-behavioral treatments are promising. Until further treatment studies have been conducted, mental health professionals are advised to draw upon "evidence-informed" materials and procedures for helping children and adolescents cope with the aftermath of disasters and acts of terrorism.

In the immediate aftermath of disasters, efforts to reduce or prevent psychological problems and stress reactions, to promote positive adaptation, and to identify children with severe reactions (who may need intensive help) seem paramount. "Best practices" for this period include reassuring children, providing information, and "normalizing" their disaster reactions. Especially important are encouraging children to express their feelings, addressing any fears, worries, or security concerns they may have, and helping them resume normal roles and routines. Clinicians also should identify children with severe reactions, so that they can receive additional help.

During the short-term recovery period, many children will exhibit subclinical levels of PTSD and difficulties coping with disaster-related experiences and their aftermath. Thus, *continued* efforts to reduce or prevent long-term psychological difficulties and promote positive adaptation are important. For large-scale community-wide disasters, efforts to deal with youth in community settings, such as schools, may be most productive from a prevention standpoint. Several intervention manuals (see Table 1) are suitable for community settings. In addition, it is desirable to refer children and adolescents who display severe PTS reactions for additional mental health services. Because disasters affect large numbers of people, intensive, individualized interventions, such as CBT, may only be feasible for children and adolescents who show marked signs of disaster-related distress or who have multiple risk factors for poor mental health outcomes (e.g., high life adversity, multiple comorbid conditions) (Vernberg, 2002).

Over the long-term recovery period, children who display chronic and persistent PTS reactions to disasters and acts of terrorism will likely need more intensive psychological interventions, such as exposure-based CBT. In light of the consistent empirical support for CBT with adults and youth with PTSD resulting from sexual abuse, such interventions represent the "best practices" for youths exposed to the trauma of a disaster and who display chronic and severe PTSD reactions.

Although is disheartening to see so little evidence on the efficacy and effectiveness of interventions for children following disasters and acts of terrorism, this reflects the inherent challenges in conducting controlled outcome research following disasters (see La Greca, 2001, 2006; La Greca et al., 2002). For example, schools are often in chaos after community-wide disasters and have more pressing priorities than conducting research. Moreover, the significant adults in children's lives, such as parents and teachers, may also be affected by the disaster and may be unaware of the extent to which children are distressed. It also is difficult to conduct controlled-outcome research without considerable resources and funding; yet, funding mechanisms are often slow or insufficient (also see La Greca et al., 2002).

Finally, it is important to emphasize that children and adolescents exposed to disasters and acts of terrorism are likely to need *more than* interventions that focus exclusively on PTSD, because their reactions are often complex and multifaceted and may include other problems (i.e., grief, depression, anxiety). Thus, additional intervention components (e.g., dealing with grief and bereavement, handling anger, promoting positive coping) are likely to be important adjuncts to PTSD-oriented interventions. Although evidence is needed, it is likely that children and adolescents with complex, comorbid postdisaster reactions may benefit from CBT treatments that focus on comorbid psychological reactions, in addition to a focus on PTSD.

REFERENCES

American Academy of Child and Adolescent Psychiatry (1998). Practice parameters for the assessment and treatment of children and adolescents with posttraumatic stress disorder. *Journal of the American Academy of Child and Adolescent Psychiatry, 37* (Suppl), 4S–26S.

American Psychiatric Association (1994). *Diagnostic and Statistical Manual of Mental Disorders,* 4th ed. Washington, DC.

Berton, M. W., & Stabb, S. D. (1996). Exposure to violence and post-traumatic stress disorder in urban adolescents. *Adolescence, 31,* 489–498.

Bolton, D., O'Ryan, D., Udwin, O., Boyle, S., & Yule, W. (2000). The long-term psychological effects of a disaster experienced in adolescence: II. General psychopathology. *Journal of Child Psychology and Psychiatry, 41,* 513–523.

Brymer, M. J., Layne, C. M., Vernberg, E. M., Steinbery, A. M., Watson, P. J., Jacobs, A. K., et al. (in press). Psychological first aid for children and adolescents. In E. Foa and J. Cohen (Eds.), *Effective Treatments for PTSD.* New York: Guilford Press.

Chemtob, C. M., Nakashima, J., & Carlson, J. G. (2002). Brief treatment for elementary school children with disaster-related posttraumatic stress disorder: A field study. *Journal of Clinical Psychology, 58,* 99–112.

Chemtob, C. M., Nakashima, J. P., & Hamada, R. S. (2002). Psychosocial intervention for postdisaster trauma symptoms in elementary school children: A controlled community field study. *Archives of Pediatric and Adolescent Medicine, 156,* 211–216.

Chemtob, C. M., Tomas, S., Law, W., & Cremniter, D. (1997). Postdisaster psychosocial intervention: A field study of the impact of debriefing on psychological distress. *American Journal of Psychiatry, 154*, 415–417.

Cohen, J. A., Mannarino, A. P., & Knudsen, K. (2005). Treating sexually abused children: 1 year follow-up of a randomized controlled trial. *Child Abuse and Neglect, 29*, 135–145.

Deblinger, E., Mannarino, A. P., Cohen, J. A., & Steer, R. A. (2006). A follow-up study of a multisite, randomized, controlled trial for children with sexual abuse-related PTSD symptoms. *Journal of the American Academy of Child and Adolescent Psychiatry, 45*, 1474–1484.

Foa, E. B., Dancu, C. V., Hembree, E. A., Jaycox, L. H., Meadows, E. A., & Street, G. P. (1999). A comparison of exposure therapy, stress inoculation training, and their combination for reducing posttraumatic stress disorder in female assault victims. *Journal of Consulting and Clinical Psychology, 67*, 194–200.

Foa, E. B., Hembree, E. A., Cahill, S. P., Rauch, S. A., Riggs, D. S., Feeny, N. C., et al. (2005). Randomized trial of prolonged exposure for posttraumatic stress disorder with and without cognitive restructuring: Outcome at academic and community clinics. *Journal of Consulting and Clinical Psychology, 73*, 953–964.

Foa, E. B., & Rothbaum, B. O. (1998). *Treating the Trauma of Rape: Cognitive-Behavioral Therapy for PTSD.* New York: Guilford Press.

Gibson, L. E. (2006a). Complicated grief: A review of current issues. Retrieved January 10, 2007, from http://redmh.org/research/specialized/grief.html.

Gibson, L. E. (2006b). A review of the published empirical literature regarding early- and later-stage interventions for individuals exposed to traumatic stress. Retrieved on January 10, 2007, from http://redmh.org/research/general/treatmt.html.

Goenjian, A. K., Karayan, I., Pynoos, R. S., Minassian, D., Najarian, L. M., Steinberg, A. M., et al. (1997). Outcome of psychotherapy among early adolescents after trauma. *American Journal of Psychiatry, 154*, 536–542.

Goenjian, A. K., Pynoos, R. S., Steinberg, A. M., Najarian, L. M., Asarnow, J. R., Karayan, I., et al. (1995). Psychiatric comorbidity in children after the 1988 earthquake in Armenia. *Journal of the American Academy of Child and Adolescent Psychiatry, 34*, 1174–1184.

Goenjian, A. K., Walling, D., Steinberg, A. M., Karayan, I., Najarian, L.M., & Pynoos, R. (2005). A prospective study of posttraumatic stress and depressive reactions among treated and untreated adolescents 5 years after a catastrophic disaster. *American Journal of Psychiatry, 162*, 2302–2308.

Green, B. L., Korol, M. S., Grace, M. C., Vary, M. G., Kramer, T. L., Gleser, G. C., et al. (1994). Children of disaster in the second decade: A 17-year follow-up of Buffalo Creek survivors. *Journal of the American Academy of Child and Adolescent Psychiatry, 33*, 71–79.

Green, B. L., Korol, M. S., Grace, M. C., Vary, M. G., Leonard, A. C., Gleser, G. C., et al. (1991). Children and disaster: Gender and parental effects on PTSD symptoms. *Journal of the American Academy of Child and Adolescent Psychiatry, 30*, 945–951.

Gurwitch, R. H., & Messenbaugh, A. K. (1998). *Healing After Trauma: Skills Manual for Helping Children.* Oklahoma City: Authors.

Gurwitch, R. H., Sitterle, K. A., Young, B. H., & Pfefferbaum, B. (2002). The aftermath of terrorism. In A. M. La Greca, W. K. Silverman, E. M. Vernberg, & M. C. Roberts (Eds.), *Helping Children Cope with Disasters and Terrorism* (pp. 327–358). Washington, DC: American Psychological Association.

Hoven, C. W., Duarte, C. S., Lucas, C. P., Wu, P., Mandell, D. J., Goodwin, R. D., et al. (2005). Psychopathology among New York city public school children 6 months after September 11. *Archives of General Psychiatry, 62*, 545–552.

Korol, M. S., Kramer, T. L., Grace, M. C., & Green, B. L. (2002). Dam break: Long-term follow-up of children exposed to the Buffalo Creek Disaster. In A. M. La Greca, W. K. Silverman, E. M. Vernberg, & M. C. Roberts (Eds.), *Helping Children Cope with Disasters and Terrorism* (pp. 241–258). Washington, DC: American Psychological Association.

La Greca, A. M. (2001). Children experiencing disasters: Prevention and intervention. In J. N. Hughes, A. M. La Greca, & J. C. Conoley (Eds.), *Handbook of Psychological Services for Children and Adolescents* (pp. 195–222). New York: Oxford University Press.

La Greca, A. M. (2006). School-based studies of children following disasters. In F. Norris, S. Galesto, D. Reissman, & P. Watson (Eds.), *Research Methods for Studying Mental*

Health After Disasters and Terrorism: Community and Public Health Approaches. New York: Guilford Press.

La Greca, A. M., & Prinstein, M. J. (2002). Hurricanes and tornadoes. In A. M. La Greca, W. K. Silverman, E. M. Vernberg, & M. C. Roberts (Eds.), *Helping Children Cope with Disasters and Terrorism* (pp. 107–138). Washington, DC: American Psychological Association.

La Greca, A. M., Sevin, S., & Sevin, E. (2001). *Helping America Cope: A Guide for Parents and Children in the Aftermath of the September 11th National Disaster.* Miami: Sevendippity. Retrieved on January 7, 2007, from http://www.7-dippity.com/index.html.

La Greca, A. M., Sevin, S., & Sevin, E. (2005). *After the Storm.* Miami: Sevendippity. Retrieved on January 7, 2007, from http://www.7-dippity.com/index.html.

La Greca, A. M., Silverman, W. K., Vernberg, E. M., & Prinstein, M. (1996). Symptoms of posttraumatic stress after Hurricane Andrew: A prospective study. *Journal of Consulting and Clinical Psychology, 64,* 712–723.

La Greca, A. M., Silverman, W. K., Vernberg, E. M., & Roberts, M. C. (2002). Children and disasters: Future directions for research and public policy. In A. M. La Greca, W.K. Silverman, E. M. Vernberg, & M.C. Roberts (Eds.), *Helping Children Cope with Disasters.* Washington, DC: American Psychological Association.

La Greca, A. M., Silverman, W. K., & Wasserstein, S. B. (1998). Children's predisaster functioning as a predictor of posttraumatic stress following Hurricane Andrew. *Journal of Consulting and Clinical Psychology, 66,* 883–892.

La Greca, A. M., Vernberg, E. M., Silverman, W. K., & Prinstein, M. (1994). *Helping Children Cope with Natural Disasters: A Manual for School Personnel.* Miami: Authors.

Lonigan, C. J., Anthony, J. L., & Shannon, M. P. (1998). Diagnostic efficacy of posttraumatic symptoms in children exposed to disaster. *Journal of Clinical Child Psychology, 27,* 255–267.

Lonigan, C. J., Shannon, M. P., Finch, A. J., Daugherty, T. K., & Taylor, C. M. (1991). Children's reactions to a natural disaster: Symptom severity and degree of exposure. *Advances in Behaviour Research and Therapy, 13,* 135–154.

Lonigan, C. J., Shannon, M. P., Taylor, C. M., Finch, A. J. & Sallee, F. R. (1994). Children exposed to disaster: II. Risk factors for the development of post-traumatic symptomatology. *Journal of the American Academy of Child Psychiatry, 33,* 94–105.

March, J. S., Amaya-Jackson, L., Murray, M. C., & Schulte, A. (1998). Cognitive-behavioral psychotherapy for children and adolescents with posttraumatic stress disorder after a single-incident stressor. *Journal of the American Academy of Child and Adolescent Psychiatry, 37,* 585–593.

Nader, K., & Mello, C. (2002). The aftermath of terrorism. In A. M. La Greca, W. K. Silverman, E. M. Vernberg, & M. C. Roberts (Eds.), *Helping Children Cope with Disasters and Terrorism* (pp. 301–326). Washington, DC: American Psychological Association.

Nolen-Hoeksema, S., & Morrow, J. (1991). A prospective study of depression and posttraumatic stress symptoms after a natural disaster: The 1989 Loma Prieta Earthquake. *Journal of Personality and Social Psychology, 61,* 115–121.

Rabalais, A. E., Ruggiero, K. J., & Scotti, J. R. (2002). Multicultural issues in the response of children to disasters. In A. M. La Greca, W. K. Silverman, E. M. Vernberg, & M. C. Roberts (Eds.), *Helping Children Cope with Disasters and Terrorism* (pp. 73–100). Washington, DC: American Psychological Association.

Robin, R. W., Chester, B., Rasmussen, J. K., Jaranson, J. M., & Goldman, D. (1997). Prevalence and characteristics of trauma and posttraumatic stress disorder in a southwestern American Indian Community. *American Journal of Psychiatry, 154,* 1582–1588.

Rose, S., Bisson, J., & Wessely, S. (2003). A systematic review of single-session psychological interventions (debriefing) following trauma. *Psychotherapy and Psychosomatics, 72,* 176–184.

Ruzek, J. I., Brymer, M. J., Jacobs, A. K., Layne, C. M., Vernberg, E. M., & Watson, P. J. (in press). Psychological first aid. *Journal of Mental Health Counseling.*

Silverman, W. K., & La Greca, A. M. (2002). Children experiencing disasters: Definitions, reactions, and predictors of outcomes. In A. M. La Greca, W. K. Silverman, E. M. Vernberg, & M. C. Roberts (Eds.), *Helping Children Cope with Disasters* (pp. 11–34). Washington, DC: American Psychological Association.

Stallard, P., Velleman, R., Salter, E., Howse, I., Yule, W., & Taylor, G. (2006). A randomised controlled trial to determine the effectiveness of an early psychological intervention with children involved in road traffic accidents. *Journal of Child Psychology and Psychiatry, 47*, 127–134.

Storm, V., McDermott, B., & Finlayson, D. (1994). *The Bushfire and Me: A Story of What Happened to Me and My Family.* Newtown, Australia: VBD Publications.

Swenson, C. C., Saylor, C. F., Powell, M. P., Stokes, S. J., Foster, K. Y., & Belter, R. W. (1996). Impact of a natural disaster on preschool children: Adjustment 14 months after a hurricane. *American Journal of Orthopsychiatry, 66*, 122–130.

Tolin, D. F., & Foa, E. B. (2006). Sex differences in trauma and posttraumatic stress disorder: A quantitative review of 25 years of research. *Psychological Bulletin, 132*, 959–992.

Vernberg, E. M. (2002). Intervention approaches following disasters. In A. M. La Greca, W. K. Silverman, E. M. Vernberg, & M. C. Roberts (Eds.), *Helping Children Cope with Disasters and Terrorism* (pp. 55–72). Washington, DC: American Psychological Association.

Vernberg, E. M., La Greca, A. M., Silverman, W. K., & Prinstein, M. (1996). Predictors of children's post-disaster functioning following Hurricane Andrew. *Journal of Abnormal Psychology, 105*, 237–248.

Vernberg, E. M., & Vogel, J. M. (1993). Interventions with children after disasters. *Journal of Clinical Child Psychology, 22*, 485–498.

Vogel, J., & Vernberg, E. M. (1993). Children's psychological responses to disaster. *Journal of Clinical Child Psychology, 22*, 464–484.

Wolmer, L., Laor, N., Dedeoglu, C., Siev, J., & Yazgan, Y. (2005). Teacher-mediated intervention after disaster: A controlled three-year follow-up of children's functioning. *Journal of Child Psychology and Psychiatry, 46*, 1161–1168.

Yule, W., Bolton, D., Udwin, O., Boyle, S., O'Ryan, D., & Nurrish, J. (2000). The long-term psychological effects of a disaster experienced in adolescence: I. The incidence and course of PTSD. *Journal of Child Psychology and Psychiatry, 41*, 503–512.

Yule, W., Udwin, O., & Bolton, D. (2002). Mass transportation disasters. In A. M. La Greca, W. K. Silverman, E. M. Vernberg, & M. C. Roberts (Eds.), *Helping Children Cope with Disasters and Terrorism* (pp. 223–240). Washington, DC: American Psychological Association.

Mood Disorders and Problems

9

Mood Disorders in Childhood

COLLEEN M. CUMMINGS and MARY A. FRISTAD

Mood disorders in childhood are associated with significant morbidity, mortality, distress, and impairment. This chapter will review current information on depression and bipolar disorder in childhood. A separate chapter in this volume will review depression and bipolar disorder as they appear in adolescence.

Although somewhat neglected in earlier research, the number of studies on childhood depressive disorders has increased significantly in recent decades. Population studies have reported prevalence rates of depression in children ranging from 0.4% to 2.5% (Anderson & McGee, 1994; Fleming & Offord, 1990). Stark et al. (1996) assert that an early-onset depressive disorder is "a risk factor for later episodes, impacts the youngster's dyads, and has potentially life-threatening consequences" (p. 59). Children's episodes of depression may have shorter durations, but they tend to recur (Kovacs et al., 1984) and can lead to a poor adult outcome, predicting a variety of disorders in adulthood, including depression, bipolar disorder, an anxiety disorder, substance abuse, conduct disorder, and antisocial personality disorder (Weissman et al., 1999). Suicide attempts in childhood are generally rare, but 76.2% of children who have attempted suicide meet DSM-III criteria for a psychiatric disorder. Of these, 37.5%, 26.2%, 7.1%, and 45.2% meet criteria for major depression, dysthymia, mania, or any mood disorder, respectively (Gould et al., 1998).

Research on bipolar disorder in children is less common. For instance, although adolescents report lifetime prevalence rates of bipolar disorder of approximately 1% (Lewinsohn et al., 1995a), similar epidemiological data are not available for children. It should be noted that Lewinsohn and colleagues' methodology involved interviewing high school students who were attending school on the days they conducted their evaluations. They did not interview parents, an important source of information when assessing psychopathology in youth, nor did they seek to interview any adolescents not in school on the days of assessment. Thus, any student

---

COLLEEN M. CUMMINGS and MARY A. FRISTAD • The Ohio State University

too impaired to attend school would have been missed using this strategy. For these two reasons, the 1% figure they published may underreport the true number of cases in the general public. In a national survey of individuals with bipolar disorder, 33% of respondents reported that they were under age 15 when symptoms of bipolar disorder first appeared, 27% were between 15 and 19, and only 39% were age 20 or older (Hirschfeld et al., 2003). In her review article, Weckerly (2002) argues that "pediatric mania represents a distinct, genetically mediated, severe subtype of BP that differs in presentation, correlates, and treatment from the adult form of the disorder" (p. 43). It is considered more severe than adult-onset bipolar disorder, often causing substantial psychosocial impairment and multiple psychiatric hospitalizations (Weckerly, 2002; Wozniak et al., 1995a).

Despite the widespread rates and sometimes devastating effects of mood disorders in children, empirically based treatments for them are few in number. We have limited knowledge about overall treatment efficacy and know even less about related treatment issues, such as comorbidity, family involvement, type of treatment (e.g., group or individual therapy), and relapse prevention.

RELEVANT TREATMENT ISSUES

Comorbidity

Comorbid conditions are the rule, not the exception, for children with mood disorders, and they pose methodological complications when conducting and evaluating treatment studies. Yorbik et al. (2004) compared comorbid conditions in children with major depressive disorder (MDD) to those of adolescents also with MDD. In the child sample, 34.8% suffered from any anxiety disorder (18.9% generalized anxiety disorder, 18.4% separation anxiety disorder), 4.5% suffered from social phobia, 14.9% had attention deficit hyperactivity disorder (ADHD), 10.0% had conduct disorder (CD), and 12.9% suffered from oppositional defiant disorder (ODD). When comorbid conditions exist, depressed youths are more likely to experience increased duration and severity of their disorder, as well as decreased response to treatment and poorer utilization of mental health resources (Birmaher et al., 1996; Lewinsohn et al., 1995b).

Children with bipolar disorder are even more likely than children with depression to have comorbid diagnoses. Wozniak and colleagues (1995b) found that 94% of a sample of children with mania also met DSM-IV-TR criteria for ADHD. Tillman et al. (2003) examined rates of comorbid DSM-IV diagnoses in children and early adolescents with bipolar disorder. They found rates of 96.8%, 22.6%, 4.3%, and 1.1% for disruptive, anxiety, tic, and sleep disorders, respectively, in their sample (Tillman et al., 2003). Comorbid disorders in youth with bipolar disorder can complicate treatment by triggering manic episodes due to either their symptom manifestation or their treatment (Lofthouse & Fristad, 2004).

Family Involvement

Children develop in complex environments and are influenced by a variety of factors, creating a dynamic, intricate, and interactive process (Cummings et al., 2000). Given this, family therapy intuitively appears to be a logical treatment choice for childhood mood disorders. However, few studies have examined the effect of family intervention on childhood mood disorders. Herring and Kaslow (2002) suggest treatment strategies that use developmentally informed models that seek to reconstruct secure attachments in families suffering from depression. The authors assert that depression affects all family members and that "one must assume a developmental, systemic, and cultural framework in which the assessment and enhancement of attachment bonds in all family members is central" (Herring & Kaslow, 2002, p. 511). Stark and colleagues (1996) propose a treatment model that includes a parent component. This component should seek to establish more positive family environments through teaching parenting skills such as behavior management techniques, strategies for parents to increase their child's self-esteem and to adjust their child's role in the family, and ways to reduce destructive conflicts (Stark et al., 1996).

Group Versus Individual Therapy

Both group and individual therapy have been studied. Each poses its own distinct advantages and disadvantages. Individual therapy allows the therapist to tailor therapy to the patient's distinct needs, making it focused and specialized (Lewinsohn & Clarke, 1999). Also, the child may not feel comfortable sharing personal information with a peer group, so the relationship with an empathic individual therapist can help address these more personal issues (Stark et al., 1996). Group therapy, however, provides a supportive atmosphere in which to practice communication and social skills. Additionally, group treatment is cost-effective, can be conducted in school-based or community health clinics, and provides care to a larger number of patients in a shorter period of time (Mufson et al., 2004). In their proposed treatment model, Stark et al. (1996) suggested a combination of group and individual therapy, citing the distinct advantages of both types.

Relapse Prevention

Relapse is common following successfully treatments. Kazdin (1997) suggested a model for continued treatment such that even after improvement, "treatment is modified rather than concluded" (p. 122). In other words, treatment may continue in a more intermittent format. However, it is difficult to test maintenance treatment results, and few such studies have been conducted (e.g., Kroll et al., 1996).

TREATMENTS FOR CHILDHOOD DEPRESSION

Nine empirically based treatment studies of depressive disorders that include children in their samples have been published. Although review of the precise research findings from each study is beyond the scope of this chapter, each treatment showed some type of significant improvement in its sample, in either reduced symptomatology, increased knowledge, or improved family functioning. Despite many differences in sample, technique, and theory, the overlap in content between therapies is striking. Below we describe the active components of these treatments.

Cognitions/Emotions/Behavior

Mood-disordered children as young as 8 to 11 report depressive cognitions similar to those found in adults (Harrington, 2005). Cognitive-behavioral therapy (CBT) seeks to identify these negative thoughts associated with depression and encourages behaving in more positive and engaging ways. Core cognitive techniques for youth include self-monitoring, cognitive restructuring, and identifying underlying assumptions. Core behavioral techniques include exposure, behavioral contingencies, self-reinforcement, activity scheduling, and relaxation training (Harrington, 2005).

Each treatment study reviewed had a significant CBT component. Vostanis et al. (1996) developed a basic CBT intervention for children to be administered individually, in which they taught children to recognize and label their emotions and to change negative cognitive attributions. Butler et al. (1980) tested a cognitive restructuring treatment, influenced by the work of Beck (1976), Ellis (1962), and Knaus (1974). The objective was to teach recognition of irrational and self-deprecating thoughts, enhance listening skills, and help children to understand the relationship between destructive thoughts and feelings that lead to depressive symptomatology (Butler et al., 1980). Stark et al. (1987) endorsed a similar self-control therapy, combining cognitive and behavioral skills training to teach children adaptive ways to self-monitor, self-evaluate performance, attribute the causes of outcomes (good and bad), and self-consequate. Thus, many cognitive-behavioral strategies frequently used in adult treatment, mainly helping individuals identify negative cognitions and change them into more adaptive thoughts and behaviors, can be successfully implemented to help children as well.

Weisz et al. (1997) tested another type of CBT—Primary and Secondary Control Enhancement Training (PASCET)—based on the premise that depression can be controlled by teaching children to apply primary control to distressing conditions that are changeable and secondary control to conditions that are not changeable. In Asarnow et al.'s (2002) 10-session CBT therapy combined with a family education component, the goal was for children to progress from skill acquisition to skill consolidation to developing a teaching role for their families.

Kroll and colleagues (1996) utilized CBT to address relapse prevention with their Continuation-Cognitive-Behavioral Therapy (C-CBT). C-CBT stresses that even though symptoms may be managed during the acute phase, the child is still vulnerable to their return several months after treatment. Therefore, it deals with ongoing risk factors for young people, such as poor peer and family relationships, subsyndromal symptoms, and self-deprecating cognitions. Children are taught to recognize harmful cognitions and stressors that may precede their own depressive episodes (Kroll et al., 1996). Relapse prevention is an important part of treatment of depression, and future research is warranted on this topic.

Jayson et al. (1998) administered a similar cognitive-behavioral treatment program to assess predictors of relapse in children and adolescents with major depression after they had received CBT. The treatment package administered was based on research findings from studies of cognitive abnormalities found in children with depression, and its aims are "the recognizing and labelling of emotions, the change of negative cognitive attributions, and the enhancement of social skills" (Vostanis & Harrington, 1994, p. 111). The researchers found that, overall, 60% of patients remitted by the end of treatment. Younger and less severely impaired youth were more likely to respond to CBT (Jayson et al., 1998).

Kahn and Kehle (1990) tested two other types of cognitive-behavioral therapies for childhood depression. Their small-group relaxation treatment condition focused on the relationships between anxiety-inducing situations, feelings of stress and tension, and depressed mood. Participants were first taught progressive relaxation skills, then modifications to some of these skills (e.g., relaxation of fewer muscle groups and relaxation through recall, counting, mental imagery, and breathing), and finally the application of these skills to specific anxiety-inducing experiences. Lecture, demonstration, discussion, practice, and feedback procedures were used in treatment. In the same treatment study, Kahn and Kehle (1990) tested an individual self-modeling treatment during which participants first identified target nondepressive behaviors, such as appropriate eye contact, expressions of positive affect (e.g., smiling, laughing, gesturing), and verbalizing positive self-attributions. Subjects then were videotaped performing these behaviors, and their therapy included observing these three-minute tapes. Kahn and Kehle's two treatment modalities emphasized first the link between anxious and depressive symptomatology, and second the importance of practicing specific nondepressive behaviors. Perhaps a combination of the two types of treatment would be an interesting next step.

Fristad and colleagues' multifamily psychoeducation groups program (MFPG) contains cognitive-behavioral components to help children diagnosed with mood disorders learn to better manage and control their symptoms (2006). For example, the "Thinking-Feeling-Doing" (T-F-D) exercise is designed to teach children the relationships between their thoughts, feelings, and behaviors and how to modify "hurtful" (e.g., negative) thoughts and behaviors into "helpful" (e.g., positive) thoughts and behaviors. Children learn impulse control strategies in the "Stop-Think-Plan-Do-Check" exercise and anger management in the "Taking Charge of the Mad, Bad, Sad Feelings" (Goldberg-Arnold & Fristad, 2003). MFPG is an example of how cognitive-behavioral components can be combined with family-based and social skills training to treat childhood mood disorders. The latter two components will be discussed.

Social Skills

Most therapies tested sought to help children with their peer relationships. In addition to using cognitive-behavioral techniques, the MFPG program emphasizes that impairment at an early age can prevent children from developing age-appropriate social skills. Thus, children are taught skills in verbal and nonverbal communication and problem solving, with role-plays frequently focusing on common peer issues (Fristad et al., 1998). Vostanis and colleagues (1996) devoted two of nine sessions to social problem solving, teaching children how to handle interpersonal problems and the importance of engaging in social activities for self-esteem. Social problem solving and the teaching of target social behaviors were included in other trials as well (Asarnow et al., 2002; Kahn & Kehle, 1990; Kroll et al., 1996).

Stark et al. (1987) specifically tested a behavioral problem-solving condition that placed a large emphasis on social relationships. Participants were taught self-monitoring, pleasant activity scheduling, and problem-solving skills. The discussion format helped children develop group problem-solving and communication skills as well as constructive ways to express their feelings to others (Stark et al., 1987). Butler et al.'s role-playing treatment (1980) also targeted the acquisition of social skills. The researchers intended that, through role-playing and discussion, children would be sensitized to their own and others' feelings and would practice social interaction skills and problem-solving approaches. As children's social relationships are so important in their development, future treatment studies targeting this aspect of childhood depression are crucial.

Family Systems

Finally, several studies specifically targeted the family environments of depressed children. The MFPG program presents mood disorders to families as biologically driven and not caused by anyone in the family, so as to avoid blame and feelings of guilt. Instead, the family is offered support and validation as they struggle to live with a child with a mood disorder (Fristad et al., 1996). Groups begin and end with parents and children meeting together, but with the bulk of each session run separately for parents and children (Fristad et al., 2003b). Within these groups, emphasis is placed on receiving social support, information, and skill building. A major objective of the program is to decrease family interaction problems, which can trigger episodes and protract recovery (Asarnow et al., 1987, 1993).

Kahn and Kehle (1990) adapted Lewinsohn and Clarke's (1984) Coping with Depression course to a younger sample partly by including a parent component. Parents were provided instruction in the cognitive and behavioral skills taught to their children, with the intention that they would understand and monitor their child's progress, offer guidance, and adapt to treatment gains.

Asarnow and colleagues (2002) tested a combined cognitive-behavioral and family education program. The researchers intended for the family education component to "enhance generalization to the real-world settings and promote a supportive family environment" (p. 225). For instance, during the family education session, the children present to their parents a videotape in which they demonstrate and practice the skills they have learned. During the family education sessions, parents are taught the conceptual rationale of the program, the important role they can play in their child's recovery, and how to help their child feel positively about what he has learned. The parents then serve as consultants and helpers to their children in putting skills into action and interacting positively with their children to provide a supportive family environment (Asarnow et al., 2002).

A family or parent component appears to be an essential part of treatment for childhood mood disorders. Once equipped with a better understanding of their child's depressive disorder, parents can play a valuable role in their child's treatment, both through recognizing and changing destructive family interaction patterns as well as through encouraging and helping their child with their new skills.

TREATMENTS FOR CHILDHOOD BIPOLAR DISORDER

Geller and Luby (1997) point out that childhood bipolar disorder differs from adult bipolar disorder in the more rapid cycling between mood episodes, the higher rates of comorbidity with ADHD, ODD, and CD, and the more chronic nature with a very early age of onset (Geller & Luby, 1997; Geller et al., 1995). Geller and colleagues (2003) assert that according to current findings, prepubertal and early adolescent bipolar disorder "resembled the severest form of late-teenage/adult-onset mania by presenting with a chronic, mixed-manic, psychotic, continuously cycling picture" (p. 47). There is some debate as to the course and outcome of bipolar disorder in children; however, Kowatch et al. (2005) conclude, "It is clear that they manifest a serious disorder and that early diagnosis and aggressive treatment are necessary for these patients to function successfully within their families, peer groups, and schools" (p. 214).

Three psychosocial treatments have been tested in children diagnosed with bipolar disorder (BPD). These are Fristad and colleagues' work (2006) with multifamily psychoeducation groups (MFPG) and individual family psychoeducation (IFP) and Pavuluri and colleagues' (2004) child- and family-focused cognitive behavioral therapy (CFF-CBT). Following are descriptions of these three types of therapies. All three studies showed significant improvements in their sample posttreatment. Examples of these improvements include increases in parental knowledge of these treatments, lower ratings of severity of symptoms, and improved family climate (Fristad, 2006; Fristad et al., 2003a, 2003b; Pavuluri et al., 2004).

Multifamily Psychoeducation Groups

MFPG consists of eight 90-minute sessions using a manual-based, multi-family group format, designed for outpatient children with any major mood disorders and their parents (Fristad et al., 2003a). The authors assert that it is not specific techniques of MFPG that are unique, but rather their integration in a psychoeducational framework. The program focuses on educating families about their child's illness and its treatment in the community, school, and mental health system; training families in communication and problem-solving strategies using CBT interventions to address management of the child's mood symptoms; and providing social support (Fristad et al., 2003a; Goldberg-Arnold & Fristad, 2003).

Each session begins with a check-in meeting of parents and children, at which time they discuss projects assigned and issues from the previous week. Parent and child groups then separate to complete their particular goals, topics, and activities. After their "lesson of the day," children receive 15–20 minutes of *in vivo* social skills training via noncompetitive group recreational activities. At the end of each session, children rejoin their parents to discuss what they have learned and their upcoming family projects (Fristad et al., 2003b).

A pivotal message of MFPG for children is "It's not your fault, but it's your challenge." Via that motto, children are reminded they are not to *blame* for their symptoms, nor are they the *cause* of their symptoms. However, they are responsible, with the help of their parents and treatment teams, for *managing* their symptoms, thus taking increased responsibility for symptom management. The "Naming the Enemy" exercise illustrates this concept in the children's group during the second session. The group leader draws two columns on a large sheet of paper, entitling them "Things I like about me," and "My symptoms." Children first generate lists of positive things they like about themselves, such as "good at math," or "likes animals," or "funny," which they place in the first column. In the second column, the children discuss and list symptoms they have experienced. The group leader than demonstrates how symptoms can cover positive traits and talents by folding the second column over the first and, additionally, how treatment can help "put the symptoms behind the child and allow their true character and strengths to come into view" (Lofthouse & Fristad, 2004, p. 83).

Individual Family Psychoeducation

Despite the advantages of group therapy, in many cases, individual therapy may be the most practical or available choice for children with bipolar disorder. Families may not feel comfortable sharing information in front of a group, clinicians may not have the resources of number of clients necessary for group therapy, or a family may want immediate treatment instead of waiting for a group session to begin (Fristad, 2006). The original format of Fristad and colleagues' IFP was delivered in 16 50-minute sessions, with 15 sessions addressing specific issues of bipolar disorder and an optional "in-the-bank" session for families to use as needed (e.g., crisis management, deal with specific issues, or additional review). In addition to content that generally mimics the MFPG content, a "Healthy Habits" component was added to improve diet, exercise, and sleep patterns to facilitate recovery and prevent relapse (Fristad, 2006). It has been modified more recently to include 24 sessions, with 9 for the parent alone, 9 for the child (with parent joining at the beginning and end), 1 for the parents, child and school professional, and 1 for parents, child, and siblings. Four "in-the-bank" sessions are available, as previously described (Leffler et al., 2006).

Child- and Family-Focused Cognitive-Behavioral Therapy

Pavuluri et al. (2004) described three features of CFF-CBT. First, CFF-CBT takes into account three sets of factors related to bipolar disorder. These are the brain's affective circuitry, characteristics of the illness, and the family, community, and school-based stressors resulting from and associated with BPD. Second, CFF-CBT combines aspects of cognitive-behavioral therapy with interpersonal psychotherapy to meet the interpersonal difficulties often faced by BPD patients. Third, CFF-CBT stresses the importance of helping parents with their frustrations and specifically works with the child's symptoms and impairments caused by BPD (Pavuluri et al., 2004).

CFF-CBT requires that children be on medication in order to participate. It utilizes the acronym RAINBOW, to list active treatment components. These include

> R = routine, A = affect regulation, I = I can do it, N = No negative thoughts, B = be a good friend and balanced lifestyle for parents, O = oh, how can we solve this problem, W = ways to get support. (Pavuluri et al., 2004, p. 532)

The RAINBOW treatment protocol is administered in 12 sessions, alternating among parent-only sessions, child-only sessions, parents and child together, and parents and siblings. In many cases, therapists also work with the school personnel, educating teachers and other school personnel about the child's illness, while informing the parents about different options to optimize school-based interventions (Pavuluri et al., 2004).

Many similarities exist among these three psychosocial treatments for pediatric bipolar disorder. For example, all three stress the importance of the disorder's effect on the entire family and seek to equip the families with powerful strategies and techniques for dealing with their son's or daughter's disorder. MFPG's motto, "It's not your fault, but it's your challenge," summarizes the philosophy of all three treatment approaches—the importance of families taking an active role in their child's treatment as well as learning the information necessary to seek out the best treatment possible. Since so few treatment programs for bipolar disorder in children currently exist, future research is essential.

CLINICAL VIGNETTE

Jason is an 11-year-old boy who began MFPG with a diagnosis of bipolar disorder-not otherwise specified (BP-NOS), ODD, and ADHD. Although Jason had performed at the gifted level on IQ tests, he had struggled with ADHD since age 3 as well as a learning disability in writing. Over the past year, his mother described symptoms of intense irritability and aggressive behavior coupled with symptoms of anhedonia, sleep difficulties, poorer academic performance, psychomotor agitation, and self-injurious behaviors, such as trying to choke himself while angry. He began trying to kiss his mother on the lips and attempted to spend thousands of dollars purchasing parts on the Internet to make a space vehicle. These behaviors escalated after the family's move to a new city. Within three weeks of moving, Jason began engaging in increasingly problematic behaviors, such as refusing to go to school, threatening his mom with a knife, and running away from the yard when angry. Jason's mother described Jason as "my black box ... you never quite know what's going on inside there."

During their initial interview, Jason's mother described a recent incident. On the way to school, Jason began throwing things at her while she was driving and tried to jump out of the moving car. His mother drove to the police station for assistance, where Jason struck a police officer, who caught him after he ran away. Jason was handcuffed and taken to the emergency room in the back of a police car. He later was released with the admonition to follow up with outpatient services. Before this incident, Jason had seen a few mental health professionals; after this incident, medication was added to his treatment regimen. Jason's parents demonstrated strong love and concern for their son, yet his behavior profoundly impacted the family life. His father expressed a desire to connect with his son more, but "It's been hard to get into Jason's world and that's been a frustration."

Throughout their participation in MFPG, Jason and his parents began to experience improvement in Jason's symptoms and the family's functioning. During the first session, Jason initially refused to join the child group. When he finally joined, the therapists noted he "seemed to derive pleasure from disrupting others and causing chaos." As sessions progressed, however, Jason began to increase his prosocial behavior. Although he still misbehaved, Jason began to share with the group some problems associated with his mood episodes and the medications he was taking. By the final session, Jason was demonstrating his knowledge of material discussed in sessions, actively participating in sessions, and often interacting appropriately with his peers.

Jason's parents actively and enthusiastically participated in group, reading their session materials and completing all projects. They discussed their son's symptoms and difficulties, such as his denial of problems and his destructive anger and irritability.

At the program's conclusion, Jason was still symptomatic, yet he and his parents appeared much better equipped to address the challenges of his disorder. At Jason's six-month follow-up interview, his mother reported that Jason was beginning to show improvements, such as less irritability and aggression and better sleeping patterns. They had made a medication adjustment and Jason had begun treatment with a new therapist whom both Jason and the family found helpful. By Jason's one-year follow-up interview, his mother stated that Jason had showed continued improvement in his moods, family relationships, schoolwork, and peer relationships. By his final 18-month follow-up, Jason's mother reported being very satisfied with his current treatment regimen. She described Jason as having made tremendous progress and expressed relief at having found an appropriate diagnosis (bipolar disorder) that allowed the family to move forward with the appropriate treatment. Jason had discontinued psychotherapy with an agreement to return if symptoms intensified, due to his outstanding progress. Although Jason still experienced some irritability, mood lability, and occasional aggressive outbursts, he had made many friends, was playing on a recreation league soccer team, was getting along better with family members, and was earning all A's in school. Overall, his mother expressed hope for Jason, stating, "I expect great things for him in the future. ... I think he's got all the tools and the skills that he needs to be successful in life, despite his having bipolar disorder ... ."

FUTURE DIRECTIONS

Many advances have been made in developing and testing psychosocial treatments for children with mood disorders. However, much work remains to be done. Different populations of affected children, different styles of therapies, and different treatment methods all need further examination (Lewinsohn & Clarke, 1999). In particular, four areas of emphasis are warranted. First, more studies are needed with young children. As summarized by Fristad et al. (2002b), "The vast majority of the published literature pertains to treatment of depressed adolescents. A limited number of studies have examined the treatment of depression in mixed-age groups ... . Few studies are available for the treatment of childhood depressive disorders ..." (pp. 230–231).

Second, much more work is needed to develop empirically proven treatments for bipolar disorder in children. In their current review of the literature on psychosocial treatments for children with bipolar disorder, Lofthouse and Fristad (2004) noted many gaps and concluded the following foci were critical: developing effective medication regimens; creating school-based interventions; determining the incremental effects of psychosocial programs in conjunction with pharmacotherapy, methods, and opportunities for transporting treatments into the community; and working with therapies for younger children with BPD.

Third, almost no progress has been made in determining the efficacy of psychosocial treatments for children of varying demographic, ethnic, and socioeconomic backgrounds (Lofthouse & Fristad, 2004, p. 84). The large majority of children who participate in and complete treatment studies are white, therefore demonstrating the crucial need for treatment studies on more ethnically diverse populations of children. Several of the studies in the current treatment review did not report demographic information such as ethnicity or socioeconomic background. Of those that did, representation of minorities in the samples ranged from only 10% of the sample to 43%. Rossello and Bernal (1999), pioneers in their studies with Latino adolescents, asserted that, "to the extent that minorities are systematically excluded from treatment research, we run the risk of constructing an ethnocentric psychological science" (p. 735).

Finally, many have identified the need for treatment research to more closely resemble clinical practice. Weisz et al. (1995) noted that specialized research clinics have many advantages over clinical settings, such as highly trained clinicians, paid research staff, and narrow inclusion criteria. However, that also leads to disadvantages. Weisz et al. (1992) concluded, "In general, research has produced extensive information on treatments that are not very much like those used in practice" (p. 577). While there clearly is a role for laboratory-based studies in the development of psychosocial treatments, future child treatment studies also should be conducted in nonlaboratory settings.

Progress in the study of empirically based treatments has been made in the past 25 years for childhood depression and in the past 5 years for childhood bipolar disorder. The treatments and components described above are very promising, yet much more research is clearly needed.

REFERENCES

Anderson, J. C., & McGee, R. (1994). Comorbidity of depression in children and adolescents. In W. M. Reynolds & H. F. Johnston (Eds.), *Handbook of Depression in Children and Adolescents* (pp. 581–601). New York: Plenum Press.

Angold, J., & Costello, E. (1987). *The Moods and Feelings Questionnaire*. Unpublished document.

Asarnow, J. R., Ben-Meir, S. L., & Goldstein, M. J. (1987). Family factors in childhood depressive and schizophrenia spectrum disorders: A preliminary report. In K. Hahlweg & M. J. Goldstein (Eds.), *Understanding Major Mental Disorder: The Contribution of Family Interaction Research* (pp. 156–175). New York: Family Process Press.

Asarnow, J. R., Goldstein, M. J., Thompson, M., & Guthrie, D. (1993). One-year outcomes of depressive disorders in child psychiatric inpatients: Evaluation of the prognostic power of a brief measure of expressed emotion. *Journal of Child Psychology and Psychiatry, 34,* 129–137.

Asarnow, J. R., Scott, C. V., & Mintz, J. (2002). A combined cognitive-behavioral family education intervention for depression in children: A treatment development study. *Cognitive Therapy and Research, 26*(2), 221–229.

Beck, A. T. (1976). *Cognitive Therapy and the Emotional Disorders.* New York: International Universities Press.

Birmaher, B., Ryan, N. D., Williamson, D. E., Brent, D. A., Kaufman, J., Dahl, R. E., et al. (1996). Childhood and adolescent depression: A review of the past 10 years, Part 1. *Journal of the American Academy of Child and Adolescent Psychiatry, 35*(11), 1427–1439.

Butler, L., Miezitis, S., Friedman, R., & Cole, E. (1980). The effect of two school-based intervention programs on depressive symptoms in preadolescents. *American Educational Research Journal, 17*(1), 111–119.

Causey, D., & Dubow, E. (1992). Development of a self-report coping measure for elementary school children. *Journal of Clinical Child Psychopathology Review, 21*(1), 47–59.

Cole, E. (1979). *Role-playing as a modality for alleviating depressive symptoms in 10–12-year-old children*. Unpublished doctoral dissertation. Ontario Institute for Studies in Education.

Cummings, E. M., Davies, P. T., & Campbell, S. B. (2000). *Developmental Psychopathology and Family Process*. New York: Guilford Press.

Ellis, A. (1962). *Reason and Emotion in Psychotherapy*. New York: Lyle Stuart.

Fleming, J. E., & Offord, D. R. (1990). Epidemiology of childhood depressive disorders: A critical review. *Journal of the American Academy of Child & Adolescent Psychiatry, 29*(4), 571–580.

Friedman, R. J., Miezitis, S., & Butler, L. F. (1977). Development and evaluation of school-based assessment and treatment approaches for depressed children: Phase I. Report to the Ministry of Education.

Friedmann, M. S., & Goldstein, M. J. (1993). Relatives' awareness of their own expressed emotion as measured by a self-report adjective checklist. *Family Process, 32*, 459–471.

Fristad, M. A. (2006). Psychoeducational treatment for school-aged children with bipolar disorder. *Development and Psychopathology, 18*(4), 1289–1306.

Fristad, M. A., Gavazzi, S. M., Centolella, D. M., & Soldano, K. W. (1996). Psychoeducation: A promising intervention strategy for families of children and adolescents with mood disorders. *Contemporary Family Therapy: An International Journal, 18*(3), 371–384.

Fristad, M. A., Gavazzi, S. M., & Mackinaw-Koons, B. (2003a). Family psychoeducation: An adjunctive intervention for children with bipolar disorder. *Biological Psychiatry, 53*, 1000–1008.

Fristad, M. A., Gavazzi, S. M., & Soldano, K. W. (1998). Multi-family psychoeducation groups for childhood mood disorders: A program description and preliminary efficacy data. *Contemporary Family Therapy: An International Journal, 20*(3), 385–402.

Fristad, M. A., Goldberg-Arnold, J. S., & Gavazzi, S. M. (2002a). Multifamily psychoeducation groups (MFPG) for families of children with bipolar disorder. *Bipolar Disorders, 4*, 254–262.

Fristad, M. A., Goldberg-Arnold, J. S., & Gavazzi, S. M. (2003b). Multi-family psychoeducation groups in the treatment of children with mood disorders. *Journal of Marital and Family Therapy, 29*(4), 491–504.

Fristad, M. A., Shaver, A. E., & Holderle, K. E. (2002b). Mood disorders in childhood and adolescence. In D. T. Marsh & M. A. Fristad (Eds.), *Handbook of Serious Emotional Disturbance in Children and Adolescents* (pp. 228–265). Hoboken, NJ: John Wiley & Sons, Inc.

Geller, B., Craney, J. L., Bolhofner, K., DelBello, M. P., Axelson, D., Luby, J., et al. (2003). Phenomenology and longitudinal course of children with a prepubertal and early adolescent bipolar disorder phenotype. In B. Geller & M. P. DelBello (Eds.), *Bipolar Disorder in Childhood and Early Adolescence* (pp. 25–50). New York: Guilford Press.

Geller, B., & Luby, J. (1997). Child and adolescent bipolar disorder: A review of the past 10 years. *Journal of the American Academy of Child and Adolescent Psychiatry, 36*(9), 1168–1176.

Geller, B., Sun, K., Zimerman, B., Luby, J., Frazier, J., & Williams, M. (1995). Complex and rapid-cycling in bipolar children and adolescents: A preliminary study. *Journal of Affective Disorders, 34*, 259–268.

Goldberg-Arnold, J. S., & Fristad, M. A. (2003). Psychotherapy for children with bipolar disorder. In B. Geller & M. P. DelBello (Eds.), *Bipolar Disorder in Childhood and Early Adolescence* (pp. 272–295). New York: Guilford Press.

Gould, M. S., King, R., Greenwald, S., Fisher, P., Schwab-Stone, M., Kramer, R., et al. (1998). Psychopathology associated with suicidal ideation and attempts among children and adolescents. *Journal of the American Academy of Child & Adolescent Psychiatry, 37*(9), 915–923.

Harrington, R. (2005). Depressive disorders. In P. J. Graham (Ed.). *Cognitive Behaviour Therapy for Children and Families* (pp. 263–281). Cambridge: Cambridge University Press.

Herring, M., & Kaslow, N. J. (2002). Depression and attachment in families: A child-focused perspective. *Family Process, 41*(3), 494–518.

Hirschfeld, R. M. A., Lewis, L., & Vornik, L. A. (2003). Perceptions and impact of bipolar disorder: How far have we really come? Results of the National Depressive and

Manic-Depressive Associations 2000 survey of individuals with bipolar disorder. *Journal of Clinical Psychiatry, 64*(2), 161–174.

Hollon, S. D., & Kendall, P. C. (1980). Cognitive self-statements in depression: Development of an Automatic Thoughts Questionnaire. *Cognitive Therapy and Research, 4*, 383–397.

Jayson, D., Wood, A., Kroll, L., Fraser, J., & Harrington, R. (1998). Which depressed patients respond to cognitive-behavioral treatment? *Journal of the American Academy of Child and Adolescent Psychiatry, 37*(1), 35–39.

Kahn, J. S., & Kehle, T. J. (1990). Comparison of cognitive-behavioral, relaxation, and self-modeling interventions for depression. *School Psychology Review, 19*(2), 196–204.

Kazdin, A. E. (1997). A model for developing effective treatments: Progression and interplay of theory, research, and practice. *Journal of Clinical Child Psychology, 26*(2), 114–129.

Knaus, W. (1974). *Rational-Emotive Education: A Manual for Elementary School Teachers.* New York: Institute for Rational Living.

Kovacs, M. (1981). Rating scales to assess depression in school-aged children. *Acta Paedopsychiatrica, 46*, 305–315.

Kovacs, M., Feinberg, T. L., Crouse-Novak, M. A., Paulauskas, S. L., & Finkelstein, R. (1984). Depressive disorders in childhood. I. A longitudinal prospective study of characteristics and recovery. *Archives of General Psychiatry, 41*(3), 229–237.

Kowatch, R. A., Fristad, M. A., Birmaher, B., Wagner, K. D., Findling, R. L., Hellander, M., et al. (2005). Treatment guidelines for children and adolescents with bipolar disorder: Child psychiatric workgroup on bipolar disorder. *Journal of the American Academy of Child and Adolescent Psychiatry, 44*(3), 213–239.

Kroll, L., Harrington, R., Jayson, D., Fraser, J., & Gowers, S. (1996). Pilot study of continuation of cognitive-behavioral therapy for major depressive disorder in adolescent psychiatric patients. *Journal of the American Academy of Child and Adolescent Psychiatry, 35*(9), 1156–1167.

Leffler, J. M., Fristad, M. A., & Walters, K. (2006). *Pilot results from Individual Family Psychoeducation (IFP)—24 session adaptation in children with bipolar disorder.* Poster session presented at the Kansas Conference in Clinical Child and Adolescent Psychology, Lawrence, KS.

Lewinsohn, P. M., & Clarke, G. N. (1984). *The Coping with Depression Course Adolescent Version: Instructor's Manual for Parent Course.* Eugene: Castalia Publishing Company.

Lewinsohn, P. M., & Clarke, G. N. (1999). Psychosocial treatments for adolescent depression. *Clinical Psychology Review, 19*(3), 329–342.

Lewinsohn, P. M., Klein, D. N., & Seeley, J. R. (1995a). Bipolar disorders in a community sample of older adolescents: Prevalence, phenomenology, comorbidity, and course. *Journal of the American Academy of Child and Adolescent Psychiatry, 34*(4), 454–463.

Lewinsohn, P. M., Rohde, P., & Seeley, J. R. (1995b). Adolescent psychopathology: III. The clinical consequences of comorbidity. *Journal of the American Academy of Child and Adolescent Psychiatry, 34*(4), 510–519.

Lofthouse, N., & Fristad, M. A. (2004). Psychosocial interventions for children with early-onset bipolar spectrum disorder. *Clinical Child and Family Psychology Review, 7*(2), 71–88.

Miezitis, S., Friedman, R. J., Butler, L. F., & Blanchard, J. (1978). Development and evaluation of school-based assessment and treatment approaches for depression children: Phase II. Report to the Ministry of Education, Ontario.

Mufson, L., Gallagher, T., Dorta, K. P., & Young, J. F. (2004). A group adaptation of interpersonal psychotherapy for depressed adolescents. *American Journal of Psychotherapy, 58*(2), 220–237.

Pavuluri, M. N., Graczyk, P. A., Henry, D. B., Carbray, J. A., Heidenreich, J., & Miklowitz, D. J. (2004). Child- and family-focused cognitive behavioral therapy for pediatric bipolar disorder: Development and preliminary results. *Journal of the American Academy of Child and Adolescent Psychiatry, 43*(5), 528–537.

Petti, T. A. (1978). Depression in hospitalized child psychiatry patients: Approaches to measuring depression. *Journal of the American Academy of Child Psychiatry, 17*, 49–69.

Piers, E. V. (1969). *Manual for the Piers-Harris Children's Self-Concept Scale.* Nashville, TN: Counselor Recordings & Tests.

Piers, E. V. (1984). *Piers-Harris Children's Self-Concept Scale: Revised Manual 1984.* Los Angeles: Western Psychological Services.

Poznanski, E. O., Grossman, J. A., Buchsbaum, Y., Banegas, M., Freeman, L., & Gibbons, R. (1984). Preliminary studies of the reliability and validity of the Children's Depression Rating Scale. *Journal of the American Academy of Child Psychiatry, 23,* 191–197.

Puig-Antich, J., & Chambers, W. (1978). *The Schedule for Affective Disorders and Schizophrenia for School Age Children (Kiddie-SADS).* New York: New York Psychiatric Institute.

Reynolds, W. M. (1987). *Reynolds Adolescent Depression Scale.* Odessa, TX: Psychological Assessment Resources, Inc.

Reynolds, W. M., Anderson, G., & Bartell, N. (1985). Measuring depression in children: A multimethod assessment investigations. *Journal of Abnormal Child Psychology, 13,* 513–526.

Rossello, J., & Bernal, G. (1999). The efficacy of cognitive-behavioral and interpersonal treatments for depression in Puerto Rican adolescents. *Journal of Consulting and Clinical Psychology, 67*(5), 734–745.

Shaffer, D., Gould, M., Brasic, J., et al. (1983). Children's Global Assessment Scale (C-GAS). *Archives of General Psychiatry, 40,* 1228–1231.

Spearing, M., Post, R., Leverich, G., Brandt, D., & Nolen, W. (1997). Modification of the Clinical Global Impressions (CGI) Scale for use in bipolar illness (BP): the CGI-BP. *Psychiatry Research, 73,* 159–171.

Stark, K. D., Napolitano, S., Swearer, S., Schmidt, K., Jaramillo, D., & Hoyle, J. (1996). Issues in the treatment of depressed children. *Applied & Preventive Psychology, 5*(2), 59–83.

Stark, K. D., Reynolds, W. M., & Kaslow, N. J. (1987). A comparison of the relative efficacy of self-control therapy and a behavioral problem-solving therapy for depression in children. *Journal of Abnormal Child Psychology, 15*(1), 91–113.

Tillman, R., Geller, B., Bolhofner, K., Craney, J. L., Williams, M., & Zimerman, B. (2003). Ages of onset and rates of syndromal and subsyndromal comorbid DSM-IV diagnoses in a prepubertal and early adolescent bipolar disorder phenotype. *Journal of the American Academy of Child and Adolescent Psychiatry, 42*(12), 1486–1493.

Vostanis, P., Feehan, C., Grattan, E., & Bickerton, W. L. (1996). A randomised controlled out-patient trial of cognitive-behavioural treatment for children and adolescent with depression: 9-month follow-up. *Journal of Affective Disorders, 40,* 105–116.

Vostanis, P., & Harrington, R. C. (1994). Cognitive-behavioural treatment of depressive disorder in child psychiatric patients: Rationale and description of a treatment package. *European Child and Adolescent Psychiatry, 3,* 111–123.

Weckerly, J. (2002). Pedriatric bipolar mood disorder. *Journal of Developmental and Behavioral Pediatrics, 23*(1), 42–56.

Weissman, M. M., Wolk, S., Wickramaratne, P., Goldstein, R. B., Adams, P., Greenwald, S., et al. (1999). Children with prepubertal-onset major depressive disorder and anxiety grown up. *Archives of General Psychiatry, 56*(9), 794–801.

Weisz, J. R., Donenberg, G. R., Han, S. S., & Weiss, B. (1995). Bridging the gap between laboratory and clinic in child and adolescent psychotherapy. *Journal of Consulting and Clinical Psychology, 63*(5), 688–701.

Weisz, J. R., Thurber, C. A., Sweeney, L., Proffitt, V. D., & LeGagnoux, G. L. (1997). Brief treatment of mild-to-moderate child depression using primary and secondary control enhancement training. *Journal of Consulting and Clinical Psychology, 65*(4), 703–707.

Weisz, J. R., Weiss, B., & Donenberg, G. R. (1992). The lab versus the clinic: Effects of child and adolescent psychotherapy. *American Psychologist, 47*(12), 1578–1585.

Weller, E. B., Weller, R. A., Rooney, M. T., & Fristad, M. A. (1999). *Children's Interview for Psychiatric Syndromes (Chips).* Washington, DC: American Psychiatric Press, Inc.

Wozniak, J., Biederman, J., Kiely, K., Ablon, J. S., Faraone, S. V., Mundy, E., et al. (1995a). Mania-like symptoms suggestive of childhood-onset bipolar disorder in clinically referred children. *Journal of the American Academy of Child and Adolescent Psychiatry, 34*(7), 867–874.

Wozniak, J., Biederman, J., Mundy, E., Mennin, D., et al. (1995b). A pilot family study of childhood-onset mania. *Journal of the American Academy of Child & Adolescent Psychiatry, 34*(12), 1577–1583.

Yorbik, O., Birmaher, B., Axelson, D., Williamson, D. E., & Ryan, N. D. (2004). Clinical characteristics of depressive symptoms in children and adolescents with major depressive disorder. *Journal of Clinical Psychiatry, 65*(12), 1654–1659.

Young, R., Biggs, J., Ziegler, V., & Meyer, D. (1978). A rating scale for mania: Reliability, validity, and sensitivity. *British Journal of Psychiatry, 133*, 429–435.

10

Empirically Supported Psychotherapies for Adolescent Depression and Mood Disorders

JOHN F. CURRY and SARA J. BECKER

Mood disorders are among the most prevalent psychiatric disorders among adolescents (Lewinsohn et al., 1993). When untreated or under-treated, adolescent mood disorders are associated with serious short- and long-term consequences such as impaired school, family, and social functioning and elevated risk of suicide attempts and completions (see Weisz et al., 2006). The substantial, persistent, and recurring costs associated with adolescent mood disorders highlight the need for effective interventions.

In this chapter we will review and, to the extent possible, compare empirically supported treatments (ESTs) for adolescent mood disorders, using the criteria developed by Chambless and Hollon (1998). We augment this set of criteria with the consideration of two key methodological issues: whether the treatment has been evaluated relative to a passive or active comparison condition and whether the treatment was analyzed using completer or intent-to-treat (ITT) analyses. In line with a recent meta-analysis by Weisz and colleagues (2006), we view comparison to an active

---

JOHN F. CURRY and SARA J. BECKER • Duke University and Duke University Medical Center

condition using ITT analyses as the most stringent test of a treatment, and comparison to a passive condition using completer analyses as the least stringent test.

ADOLESCENT MOOD DISORDERS

Following current diagnostic categorization, there are two major branches of mood disorders; depressive (unipolar) disorders and bipolar disorders (American Psychiatric Association, 1994). Depressive disorders include major depressive disorder (MDD), dysthymic disorder (DD), and depressive disorder-not otherwise specified (D-NOS). Full manifestation of depressive symptomatology occurs in MDD, while partial manifestation is characteristic of DD and of DD-NOS. Bipolar disorders (BD), characterized both by manic or hypomanic and by depressive episodes, include those with full manic symptomatology (Bipolar I) and those with partial manic (hypomanic) symptomatology (Bipolar II). In addition, cyclothymic disorder is marked by partial depressive and partial manic episodes (cycles of dysthymia and hypomania). Bipolar disorder-not otherwise specified (BD-NOS), like its depressive counterpart, is a partial syndrome that fails to meet criteria for the other bipolar disorders.

Current prevalence estimates suggest that approximately 2.5% of adolescents meet criteria for MDD and about 0.50% for DD at any given time (Lewinsohn et al., 1993). Epidemiological studies suggest, however, that the lifetime prevalence for MDD approaches 20% by late adolescence (see Birmaher et al., 1996), indicating that almost one in five American adolescents has experienced a full depressive episode during their lives. There is less clarity around prevalence estimates of BD due to the lack of large-scale epidemiological studies and controversy around the core symptoms of BD in this age cohort (Pavuluri et al., 2005). The only community study investigating the occurrence of BDs in teens aged 14 to 18 years (Lewinsohn et al., 1995) found a lifetime prevalence of 1% using DSM-IV criteria, with a minority meeting the criteria for a full manic episode.

Unipolar depressive episodes range in severity from mild to markedly severe. At one extreme, MDD borders on adjustment disorder with depressed mood, while at the other extreme, MDD can be characterized by severe functional impairment, such as inability to attend school or work or serious suicidal behavior. Bipolar episodes also vary significantly in severity and level of impairment in academic, family, and social settings. Among adolescents, unipolar and bipolar depressive disorders have been linked to increased risk of other psychiatric disorders (Angold & Costello, 1993), alcohol and drug use (Deykin et al., 1987), and suicide (Brent et al., 1998). Moreover, severe unipolar and bipolar depression may be associated with psychotic symptoms, such as delusions or hallucinations. Given the range of severity of depressive disorders, the negative outcomes of adolescent mood disorders, and the potential for psychotic symptoms, medication for affective disorders is necessary in many cases. Therefore, we review combined psychotherapeutic and medical treatments as well as psychotherapeutic interventions, alone, in the present chapter.

THE THERAPEUTIC RELATIONSHIP

All psychotherapies are embedded in a relationship between the identified patient and the therapist. For adolescent patients, there is also a relationship between the parents and the therapist. In the context of the therapeutic relationship, the therapist must forge a working alliance with the patient, so that there is some agreement on the goals of the treatment and a sense of working together toward such goals. Nonspecific therapeutic factors, such as empathy and installation of hope, are those that have a positive impact on outcome but are not limited to any one theoretical approach to treatment. Such factors are essential to each of the treatments that we next review.

EMPIRICALLY SUPPORTED PSYCHOLOGICAL TREATMENTS FOR ADOLESCENT DEPRESSION

Two ESTs for adolescent depression have garnered considerable empirical support: interpersonal psychotherapy (IPT) and cognitive-behavioral therapy (CBT). In addition, combined CBT-and-fluoxetine is an empirically supported intervention for moderate to severe nonpsychotic MDD in adolescents. Attachment-based family therapy (ABFT) has initial (pilot) support as a promising intervention for depression among adolescents, while family and coping skills (FACS) therapy has limited pilot data in support of its use with depressed, substance-abusing teens.

Interpersonal Psychotherapy

IPT has been modified for adolescents (IPT-A) by Mufson and her colleagues at Columbia University (1994) and was adapted for Puerto Rican teens by Rossello and Bernal (1999). These two protocols are not identical, but both are derived from IPT as a treatment for adult depression (Klerman et al., 1984). IPT does not assume that interpersonal difficulties cause a depressive episode but, rather, that such an episode is embedded in an interpersonal context. In IPT the therapist conducts a systematic review of symptoms, assigns a diagnosis and a "sick role" to the patient, and then proceeds to conduct an interpersonal inventory of significant relationships in the life of the patient. Episodes of depression are then related to one of four core interpersonal problem areas: loss or grief; role transition; role disputes; or interpersonal deficits. Example behaviors typical of these four problem areas, respectively, might include grieving the death of a parent, struggling with the transition into high school, experiencing recurring conflicts with parents, and having pervasive social problems with same-age peers. Compared to IPT for adults with depression, IPT-A modifications for adolescents include limiting the "sick role" so as to prevent avoidant behavior, involvement of the therapist with parents and school personnel, use of brief telephone contacts between sessions, dealing with intergenerational and acculturation conflicts, and working with single-parent families.

In an initial study of IPT, Mufson and colleagues (1999) randomized 48 primarily female (72%) and Hispanic (71%) adolescents with nonpsychotic MDD to 12 weeks of IPT-A or clinical monitoring (CM). IPT-A sessions were weekly; CM sessions were biweekly or monthly. Twenty-one of 24 IPT-A teens completed treatment, while almost half of the CM teens dropped out. Statistical analyses were conducted using ITT analyses: Data from all teens who entered the trial were used in the analyses, and missing data were handled by carrying forward the adolescent's last observed scores. Seventy-five percent of IPT-A teens reached criteria for remission, as opposed to 46% of CM teens. There was no difference between treatments on global functioning.

In a further test of IPT-A (Mufson et al., 2004), 63 predominantly Hispanic and female teens were treated in school-based clinics at five sites in New York. Depressive diagnoses were mixed, with 57% experiencing MDD, and the remainder experiencing DD, D-NOS, or adjustment disorder with depressed mood. Treatment was administered by school clinicians, primarily social workers. Teens were randomly assigned to IPT-A or to Treatment as Usual (TAU), primarily supportive counseling for 12 to 16 weeks. Outcomes for IPT-A were superior to those for TAU across a range of measures, including self-reported and interviewer-rated depression and global functioning.

Rossello and Bernal (1999) assigned 71 Puerto Rican teens with MDD to IPT, CBT, or a waitlist (WL) control for 12 weeks. Using completer analyses, both active treatments led to better results than WL on self-reported, but not on parent-reported, levels of adolescent depression. IPT, but not CBT, also improved self-esteem and social adaptation relative to the WL condition.

Based on this literature, IPT has demonstrated superiority to no treatment, to CM, and, for a sample with mixed diagnoses and levels of severity, to TAU on a range of self-reported and interviewer-rated measures. Results on parent-report measures were given in only one study and did not differentiate between IPT-A and the comparison condition, while results on general functioning have been mixed. Of the comparison conditions, TAU was the only active condition and thus provided the most stringent test of the treatment. IPT has not yet been tested against pill placebo, antidepressant medication, or combined treatment.

Cognitive-Behavioral Therapy (CBT)

CBT has been the most broadly tested psychotherapy for adolescent MDD and has accumulated the most supportive evidence. As outlined by Lewinsohn and Clarke (1999), different CBT interventions rely on different techniques to effect change. The various techniques used in CBT can be classified as targeting primarily behavioral, primarily cognitive, or primarily affect management skills. Behavioral techniques include increased engagement in pleasant activities and enhanced problem-solving or social skills. Primarily cognitive techniques include identifying and modifying distorted automatic thoughts and beliefs. Adolescents with impulse control problems or affective lability may also benefit from a third set of skills, affect management strategies. Under these are included relaxation methods and methods that combine affect monitoring with active self-soothing or distraction techniques.

Despite the reliance upon different techniques across various CBT interventions, there appear to be two major theoretical approaches within the broader umbrella of CBT. One approach, identified with the cognitive therapy (CT) of Beck and his colleagues (Beck et al., 1979), is based on a model in which cognitive processes are the major maintaining variables associated with depressive disorder. In this model the task of the therapist is to assist the patient to monitor mood; to see the connections between mood and cognition; and to identify, challenge, and modify automatic thoughts, assumptions, and core beliefs that sustain MDD. A second approach is more behavioral and more heterogeneous. Identified with Lewinsohn and colleagues (1990), this approach is based on the assumption that behavior and thoughts sustain depressed mood, so that changes in either domain can serve as the engine of therapeutic progress.

Brent and colleagues (1997) adapted CT for teens by including psychoeducation, problem solving, affect regulation, and social skills training. They randomized 107 adolescents with MDD to CT or to one of two active comparative psychotherapies: systemic behavioral family therapy (SBFT) or nondirective supportive therapy (NST). The sample was 76% female and 83% Caucasian. At the end of 12 to 16 weeks of treatment, ITT analysis showed that 60% of CT versus 38% of SBFT and 39% of NST adolescents were remitted, significant differences favoring CT.

Follow-up analyses (Birmaher et al., 2000) showed that 84% of adolescents recovered within two years, with no differences across treatments. Combined with results of the initial study, these data suggest that CBT was faster in reducing depressive symptoms than the two active comparison treatments. However, across treatments, 30% suffered a relapse during this two-year period, and many adolescents received additional treatment during that time (49% of CT, 37% of SBFT, and 40% of NST).

The second stream of research has built upon Lewinsohn's multifactorial model of MDD. Lewinsohn and colleagues (1990) designed the Adolescent Coping with Depression Course (CWD-A), a course of CBT that is group-administered and psychoeducational in nature. Depressed adolescents receiving CWD-A participate in highly structured groups of two hours' duration that meet biweekly. Multiple skills are taught, including mood monitoring, relaxation, cognitive restructuring, problem-solving, communication, and social engagement skills.

In their original study, Lewinsohn and colleagues (1990) randomly assigned 69 adolescents to CWD-A, CWD-A plus a weekly parent psychoeducation group, or waitlist (WL) for seven weeks. This study based results upon the 59 completers. Only 5.3% of WL adolescents responded, compared to 47.6% of CWD-A plus parent group and 42.9% of CWD-A-alone adolescents. Results indicated that both treated conditions improved significantly more than did the WL group but that the addition of a parent group did not enhance outcome. Also of note, treated adolescents improved according to interviewer-rated and self-reported measures, but not according to parent-reported measures.

In a replication and extension study, Clarke and colleagues (1999) similarly randomized 123 adolescents to one of the same three conditions. The sample was 71% female, and all had MDD or DD. Treatment was extended to 8 weeks, and 96 adolescents who completed treatment served as the study sample. Responders included 65% and 69% of the two active treatment groups, contrasted with 48% of the WL adolescents. As in the previous study, parent groups did not enhance outcome, nor did parent measures reveal significant differences for the different adolescent conditions. These authors explored the protective value of continuation care against relapse by testing three posttreatment conditions: annual assessment; assessments every four months; or booster sessions and assessments every four months. There was no differential effect of these conditions on relapse, but booster sessions led to continued improvement in teens who were still depressed at termination of acute treatment.

In summary, these two sets of CBT studies demonstrated that CBT was better than no treatment, was faster than two alternative psychotherapies, and was feasible for the treatment of MDD as well as for less severe disorders. The CT study contained a more stringent test of CBT due to the use of an ITT design and active comparison conditions. These two research projects led to several key questions: how to increase the percentage of adolescents remitted by the end of acute treatment, how to reduce the high risk of relapse, and whether CBT can work in the broader clinical arena of practice settings and clinics.

A limitation of psychotherapy research has been its relative isolation from developments in pharmacotherapy research. The work of Emslie and colleagues (1997) indicated that fluoxetine was efficacious in the acute treatment of adolescent MDD. While other evidence for positive effects of certain antidepressants is beyond the scope of this chapter, it should be noted that data have accumulated in the past decade to support the use of certain selective serotonin reuptake inhibitors in treating depressed teens. Despite these data, as of 1998, CBT studies had not compared CBT to active medication or to pill placebo, and they had not provided a test of combined CBT plus medication for adolescent MDD. Since neither CBT nor fluoxetine had exceeded about a 60% response rate during the acute period of treatment, there was considerable room for improvement in both psychosocial and pharmacological response rates.

The Treatment for Adolescents with Depression Study (TADS)

TADS was initiated in 1998 to address effective treatment for adolescent MDD, given the knowledge base at the time [see the Treatment for

Adolescents with Depression Study (TADS) Team, 2003]. TADS was designed as a hybrid between efficacy and effectiveness studies and was intended to answer questions about the durability of treatment effects and the relative advantages of psychosocial and pharmacological treatment. Like an efficacy study, TADS included a pill placebo control during acute treatment, independent evaluators uninformed of treatment assignment, and training and ongoing supervision of CBT therapists and pharmacotherapists. Like an effectiveness study, TADS had fewer exclusion criteria than most prior efficacy studies, was conducted across multiple sites (13), and had CBT and pharmacotherapy conducted by therapists ranging widely in experience and degree of specialized training.

In TADS, 439 adolescents with MDD were randomly assigned to receive CBT, fluoxetine (FLX), both CBT and fluoxetine (COMB), or medical management with a pill placebo (PBO) for 12 weeks of acute treatment. The placebo condition was unblinded at week 12, and nonresponders to placebo were given their active treatment of choice. Other subjects who had at least partially responded continued in treatment for Stages II (6 weeks) and III (18 weeks) and were then followed for a year openly. TADS CBT combined the two prior streams of American CBT for adolescents: Skills training from the Lewinsohn model was embedded in individual psychotherapy sessions that followed a CT structure from the Beck model. Each session included reviewing homework, setting an agenda, skill training, continuing work on the agenda, and deciding on a new homework. Parents were more involved in TADS CBT than in prior models, attending both psychoeducation and conjoint interactive sessions. The TADS CBT model has been described extensively in a special issue of *Cognitive & Behavioral Practice* (Vol. 12, No. 2, 2005). TADS CBT included certain skills that were designated to be included in the treatment of every depressed adolescent (mood monitoring, goal setting, increasing pleasant activities, problem solving, cognitive restructuring) and other optional skills for use as determined by therapists (assertion, social engagement, relaxation, affect regulation, and several family-specific skills).

TADS subjects were 54% female and ethnicity was 74% Caucasian, 12.5% African-American, and 9% Hispanic. TADS adolescents had persistent and pervasive MDD. Mood disturbance must have been present for at least six weeks prior to intake and must have been associated with functional impairment in two of three settings (family, school, peers). At baseline, 98% of TADS adolescents were in the moderate to severe range of MDD.

At the end of acute treatment (week 12), ITT random regression analyses showed that only the slope of improvement for COMB adolescents was significantly different (faster) than that of PBO adolescents (The TADS Team, 2004). Based on independent evaluator ratings of improvement in MDD symptoms, 71% of COMB, 61% of FLX, 43% of CBT, and 35% of PBO adolescents were much or very much improved (*responders*). The two medication-containing conditions were significantly more responsive than CBT or PBO, which did not statistically differ. Similarly, with *remission* from episode (as opposed to *response* to treatment) defined as a score of 28 or lower on the Children's Depression Rating Scale-Revised (Poznanski & Mokros, 1995), only COMB was significantly superior to PBO. By the end of acute treatment, 37% of COMB adolescents fell in the normal range on this outcome measure, compared to 23% of FLX, 16% of CBT, and 17% of PBO adolescents (Kennard et al., 2006).

Acute treatment results supported COMB as the most effective intervention, across measures of response, suicidal ideation, and remission. FLX was effective on most, but not all, measures of improvement. CBT alone was not significantly better than medical management with PBO in this sample of moderately to severely depressed teens. However, CBT as a part of COMB contributed to a high response rate, a lowering of suicidal ideation, and remission in a sample that had more global functional impairment than samples treated in prior CBT studies.

Summary

IPT and CBT constitute two ESTs for adolescent depression. Both have demonstrated efficacy compared to no or minimal intervention in well-designed studies by more than one research group. Of the two interventions, CBT has been studied more extensively and has been tested using more stringent criteria. However, the evidence for CBT relative to active comparison conditions is somewhat mixed. In the study by Brent et al. (1997), CT was superior acutely (by 16 weeks) to two active comparison interventions in a clinically depressed sample. In the TADS sample, 12 weeks of CBT alone was not superior to PBO, although CBT in combination with FLX proved to be efficacious. The inability of TADS to replicate Brent's findings may have been attributable to characteristics of the TADS sample or to characteristics of the treatment package or implementation process. Continued research is needed to further determine the indicators and limitations of CBT, IPT, or other psychotherapies for depressed teens.

PROMISING INTERVENTIONS FOR ADOLESCENT DEPRESSION

There are two models of intervention with supportive pilot data for treating depressed adolescents, but both are targeted to specific subgroups. Diamond and colleagues (2002) developed attachment-based family therapy (ABFT), a treatment that focuses on reframing adolescent depression in terms of family relationships. Treatment proceeds to improve parent-child relationships by rekindling attachment and promoting competence in the teenager. In a pilot study, 32 adolescents with MDD, primarily female and African-American, were randomized to receive ABFT or a six-week WL condition. Thirteen of the 16 ABFT teens were below diagnostic threshold after 12 weeks of treatment. By week 6, more ABFT than WL teens had normal scores on self-reported depression. This treatment shows promise for cases in which depression is associated with attachment issues.

Curry and colleagues (2003) developed family and coping skills (FACS) therapy to treat dually diagnosed adolescents. Treatment consists of adolescent skill-building group therapy and concurrent individual family therapy. The group component is based on the Adolescent Coping with Depression course (Clarke et al., 1990) augmented by skills specific to substance abuse treatment, such as drug refusal, assertion, and consequential thinking. Family therapy is based on an adaptation of systems behavioral family therapy (Robin & Foster, 1989). FACS therapy also includes parent psychoeducation, urine drug screens for participating adolescents, and as-needed individual therapy sessions. A pilot study involved 13 adolescents with both a depressive and a substance use disorder. Pre- to posttreatment comparisons indicated that participants improved in both major domains targeted by the treatment: depressive symptoms and symptoms of substance abuse. To date, this treatment has not been compared to alternative interventions and cannot be considered an EST.

PROMISING PSYCHOSOCIAL TREATMENTS FOR ADOLESCENT BIPOLAR DISORDER

While there are no psychosocial treatments for adolescent bipolar disorder (BD) meeting the criteria of an EST, group psychoeducation, CBT, and family-focused treatment (FFT) each has supportive evidence in combination with pharmacotherapy. Pharmacological treatment with mood stabilizers, antipsychotics, and/or antidepressants is currently the cornerstone of outpatient treatment for adolescents with BD. As with adults, relapse rates among adolescents taking a mood stabilizer approach 50% and are greatly affected by long-term compliance (Pavuluri et al., 2005). In an open-label, randomized trial, Kowatch and colleagues (2000) found that 31% of adolescents with BD failed to comply with any mood stabilizer over a six-week period of open treatment. Poor compliance is exacerbated when there is a chaotic family environment, because first-degree relatives are typically responsible for the adolescent's care. Thus, psychosocial interventions have been developed as adjuncts to medication to increase adherence to medication, prevent relapse, and enhance skills for coping with environmental stressors.

Group Psychoeducation

Fristad and colleagues (1998) developed Multi-Family Psychoeducation Groups (MFPGs) as a six-week adjunct to pharmacological treatment for children and adolescents with bipolar and depressive spectrum disorders. Building on models of psychoeducation in the treatment of adult BD, MFPGs are intended to educate families about mood disorders and provide opportunities to share coping strategies. Each session consists of time with a group of families followed by breakout sessions with separate groups of parents and adolescents. Parent breakout sessions focus on education about topics such as mood symptoms and disorders, treatment options (medication, therapy, environmental changes), and healthy family responses to the disorder. Adolescent breakout sessions place more emphasis on the acquisition of skills such as monitoring mood changes, managing symptoms, and promoting positive interpersonal relationships. Pilot data from three families of children and six families of adolescents indicate that participation in MFPGs was associated with positive attitudinal shifts, accrued knowledge, improved family climate, and enhanced social support. Similar results were found in a randomized trial comparing MFPGs to a waitlist condition in children aged 8 to 12 years (Fristad et al., 2002). The influence of MFPGs on the course of BD in children and adolescents is under investigation.

Cognitive-Behavioral Therapy

Danielson and colleagues (2004) developed a time-limited CBT protocol for BD adolescents aged 11 to 18 years. Combination treatment with CBT and medication is believed to be well suited for the treatment of BD adolescents due to its success among adults with BD and adolescents with unipolar depression. In the adult BD population, several CBT manuals have been developed, and, to varying degrees, treatment using these approaches has been associated with fewer bipolar episodes, fewer days per bipolar episode, fewer hospitalizations, less subsyndromal mood symptoms, better coping with manic prodromes, and higher social functioning (as reviewed by Zaretsky, 2003).

The CBT protocol for adolescent BD builds upon the TADS protocol for MDD and consists primarily of individual work, with families incorporated in psychoeducation and conjoint interactive sessions. The treatment has seven key components intended to target problem areas specific to BD: psychoeducation, medication compliance, mood monitoring, identifying and modifying unhelpful thinking, stressor/trigger identification, sleep monitoring, and family communication. The protocol progresses through 12 sessions of acute treatment, followed by a 12-week maintenance phase, and then semiannual check-ins to facilitate the early detection of mood episodes. No data on this model have been reported, although a clinical study is underway.

Family-Focused Treatment

Family-focused treatment for adolescents (FFT-A) was designed by Miklowitz and colleagues (2004) and is intended for use with adolescent patients, aged 13 to 17 years, who meet diagnostic criteria for BD. FFT-A aims to promote a family environment conducive to long-term mood stability through education about BD, acceptance of the disorder, compliance with long-term medication, and management of environmental stressors. The treatment typically consists of 20 family sessions, with three primary components: psychoeducation, communication enhancement, and problem-solving skills training. In a 12-month, open trial of 20 adolescent BD patients and their families, FFT-A and medication was associated with symptomatic improvement in mania (46%), depression (36%), and behavioral problems. These rates of improvement are similar to those reported in two randomized controlled trials of FFT in adults by Miklowitz and colleagues (2000, 2003). In these studies, combination treatment with FFT was related to lower relapse rates, less severe manic and depressive symptoms, and better medication adherence than pharmacological treatment with a brief crisis management intervention. An ongoing, large-scale randomized clinical trial comparing FFT-A plus medication to an enhanced-care condition plus medication will clarify the efficacy of FFT-A.

Child and family-focused CBT (CFF-CBT) was developed by Pavuluri and colleagues (2004) primarily for children, aged 8 to 12 years, diagnosed with BD. However, an exploratory investigation of 34 youth, aged 5 to 17 years, indicates that the treatment may be useful across a wide range of ages. The treatment builds upon principles from Miklowitz and colleagues' (2004) FFT-A model to address developmental issues and problems specific to early-onset BD. Over 12 sessions, CFF-CBT works to teach children, their parents, and siblings principles from the mnemonic "RAINBOW": R for Routine, A for Affect regulation, I for "I can do it!", N for No negative thoughts & live in the Now, B for Be a good friend and Balanced lifestyle for parents, O for Oh, how can we solve the problem?, and W for Ways to get support. Results of the exploratory investigation suggest that CFF-CBT and medication is related to reductions in mania, depression, aggression, ADHD, and sleep disorder, as measured by therapist ratings. High treatment integrity, adherence, and parent satisfaction ratings were achieved at the end of the study. Conclusions based on these findings are limited by the study's open design as well as the reliance on therapist ratings to assess symptomatic improvement.

Summary

Group psychoeducation, CBT, and FFT each have supportive evidence in combination with pharmacotherapy for the outpatient management of adolescent BD. In addition, other psychosocial treatments that are currently being tested in the adult BD population may subsequently show benefit for BP youth. Considering the chronic nature and negative outcomes associated with pediatric BD, tests of psychosocial interventions should pay particular attention to their effect on relapse rates and functional impairment.

Effective treatment of BD is complicated by the controversy surrounding the core symptoms of a BD diagnosis, the high degree of overlap with other childhood disorders, and the limited data on treatment outcomes. Priorities for future research should include external validation of BD symptoms, differentiation from other psychiatric diagnoses, and conduct of double-blind, randomized controlled trials.

SUMMARY OF CURRENT PSYCHOSOCIAL TREATMENTS FOR ADOLESCENT MOOD DISORDERS

To date, there are two ESTs for adolescent depression and a number of promising treatments for adolescent unipolar and bipolar depressive disorders. Both of the ESTs for adolescent depression, CBT and IBT, have demonstrated effectiveness relative to a no-treatment comparison condition in more than one study conducted by different research groups. Of the two interventions, CBT has a broader evidence base and has demonstrated effectiveness using more stringent criteria. Indeed, of the few studies of adolescent mood disorders using ITT analyses and active comparison conditions, two were the Brent study and the TADS, which both tested CBT. In the Brent study, CBT demonstrated superiority relative to two active comparison conditions, while in the TADS CBT did not separate from the active placebo condition on any of the outcome measures. The mixed results of these two studies may be attributable to differences in the characteristics of the samples or to differences in treatment design or implementation. IPT has also garnered good support as an intervention for adolescent depression, including one study against an active comparison. Other studies of treatments for adolescent depression have generally used passive control conditions using completer analyses, while studies of treatments for adolescent bipolar disorder have tended to use simple pre- to posttest comparisons. Differences in the evidence base for psychosocial interventions for adolescent unipolar versus bipolar affective disorders reflect the relative maturity of the research fields.

The past decade has witnessed very significant advances in the development and testing of treatments for adolescent mood disorders, but clear areas of improvement remain. There is a need for additional studies evaluating specific interventions relative to active conditions that control for patient expectations and other nonspecific therapy factors. In addition, more studies using ITT analyses are required in order to ensure that treatment results are not inflated by the exclusion of patients who discontinue treatment. The studies reviewed here also highlight a need for the inclusion of a broader range of treatment outcomes than the reduction of symptoms. Such outcomes might include functioning in school, at home, and with peers, satisfaction with quality of life, prevention of subsequent disorders, and effect on comorbid conditions.

Beyond these design considerations, the existing evidence base raises a number of key clinical questions. Important questions include how to increase response rates beyond the acute phase of treatment, how to protect against relapse, and how to increase the acceptance and effectiveness of ESTs in the broader community. Another vital question includes the indications and, conversely, the limitations of psychosocial treatment alone, or in combination with medication, for adolescent mood disorders varying in severity and duration. Two final areas of priority for future work include identification of moderators and mediators of treatment outcome. Research in these areas is needed in order to answer the important questions of by what mechanism treatment works and for whom.

TREATMENT OF AN ADOLESCENT WITH MAJOR DEPRESSION

Emily was a 16-year-old Caucasian female who was referred for outpatient treatment of depression following a brief psychiatric hospitalization for suicidal risk. She had been hospitalized through the emergency department of a local hospital after telling her coach of a suicide attempt that was disrupted by the unexpected arrival of a friend. During hospitalization, she reported having been depressed for two years, with symptoms of suicidal thoughts, insomnia, decreased appetite, low energy, and loss of interest in activities. During hospitalization, she was started on an antidepressant medication, which she continued to take as an outpatient.

Emily's treatment consisted of 20 sessions over five months. Two of these were with Emily and her parents, two were with only her parents, and the remaining 16 were with Emily. Initially, it was important to allow her sufficient time to tell her story and to feel understood by the therapist. The initial session was also used to explain to Emily the cognitive-behavioral model of depression, how CBT works, and what sessions would be like. This young woman was treated with the TADS CBT approach, in which a session agenda is set, homework is given and reviewed, skills training occurs, and time is allowed to work on problems that teens bring to the meetings.

The second session, held during the same week, was a meeting with Emily and her parents. The focus was to allow the parents to express their concerns and observations, and for both parents and Emily to establish treatment goals. Sessions 3 to 6 focused on helping her to monitor her mood daily, so that she could begin to see the connections between how she felt and what she was doing or what she was thinking. She began to report a considerable degree of anxiety. She noticed that schoolwork was a major source of this stress, since she felt far behind academically, worried that she would never catch up, and realized that she was a perfectionist in academic and other domains. Since her anxiety became apparent early in treatment, and was contributing to her sleep difficulty, the skill of relaxation was brought to bear early in treatment. Using imagery methods, she learned relaxation skills during sessions 4 to 6.

Relaxation and stimulus control were then used to improve her sleep pattern. She would complete her homework in a room other than her bedroom and then do another relaxing activity such as reading, only going to bed when she felt drowsy. Simultaneously, since academic stress was a major factor, school consultation involved phone calls with her school counselor, who intervened with teachers to offer assistance and to reduce any extra required work. Emily had difficulty accepting help or reduced expectations, because it conflicted with her perfectionism, indicating a need for more cognitive work.

By the seventh session, she was reporting that relaxation was helping considerably, and the skill training aspect of sessions shifted to problem-solving skills and cognitive restructuring. Sessions 7 through the end of treatment all involved some degree of cognitive restructuring of her expectations of self and others, and of her self-schema. In session 8, a method of problem-solving was taught and applied to the problem of excessive homework and schoolwork. After reviewing advantages and disadvantages of several options for dealing with academic pressure, Emily decided to do whatever work she could do within a given time period and to hand this in, even if it were not "perfect." In the cognitive restructuring process, reverse role-plays, in which she took the role of someone helping a "perfection-istic" friend, proved to be useful in enabling her to get a perspective on the unrealistic nature of her beliefs. She began to accept help from teachers and to set reasonable expectations.

As incidents of suicidal impulses occurred, it became clear that Emily's anxiety escalated quickly. She experienced this as a sudden, overwhelming loss of control. Thus, skill training was broadened to include affect regulation skills. Using a method originally developed by Rotheram (1987) and used by Brent et al. (1997), Emily was taught to use the mood monitor to rate gradations in feeling "stressed" and to note the point in affective escalation at which she still had control. Then she and the therapist outlined steps to take when she reached this point, including self-statements and simple pleasant activities.

By late in treatment, she was using a record of daily thoughts to capture negative cognitions and formulate more realistic counter-thoughts. By session 16, she reported that her mood was much improved, as were the associated symptoms. Further work could have been done on her self-schema, particularly on dysfunctional attitudes that affected her peer relationships. However, because she was moving to a new town, treatment was terminated by consensus after 20 sessions.

REFERENCES

American Psychiatric Association (1994). *Diagnostic and Statistical Manual of Mental Disorders*, 4th ed. Washington, DC.

Angold, A., & Costello, E. J. (1993). Depressive comorbidity in children and adolescents: Empirical, theoretical, and methodological issues. *American Journal of Psychiatry, 150,* 1779–1791.

Beck, A. T., Rush, A. J., Shaw, B. F., & Emery, G. (1979). *Cognitive Therapy of Depression.* New York: Guilford Press.

Birmaher, B., Brent, D. A., Kolko, D. J., Baugher, M., Bridge, J., Holder, D., et al. (2000). Clinical outcome after short-term psychotherapy for adolescents with major depressive disorder. *Archives of General Psychiatry, 57,* 29–36.

Birmaher, B., Ryan, N. D., Williamson, D. E., Brent, D. A., Kaufman, J., Dahl, R. E., et al. (1996). Childhood and adolescent depression: A review of the past 10 years. Part I. *Journal of the American Academy of Child & Adolescent Psychiatry, 35,* 1427–1439.

Brent, D. A., Holder, D., Kolko, D. J., Birmaher, B., Baugher, M., Roth, C., et al. (1997). A clinical psychotherapy trial for adolescent depression comparing cognitive, family, and supportive therapy. *Archives of General Psychiatry, 54,* 877–885.

Brent, D. A., Perper, J. A., Goldstein, C. E., Kolko, D. J., Allan, M. J., Allman, C. J., et al. (1988). Risk factors for adolescent suicide. A comparison of adolescent suicide victims with suicidal inpatients. *Archives of General Psychiatry, 45,* 581–588.

Chambless, D. L., & Hollon, S. D. (1998). Defining empirically supported therapies. *Journal of Consulting and Clinical Psychology, 66,* 7–18.

Clarke, G. N., Lewinsohn, P. M., & Hops, H. (1990). *Adolescent Coping with Depression Course.* Eugene, OR: Castalia Press.

Clarke, G. N., Rohde, P., Lewinsohn, P. M., Hops, H., & Seeley, J. R. (1999). Cognitive-behavioral treatment of adolescent depression: Efficacy of acute group treatment and booster sessions. *Journal of the American Academy of Child and Adolescent Psychiatry*, *38*, 272–279.

Curry, J. F., Wells, K. W., Lochman, J. E., Craighead, W. E., & Nagy, P. D. (2003). Cognitive behavioral intervention for depressed, substance abusing adolescents: Development and pilot testing. *Journal of the American Academy of Child and Adolescent Psychiatry*, *42*, 656–665.

Danielson, C. K, Feeny, N. C., Findling, R. L, & Youngstrom, E. A. (2004). Psychosocial treatment of bipolar disorders in adolescents: A proposed cognitive-behavioral intervention. *Cognitive and Behavior Practice*, *11*, 283–297.

Deykin, E. Y., Levy, J. C., & Wells, V. (1987). Adolescent depression, alcohol and drug abuse. *American Journal of Public Health*, *77*, 178–182.

Emslie, G. J., Rush, A. J., Weinburg, W. A., Kowatch, R. A., Hughes, C. W., Carmody, T., et al. (1997). A double-blind, randomized, placebo-controlled trial of fluoxetine in children and adolescents with depression. *Archives of General Psychiatry*, *54*, 1031–1037.

Fristad, M. A., Gavazzi, S. M., & Soldano, K. W. (1998). Multi-family psychoeducation groups for childhood mood disorders: A program description and preliminary efficacy data. *Continuous Family Therapy*, *20*, 385–402.

Fristad, M. A., Goldberg-Arnold, J. S., & Gavazzi, S. M. (2002). Multifamily psychoeducation groups (MFPG) for families of children with bipolar disorder. *Bipolar Disorders*, *4*, 254–262.

Kennard, B., Silva, S.G., Vitiello, B., Curry, J., Kratochvil, C., Simons, A., Hughes, J., Feeny, N., Weller, E., Sweeny, M., Reinecke, M., Pathak, S., Ginsburg, G., Emslie, G., March, J., and The TADS Team (2006). Remission and residual symptoms after short-term, treatment in the Treatment for Adolescents with Depression Study (TADS). *Journal of the American Academy of Child and Adolescent Psychiatry*, *45*, 1404–1411.

Klerman, G. L., Weissman, M. M., Rounsaville, B. J., & Chevron, E. S. (1984). *Interpersonal Psychotherapy for Depression*. New York: Basic Books.

Kowatch, R. A., Suppes, T., Carmody, T. J., Bucci, J. P., Hume, J. H., Kromelis, M., et al. (2000). Effect size of lithium, divalproex sodium, and carbamazepine in children and adolescents with bipolar disorder. *Journal of the American Academy of Child and Adolescent Psychiatry*, *39*, 713–720.

Lewinsohn, P. M., & Clarke, G. N. (1999). Psychosocial treatments for adolescent depression. *Clinical Psychology Review*, *19*, 329–342.

Lewinsohn, P. M., Clarke, G. N., Hops, H., & Andrews, J. (1990). Cognitive-behavioral treatment for depressed adolescents. *Behavior Therapy*, *21*, 385–401.

Lewinsohn, P. M., Hops, H., Roberts, R. E., Seeley, J. R., & Andrews, J. A. (1993). Adolescent psychopathology: I. Prevalence and incidence of depression and other DSM-III-R disorders in high school students. *Journal of Abnormal Psychology*, *102*, 133–144.

Lewinsohn, P. M., Klein, D. N., & Seeley, J. R. (1995). Bipolar disorders in a community sample of older adolescents: prevalence, phenomenology, comorbidity, and course. Journal of the American Association of Child and Adolescent Psychiatry, 34, 454–463.

Miklowitz, D. J., George, E. L., Axelson, D. A., Kim, E. Y., Birmaher, B., Schneck, C., et al. (2004). Family-focused treatment for adolescents with bipolar disorder. *Journal of Affective Disorders*, *82S*, S113–S128.

Miklowitz, D., Goldstein, M., Nuechterlein, K., Snyder, K., & Mintz, J. (2003). A randomized study of family-focused psychoeducation and pharmacotherapy in the outpatient management of bipolar disorder. *Archives of General Psychiatry*, *60*, 904–912.

Miklowitz, D., Simoneau, T. L., George, E. L., Richards, J. A., Kalbag, A., Sachs-Ericsson, N., et al. (2000). Family-focused treatment of bipolar disorder: 1-year effects of a psychoeducational program in conjunction with pharmacotherapy. *Biological Psychiatry*, *48*, 430.

Mufson, L., Dorta, K. P., Wickramaratne, P., Nomura, Y., Olfson, M., & Weissman, M. M. (2004). A randomized effectiveness trial of interpersonal psychotherapy for depressed adolescents. *Archives of General Psychiatry*, *61*, 577–584.

Mufson, L., Moreau, D., & Weissman, M. M. (1994). Modification of interpersonal psychotherapy with depressed adolescents (IPT-A): Phase I and II studies. *Journal of the American Academy of Child and Adolescent Psychiatry*, *33*, 695–705.

Mufson, L., Weissman, M. M., Moreau, D., & Garfinkel, R. (1999). Efficacy of interpersonal psychotherapy for depressed adolescents. *Archives of General Psychiatry, 56*, 573–579.

Pavuluri, M. N., Birmaher, B., & Naylor, M. W. (2005). Pediatric bipolar disorder: A review of the past 10 years. *Journal of the American Academy of Child and Adolescent Psychiatry, 44*, 846–871.

Pavuluri, M. N., Graczyk, P. A., Henry, D. B., Carbray, J. A., Heidenreich, J., & Miklowitz, D. M. (2004). Child- and family-focused cognitive-behavioral therapy for pediatric bipolar disorder: development and preliminary results. *Journal of the American Academy of Child and Adolescent Psychiatry, 43*, 528–537.

Poznanski, E. O., & Mokros, H. B. (1996). *Manual for the Children's Depression Rating Scale-Revised.* Los Angeles: Western Psychological Services.

Reynolds, W. M. (1987). *Professional Manual for the Suicidal Ideation Questionnaire.* Lutz, FL: Psychological Assessment Resources, Inc.

Robin, A. L., & Foster, S. L. (1989). *Negotiating Parent-Adolescent Conflict: A Behavioral Family Systems Approach.* New York: Guilford Press.

Rossello, J., & Bernal, G. (1999). The efficacy of cognitive-behavioral and interpersonal treatments for depression in Puerto Rican adolescents. *Journal of Consulting and Clinical Psychology, 67*, 734–745.

Rotheram, M. (1987). Evaluation of imminent danger for suicide among youth. *American Journal of Orthopsychiatry, 57*, 102–110.

The Treatment for Adolescents with Depression Study (TADS) Team (2003). Treatment for Adolescents with Depression Study (TADS): Rationale, design, and methods. *Journal of the American Academy of Child and Adolescent Psychiatry, 42*, 531–542.

The Treatment for Adolescents with Depression Study (TADS) Team (2004). Fluoxetine, cognitive-behavioral therapy, and their combination for adolescents with depression. *Journal of the American Medical Association, 292*, 807–820.

Weisz, J.R., McCarty, C.A., & Valeri, S.M. (2006). Effects of psychotherapy for depression in children and adolescents: A meta-analysis. *Psychological Bulletin, 132*, 132–149.

Werry, J. S., McClellan, J. M., & Chard, L. (1991). Childhood and adolescent schizophrenic, bipolar, and schizoaffective disorders: A clinical and outcome study. *Journal of the American Academy of Child and Adolescent Psychiatry, 30*, 457–465.

Wood, A., Harrington, R., & Moore, A. (1996). Controlled trial of a brief cognitive-behavioral intervention in adolescent patients with depressive disorders. *Journal of Child Psychology and Psychiatry and Allied Disciplines, 37*, 737–746.

Zaretsy, A. (2003). Targeted psychosocial interventions for bipolar disorder. *Bipolar Disorders, 5*, 80–87.

11

Evidenced-Based Therapies for Adolescent Suicidal Behavior

ANTHONY SPIRITO and CHRISTIANNE ESPOSITO-SMYTHERS

Rates of attempted and completed suicide rise precipitously during adolescence (Kessler et al., 1999). Within a 12-month period, approximately 17% of adolescents in the United States seriously consider attempting suicide, 16.5% develop a suicide plan, 8.5% attempt suicide, and 2.9% of adolescents attempt suicide in a manner requiring emergency medical treatment (Centers for Disease Control and Prevention, 2004). These rates translate into approximately 2 million attempts per year, of which about 700,000 receive emergency medical treatment (Shaffer & Pfeffer, 2001).

Although there are important differences between those adolescents who attempt and those who complete suicide, a previous suicide attempt is one of the best predictive risk factors for eventual completed suicide by an adolescent. In one study (Lecomte & Fornes, 1998), one-third of youth who died by suicide had previously attempted suicide at least once. Thus, it is clear that effective treatment of adolescents who attempt suicide, the focus of this chapter, is an important facet of addressing the public health problem of youth suicide.

ANTHONY SPIRITO and CHRISTIANNE ESPOSITO-SMYTHERS • Center for Alcohol and Addiction Studies, Bradley/Hasbro Children's Research Center, and Department of Psychiatry and Human Behavior, Brown University

TREATMENT ISSUES WITH ADOLESCENT SUICIDE ATTEMPTERS

Several issues are pertinent to treatment of this high-risk population. First, adolescents who attempt suicide vary greatly in terms of treatment attendance. Follow-up studies of these adolescents have typically found poor adherence with outpatient treatment (Boergers & Spirito, 2003). Therapy dropout among adolescent suicide attempters occurs earlier and at a higher rate compared to adolescents in therapy for other problems (median session attendance = 3 sessions vs. 11 sessions) (Trautman et al., 1993). One factor that undoubtedly affects treatment attendance is that families who enter into treatment often have multiple sources of stress and adverse conditions in their lives that make participation in treatment a burden, consistent with the "burden of treatment model" (Kazdin, 1996). Thus, efforts must be made early on to problem-solve through obstacles to treatment participation. Specific steps to encourage families to come to counseling regularly and complete the full treatment program have been tested by Spirito et al. (2001), who presented the following rationale: *It takes time for the family to know the therapist and feel comfortable sharing information. It also takes time for the therapist to get to know the child and family. Furthermore, families have usually struggled for a few years so it takes time for therapy to produce desired changes.* Terminating treatment early can also lead to a relapse of suicidal behavior. The importance of completing the full course of treatment to obtain the best treatment outcomes is emphasized. Finally, it is also important to build a strong therapeutic alliance with both the adolescent and family, because it has been shown to have a positive effect on youth treatment retention and treatment outcome (Chatoor & Krupnick, 2001).

Second, suicidal behavior rarely occurs in the absence of psychopathology (Shaffer et al., 1996). Further, adolescent suicide attempters possess great diagnostic heterogeneity. A diagnosis of a mood disorder has consistently been identified as the most powerful diagnostic predictor of suicide completions, attempts, and ideation in adolescents (Brent et al, 1993; Shaffer et al., 1996). Anxiety, disruptive behavior, and substance use disorders, which are covered in other chapters of this book, have also been linked with adolescent suicidal behavior (Brent et al., 1993; Shaffer et al., 1996). Comorbid psychiatric disorders further increase risk for suicidality. Rates of suicide attempts in depressed adolescents increase when they are diagnosed with a comorbid anxiety, disruptive behavior (oppositional defiant or conduct disorder), and/or substance use disorder (Brent et al., 1993; Shaffer et al., 1996). Thus, treatment of suicidal behavior must, by necessity, address to some degree the symptomatology associated with the accompanying psychiatric disorder.

Third, there exists evidence for at least two distinct types of suicide attempters based on (1) degree of premeditation prior to the suicide attempt and (2) patterns of co-occurring psychopathology. The two types are impulsive suicide attempters with predominant externalizing symptoms and nonimpulsive suicide attempters with predominant internalizing symptoms. Relative to impulsive attempters, nonimpulsive attempters were found to have higher levels of depression and hopelessness and a trend toward greater suicidal ideation (Brown et al., 1991). Further, anger turned inward was associated with hopelessness only in the nonimpulsive group. Thus, treatment must be flexible enough to address these different presentations.

TREATMENT LITERATURE

To date, no psychosocial or psychopharmacological treatments have been designed specifically to address suicidal behavior that meet the criteria to be classified as an empirically supported treatment (Chambless, 1996). Below we review the few studies conducted on adolescents with suicidal behavior that have used individual, family, and group therapy, as well as several studies of treatment programs. Only studies with experimental or quasi-experimental designs are reviewed. In the section on individual therapy, we describe a case example in which selected cognitive-behavioral techniques are implemented.

Individual Psychotherapy Literature

Rathus and Miller (2002) adapted Linehan's (1993) dialectical behavior therapy (DBT) for use with suicidal adolescents. The focus of DBT is to improve distress tolerance, emotional regulation, and interpersonal effectiveness. Using a quasi-experimental design, they compared treatment efficacy of DBT to treatment-as-usual (TAU) for suicidal adolescents. The DBT group, which had more severe baseline symptomatology than the TAU group, had fewer psychiatric hospitalizations and higher rates of treatment completion than the TAU group. No differences in repeat suicide attempts were found. About 40% reattempted over the course of treatment.

Donaldson et al. (2005) conducted the only randomized trial to date of individual therapy. In this trial, CBT was compared to a problem-oriented supportive therapy designed to mimic standard care with adolescent suicide attempters. Both treatments were delivered in an individual format with conjoint parent-adolescent sessions. Adolescents were randomized to either 10 sessions of CBT or the problem-oriented supportive treatment. Seven different therapists provided both treatments to control for therapist effects. The groups were equivalent across baseline variables as well as percent placed on medication during the study. More than half of the sample had made multiple suicide attempts. Participants in both conditions reported significant reductions in suicidal ideation and depression at three-month follow-up, but there were no between-groups differences. At 6 months, both groups retained improvement over baseline; however, levels of suicide ideation and depression were slightly higher than at – three-month follow-up.

Family Therapy

One experimental study and one quasi-experimental study of family therapy have been published in the literature. In a highly structured six-session outpatient family therapy program called "SNAP" (Successful Negotiation/Acting Positively), problem-solving skills were taught and practiced using role-playing, modeling, and feedback. Negotiating, active listening skills, and strategies for managing affective arousal were also taught. Although a randomized trial was not conducted, SNAP reduced overall symptom levels among female minority adolescent suicide attempters (Rotheram-Borus et al., 1994).

Harrington and colleagues (1998) provided treatment to adolescents who had attempted suicide by overdose. Patients were randomly assigned to either routine care (M = 3.6 sessions) or routine care plus a four-session home-based family intervention (M = 3.2 sessions). The family sessions focused on discussion of the suicide attempt, communication skills, problem solving, and psychoeducation on adolescent development. The additional home-based family intervention resulted in reduced suicidal ideation at six-month follow-up, but only for adolescents without major depression. There were no differences in rate of suicide reattempts.

Both of these studies included communication and problem solving in their work with families. Examples of these techniques are described in more detail below.

Communication Training

Communication sessions typically begin with a review of both negative and positive communication habits (Robin & Foster, 1989) followed by a discussion about the communication style used by the adolescent and his or her parents. The negative/hurtful effects of negative communication behavior (e.g., anger, resentment, low self-esteem, etc.) are also reviewed. To decrease defensiveness, the therapist notes that most people use negative communication behavior when upset or frustrated. However, it is important to recognize these patterns and alter them.

One specific set of procedures for improving family communication was developed by Clarke et al. (1990). In this approach, "active listening" skills are introduced as the first step in improving communication. Clarke et al. (1990) presented three rules of active listening: (1) Restate the sender's message in your own words; (2) begin restatements with phrases such as "I hear you saying that ...," or "You said you feel ..."; and (3) be neutral about the other person's views (think of them as neither good nor bad).

The therapist first demonstrates the use of active listening skills by having the adolescent state a problem and then restates the adolescent's message using the techniques described above. Active listening skills are then role-played by family members. The adolescent is asked to describe a minor problem, and the parent, with the therapist's guidance, is asked to demonstrate the use of active listening skills. Then the adolescent is asked to practice active listening skills in response to a minor problem described by his or her parent. Reactions from the adolescent and parents are elicited and the importance of using active listening skills discussed.

The therapist shares that it is very difficult to use active listening skills, which are essential to effective communication, when upset. Therefore, it is important that all parties involved are calm before engaging in discussions. Further, the therapist discusses the importance of not forcing anyone to engage in a discussion who is not ready and/or is upset. If a discussion that initially starts off in a calm tone becomes heated, family members are instructed to separate and allow adequate time to calm down. Family members only reengage in the discussion when everyone involved is ready.

Family Problem Solving

Family problem solving is the other major commonality between these two studies. In family problem-solving sessions, the therapist first facilitates discussion regarding how solving problems together can be difficult because everyone in the family may have different feelings and ideas about the problem. Clarke et al. (1990) suggest that the therapist first provide the family with rules for selecting a problem. These rules include being specific, describing what the other person is doing or saying that is problematic, avoiding name-calling when describing the problem, expressing feelings in reaction to the problem (not the person), admitting responsibility for the problem when appropriate, avoiding blaming others, and being brief in providing input. After the rules have been established, the therapist assists the family in establishing a problem-solving system and teaches the problem-solving steps. (See case study for details regarding our problem-solving technique.)

Group Therapy

There has been one study of group therapy with adolescent suicide attempters. Wood et al. (2001) randomized 12- to 16-year-old adolescents who had deliberately harmed themselves on at least two occasions within a year to group therapy plus routine care or routine care alone. The group therapy approach utilized techniques from a variety of theoretical orientations, including cognitive-behavioral techniques previously used with depressed or suicidal adolescents and their families (Harrington et al., 1998) and DBT techniques. Adolescents randomized to the group intervention attended six structured "acute" group sessions, followed by weekly process-oriented long-term group therapy that could continue until the patient felt ready to terminate sessions. Those randomized to this condition attended a median of eight group sessions. They were also permitted to attend individual sessions as needed with the group therapist (median of 3). Adolescents in routine care alone attended a median of four sessions. Adolescents who received group therapy plus routine care compared to routine care alone were less likely to make more than one repeat suicide attempt (2/32 vs. 10/31; odds ratio 6.3), had better school attendance, and had a lower rate of behavior problems. The interventions did not differ in their effects on depression or global outcome. Interestingly, more sessions of routine care were associated with a worse outcome.

The six structured group therapy sessions covered specific topics. The first session discussed issues in relationships. The second session reviewed school problems including bullying and peer relationships. A problem-solving approach was used in attempting to resolve the issues discussed. The third session discussed family problems and used role-plays and writing letters to parents as a means to stimulate discussion. Session 4 presented anger management strategies to the adolescents, and session 5 discussed the relationship between depression and self-harm. The final session envisioned the future and helped the adolescents set goals and make plans for their lives.

Treatment Programs

Rudd et al. (1996) conducted a randomized trial comparing an experimental problem-solving–based day treatment program to standard care in the community for older adolescents and young adults (42% ideators, 58% attempters). Those in the experimental program received group therapy that primarily focused on psychoeducation, problem-solving, and experiential-affective techniques over the course of two weeks. The experimental program resulted in improvements in suicidal ideation and behavior, but the comparison group had comparable improvement. However, further analyses revealed that patients with comorbid symptomatology experienced the most improvement with the problem-solving–based experimental day treatment program (Joiner et al., 2001).

Huey et al. (2004) randomized adolescents presenting with psychiatric emergencies to either psychiatric hospitalization or multisystemic therapy (MST). MST is a family-focused home-based intervention that addresses home, school, and community factors related to youth difficulties, with a particular emphasis on parenting skills. A variety of behavioral interventions are typically delivered in MST based on a set of nine treatment principles and ongoing supervision. Caseloads are low for each therapist, and treatment ranges from three to six months, with daily sessions when necessary. At one-year follow-up, the MST group had significantly lower rates of suicide attempts than the hospitalized adolescents. Depressed mood, hopelessness, and suicidal ideation improved for both groups over follow-up, but there were no differences between the two groups on these variables.

CASE EXAMPLE

Because individual therapy is the most common treatment modality, below we describe a case using a CBT protocol. Both CBT and DBT studies have been described in the research literature (Donaldson et al., 2005; Rathus & Miller, 2002). Although neither of these studies demonstrated a differential treatment effect, the CBT and DBT protocols have many common components. Individual sessions include instruction in problem-solving, cognitive restructuring, and affect regulation skills to remediate coping skill deficits, cognitive distortions, affect regulation deficits, and problematic social behavior exhibited by suicidal adolescents. Moreover, these treatment techniques target many of the same cognitive distortions and skill deficits commonly found to underlie other forms of co-occurring psychopathology exhibited by suicidal adolescents (e.g., depression, substance abuse).

In the case described below, the primary skills in the protocol that are taught to specifically address suicidality are reviewed. All individual sessions in this treatment protocol follow the same format. They begin with a medication adherence check, if applicable, followed by an assessment of suicidal thoughts or behavior experienced since the last session. A verbal no-suicide contract is also reviewed with all adolescents. The adolescent is asked whether he or she can promise to keep him- or herself safe until the next treatment session. The session then follows a typical cognitive-behavioral format. First, the adolescent is asked to identify an agenda item for the session, homework from the prior session is reviewed, a new skill is introduced or a previously taught skill reviewed, the skill is practiced, the agenda item is discussed with efforts directed toward incorporating the use of skills learned previously in treatment, and a personalized homework assignment is created.

Jane was a 15-year-old female from a middle-class family. She lived with her biological parents and younger brother. Jane was referred to our treatment program from a psychiatric inpatient unit where she was hospitalized for a suicide attempt. She had reportedly taken a nonlethal overdose of Tylenol. Jane reported a history of recurrent depressive episodes for the prior two years and nonsuicidal self-injurious behavior. At the time of intake, she met criteria for major depressive disorder, severe, recurrent, and reported clinically significant suicidal ideation. Jane had attended counseling with treatment providers in the community on and off for the prior two years, during which she received pharmacotherapy and nondirective supportive therapy. She reported only brief periods of relief during her prior counseling sessions. Below, we describe in detail sessions focusing on three key skills in our cognitive-behavioral protocol: problem solving, cognitive restructuring, and affect regulation.

In the first session, the therapist met alone with the adolescent to engage in rapport building and conduct safety assessments. The therapist then worked with Jane to create a personal "reasons to live list" and a coping card. Jane generated several reasons to live, including "to have a family of my own" and "to see my little brother grow up." For the coping card, she generated a list of strategies that she could use to help cope with difficult situations as well as the names and numbers of adults that she could contact if she felt unsafe and believed that she might hurt herself. Her coping strategies included engaging in activities that helped her to self-soothe such as listening to her favorite CD, taking her dog for a walk, going for a run, calling a friend, and writing in her journal. She also listed the names and numbers of adults whom she could call, including the therapist, as well as the 24-hour hotline number for a local crisis service.

Problem Solving

Deficits in problem solving include limited flexibility, difficulty generating alternative solutions, and limited ability to identify positive consequences of potential solutions. Although there are several approaches to problem-solving training, we use the "SOLVE" system (Donaldson et al., 2003), which covers the basic steps and has been easily implemented with adolescent suicide attempters. We begin with the generation of a list of triggers for suicidality. After a list has been generated by the adolescent, which tends to range from two to five events, the therapist teaches the adolescent the SOLVE system. Each letter in the word SOLVE stands for a different step of the problem-solving process: S stands for "Select a problem," O for "generate Options," L for rate the "Likely outcome" of each option, V for choose the "Very best option," and E for "Evaluate" how well each option worked. A worksheet is used to assist in the SOLVE process. Often, the adolescent will have initial difficulties generating "Options." The therapist may need to model the skills to help the adolescent accept and use these new behaviors. The following is an example of the SOLVE system used with Jane.

> **Therapist:** Okay, so let's practice the SOLVE system using the stressor that led to your suicide attempt. S stands for "Select" a problem. How would you define your problem?
>
> **Jane:** Fight with my parents?
>
> **Therapist:** Yes, that is right. Let's write that down on your worksheet where it says "Select a Problem." Now, the second step begins with O and stands for generate "Options." It is important to list ALL possible options to deal with the problem, not just the ones you think would work. The bigger the list you make, the better the chance you have of solving the problem. So, let's get started. I want you to write down each option that you generate on the numbered lines 1–8 on your worksheet. What is the first option that you can think of?
>
> **Jane:** Go to my room and listen to music.
>
> **Therapist:** Yes, now let's write that down on the first line here. What else?
>
> **Jane:** Call a friend.
>
> **Therapist:** Good, what else?
>
> **Jane:** Go to sleep.
>
> **Therapist:** Good, what else?
>
> **Jane:** Take a walk.
>
> **Therapist:** You are doing great. What other options do you have?
>
> **Jane:** I can't think of anymore.
>
> **Therapist:** What about attempting suicide?
>
> **Jane:** You want me to write that down?
>
> **Therapist:** Yes, it is an option. Go ahead and write it down. Remember, we want to list all possible options at this stage, and attempting suicide is an option. What else?
>
> **Jane:** I can't really think of anything else.
>
> **Therapist:** Can I share a few options that other teenagers have shared with us when faced with the same situation?

> **Jane:** Sure.
>
> **Therapist:** Okay, what about trying to talk things through with your parents after you and your parents have cooled down?
>
> **Jane:** That won't work, they never listen to me.
>
> **Therapist:** Remember, this is the time to list all possible options, not to decide how good they are. I also want you to keep in mind that one of the things that we will be doing with our time together is to help improve the communication between you and your parents. How about using the coping card that we just created together?
>
> **Jane:** Yes, I could do that.
>
> **Therapist:** Good, so let's write that down too. Now, the next step is to rate the "Likely outcome" of each option. Think about whether things would get better or worse with each option and then rate each option as positive, negative, or even both. So, let's go ahead and rate each option. Would going to your room and listening to music lead to a good or bad outcome?
>
> **Jane:** It would cool me down, so I think it would be positive.
>
> **Therapist:** Okay, so let's put a "+" in the box next to that option. What about the next option?

The therapist should have the adolescent rate each option. Some options may be rated as positive and negative because they could potentially be associated with both outcomes. It is useful for the therapist to ask the adolescent to list a suicide attempt as an option if he or she does not introduce it. This demonstrates that it is safe to talk about suicidal thoughts and behavior in session. It also helps to open lines of communication around the suicide attempt and provides the therapist with the opportunity to begin to address any cognitive distortions surrounding this behavior.

> **Therapist:** Now what about attempting suicide? How would you rate that option?
>
> **Jane:** Well, probably positive because if I was dead I would not have any more problems with my parents.
>
> **Therapist:** Okay, that is true. You would not be around anymore, so you would not have any more problems. In what ways is suicide a negative outcome?
>
> **Jane:** It would not matter because I would not be here anymore.
>
> **Therapist:** Okay ... but what about the other people who are left behind that care about you? Would they view your suicide as something positive?
>
> **Jane:** No, I guess not.
>
> **Therapist:** How would they feel?
>
> **Jane:** They would probably be very upset, especially my little brother.
>
> **Therapist:** So, those you left behind would be in a great deal of pain, especially your little brother. In fact, you would never have the opportunity to spend time with your little

brother again or see him grow up. What other things would you miss out on?

Jane: I would never graduate from high school.

Therapist: That is true. You would never get the chance to finish high school. What else?

Jane: I would never get married or have a family.

Therapist: Yes, you are right. You would never get the chance to meet a great guy, get married, or have little ones of your own. In fact, you would lose out on all the things that you listed on your "reasons to live" list that you created in last week's session. Death is permanent. It is not something that you can change your mind about later. And is fighting with your parents a problem that can NEVER be worked out? Before you answer, think about whether there have been times in past when you felt that same way after an argument only to work thinks out later.

Jane: I guess that it may be possible to work things out.

Therapist: Good. I think so, too. If your parents were not willing to work on problems with you, they likely would not be here today. So, back to my question: Is committing suicide associated with any negative outcomes?

Jane: Yes. I guess that it is.

Therapist: Okay, so let's put a "—" in the box next to suicide.

After each option is rated, the therapist helps the adolescent select the "Very best option" or combination of options to try out. Lastly, the adolescent is told that after he or she gives the option(s) a try, he or she should then evaluate how well it worked. If it worked out well, then the problem is solved. If it did not work, the adolescent is instructed to go back to the list of "Options," weigh them, and pick the next "Very Best One" to try. The adolescent can keep doing this until the problem is solved.

After the exercise is complete, the therapist reframes the suicide attempt as a failure in problem solving. The therapist points out that many teenagers who attempt suicide do not think that they have other options, so they pick the only option that they think that have, which is to hurt themselves. The therapist emphasizes that the more adolescents practice coming up with a long list of "Options," the more potential solutions they have to choose from when they have a problem, and the less likely they will feel stuck or that the only thing left to do is to hurt themselves. This explanation helps provide adolescents with an adaptive way to understand the suicide attempt and obtain a better sense of control over future problems that arise.

Cognitive Restructuring

Much of the cognitive distortion in suicidal adolescents stems from co-occurring psychiatric disorders such as mood, anxiety, and conduct disorders. We use a modified version of rational emotive therapy (Bernard & Joyce, 1984) in teaching cognitive restructuring created by McClung

(2000). We call it the ABCDE method to help adolescents better remember the steps in cognitive restructuring. We introduce this method as a skill that helps adolescents deal with negative beliefs or thoughts that they may experience when problems arise. The experience of negative thoughts in and of themselves is normalized for the adolescent, but it is noted that they become problematic when they occur too frequently. This is typically what happens when suicidal thoughts emerge. Adolescents are guided to address and change irrational thoughts through the ABCDE method.

The adolescent is provided with a worksheet developed for this exercise. Each letter of the ABCDE method stands for a different step of thought changing process. "A" stands for "Activating Event" or the problem. The "B" stands for "Beliefs." The therapist shares that it is the "Beliefs" associated with the "Activating Event" that cause people to feel bad. These beliefs are typically negative and occur so quickly that people do not even know that they have them. Many of these beliefs are "irrational or untrue." The "C" stands for "Consequences" or feelings associated with the negative "Beliefs." The "D" stands for "Dispute," or argue. To feel better, it is important to argue against negative and irrational beliefs. The last step "E" stands for "Effect." If you are "Effecting" something, you are changing it. While people may not be able to change the fact that an activating event occurred, they can change their negative beliefs about it. This, in turn, will help them to feel better and make better and safer decisions. The following is an example of the ABCDE method used with Jane.

> **Therapist:** Okay Jane. So let's give the ABCDE method a try using the fight with your parents as the "Activating Event." Why don't you go ahead and write that down on the line next to "Activating Event." Now let's skip the 2nd step for a minute and go to the 3rd step. The 3rd step is to identify "Consequences or Feelings" related to the "Activating Event." How did you feel after the fight with your parents?
>
> **Jane:** Hopeless.
>
> **Therapist:** Okay, let's write this feeling down next to "Consequences." Now, let's go back to the 2nd step, which is to identify "Beliefs." What were you thinking after the fight with your parents that led you to feel hopeless?
>
> **Jane:** I hate my life.
>
> **Therapist:** Good, let's write that down as your first belief. What else?
>
> **Jane:** My parents don't care about me.
>
> **Therapist:** Okay, let's write that down too. Now, the next step is to take a look at these beliefs and dispute them if needed. I want you to ask yourself two questions as you evaluate them. The questions are (1) Is this belief true? And if it is true, (2) is this belief helpful? If the answer is "no" to either of these questions, then it is important to dispute them. So, let's get started. Is it true that you hate your life?
>
> **Jane:** Yes, it is true.

Therapist: So, you hate everything about your life including your little brother, your friends, your room that you told me you decorated so nicely, and everything else?

Jane: Well, maybe not everything.

Therapist: So what is a more accurate statement?

Jane: I don't hate everything about my life?

Therapist: Okay, that is better. But what was it that you really disliked in the moment?

Jane: Fighting with my parents?

Therapist: Right, so a more accurate statement may be, "I don't like fighting with my parents." Why don't you go ahead and write that down. And what about your next thought, "My parents don't care about me"? Is that true?

Jane: It feels that way. We are always fighting.

Therapist: Okay, I want you to turn over your worksheet for a minute and go to the place that says "Evidence For Belief" and "Evidence Against Belief" at the top of the page. What is some evidence you have that your parents don't care about you?

Jane: We are always fighting and they never let me do anything that I want.

Therapist: Okay, write these beliefs down under the "Evidence For Belief" column. Now, what about "Evidence Against" this belief? Can you think of any?

Jane: No, not really.

Therapist: Well, do you think that your parents would bring you here if they did not care about you or to any doctors for that matter?

Jane: Probably not.

Therapist: Okay, so let's write down, "They get me help when I need it." And are you still living at home? And do your parents buy you food and clothes and other things that you need?

Jane: Well, yes. But they have to … they are my parents.

Therapist: Unfortunately, you have probably heard about some parents that don't care for their children. Some kids are in the custody of the Department of Children, Youth, and Families because their parents don't take care of them. So, why don't you write down "They provide me with a home, food, and other things that I need" in the "Evidence Against Belief" column. Now, you told me that you were on the swim team last semester. Did your parents drive you to practices and come to your meets?

Jane: Yes.

Therapist: Would they do that if they did not care about you?

Jane: Probably not.

Therapist: Okay, so let's write that down, too. Now, let's take a look at the things that you have listed under your "Evidence For Belief" column. Is it true that you are ALWAYS arguing with your parents and that there are not any times that you get along?

Jane: I guess that we are not always arguing.

> **Therapist:** Okay, do you know of any teenager that does not argue with her parents?
>
> **Jane:** Well, no.
>
> **Therapist:** Okay, so is it possible that arguing is something that occurs between all teenagers and their parents and that it does not necessarily mean that they don't care about you?
>
> **Jane:** Yes, it is possible.
>
> **Therapist:** Okay, so why don't you write down "All kids argue with their parents" under the "Evidence Against Belief" column. Now, is it true that they NEVER let you do anything that you want?
>
> **Jane:** It feels that way.
>
> **Therapist:** But is that true? They never let you out of the house?
>
> **Jane:** No, it is not true.
>
> **Therapist:** And what reasons do they give you for not letting you do things?
>
> **Jane:** They don't trust my friends.
>
> **Therapist:** Hmmm ... so they don't want anything bad to happen to you?
>
> **Jane:** I guess not, but it is not fair.
>
> **Therapist:** I hear what you are saying and that is something that we can work on with your parents in other sessions. But for now, would it be true to say that it is possible that they may not let you do what you want because they don't want to see anything bad happen to you?
>
> **Jane:** Yes, it is possible.
>
> **Therapist:** Okay, so let's write this down under the "Evidence Against Belief" column. Now, let's take a look at your two columns. Taking into account all of this information, is it really true that your parents don't care about you?
>
> **Jane:** No, I guess not, but it feels that way.
>
> **Therapist:** Okay, so what is a more accurate belief?
>
> **Jane:** My parents do care about me but they don't always show it?
>
> **Therapist:** Okay, that is much better. Flip the page back over and let's write that down under your disputes.

As is evident, when adolescents begin to use this method, the therapist will need to provide much guidance in disputing through Socratic questioning. Questions that we commonly use include: Is this belief true? (which may be followed by the generation of an Evidence For Belief/Evidence Against Belief list if needed); does this belief help you feel the way that you want?; what would your friend say if he/she heard this belief?; and is there another explanation for this event? After the adolescent becomes more comfortable with the ABCDE method, we also present the adolescent with a list of cognitive distortions (e.g., black/white thinking, predicting the worst, missing the positive, feelings as facts, jumping to conclusions, expecting perfection; see Beck et al., 1979), which we have adapted to include simpler language and call "Thinking Mistakes." We ask the adolescent to identify any thinking mistakes in his or her beliefs and then use disputing to rework the irrational belief.

The therapist also helped Jane reframe the suicide attempt by noting that at the time of the suicide attempt, she likely only had negative beliefs running through her head. So, in addition to not seeing any other "options" to suicide, she had all of these negative beliefs running through her head and did not dispute any of them, which left her feeling suicidal. The therapist also shared with Jane that the more she practices disputing negative beliefs, the more positive beliefs will run through her head. It is important to remember that it took quite a lot of practice before Jane became proficient at these skills.

There are a number of other cognitive techniques specifically useful for suicidal persons that can be integrated into the cognitive restructuring module (Freeman & Reinecke, 1993). Decatastrophizing involves having the therapist help the adolescent decide whether he or she is overestimating the catastrophic nature of the suicide attempt precipitant. Questions include "What would be the worst thing that will arise if ___ occurs again? If ___ does occur, how will it affect your life in 3 months, 6 months? What is the most likely thing to happen? How will you handle it?" Scaling the severity of stressful events involves having the adolescent scale the suicidal precipitant or anticipated future stressful events (e.g., scale from 0 to 100). Scaling helps the adolescent view events on a continuum, rather than in a dichotomous (black/white) fashion.

Affect Regulation

Affect regulation techniques that are used include training adolescents to recognize stimuli that provoke negative emotions and learning to reduce physiological arousal via self-talk and relaxation. In the initial affect management session, we review with the adolescent that negative activating events can trigger negative or untrue beliefs. These beliefs then cause negative feelings such as depression and anger. In addition to negative feelings, these negative beliefs can also cause our body to start feeling out of control. We might experience muscle tightness, a faster heart rate, sweating, or shortness of breath. The more our body feels out of control, the harder it is to use problem solving or dispute negative beliefs. Therefore, it is important to learn ways to keep our bodies from spiraling out of control.

The therapist then shows the adolescent a series of feelings cards and asks him or her to choose the card that best describes how he or she was feeling when the event that triggered the suicide attempt occurred. Next, the therapist presents the adolescent with a list of physiological and behavioral symptoms associated with negative affect, referred to as "body talk," and asks him or her to circle those symptoms he or she experienced when feeling the way described on the selected feeling card. The adolescent is then introduced to the concept of a "feelings thermometer" (e.g., see Rotheram-Borus et al., 1994). The bottom of the thermometer has a rating of "1" and stands for "calm and cool," and the top is "10" and stands for "extremely upset" or whatever the predominant feeling was for the adolescent at the time of the suicide trigger.

The following is an example of the subsequent portion of the emotion regulation session with Jane.

> **Therapist:** Okay, so you have selected "hopeless" as the main feeling that you experienced at the time of your suicide attempt. So let's list "hopelessness" at the top of your emotions thermometer above the number "10." Now, what I would like you to do is to fill in the lines by each rating on the feelings thermometer with the "body talk" you circled on your worksheet. "Body talk" symptoms do not occur all at once but successively, like a set of dominos. So, I want you to think back to the night of your fight with your parents. Of all of the body talk that you circled, what was the first body talk symptom that you noticed?
> **Jane:** I started to crack my knuckles.
> **Therapist:** Okay, good, so why don't you write this on the line by #1. What next?
> **Jane:** I started to yell at my parents.
> **Therapist:** Okay, so where would that fall on the thermometer?
> **Jane:** Probably around #3.
> **Therapist:** Good, write that down by #3. Then what?
> **Jane:** I ran upstairs and slammed my bedroom door.
> **Therapist:** Okay, where should that go?
> **Jane:** Probably around #7.
> **Therapist:** Then what?
> **Jane:** I started to cry.
> **Therapist:** Okay, when did that occur?
> **Jane:** Around #9.

After all of the "body talk" symptoms were listed on the thermometer, the therapist asked Jane to identify and insert any negative beliefs that she might have experienced next to the appropriate rating.

> **Therapist:** Now, what I would like you to do next is to list negative beliefs that you might have had on the feelings thermometer. Can you think of any negative beliefs that you might have experienced when you first started to argue with your parents?
> **Jane:** "It's not fair."
> **Therapist:** Good, where should that go?
> **Jane:** Around #4.
> **Therapist:** What else?
> **Jane:** "I can't stand my parents."
> **Therapist:** Okay, please write that in on the appropriate line. What else?
> **Jane:** "I hate my life."
> **Therapist:** And where should that go?
> **Jane:** That was probably around #8.

After the adolescent has filled in lines #1 through #10 on the thermometer, the session proceeds as follows.

> **Therapist:** Okay Jane. Now the next step is to identify your personal danger zone—that is the point on your thermometer where your body spirals so far out of control that it is hard to calm back down, leaving you at risk for unsafe or suicidal behavior. Where would that be?
>
> **Jane:** Probably when I start thinking about how much I hate my life.
>
> **Therapist:** Good, so what I would like you to do is to begin to recognize the early "body talk" that precedes this thought so that you can work on decreasing it before you hit your danger zone. You can do this by creating a "stay cool" plan to use when you begin to notice early "body talk" and negative beliefs. This includes things that you can do and things that you can say to yourself to help yourself calm down. So let's go ahead and work on a stay cool plan. Let's try to list at least three things that you can do when you begin to notice your early body talk.
>
> **Jane:** I can walk away when I start to get upset, listen to my music, maybe take a walk, or go online.
>
> **Therapist:** Yes, those are all good things that can help you keep your cool. And what about things that you can tell yourself? You can use the disputes that we came up with last week if that would be helpful.
>
> **Jane:** I can remind myself that all kids argue with their parents.
>
> **Therapist:** Good, let's write that down. What else?
>
> **Jane:** That there are good things about my life and things will get better.
>
> **Therapist:** Those are two great beliefs. Why don't you write down both of them?

Finally, before the adolescent leaves the session, the parents are briefed on the session content so that they are aware of the child's coping plan and can provide their support.

When an adolescent reports instances of suicidal or self-injurious behavior during the course of treatment, we conduct a functional analysis of this behavior with the adolescent. This functional analysis combines the use of problem solving, cognitive restructuring, and other affect regulation techniques. It is more fully described by Linehan (1993).

FUTURE RESEARCH

The treatment outcome literature on adolescent suicide attempters is small, because of both the difficulties inherent in treating this population and investigator concerns about liability in clinical trials with such high-risk patients (Pearson et al., 2001). Adolescents with a history of suicidal behavior have a high likelihood of continued suicidality during a research protocol. This latter factor typically results in patients being removed from clinical trials. If removal from a trial due to continued suicidality is the standard in research with suicide attempters, a substantial percentage may never complete treatment trials, making it difficult to accrue knowledge. Thus, it is important to keep suicidal adolescents in treatment protocols so that the results of these studies will be more relevant to community care.

Even if therapy has been successful, adolescent suicide attempters remain vulnerable to a sudden resurgence of suicidal feelings (Beck, 1996). The therapist should forewarn the adolescent and parents of the potential for resurgence of suicidality. Identifying subclinical levels of sadness or pessimism that can be managed before they reach crisis proportions, via individual efforts or booster sessions, is a priority. Therefore, research protocols may need to include both scheduled and as-needed booster sessions over a four- to six-month period. Although these sessions complicate the research design, they greatly enhance the relevance of the research for clinicians managing these patients.

Finally, when enrolled in trials immediately following a suicide attempt, many of these adolescents will be on one or more medications. Consequently, it is difficult to test the effectiveness of psychosocial treatments alone. Thus, combined psychosocial/ psychopharmacological treatments, with a standard algorithm guiding medication use, may be the research designs best suited to address the clinical and ethical realities of studying such a high-risk population.

REFERENCES

Beck, A. T. (1996). Beyond belief: A theory of modes, personality, and psychopathology. In P. Salkovskis (Ed.), *Frontiers of Cognitive Therapy* (pp. 1–25). New York: Guilford Press.

Beck, A. T., Rush, A. J., Shaw, B. F., & Emery, G. (1979). *Cognitive Therapy of Depression.* New York: Guilford Press.

Bernard, M. E., & Joyce, M. R. (1984). *Rational Emotive Therapy with Children and Adolescents: Theory, Treatment Strategies, Preventative Methods.* New York: John Wiley & Sons.

Boergers, J., & Spirito, A. (2003). The outcome of suicide attempts among adolescents. In A. Spirito & J. Overholser (Eds.), *Evaluating and Treating Adolescent Suicide Attempters: From Research to Practice* (pp. 261–276) San Diego: Academic Press.

Brent, D. A., Perper, J., Moritz, G., Allman, C., Friend. A., Roth, C., et al. (1993). Psychiatric risk factors for adolescent suicide: A case-control study. *Journal of the American Academy of Child and Adolescent Psychiatry, 32,* 521–529.

Brown, L. K., Overholser, J., Spirito, A., & Fritz, G. K. (1991). The correlates of planning in adolescent suicide attempts. *Journal of the American Academy of Child and Adolescent Psychiatry, 30,* 95–99.

Centers for Disease Control and Prevention (CDC) (2004). Youth Risk Behavior Surveillance— United States, 2003. *Morbidity and Mortality Weekly Report,* 53(SS-2).

Chambless, D. (1996). In defense of dissemination of empirically supported psychological interventions. *Clinical Psychology: Science and Practice, 3,* 230–235.

Chatoor, I., & Krupnick, J. (2001). The role of non-specific factors in treatment outcome of psychotherapy studies. *European Child and Adolescent Psychiatry, 10,* 19–25.

Clarke, G., Lewinsohn, P., & Hops, H. (1990). *Adolescent Coping with Depression Course.* Eugene, OR: Castalia Publishing Company.

Donaldson, D., Spirito, A., & Esposito-Smythers, C. (2005). Treatment for adolescents following a suicide attempt: Results of a pilot trial. *Journal of the American Academy of Child and Adolescent Psychiatry, 44,* 113–120.

Donaldson, D., Spirito, A., & Overholser, J. (2003). Treatment of adolescent suicide attempters. In A. Spirito & J. Overholser (Eds.), *Evaluating and Treating Adolescent Suicide Attempters: From Research to Practice* (pp. 295–321). San Diego: Academic Press.

Freeman, A., & Reinecke, M. (1993). *Cognitive Therapy for Suicidal Behavior.* New York: Springer-Verlag.

Harrington, R., Kerfoot, M., Dyer, E., McNiven, F., Gill, J., Harrington, V., et al. (1998). Randomized trial of a home-based family intervention for children who have deliberately poisoned themselves. *Journal of the American Academy of Child and Adolescent Psychiatry, 37,* 512–518.

Huey, S., Henggeler, S. W., Rowland, M. D., Halliday-Boykins, C. A., Cunningham, P. B., Pickrel, S. G., et al. (2004). Multisystemic therapy effects on attempted suicide by youths presenting psychiatric emergencies. *Journal of the American Academy of Child and Adolescent Psychiatry, 43,* 183–190.

Joiner, T., Voelz, Z., & Rudd, M. D. (2001). For suicidal young adults with comorbid depression and anxiety disorders, problem-solving treatment may be better than treatment as usual. *Professional Psychology: Research and Practice, 32,* 278–282.

Kazdin, A. E. (1996). Dropping out of child psychotherapy: Issues for research and practice. *Clinical Child Psychology and Psychiatry, 1,* 133–156.

Kessler, R., Borges, G., & Walters, E. (1999). Prevalence of and risk factors for lifetime suicide attempts in the National Comorbidity Survey. *Archives of General Psychiatry, 56,* 617–626.

LeComte, D., & Fornes, P. (1998). Suicide among youth and young adults, 15 through 24 years of age: A report of 392 cases from Paris, 1989–1996. *Journal of Forensic Sciences, 43,* 964–968.

Linehan, M. (1993). *Cognitive Behavior Therapy of Borderline Personality Disorder.* New York: Guilford Press.

McClung, T. (2000). *Rational Emotive Therapy Adapted for Adolescent Psychiatric Inpatients.* Unpublished manual, West Virginia University School of Medicine.

Pearson, J., Stanley, B., King, C., & Fisher, C. (2001). Intervention research with persons at high risk for suicidality: Safety and ethical considerations. *Journal of Clinical Psychiatry, 62,* 17–26.

Rathus, J. H., & Miller, A. L. (2002). Dialectical Behavior Therapy adapted for suicidal adolescents. *Suicide and Life-Threatening Behavior, 32,* 146–157.

Robin, A. L., & Foster, S. L. (1989). *Negotiating Parent-Adolescent Conflict: A Behavioral-Family Systems Approach.* New York: Guilford Press.

Rotheram-Borus, M. J., Piacentini, J., Miller, S., Graae, F., & Castro-Blanco, D. (1994). Brief cognitive-behavioral treatment for adolescent suicide attempters and their families. *Journal of the American Academy of Child & Adolescent Psychiatry, 33,* 508–517.

Rudd, M. D., Rajab, M. H., Orman, D. T., Stulman, D. A., Joiner, T., & Dixon, W. (1996). Effectiveness of an outpatient intervention targeting suicidal young adults: Preliminary results. *Journal of Consulting and Clinical Psychology, 64,* 179–190.

Shaffer, D., Gould, M. S., Fisher, P., Trautman, P., Moreau, D., Kleinman, M., & et al. (1996). Psychiatric diagnoses in child and adolescent suicide. *Archives of General Psychiatry, 53,* 339–348.

Shaffer, D., & Pfeffer, C. (2001). Practice parameters for the assessment and treatment of children and adolescents with suicidal behavior. *Journal of the American Academy of Child and Adolescent Psychiatry, 40* (Suppl 7), 245–515.

Spirito, A., Boergers, J., Donaldson, D., Bishop, D., & Lewander, W. (2001). An intervention trial to improve adherence to community treatment by adolescents after a suicide attempt. *Journal of the American Academy of Child and Adolescent Psychiatry, 41,* 435–442.

Trautman, P. D., Stewart, N., & Morishima, A. (1993). Are adolescent suicide attempters noncompliant with outpatient care? *Journal of the American Academy of Child and Adolescent Psychiatry, 32,* 89–94.

Wood, A., Trainor, G., Rothwell, J., Moore, A., & Harrington, R. (2001). Randomized trial of group therapy for repeated deliberate self-harm in adolescents. *Journal of the American Academy of Child and Adolescent Psychiatry, 40,* 1246–1253.

Disruptive Behavior Disorders and Related Problems

12

Evidence-Based Treatments for Attention-Deficit/ Hyperactivity Disorder (ADHD)

BETSY HOZA, NINA KAISER, and ELIZABETH HURT

Childhood attention-deficit/hyperactivity disorder (ADHD) has a 3–7% prevalence rate among elementary-school children (American Psychiatric Association, 2000). The course of the disorder is chronic, persisting beyond childhood in a majority of cases (Biederman et al., 1996). Although inattentive and hyperactive/impulsive symptoms define the disorder, the impairments caused by these symptoms pervade many domains of functioning—such as the academic and social domains, as well as the domain of parent-child relationships, among others. Not surprisingly, effective treatments for ADHD therefore target not only core symptoms of the disorder (i.e., hyperactivity/impulsivity and inattention) but also these associated functional deficits.

The most widely used treatment for ADHD is pharmacotherapy primarily with stimulant medication. In fact, as previously argued, the efficacy of stimulant medication is established, thus making this the treatment to which other therapies should be compared (Pelham et al., 1998). Yet medication does not by itself adequately address the functional impairments associated with ADHD. Specifically, combined treatment using both behavior therapy and medication management is considered the treatment of choice for functional problems extending beyond core ADHD symptoms (oppositional/aggressive behavior, internalizing symptoms, social skills, parent-child relationships, and academic functioning; MTA Cooperative

BETSY HOZA • University of Vermont, **NINA KAISER and ELIZABETH HURT** • Purdue University

Group, 1999). In addition, children receiving combined treatment can be maintained on significantly lower total daily doses of medication than those receiving only medication, a noteworthy finding given that medication side effects are usually dose-related (MTA Cooperative Group, 1999). Finally, not all children respond to stimulant medications (Pelham et al., 1998) and not all parents view drug treatments as an acceptable choice for their children (Pelham et al., 2006).

In light of these considerations, there is ongoing interest in evidence-based psychosocial treatments for ADHD, used both alone and in combination with medication. Our goal is to review the most recent evidence for psychosocial treatments, focusing primarily on studies conducted in the past 10 years. We select this time frame because earlier literature already has been adequately summarized (see Pelham et al., 1998) and this time frame overlaps only minimally with Pelham et al.'s prior review.

To set the stage for the current chapter, we briefly review the conclusions of Pelham et al. (1998), who summarized the evidence-based psychosocial treatment literature for ADHD through approximately the mid-1990s. We select this article as a starting point because we structure our review in a somewhat similar fashion and use a similar conceptual approach. At the same time, we wish to acknowledge other excellent recent reviews that space will not permit us to describe (e.g., Barkley, 2002; Chronis et al., 2006; Smith et al., 2000); we refer the reader to these other useful sources.

Setting the Stage: Pelham et al.'s (1998) Conclusions as a Starting Point

Pelham and colleagues (1998) limited their review predominantly to short-term behavioral interventions for ADHD used alone and opted to evaluate these interventions according to the criteria outlined by Lonigan et al. (1998). Studies were subgrouped according to type of intervention (parent training vs. school intervention), level of evidence (well-established vs. probably efficacious), and design type (group vs. single-subject). Their conclusion was that "Behavioral parent training for ADHD just barely meets criteria for well-established treatment," and only if flexible interpretations of criteria are used; "[h]owever, behavioral parent training solidly meets criteria for probably efficacious treatment" (Pelham et al., 1998, p. 192). Classroom behavioral interventions, on the other hand, "clearly [meet] criteria for well-established treatment" (Pelham et al., 1998, p. 192). Conclusions based on their review, therefore, indicated behavioral parent training and behavioral classroom interventions to be the nonpharmacological treatments with the greatest empirical support.

Our goal for this chapter was to pick up when and where Pelham et al. (1998) left off and, at the same time, expand upon their methodology in several ways. Specifically, we wanted to document our criteria for including and excluding studies in our review as specifically as possible, as we were not always able to identify criteria for final inclusion/exclusion decisions in their review. Second, we wanted to report results separately by domain of outcome to facilitate evaluation of whether certain treatments or combinations of treatments better address problems in one domain as compared to another. The domains we summarize include: core ADHD symptoms, behavior, child internalizing symptoms, academic performance, social/peer functioning, and parenting practices or qualities of the parent-child relationship. Our selection of these specific domains is not meant to imply that other domains (e.g., parental psychopathology such as depression, parenting stress) are unimportant but, rather, that these domains were of most interest to us.

Our Criteria for Identifying Evidence-Based Treatments (1995 to Present)

Identifying criteria to use in determining whether treatments are evidence-based is not an easy task. Even among skilled researchers working toward similar goals, criteria tend to differ somewhat across workgroups (e.g., see Chambless & Ollendick, 2001). Our goal was not to review available criteria for evaluating evidence-based treatments, as a thorough and interesting discussion may be found elsewhere (see Roberts & James, Chapter 2). Instead, our goal was to draw from commonalities of previous work in establishing a list of criteria for evaluating the childhood ADHD literature. We based our decisions regarding which articles to include in the current review on recommendations from prior task forces that appropriate control groups be used and that samples be well defined (see Chambless & Ollendick, 2001, for a review), but also considered limitations of prior work (e.g., failure to consider evidence by different domains of outcome) that we judged to be especially pressing. Using these broad principles, our criteria for inclusion in the present review included the following: (1) Participants clearly met diagnostic criteria for ADHD (i.e., the study included either a sample clinically diagnosed with ADHD using DSM-IV criteria or an analogue sample selected using appropriate parent and/or teacher cutoffs on dimensional measures of ADHD symptoms; thus, we excluded studies failing to provide information permitting the reader to understand the diagnostic process); (2) the study included application of a psychosocial treatment based on well-researched psychological theories and examination of treatment effects as a primary purpose of the paper. We excluded alternative treatments such as biofeedback, dietary supplementation, yoga, etc., as well as tests of a specific technique (e.g., time out) or of an environmental manipulation that did not constitute a complete treatment (e.g., changing a child's seat location in the classroom). In addition, we included studies involving a pharmacological treatment only if the pharmacological treatment was the control group to which a psychosocial treatment was compared, or if the pharmacological treatment was part of a multimodal intervention that also involved a psychosocial treatment; (3) the study included a control condition (pill or psychological placebo, alternative treatment, waitlist control group, no-treatment control group, or treatment reversal); (4) the study assessed outcomes from one or more of our six key domains: ADHD symptoms (e.g., rating scales completed by adult informants assessing inattention, hyperactivity, and/or impulsivity or behavior counts assessing frequencies of behaviors that are DSM-IV ADHD symptoms, such as fidgeting); behavior (oppositional or aggressive behavior, general behavioral problems, conduct problems, and any other behaviors that were not explicitly ADHD symptoms); social/peer functioning (including assessments of social skills such as sportsmanship), academic functioning, parenting practices/parent-child relationship measures, and child internalizing symptoms [Of note, child self-report measures were included only in domains of functioning in which children are thought to be valid reporters (e.g., internalizing symptoms but not ADHD symptoms)]; (5) the study included only children of preschool or school age (in order to ensure comparability of interventions across studies);[1] and (6) the study reported either the data necessary to compute effect sizes for posttreatment differences between treatment and control conditions or contact information for the authors was provided in the original article and the authors responded to our request for this information.

These review parameters yielded a total of 24 studies, all of which were published between 1995 and 2005. Three studies employed a parent training treatment, seven studies employed a classroom intervention, and two studies involved a summer treatment program. These 12 studies included both single-component treatments and multicomponent treatments. In other words, interventions comprised of multiple strategies or techniques of a single therapy type (e.g., behavior modification) but occurring within a single treatment context were considered unimodal therapies. We also identified 12 studies (16 articles)[2] examining the incremental benefit achieved by combining multiple types of therapy. In order for a study to be considered an "incremental benefit" study, two distinct forms of active intervention had to be included (e.g., medication, behavior modification), and the use of one active treatment had to be compared to the use of two or more active treatments. In other words, incremental benefit studies examined whether multiple treatments administered together outperformed one or a smaller subset of treatments.

---

[1] Initially, we also included studies meeting our other review criteria but focusing on adolescent populations; however, this strategy provided us with only one study involving adolescents (Barkley et al., 2001). Given the differences in treatment strategies targeting adolescents with ADHD versus those targeting younger children diagnosed with the disorder, we opted to eliminate this study from the current review and to refer the reader instead to the original article.

[2] Please note that when a single study generated multiple publications yielding pertinent outcome data, we grouped these publications together and treated them as a single study. For example, Abikoff and colleagues produced four separate articles reporting on various treatment outcomes from a single study (Abikoff et al., 2004a, b; Hechtman et al., 2004a, b); similarly, we aggregated data from two articles generated by the MTA (MTA Cooperative Group, 1999; Wells et al., 2000). To emphasize that multiple articles may provide data from a single study, we hereafter refer the reader to this footnote each time such a result is cited.

The reader should also note that two additional studies (Hoza et al., 2005; Pelham et al., 2000) employed nonidentical subsets of the MTA sample; however, as outcomes for the subset of children participating in these studies potentially could differ from those for the entire sample, we treated these articles as separate studies in the current review.

Sometimes, within these studies, additional comparisons were possible given the study design. For example, an incremental benefit study also may have included a comparison to a no-treatment, treatment withdrawal, or waitlist control condition. However, because these comparisons were not the primary goal of the study, and because they were not the comparisons of interest to our review, they are not discussed here.

The studies reviewed here fell into three classes of study design: (1) group studies examining between-subjects treatment effects; (2) group studies examining within-subjects treatment effects; and (3) case studies describing one or more single-subject designs. Whenever feasible, we assessed the magnitude of treatment effects by computing Cohen's d effect sizes indexing posttreatment differences for between-subjects studies[3] comparing the psychosocial treatment group or condition and the control and/or alternative treatment group(s) or condition(s) for each relevant outcome variable. For within-subjects studies, data were averaged across multiple repetitions of the same condition, if applicable. Within each study, regardless of design type, we averaged effect sizes across all dependent measures within the same outcome domain in order to produce one overall effect size for that domain. In some instances, results for different measures within a domain produced discrepant results. Thus, our results are not necessarily parallel to those reported by the original authors. Further, the reader should note that in order to facilitate ease of comparison across outcome domains, we manipulated the direction of effect sizes such that positive effect sizes indicate improved functioning on the part of the treatment group or condition relative to the control or alternative treatment group/condition (i.e., lower ADHD symptoms, better behavior, more positive peer relations, better academic performance, more positive parenting practices or better parent-child relationships, and lower internalizing symptoms). Finally, following Cohen (1988), in evaluating effect sizes, we categorized values below 0.20 as nonimportant, those ranging from 0.20 to <0.50 as "small" in magnitude, those from 0.50 to <0.80 as "moderate" in magnitude, and values at or above 0.80 as "large." For case study designs using visual inspection of graphs to draw conclusions, we indicated for each domain whether improvement, deterioration, or no change was observed, in the absence of a method to otherwise quantify these effects. For case studies reporting on multiple dependent variables within a single domain or including more than one participant, we provided the qualitative label applying to the majority of dependent variables within

---

[3] Please note that Barkley et al. (2000) provided only posttreatment group means adjusted for pretreatment scores; thus, for this article alone, we computed effect sizes using adjusted means. All other between-groups effect sizes were computed using unadjusted posttreatment scores on the relevant outcome measures. Importantly, this approach was taken regardless of whether or not authors reported pretreatment differences between groups and/or used a strategy to control for these differences (e.g., conducting covariance analysis or comparing pre-post change across groups as opposed to comparing only data gathered at the end of treatment). This approach was taken because not all studies reported adjusted means when pretreatment differences were found and we preferred a uniform method of computing effect sizes across all between-subjects studies. We acknowledge that this method is not without limitations.

the domain (e.g., a study reporting improvement on two of three behavioral variables for a single child would be categorized as demonstrating improvement in the behavioral domain).

What Conclusions Can We Draw About Current Evidence-Based Psychosocial Treatments for Childhood ADHD?

Using the above approach, in this section we summarize our conclusions about the current state of evidence-based psychosocial treatments for ADHD. In so doing, we present our conclusions by type of treatment (parent training, classroom interventions, summer treatment programs) and offer the reader tables (as deemed useful) that organize the literature both by type of study design (between-subjects, within-subjects, single-subject designs) and by outcome domain (core ADHD symptoms, behavior, child internalizing symptoms, academic functioning, social/peer functioning, and parenting practices/parent-child relationship measures). Because we do not adhere to nor advocate for one specific definition of what constitutes sufficient evidence to consider a therapy to be "evidence-based" (see Roberts & James, Chapter 2, for a discussion of various criteria), we draw our conclusions based on the effect sizes calculated for studies that met our inclusion criteria outlined above.

Parent Training Studies

Three parent training studies using a between-subjects design met our criteria for inclusion (see Table 1). (Of note: Studies involving parent training as one component of a multimodal intervention examining incremental benefit of unimodal versus multimodal treatment were not considered in this section but, rather, are discussed briefly in a subsequent section on incremental benefit.) All studies meeting our criteria were relatively short-term studies ($\leq$12 sessions); two studies included preschoolers, and one included elementary-school children. Two of the studies used the Triple P–Positive Parenting Program, administered in either an individual (Bor et al., 2002) or a group (Hoath & Sanders, 2002) format and geared toward teaching 17 core skills to parents. These skills included both child competence-building skills (e.g., praise, attention, behavior charts) and behavior management skills (e.g., establishing rules, appropriate instructions, time out). Enhancements to parent training in the form of parent-targeted coping skills training were included also in both of these studies. The third study (Sonuga-Barke et al., 2001) also employed a structured approach, similarly geared toward teaching behavioral management strategies to parents.

As shown in Table 1, when these parent training interventions, either involving standard parent training or with enhancements, were compared to control groups such as a waitlist group or parent support in preschool- or elementary-aged children, studies generally yielded positive

Table 1. Studies Employing Behavioral Parent Training

A1: Parent Training Studies Employing Between-Subjects Designs: ADHD Symptom and Behavior Domains

Study	N	Diagnostic Procedures	Treatment Length	Treatment Components*	Control Conditions*	Symptom Measure**	Mean ES (Range)	Behavior Measure**	Mean ES (Range)
Bor et al. (2002)	63[p]	b, d	12 sessions for enhanced PT; 10 sessions for standard (on average)	2, 3 2	2 20 20	d d d	−0.65 0.04 0.68	d, i, t d, i, t d, i, t	−0.19 (−0.55, 0.38) 0.73 (0.40, 1.14) 0.89 (−0.03, 1.46)
Hoath & Sanders (2002)	21[s]	a, c	5 in-person sessions and 4 follow-up phone consultations	2, 3	20	d, k	0.58 (0.47, 0.67)	d, k	0.25 (0.03, 0.61)
Sonuga-Barke et al. (2001)	78[p]	b, d	8 sessions	2	5 20	b, t b	0.70 0.97	b b, t	0.66 (0.55, 0.77) 0.18 (0.10, 0.26)

A2: Parent Training Studies Employing Within-Subjects Designs: ADHD Symptom and Behavior Domains: None

A3: Parent Training Studies Employing Single-Subject Designs: ADHD Symptom and Behavior Domains: None

(Continued)

Table 1. *(Continued)*

B1: Parent Training Studies Employing Between-Subjects Designs: Parenting/Parent-Child Relationship and Child Internalizing Domains

Study	N	Diagnostic Procedures	Treatment Length	Treatment Components*	Control Conditions*	Parenting Measure**	Mean ES (Range)	Internalizing Measure**	Mean ES (Range)
Bor et al. (2002)	63[p]	b, d	12 sessions for enhanced PT; 10 sessions for standard (on average)	2, 3 2	2 20 20	e, i e, i e, i	0.36 (0.30, 0.41) 0.68 (0.27, 1.09) 0.28 (−0.22, 0.77)	NA	NA
Hoath & Sanders (2002)	21[s]	a, c	5 in-person sessions and 4 follow-up phone consultations	2, 3	20	e	0.52 (0.37, 0.76)	NA	NA

B2: Parent Training Studies Employing Within-Subjects Designs: Parenting/Parent-Child Relationship and Child Internalizing Domains: None

B3: Parent Training Studies Employing Single-Subject Designs: Parenting/Parent-Child Relationship and Child Internalizing Domains: None

C1: Parent Training Studies Employing Between-Subjects Designs: Academic and Social/Peer Domains: None

C2: Parent Training Studies Employing Within-Subjects Designs: Academic and Social/Peer Domains: None

C3: Parent Training Studies Employing Single-Subject Designs: Academic and Social/Peer Domains: None

NA = Not applicable. Under N: [p] = preschool; [s] = school-age. *Treatment components and control conditions: 1 = Stimulant medication or medication assessment/referral; 2 = parent training; 3 = parent-targeted partner-support and/or coping skills training; 4 = family problem-solving or communication therapy; 5 = support group; 6 = child-targeted social skills training; 7 = child-targeted self-control/anger management training; 8 = individual child-targeted psychotherapy; 9 = behavioral summer treatment program; 10 = child-focused academic organizational skills training; 11 = individualized academic assistance/remediation/tutoring; 12 = behaviorally trained individual paraprofessional support; 13 = school consultation and/or teacher psychoeducation; 14 = Daily Report Card; 15 = token reinforcement; 16 = token response cost; 17 = delayed reward; 18 = time out; 19 = peer attention/feedback/positive reinforcement; 20 = waitlist control; 21 = attention control; 22 = community care; 23 = treatment withdrawal; 24 = no intervention; 25 = adult-administered positive reinforcement/praise; 26 = sports skills training. **Diagnostic and outcome measures: a = clinical diagnosis by pediatrician or mental health professional; b = clinician-administered interview with parent, child, and/or teacher; c = clinician ratings; d = parent ratings; e = parent ratings of parenting practices/strategies; f = child ratings of parenting practices/strategies; g = parent ratings of parent-child relationship; h = child ratings of parent-child relationship; i = parent-child relationship observations; j = counselor ratings; k = teacher ratings; l = classroom observations; m = observer ratings; n = academic productivity; o = academic performance; p = cognitive tests; q = achievement tests; r = peer ratings or nominations; s = child self-ratings; t = behavior counts. For case studies, IM = improved; NC = no change; DT = deteriorated. The range of effect sizes is designated by (lower bound, upper bound).

effect sizes favoring parent training, with effect sizes most frequently falling in the moderate range. Indeed, 7 of 13 comparisons yielded moderate-sized effects, with fairly consistent results seen in all three domains for which data were available: core symptoms, behavior, and parenting practices/parent-child relationships. These results are consistent with prior reviews indicating that parent training is an effective treatment for childhood ADHD (e.g., Pelham et al., 1998). One multicomponent parent training study demonstrated a small incremental benefit of adding parent coping skills training to standard parent training, but only for one of three domains considered—the parenting practices/parent-child relationship domain (Bor et al., 2002).

Of note, there were no parent training studies using a primarily within-subjects or single-subject design that met our inclusion criteria. Also, none reported internalizing symptoms, academic measures, or social/peer measures as outcomes.

Classroom Studies

Only one between-subjects classroom study and one within-subjects classroom study met our criteria. The between-subjects study (Miranda et al., 2002) employed elementary school-aged children undergoing a four-month multicomponent classroom intervention as compared to a no-treatment control group. Specifically, teachers received education about ADHD as well as training in both behavior modification and instructional management for ADHD. The behavior modification training included both strategies for increasing positive behaviors (e.g., positive reinforcement, token systems) as well as procedures for decreasing inappropriate behaviors (e.g., time out, response cost). The instructional management included strategies such as how to optimally arrange the physical environment, and methods for giving instructions and feedback. Finally, teachers were trained in strategies to promote child self-instruction and self-evaluation and, importantly, how to combine self-evaluation strategies with a reinforcement system geared toward promoting the child's appropriate use of self-evaluation skills. In contrast, the one within-subjects classroom study that met our criteria (Strayhorn & Bickel, 2002) examined behavior of elementary-aged children involved in an 11-month (on average) individual tutoring intervention (with an adult tutor) relative to their own behavior pre- and postintervention during regular classroom instruction. Importantly, this individual tutoring program incorporated almost continuous use of social reinforcement, although the incremental value of this aspect of the intervention was not evaluated separately. Together, these between-subjects and within-subjects studies generally provide support for the interventions employed with four of five averaged (if applicable) effect sizes falling in the moderate to large range—specifically in the symptoms, behavior (in one of two instances), and academic domains. There were no data from the between- or within-subjects categories for the internalizing, social/peer, or parenting/parent-child relationship domains.

Single-subject design classroom studies were greater in number. Five studies employing single-subject designs involving a total of 30 children met our inclusion criteria; four of these studies examined elementary school-aged children and one employed preschoolers. The length of treatment for the single-subject design studies varied as indicated in Table 2. As a group, these studies utilized several different types of treatments including consequences for appropriate and inappropriate behavior delivered by teachers (Anhalt et al., 1998; McGoey & DuPaul, 2000); school home note programs (i.e., daily report cards) delivered with or without accompanying response cost (Kelley & McCain, 1995); and a variety of interventions involving classroom peers: for example, group-based rewards and consequences (Anhalt et al., 1998); classwide peer tutoring (DuPaul et al., 1998); and peer prompting and reinforcement of appropriate behavior (Flood et al., 2002). Although these studies were somewhat harder to quantify due to investigators' use of visual inspection of graphs to draw conclusions regarding treatment effects, they generally yielded results in concert with the between-subjects and within-subjects designs. Specifically, these classroom interventions, as compared to treatment withdrawal or usual classroom procedures, generally (though not uniformly) yielded improvements in the core symptoms, behavioral, and social/peer domains. The only study employing a measure from the academic domain yielded no substantive change (DuPaul et al., 1998). There were no data for the parenting practices/parent-child relationships and internalizing domains.

The overall conclusion for classroom studies thus was quite consistent with prior reviews (e.g., Pelham et al., 1998) in indicating beneficial effects of classroom-based treatments. This was true regardless of design type (between-subjects, within-subjects, single-subject) and for most domains for which data were available.

Summary for Parent Training and Classroom Interventions

The literature described to this point primarily addressed the question of whether parent training and classroom interventions benefit families of children with ADHD relative to waitlist, no-treatment, or treatment withdrawal (for within-subjects designs) control groups. The evidence, reviewed here, as in prior reviews (e.g., Pelham et al., 1998), generally supports parent training and classroom interventions in the treatment of childhood ADHD. Further, most of these interventions could be broadly characterized as behavioral in nature. Specifically, common characteristics of effective parent training and classroom approaches appear to include: educating parents and teachers about ADHD; teaching parents and teachers strategies for praising and attending to positive child behaviors and consistently using appropriate consequences (e.g., time out, loss of privileges) for negative behavior; and helping parents and teachers structure the home and classroom environments and set clear expectations through the use of clear instructions, rules, and establishment of guidelines and structure for planned activities. In addition, incorporating classroom peers into interventions to facilitate positive peer contact, help

Table 2. Studies Employing Classroom Interventions

A1: Classroom Intervention Studies Employing Between-Subjects Designs: Symptom and Behavior Domains

Study	N	Diagnostic Procedures	Treatment Length	Treatment Components*	Control Conditions*	Symptom Measure**	Mean ES (Range)	Behavior Measure**	Mean ES (Range)
Miranda, et al. (2002)	50[s]	b, d, k	8 sessions (3 hours each)	13, 15, 16, 17, 18, 25	24	d, k	0.55 (−0.08, 0.91)	k	−0.09

A2: Classroom Intervention Studies Employing Within-Subjects Designs: Symptom and Behavior Domains

Study	N	Diagnostic Procedures	Treatment Length	Treatment Components*	Control Conditions*	Symptom Measure**	Mean ES (Range)	Behavior Measure**	Mean ES (Range)
Strayhorn & Bickel (2002)	30[s]	k	Average of 68 tutoring sessions	11, 19	23	k	1.43 (1.03, 1.83)	k	0.97 (0.86, 1.08)

A3: Classroom Intervention Studies Employing Single-Subject Designs: Symptom and Behavior Domains

Study	N	Diagnostic Procedures	Treatment Length	Treatment Components*	Control Conditions*	Symptom Measure**	Effect	Behavior Measure***	Effect
Anhalt et al. (1998)	1[s]	k	Unspecified treatment duration; 43 observation days	13, 15, 16, 19, 25	23	k	IM	k, t	IM
DuPaul et al. (1998)	18[s]	b, d, k	4 to 8 weeks	11, 13, 15, 19	23	t	NC	t	IM

(Continued)

Table 2. (Continued)

Study	N	Diagnostic Procedures	Treatment Length	Treatment Components*	Control Conditions*	Symptom Measure**	Effect	Behavior Measure**	Effect
Flood et al. (2002)	2[s]	a, d, t	Unspecified	19	23	NA		t	IM
Kelley & McCain (1995)	5[s]	d, k, t	32 to 50 school days	14, 16	14	NA		t	IM
					23			t	IM
McGoey & DuPaul (2000)	4[p]	b, d, k	Unspecified treatment duration; 36 to 40 observations	14	23			t	IM
				16	23	k	IM	k, t	IM
					15	k	NC	k, t	NC
				15	23	k	IM	k, t	IM

B1: Classroom Intervention Studies Employing Between-Subjects Designs: Parenting/Parent-Child Relationship and Child Internalizing Domains: None

B2: Classroom Intervention Studies Employing Within-Subjects Designs: Parenting/Parent-Child Relationship and Child Internalizing Domains: None

B3: Classroom Intervention Studies Employing Single-Subject Designs: Parenting/Parent-Child Relationship and Child Internalizing Domains: None

C1: Classroom Intervention Studies Employing Between-Subjects Designs: Academic and Social/Peer Domains

Study	N	Diagnostic Procedures	Treatment Length	Treatment Components*	Control Conditions*	Academic Measure**	Mean ES (Range)	Social/Peer Measure**	Mean ES (Range)
Miranda et al. (2002)	50[s]	b, d, k	8 sessions (3 hours each)	13, 15, 16, 17, 18, 25	24	o	0.66 (0.45, 0.96)	NA	

Table 2. (Continued)

C2: Classroom Intervention Studies Employing Within-Subjects Designs: Academic and Social/Peer Domains: None

C3: Classroom Intervention Studies Employing Single-Subject Designs: Academic and Social/Peer Domains

Study	N	Diagnostic Procedures	Treatment Length	Treatment Components*	Control Conditions*	Academic Measure**	Effect	Social/Peer Measure**	Effect
DuPaul, et al. (1998)	18[s]	b, d, k	4 to 8 weeks	11, 13, 15, 19	23	o	NC	NA	NA
McGoey & DuPaul (2000)	4[p]	b, d, k	Unspecified treatment duration; 36 to 40 observations	16	23	NA		k	IM
					15			k	NC
				15	23			k	IM

NA = Not applicable. Under N: [p] = preschool; [s] = school-age. *Treatment components and control conditions: 1 = stimulant medication or medication assessment/referral; 2 = parent training; 3 = parent-targeted partner support and/or coping skills training; 4 = family problem-solving or communication therapy; 5 = support group; 6 = child-targeted social skills training; 7 = child-targeted self-control/anger management training; 8 = individual child-targeted psychotherapy; 9 = behavioral summer treatment program; 10 = child-focused academic organizational skills training; 11 = individualized academic assistance/remediation/tutoring; 12 = behaviorally trained individual paraprofessional support; 13 = school consultation and/or teacher psychoeducation; 14 = Daily Report Card; 15 = token reinforcement; 16 = token response cost; 17 = delayed reward; 18 = time out; 19 = peer attention/feedback/positive reinforcement; 20 = waitlist control; 21 = attention control; 22 = community care; 23 = treatment withdrawal; 24 = no intervention; 25 = adult-administered positive reinforcement/praise; 26 = sports skills training. **Diagnostic and outcome measures: a = clinical diagnosis by pediatrician or mental health professional; b = clinician-administered interview with parent, child, and/or teacher; c = clinician ratings; d = parent ratings; e = parent ratings of parenting practices/strategies; f = child ratings of parenting practices/strategies; g = parent ratings of parent-child relationship; h = child ratings of parent-child relationship; i = parent-child observations; j = counselor ratings; k = teacher ratings; l = classroom observations; m = observer ratings; n = academic productivity; o = academic performance; p = cognitive tests; q = achievement tests; r = peer ratings or nominations; s = child self-ratings; t = behavior counts. For case studies, IM = improved; NC = no change; DT = deteriorated. The range of effect sizes is designated by (lower bound, upper bound).

both peers and target children become invested in improved behavioral and academic performance, and provide more one-on-one time for children in need of additional assistance in the classroom, appeared beneficial. We next turn to a discussion of summer program interventions in the treatment of childhood ADHD.

Summer Program Studies

Two studies utilizing summer treatment programs met our inclusion criteria (Chronis et al., 2004; Coles et al., 2005). Both of these studies employed the Pelham Summer Treatment Program (STP; Pelham et al., 1997, 2005b; Pelham & Hoza, 1996), a multicomponent behavioral intervention involving a point system with both reward and response-cost components, social skills training, academic remediation or enrichment (depending on the child), among other components (for a complete description, see Pelham et al., 2005b). The Chronis et al. study used a BAB treatment withdrawal design to investigate the effects of withdrawing all behavioral treatment components for two days on the children attending the STP; treatment was then reinstated. The Coles et al. study employed single-case designs with four individual children attending the summer program to examine treatment withdrawal on two occasions for one week with multiple repeats (BABAB design). Both studies provided support for the STP treatment package in the behavioral and academic domains.

Multimodal Incremental Benefit Studies

Despite the evidence for the unimodal treatments described above, an equally important question has to do with whether combining multiple effective treatments leads to incremental benefit over and above the use of the treatments administered alone. An important point in addressing this question is that the comparison being made is quite different—in a sense, the "bar is set higher"—as favorable evaluation of a treatment requires improvement above and beyond improvement already attained with another effective treatment(s). We examine this question primarily in the context of multimodal interventions.

Nine multimodal incremental benefit studies using a between-subjects design met our criteria (Abikoff and colleagues—see footnote 2 for a listing of multiple articles from this study; Barkley et al., 2000; Ercan et al., 2005; Hoza et al., 2005; Klein & Abikoff, 1997; MTA Cooperative Group—see footnote 2 for multiple articles from this study; Pelham et al., 2000; Pfiffner & McBurnett, 1997; Tutty et al., 2003), as did two involving a within-subjects design (Kolko et al., 1999; Pelham et al., 2005a), and one using single-case designs (Reitman et al., 2001). All of these studies employed elementary school-aged children as participants. The length of treatment varied widely and ranged from 4 weeks to 24 months. Eight of these studies included medication used alone (i.e., an already established treatment) as a comparison condition in examining the incremental benefit of psychosocial treatment over and above the effects of medication (Abikoff and colleagues—studies listed in footnote 2; Ercan et al., 2005;

Hoza et al., 2005; Klein & Abikoff, 1997; Kolko et al., 1999; MTA Cooperative Group—articles listed in footnote 2; Pelham et al., 2005a; Reitman et al., 2001). Conversely, seven studies allowed for an examination of behavioral treatment versus a combined behavioral and medication intervention, hence examining the incremental benefit of medication over and above the effects of behavioral treatment (Hoza et al., 2005; Klein & Abikoff, 1997; Kolko et al., 1999; MTA Cooperative Group—articles listed in footnote 2; Pelham et al., 2000, 2005a; Reitman et al., 2001). Two studies made comparisons among varying combinations of psychosocial treatments (Barkley et al., 2000; Pfiffner & McBurnett, 1997) and one compared medication plus psychosocial treatment to medication plus community care (Tutty et al., 2003).[4]

These studies, however, provided conflicting data regarding the incremental benefit of multimodal interventions over unimodal approaches. For example, some studies comparing both medication and psychosocial treatment to medication treatment alone did not provide support for incremental benefit in any domains for which data were available using our averaged effect sizes approach (if applicable) (Abikoff and colleagues—articles listed in footnote 2; Ercan et al., 2005; Hoza et al., 2005; Kolko et al., 1999; MTA Cooperative Group—articles listed in footnote 2), whereas other studies found support in some domains but not others (Klein & Abikoff, 1997; Pelham et al., 2005a), and one study found support in all domains considered (Reitman et al., 2001). When comparing treatment involving both medication and psychosocial treatment to psychosocial treatment alone, evidence for incremental benefit was almost uniformly apparent in the core symptoms and behavioral domains (Klein & Abikoff, 1997; MTA Cooperative Group, 1999; Pelham et al., 2000, 2005a; Kolko et al., 1999; Reitman et al., 2001), but not for parenting practices/parent-child relationships or internalizing domains (Klein & Abikoff, 1997; MTA Cooperative Group—articles listed in footnote 2).Pelham et al. (2005a) was the only study demonstrating the incremental benefit of adding medication to psychosocial treatment in the academic domain; the other three studies providing data yielded unimportant effect sizes (Klein & Abikoff, 1997; MTA Cooperative Group, 1999; Pelham et al., 2000). Results in the social domain were more promising, with most studies supporting the addition of medication to psychosocial interventions (Hoza et al., 2005; Kolko et al, 1999; MTA Cooperative Group, 1999; Pelham et al., 2000, 2005a). Finally, comparisons of multimodal interventions to unimodal interventions in studies not involving medication (i.e., examining psychosocial treatments singularly and/or in combinations) yielded similarly mixed

---

[4] Space limitations prevented our inclusion of the table listing multimodal studies examining incremental benefit. Because we felt it was important for the reader to understand the scope of treatments and measures included in these studies, codes for all treatments and measures from these studies, as well as studies listed in Tables 1, 2, and 3, are included in our table note at the bottom of each table (i.e., all three tables use the same comprehensive list of codes). This represents our attempt at providing information to the reader about the entire scope of treatments and measures used across the collection of studies discussed in this review without exceeding our page limitation. It also explains why some of the codes appearing in the table note are not used in the tables.

Table 3. Studies Employing Summer Treatment Program

A1: Summer Treatment Program Studies Employing Between-Subjects Designs: Symptom and Behavior Domains: None

A2: Summer Treatment Program Studies Employing Within-Subjects Designs: Symptom and Behavior Domains

Study	N	Diagnostic Procedures	Treatment Length	Treatment Components*	Control Conditions*	Symptom Measure**	Mean ES (Range)	Behavior Measure**	Mean ES (Range)
Chronis et al. (2004)	44[s]	a, b, d, k	8 weeks	9 (2, 6, 14, 15, 16, 18, 25, 26)	23 (26)	NA		t	0.79 (0.39, 1.85)

A3: Summer Treatment Program Studies Employing Single-Subject Designs: Symptom and Behavior Domains

Study	N	Diagnostic Procedures	Treatment Length	Treatment Components*	Control Conditions*	Symptom Measure**	Effect	Behavior Measure**	Effect
Coles et al. (2005)	4[s]	a, b, d, k	8 weeks; b-mod admin during weeks 1, 2, 4, 6–8	9 (2, 6, 7, 14, 15, 16, 18, 25)	23	NA		t	IM

B1: Summer Treatment Program Studies Employing Between-Subjects Designs: Parenting/Parent-Child Relationship and Child Internalizing Domains: None

B2: Summer Treatment Program Studies Employing Within-Subjects Designs: Parenting/Parent-Child Relationship and Child Internalizing Domains: None

B3: Summer Treatment Program Studies Employing Single-Subject Designs: Parenting/Parent-Child Relationship and Child Internalizing Domains: None

C1: Summer Treatment Program Studies Employing Between-Subjects Designs: Academic and Social/Peer Domains: None

Table 3. (Continued)

C2: Summer Treatment Program Studies Employing Within-Subjects Designs: Academic and Social/Peer Domains

Study	N	Diagnostic Procedures	Treatment Length	Treatment Components*	Control Conditions*	Academic Measure**	Mean ES (Range)	Social/Peer Measure**	Mean ES (Range)
Chronis et al. (2004)	44[s]	a, b, d, k	8 weeks	9 (2, 6, 14, 15, 16, 18, 25, 26)	23 (26)	t	0.78 (0.62, 0.94)	NA	NA

C3: Summer Treatment Program Studies Employing Single-Subject Designs: Academic and Social/Peer Domains

Study	N	Diagnostic Procedures	Treatment Length	Treatment Components*	Control Conditions*	Academic Measure**	Effect	Social/Peer Measure**	Effect
Coles et al. (2005)	4[s]	a, b, d, k	8 weeks; b-mod admin during weeks 1, 2, 4, 6–8	9 (2, 6, 7, 14, 15, 16, 18, 25)	23	n	IM	NA	NA

NA = Not applicable. Under N: [p] = preschool; [s] = school-age. *Treatment components and control conditions: 1 = stimulant medication or medication assessment/referral; 2 = parent training; 3 = parent-targeted partner support and/or coping skills training; 4 = family problem-solving or communication therapy; 5 = support group; 6 = child-targeted social skills training; 7 = child-targeted self-control/anger management training; 8 = individual child-targeted psychotherapy; 9 = behavioral summer treatment program; 10 = child-focused academic organizational skills training; 11 = individualized academic assistance/remediation/tutoring; 12 = behaviorally trained individual paraprofessional support; 13 = school consultation and/or teacher psychoeducation; 14 = Daily Report Card; 15 = token reinforcement; 16 = token response cost; 17 = delayed reward; 18 = time out; 19 = peer attention/feedback/positive reinforcement; 20 = waitlist control; 21 = attention control; 22 = community care; 23 = treatment withdrawal; 24 = no intervention; 25 = adult-administered positive reinforcement/praise; 26 = sports skills training. **Diagnostic and outcome measures: a = clinical diagnosis by pediatrician or mental health professional; b = clinician-administered interview with parent, child, and/or teacher; c = clinician ratings; d = parent ratings; e = parent ratings of parenting practices/strategies; f = child ratings of parenting practices/strategies; g = parent ratings of parent-child relationship; h = child ratings of parent-child relationship; i = parent-child relationship; j = counselor ratings; k = teacher ratings; l = classroom observations; m = observer ratings; n = academic productivity; o = academic performance; p = cognitive tests; q = achievement tests; r = peer ratings or nominations; s = child self-ratings; t = behavior counts. For case studies, IM = improved; NC = no change; DT = deteriorated. The range of effect sizes is designated by [lower bound, upper bound].

results (Barkley et al., 2000; Pfiffner & McBurnett, 1997). Given the difficulty in deriving meaningful interpretations from this multimodal incremental benefit literature, we use this literature primarily to outline key
issues for future research.

DISCUSSION

Our conclusions regarding parent training and classroom interventions
for childhood ADHD echo those of prior reviews in supporting these
approaches to treatment, especially as compared to waitlist, no-treatment,
or treatment withdrawal control strategies. Based on an examination
of effect sizes and single-subjects' graphs for the studies summarized
herein, we feel the data support these treatments as effective for childhood
ADHD. Critical components of these treatments appear to be behavioral management strategies implemented by key adults in the child's
life (parents, teachers) and designed to promote child competence and
positive interactions between the child and these caregivers; clear instructions, predictable rules and structure; and consequences (such as time
out) for negative behaviors. The reader should note that there are many
well-established, widely available behavioral treatment manuals focused
on these skills and that these conclusions apply to any of these programs
applying these evidence-based principles, not just the specific programs
described herein. Examples of such excellent manuals include those by
Barkley (1997) and McMahon and Forehand (2003), among others.

Studies published over the past decade also provide evidence that
incorporating classroom peers into interventions for children with ADHD
in a variety of capacities (e.g., as group members for group-based contingencies, as peer tutors, and to assist in prompting and reinforcing
appropriate behaviors in target children) may facilitate improvement and
also prove a valuable resource for teachers. This is especially likely to
be true when resources limit the amount of one-on-one attention that
teachers themselves can realistically provide. This approach holds promise
especially if used as part of a comprehensive classroom intervention incorporating other effective strategies such as reinforcement and response cost.

Finally, a limited literature meeting our inclusion criteria has emerged
recently examining the Pelham summer treatment program (Pelham et al.,
1997) as a treatment for childhood ADHD (Chronis et al., 2004; Coles
et al., 2005). Because the number of STP studies meeting our inclusion
criteria was quite small (two studies employing a total of 48 children), one
should draw conclusions with caution. Nonetheless, preliminary evidence
suggests this is a promising approach worthy of further investigation.

Issues in Assessing the Multimodal Incremental Benefit Literature

Studies comparing multimodal treatments to established unimodal interventions also were examined, and our intent was to draw conclusions from

these comparisons to guide the field as to what combinations of interventions might best address problems in each of the outcome domains we reviewed. Our efforts in this regard yielded conflicting evidence regarding the incremental benefit of multimodal interventions. Of note, we found this task to be surprisingly onerous, as the multimodal studies we intended to compare seemed of limited comparability in many cases upon closer examination. Below we briefly discuss some of the issues that make us reluctant to draw definitive conclusions at the present time.

Most of the multimodal studies examined were package interventions involving a large number of treatment components administered simultaneously. Dismantling of these complex packages typically was not undertaken, with the package as a whole administered or withdrawn. The mixed findings across studies may reflect comparisons of treatment packages comprised of components of varying utility, consequently yielding results that do not converge. However, these results are nonetheless puzzling since most of these component interventions in each instance are evidence-based.

In a related fashion, some studies examined different doses of medication relative to and in combination with behavioral treatment (Kolko et al., 1999; Pelham et al., 2005a). These studies nicely demonstrated that results for unimodal versus multimodal comparisons differ widely as a function of medication dose of the comparison group. For example, in Pelham et al. (2005a), effect sizes for combined treatment (low dose of medication plus a summer treatment program) versus medication alone on the frequency of conduct problems exhibited yielded effect sizes ranging from 0 to +0.52, depending on the medication dose of the comparison group. The "take-home message" is that the selection of doses of medication (and behavior therapy) will affect the conclusions of the study. This makes it exceedingly difficult to draw global conclusions regarding the usefulness of multimodal interventions on a general level.

Another factor that may have contributed to these conflicting results is that even when a similar type or dose of component treatment *was* used across studies, outcome measures may have differed. Because of this, it remains unclear whether the source of discrepancy was attributable to the treatment package administered or to the outcome measurement strategy employed. In addition, studies often included multiple measures within the same domain; in these instances, we averaged effect sizes within domain for each study. However, these effect sizes for comparisons within the same domain often were quite discrepant depending on the measure employed. The question of how to appropriately aggregate findings from studies with multiple outcomes within a domain and different doses of treatment remains an important question for future research.

Despite these difficulties in interpreting the multimodal incremental benefit literature, we offer several conclusions based not only on this literature, but on our clinical experiences as well. First, we believe that multimodal interventions involving both stimulant medication and behavior modification may be most likely to provide a comprehensive intervention for ADHD. Whereas medication helps reduce symptoms that interfere with learning as well as behaviors that prove aversive to peers and adults, behavior modification helps promote skill development and effortful control of behavior. Further, the combination of medication and behavior modification allows lower doses of medication to be used, as well as lower "doses" of behavior modification, thus reducing medication-related side effects and the implementation burden on parents and teachers.

Second, the multimodal intervention that is most likely to be effective for a given child may be the one specifically geared toward that child's specific problem profile. Hence, clinicians would be wise to incorporate into their practice evidence-based treatments that allow some flexibility geared toward tailoring treatment plans toward the individual needs of children. Given the heterogeneity and chronicity of ADHD, a one-size-fits-all approach is unlikely to prove beneficial, and different modes of treatment are likely to be needed at different points in time even for the same child.

Third, there is a lack of evidence for the long-term persistence of treatment effects over time, regardless of the type of treatment, once the actual treatments have been stopped. For example, in the MTA study, treatment group differences that were evident at 14 months (end-of-treatment) had diminished by 24 months (MTA Cooperative Group, 2004) and were nonsignificant by 36 months (Jensen, 2005). Hence, the most important ingredient for successful treatment of childhood ADHD is likely to be continuing use of effective treatments, just as it is for chronic medical diseases (such as diabetes).

SUMMARY

This chapter reviewed empirical studies published in the past 10 years on psychosocial treatments for childhood ADHD meeting our specific inclusion criteria. Evidence was reviewed primarily for unimodal treatments given the problems we encountered in evaluating incremental benefit of multimodal interventions. Conclusions for unimodal treatment studies conducted over the past 10 years were generally consistent with conclusions of reviews summarizing earlier literature (e.g., Pelham et al., 1998) in finding support for both behavioral parent training and classroom interventions as effective strategies in treating childhood ADHD. Preliminary support for summer program interventions also was presented. Results of multimodal incremental benefit studies were difficult to interpret due to varying study designs, conflicting evidence arising from multiple outcome measures within the same domain, and the mixed results that characterized this literature. Results were discussed relative to these issues, and implications for future research were explored.

REFERENCES

Abikoff, H., Hechtman, L., Klein, R. G., Gallagher, R., Fleiss, K., Etcovitch, J., et al. (2004a). Social functioning in children with ADHD treated with long-term methylphenidate and multimodal psychosocial treatment. *Journal of the American Academy of Child and Adolescent Psychiatry, 43*, 820–829.

Abikoff, H., Hechtman, L., Klein, R. G., Weiss, G., Fleiss, K., Etcovitch, J., et al. (2004b). Symptomatic improvement in children with ADHD treated with long-term methylphenidate and multimodal psychosocial treatment. *Journal of the American Academy of Child and Adolescent Psychiatry, 43*, 802–811.

American Psychiatric Association (2000). *Diagnostic and Statistical Manual of Mental Disorders,* 4th ed. (rev. ed.). Washington, DC.

Anhalt, K., McNeil, C. B., & Bahl, A. B. (1998). The ADHD Classroom Kit: A whole-classroom approach for managing disruptive behavior. *Psychology in the Schools, 35*, 67–79.

Barkley, R. A. (1997). *Defiant Children: A Clinician's Manual for Assessment and Parent Training,* 2nd ed. New York: Guilford Press.

Barkley, R. A. (2002). Psychosocial treatments for attention-deficit/hyperactivity disorder in children. *Journal of Clinical Psychiatry, 63* (Suppl 12), 36–43.

Barkley, R. A., Edwards, G., Laneri, M., Fletcher, K, & Metevia, L. (2001). The efficacy of problem-solving communication training alone, behavior management training alone, and their combination for parent-adolescent conflict in teenagers with ADHD and ODD. *Journal of Consulting and Clinical Psychology, 69*, 926–941.

Barkley, R. A., Shelton, T. L., Crosswait, C., Moorehouse, M., Fletcher, K., Barrett, S., et al. (2000). Multi-method psycho-educational intervention for preschool children with disruptive behavior: Preliminary results at post-treatment. *Journal of Child Psychology and Psychiatry, 41*, 319–332.

Biederman, J., Faraone, S., Milberger, S., Curtis, S., Chen, L., Marrs, A., et al. (1996). Predictors of persistence and remission of ADHD into adolescence: Results from a four-year prospective follow-up study. *Journal of the American Academy of Child and Adolescent Psychiatry, 35*, 343–351.

Bor, W., Sanders, M. R., & Markie-Dadds, C. (2002). The effects of the Triple P-Positive Parenting Program on preschool children with co-occurring disruptive behavior and attentional/hyperactive difficulties. *Journal of Abnormal Child Psychology, 30*, 571–587.

Chambless, D. L., & Ollendick, T. H. (2001) Empirically supported psychological interventions: Controversies and evidence. *Annual Review of Psychology, 52*, 685–716.

Chronis, A. M., Fabiano, G. A., Gnagy, E. M., Onyango, A. N., Pelham, W. E., Lopez-Williams, A., et al. (2004). An evaluation of the Summer Treatment Program for children with attention-deficit/hyperactivity disorder using a treatment withdrawal design. *Behavior Therapy, 35*, 561–585.

Chronis, A. M., Jones, H. A., & Raggi, V. L. (2006). Evidence-based psychosocial treatments for children and adolescents with attention-deficit/hyperactivity disorder. *Clinical Psychology Review, 26*, 486–502.

Cohen, J. (1988). *Statistical Power Analysis for the Behavioral Sciences,* 2nd ed. Hillsdale, NJ: Lawrence Erlbaum Associates.

Coles, E. K., Pelham, W. E., Gnagy, E. M., Burrows-MacLean, L., Fabiano, G. A., & Chacko, A., et al. (2005). A controlled evaluation of behavioral treatment with children with ADHD attending a summer treatment program. *Journal of Emotional and Behavioral Disorders, 13*, 99–112.

DuPaul, G. J., Ervin, R. A., Hook, C. L., & McGoey, K. E. (1998). Peer tutoring for children with attention deficit hyperactivity disorder: Effects on classroom behavior and academic performance. *Journal of Applied Behavior Analysis, 31*, 579–592.

Ercan, E. S., Varan, A., & Deniz, U. (2005). Effects of combined treatment on Turkish children diagnosed with attention-deficit/hyperactivity disorder: A preliminary report. *Journal of Child and Adolescent Psychopharmacology, 15*, 203–219.

Flood, W. A., Wilder, D. A., Flood, A. L., & Masuda, A. (2002). Peer-mediated reinforcement plus prompting as treatment for off-task behavior in children with attention deficit hyperactivity disorder. *Journal of Applied Behavior Analysis, 35*, 199–204.

Hechtman, L., Abikoff, H., Klein, R. G., Greenfield, B., Etcovitch, J., Cousins, L., et al. (2004a). Children with ADHD treated with long-term methylphenidate and multimodal psychosocial treatment: Impact on parental practices. *Journal of the American Academy of Child and Adolescent Psychiatry, 43*, 830–838.

Hechtman, L., Abikoff, H., Klein, R. G., Weiss, G., Respitz, C., Kouri, J., et al. (2004b). Academic achievement and emotional status of children with ADHD treated with long-term methylphenidate and multimodal psychosocial treatment. *Journal of the American Academy of Child and Adolescent Psychiatry, 43*, 812–819.

Hoath, F. E., & Sanders, M. R. (2002). A feasibility study of Enhanced Group Triple P-Positive Parenting Program for parents of children with attention-deficit/hyperactivity disorder. *Behaviour Change, 19*, 191–206.

Hoza, B., Gerdes, A. C., Mrug, S., Hinshaw, S. P., Bukowski, W. M., Gold, J. A., et al. (2005). Peer-assessed outcomes in the Multimodal Treatment Study of Children with Attention Deficit Hyperactivity Disorder. *Journal of Clinical Child and Adolescent Psychology, 34*, 74–86.

Jensen, P. S. (2005). Do children with ADHD get better? An MTA perspective. In L. E. Arnold (Chair), *New ADHD Insights from MTA Data Through 36 Months*. Symposium conducted at the joint annual meeting of the American Academy of Child and Adolescent Psychiatry and the Canadian Academy of Child and Adolescent Psychiatry, Toronto, Canada.

Kelley, M. L., & McCain, A. P. (1995). Promoting academic performance in inattentive children: The relative efficacy of school-home notes with and without response cost. *Behavior Modification, 19*, 357–375.

Klein, R. G., & Abikoff, H. (1997). Behavior therapy and methylphenidate in the treatment of children with ADHD. *Journal of Attention Disorders, 2*, 89–114.

Kolko, D. J., Bukstein, O. G., & Barron, J. (1999). Methylphenidate and behavior modification in children with ADHD and comorbid ODD or CD: Main and incremental effects across settings. *Journal of the American Academy of Child and Adolescent Psychiatry, 38*, 578–586.

Lonigan, C. J., Elbert, J. C., & Johnson, S. B. (1998). Empirically supported psychosocial interventions for children: An overview. *Journal of Clinical Child Psychology, 27*, 138–145.

McGoey, K. E., & DuPaul, G. J. (2000). Token reinforcement and response cost procedures: Reducing the disruptive behavior of preschool children with attention-deficit/hyperactivity disorder. *School Psychology Quarterly, 15*, 330–343.

McMahon, R. J., & Forehand, R. L. (2003). *Helping the Noncompliant Child:Family-Based Treatment for Oppositional Behavior*, 2nd ed. New York: Guilford Press.

Miranda, A., Presentación, M. J., & Soriano, M. (2002). Effectiveness of a school-based multi-component program for the treatment of children with ADHD. *Journal of Learning Disabilities, 35*, 546–562.

MTA Cooperative Group (1999). A 14-month randomized clinical trial of treatment strategies for attention-deficit/hyperactivity disorder. *Archives of General Psychiatry, 56*, 1073–1086.

MTA Cooperative Group (2004). National Institute of Mental Health multimodal treatment study of ADHD follow-up: 24-month outcomes of treatment strategies for attention-deficit/hyperactivity disorder. *Pediatrics, 113*, 754–761.

Pelham, W. E., Burrows-MacLean, L., Gnagy, E. M., Fabiano, G. A., Coles, E. K., Tresco, K. E., et al. (2005a). Transdermal methylphenidate, behavioral, and combined treatment for children with ADHD. *Experimental and Clinical Psychopharmacology, 13*, 111–126.

Pelham, W. E., Erhardt, D., Gnagy, E. M., Greiner, A. R., Arnold, L. E., Abikoff, H. B., et al. (2006). *Parent and Teacher Evaluation of Treatment in the MTA: Consumer Satisfaction and Perceived Effectiveness*. Manuscript submitted for publication.

Pelham, W. E., Fabiano, G. A., Gnagy, E. M., Greiner, A. R., & Hoza, B. (2005b). The role of summer treatment programs in the context of comprehensive treatment for attention-deficit/hyperactivity disorder. In E. D. Hibbs & P. S. Jensen (Eds.), *Psychosocial Treatments for Child and Adolescent Disorders: Empirically Based Strategies for Clinical Practice*, 2nd ed. (pp. 377–409). Washington, DC: American Psychological Association.

Pelham, W. E., Gnagy, E. M., Greiner, A. R., Hoza, B., Hinshaw, S. P., Swanson, J. M., et al. (2000). Behavioral versus behavioral and pharmacological treatment in ADHD children attending a summer treatment program. *Journal of Abnormal Child Psychology, 28*, 507–525.

Pelham, W. E., Greiner, A. R., & Gnagy, E. M. (1997). *Summer Treatment Program Manual*. Buffalo, NY: Comprehensive Treatment for Attention Deficit Disorders, Inc.

Pelham, W. E., & Hoza, B. (1996). Intensive treatment: A summer treatment program for children with ADHD. In E. D. Hibbs & P. S. Jensen (Eds.), *Psychosocial Treatments for Child and Adolescent Disorders: Empirically Based Strategies for Clinical Practice* (pp. 311–340). Washington, DC: American Psychological Association.

Pelham, W. E., Wheeler, T., & Chronis, A. (1998). Empirically supported psychosocial treatments for attention deficit hyperactivity disorder. *Journal of Clinical Child Psychology, 27,* 190–205.

Pfiffner, L. J., & McBurnett, K. (1997). Social skills training with parent generalization: Treatment effects for children with attention deficit disorder. *Journal of Consulting and Clinical Psychology, 65,* 749–757.

Reitman, D., Hupp, S. D. A., O'Callaghan, P. M., Gulley, V., & Northup, J. (2001). The influence of a token economy and methylphenidate on attentive and disruptive behavior during sports with ADHD-diagnosed children. *Behavior Modification, 25,* 305–323.

Roberts, M. C., & James, R. (this volume; 2008). Criteria for evidence-based therapies: What is necessary? What is sufficient? In. R. G. Steele, T. D. Elkin, & M. C. Roberts (Eds.), *Handbook of Evidence-Based Therapies for Children and Adolescents.* NY: Springer.

Smith, B. H., Waschbusch, D. A., Willoughby, M. T., & Evans, S. (2000). The efficacy, safety, and practicality of treatments for adolescents with attention-deficit/hyperactivity disorder. *Clinical Child and Family Psychology Review, 3,* 243–267.

Sonuga-Barke, E. J. S., Daley, D., Thompson, M., Laver-Bradbury, C., & Weeks, A. (2001). Parent-based therapies for preschool attention-deficit/hyperactivity disorder: A randomized, controlled trial with a community sample. *Journal of the American Academy of Child & Adolescent Psychiatry, 40,* 402–408.

Strayhorn, J. M., & Bickel, D. D. (2002). Reduction in children's symptoms of attention deficit hyperactivity disorder and oppositional defiant disorder during individual tutoring as compared with classroom instruction. *Psychological Reports, 91,* 69–80.

Tutty, S., Gephart, H., & Wurzbacher, K. (2003). Enhancing behavioral and social skill functioning in children newly diagnosed with attention-deficit hyperactivity disorder in a pediatric setting. *Developmental and Behavioral Pediatrics, 24,* 51–57.

Wells, K. C., Epstein, J. N., Hinshaw, S. P., Conners, C. K., Klaric, J., Abikoff, H. B., et al. (2000). Parenting and family stress treatment outcomes in attention deficit hyperactivity disorder (ADHD): An empirical analysis in the MTA study. *Journal of Abnormal Child Psychology, 28,* 543–553.

13

Evidence-Based Therapies for Oppositional Behavior in Young Children

ROBERT J. MCMAHON and JULIE S. KOTLER

The primary purpose of this chapter is to present and critically evaluate current evidence-based interventions for oppositional behavior (OB) in young children. Children with OB are typically described by parents and teachers as argumentative, disobedient, disruptive, demanding, and defiant. We have operationalized "young children" as including children between the ages of 3 and 8, thus encompassing the preschool and early school-age periods. Although OB can be manifested in a variety of child disorders, this chapter focuses on OB manifested in the broader context of "conduct problems" [i.e., oppositional defiant disorder (ODD) and/or conduct disorder], as that is the area for which evidence-based treatments exist (see McMahon et al., 2006). Likewise, the focus of this chapter is on family-based interventions, as this is the locus of most of the evidence base for treatment of OB in young children.

The first section of this chapter consists of a description of OB, including diagnostic issues, epidemiology, contextual influences (including the family, peer group, and neighborhood), and developmental pathways. The second section of the chapter provides a description of family-based interventions for OB and a discussion of several cross-cutting issues concerning such family-based interventions. The chapter concludes with a brief case example and suggestions for the enhancement of the clinical utility of these interventions.

ROBERT J. MCMAHON and JULIE S. KOTLER • University of Washington

OPPOSITIONAL BEHAVIOR IN YOUNG CHILDREN

Diagnostic Criteria

In the *Diagnostic and Statistical Manual of Mental Disorders* (DSM-IV-TR;
American Psychiatric Association, 2000), the diagnostic category that is
most relevant to OB is ODD, which is defined as a "recurrent pattern of
negativistic, defiant, disobedient, and hostile behavior toward authority
figures" (p. 91). At least a six-month duration is needed, and four of the
following eight behaviors must be present: losing temper, arguing with
grownups, defying or not complying with grownups' rules or requests,
deliberately doing things that annoy other people, blaming others for own
mistakes, being touchy or easily becoming annoyed by others, exhibiting
anger and resentment, and showing spite or vindictiveness. The behaviors
must have a higher frequency than is generally seen in other children
of similar developmental level and age and must lead to meaningful
impairment in academic and social functioning.

There is a paucity of data concerning the diagnostic criteria for ODD
(and conduct disorder) as it might be applied to children younger than age
7 (Angold & Costello, 2001), although the ability to identify an externalizing
broad-band syndrome of conduct problems (including OB) is well established in these younger children (e.g., Campbell, 1995). There is increasing
evidence that the DSM diagnosis of ODD can be reliably made in preschool-
aged children and that the diagnosis has concurrent and predictive validity
(e.g., Speltz et al., 1999). Some of the ODD symptoms pertaining to affective
reactivity (i.e., blaming others, being touchy or easily annoyed, displaying
anger and resentment) may be especially predictive of later risk for both
externalizing and internalizing problems (Speltz et al., 1999).

Noncompliance

One key manifestation of OB is noncompliance (i.e., excessive disobe-
dience to adults) (McMahon & Forehand, 2003). Noncompliance is a
keystone behavior in the development of more serious forms of conduct
problems: (1) It appears early in the progression of conduct problems and
continues to be manifested in subsequent developmental periods (e.g.,
Chamberlain & Patterson, 1995; McMahon & Forehand, 2003); (2) low
compliance is associated with referral for services in children with conduct
problems (Dumas, 1996); and (3) when noncompliance is targeted, there
is often concomitant improvement in other conduct problem behaviors as
well (e.g., Wells et al., 1980a). In Patterson's comprehensive theoretical
model for the development and maintenance of conduct problems (see
below; Chamberlain & Patterson, 1995; Patterson et al., 1992), early
childhood noncompliance is the precursor of severe manifestations of
conduct problem behaviors later in childhood and adolescence and plays a
role in subsequent academic and peer relationship problems. Walker and
Walker (1991) have stressed the role of compliance and noncompliance in
the classroom.

Epidemiology

OB is among the most frequently occurring child behavioral problems. However, accurately determining the prevalence of OB has proven to be quite difficult as a function of the numerous changes in diagnostic criteria for ODD over DSM revisions, whether an impairment criterion is included, the informant (i.e., youth, parent, teacher, clinician), and the method of combining information from informants (Essau, 2003). Prevalence rates generally range from 2% to 10% for ODD in nonclinical samples (e.g., Essau, 2003; Nock et al., 2007). More boys than girls are diagnosed with ODD prior to adolescence (DSM-IV-TR, 2000).

There is an asymmetrical relationship between early OB and the later development of more serious forms of conduct problems (e.g., conduct disorder). Although most children with OB do not go on to receive a diagnosis of conduct disorder, the large majority of youth who do eventually receive this diagnosis manifested OB (and ODD) previously (Hinshaw & Lee, 2003).

ADHD is one of the most common comorbid conditions, and its presence is predictive of more negative outcomes (e.g., Speltz et al., 1999). Preschool-aged children with ODD, especially if it is comorbid with ADHD, are at risk not only for the later development of more serious conduct problems (e.g., diagnosis of conduct disorder) but also for anxiety, mood, and/or substance use disorders (e.g., Nock et al., 2007; Speltz et al., 1999).

Conceptualizations

The most comprehensive family-based formulation for the development of child OB has been the coercion model developed by Patterson (e.g., Patterson et al., 1992). The model describes "basic training" in OB behaviors that occurs in the context of an escalating cycle of coercive parent-child interactions beginning prior to school entry. The proximal cause for entry into the coercive cycle is thought to be ineffective parental management strategies, particularly in regard to child compliance with parental directives during the preschool period. Types of parenting practices that have been closely associated with the development of child OB (and other forms of conduct problems) include inconsistent discipline; irritable, explosive discipline; low supervision and involvement; and inflexible, rigid discipline (Chamberlain et al., 1997). Other family risk factors that may impact parenting practices include maladaptive social cognitions, personal (e.g., antisocial behavior, substance use, depression) and interparental (e.g., marital problems) distress, and social isolation (e.g., insularity) (McMahon et al., 2006). Coercive interactions with siblings can also play a role in the development and maintenance of OB (e.g., Garcia et al., 2000).

Various child characteristics, such as comorbid disorders (e.g., ADHD, mood and anxiety disorders) and developmental phenomena (e.g., temperament, executive functions, emotion regulation, language development, social cognition), can also play a role in the development and maintenance of the coercive cycle (Greene et al., 2004; McMahon et al., 2006). There is support for a cumulative risk conceptualization of ODD, in which an increasing number of risks in the domains of parenting practices, child characteristics, attachment, and family adversity increase the likelihood of the development of ODD (Greenberg et al., 2001).

Developmental Pathways

Hinshaw and Lee (2003) suggest that at least three developmental pathways have childhood onset of conduct problems (including OB) as a common starting point: (1) "early starters" (who persist in high levels of conduct problem behavior throughout the developmental period and into adulthood), (2) "desisters", and (3) "low-level chronics" (who engage in relatively low but persistent levels of conduct problems throughout the developmental period and into adulthood) (e.g., Moffitt et al., 2002). It is estimated that 50% of children who demonstrate high levels of CP behavior during the preschool period will not follow the early-starter progression of increasingly severe conduct problems as they get older (Campbell, 1995).

FAMILY-BASED INTERVENTIONS FOR OPPOSITIONAL BEHAVIOR IN YOUNG CHILDREN

Approaches to treating children with CP in the family have typically been based on a social learning-based "parent training" (PT) model of intervention (e.g., Miller & Prinz, 1990). PT can be defined as an approach to treating child behavioral problems (including OB) by using "... procedures in which parents are trained to alter their child's behavior in the home. The parents meet with a therapist or trainer who teaches them to use specific procedures to alter interactions with their child, to promote prosocial behavior, and to decrease deviant behavior" (Kazdin, 1995, p. 82). PT has been applied to a broad array of child problems and populations but has been primarily employed in the treatment of preadolescent children who exhibit overt conduct problem behaviors (e.g., temper tantrums, aggression, and excessive noncompliance), and it is in this area that PT has the greatest empirical support. This chapter focuses on PT interventions for preschool- and early-school-aged (3–8 years old) children who engage in excessive levels of OB.

The underlying assumption of social learning–based PT models is that some sort of parenting skills deficit has been at least partly responsible for the development and/or maintenance of the conduct-problem behaviors. The core elements of the PT approach include that (1) intervention is conducted primarily with the parents, with relatively less therapist-child contact; (2) therapists refocus parents' attention from a preoccupation with conduct-problem behavior to an emphasis on prosocial goals; (3) the content of these programs typically includes instruction in the social learning principles underlying the parenting techniques; training in defining, monitoring, and tracking child behavior; training in positive reinforcement procedures including praise and other forms of positive parent attention and token or point systems; training in extinction and mild punishment procedures such as ignoring, response cost, and time out in lieu of physical punishment; training in giving clear instructions or commands; and training in problem solving; and (4) therapists make extensive use of didactic instruction, modeling, role-playing, behavioral rehearsal, and structured homework exercises to promote effective parenting (Dumas, 1989; Kazdin, 1995; Miller & Prinz, 1990). PT interventions have been successfully utilized in the clinic and home settings, have been implemented with individual families or with groups of families, and have involved some or all of the instructional techniques listed above.

We present several PT programs as examples of state-of-the-art family-based interventions for young oppositional children. Descriptions of the clinical procedures utilized in these programs are widely available (e.g., therapist manuals, videotapes for therapist training, and/or books for parents), and each of the programs has been extensively evaluated.

The Hanf Model of Parent Training

The first three PT programs described in this chapter have their origins in the pioneering work of Constance Hanf (e.g., 1969) nearly 40 years ago. They are (1) "Helping the Noncompliant Child" (HNC; McMahon & Forehand, 2003), (2) "Parent-Child Interaction Therapy" (PCIT; e.g., Brinkmeyer & Eyberg, 2003), and (3) "The Incredible Years: Early Childhood BASIC Parent Training Program" (BASIC; Webster-Stratton, 2005).

In general, these programs focus on treating noncompliance and other OB in preadolescent children, especially those of preschool and early school age. HNC and PCIT are typically administered via individual contact with a therapist or trainer, whereas BASIC is designed primarily to work with parents in a group setting. Characteristic of all Hanf-based PT programs, therapists make extensive use of modeling and role-play during sessions (in addition to didactic instruction and discussion) to teach parents the skills of attends, rewards, ignoring, clear instructions, and time out and the use of home practice assignments and exercises. Similar to Hanf, two of the programs (HNC, PCIT) describe behavioral performance criteria that the parent must meet for each parenting skill.

Helping the Noncompliant Child

The HNC program (McMahon & Forehand, 2003) is specifically designed to treat noncompliance in younger children (3–8 years of age). It consists of two phases. During the differential-attention phase of treatment (Phase I), the parent learns to break out of the coercive cycle of interaction by increasing the frequency and range of positive attention to the child and ignoring minor inappropriate behaviors. The primary goal is to establish a positive, mutually reinforcing relationship between parent and child.

The parent is first taught to attend to and describe the child's appropriate behavior while eliminating commands, questions, and criticisms. The second segment of Phase I consists of teaching the parent to use verbal and physical attention contingent upon compliance and appropriate behaviors and to actively ignore minor inappropriate behaviors. Assigned homework includes daily 10-minute practice sessions with the child using the skills taught in the clinic, and the parent is required to develop programs for use outside the clinic to increase at least three child behaviors using the new skills.

In Phase II (Compliance Training), the primary parenting skills are taught in the context of the clear instructions sequence. This involves teaching the parent to use appropriate commands and a time-out procedure to decrease noncompliant behavior exhibited by the child. The parent is taught to give direct, concise, single instructions, to allow the child sufficient time to comply, and to provide positive attention for child compliance. If compliance is not initiated, the parent learns to implement a three-minute time-out procedure. Following time out, the command that originally elicited noncompliance is repeated. Parents are also taught to use permanent "standing rules" as an occasional supplement to this sequence.

Progression to each new skill in the HNC program is determined by the use of behavioral and temporal (number of sessions) criteria. These criteria ensure that the parent has attained an acceptable degree of competence in a skill before being taught additional parenting techniques and allow for the individualization of the program by allocating training time more efficiently.

Parent-Child Interaction Therapy

A second PT program modeled after the Hanf approach is PCIT (e.g., Brinkmeyer & Eyberg, 2003). In addition to being grounded in social learning theory, PCIT has been influenced by attachment theory. Thus, compared to other Hanf-based models of parenting training, PCIT could be described as being somewhat more explicit in its focus on the enhancement of a nurturing parent-child relationship (although the intervention does not differ substantially from other Hanf-based parenting training approaches). PCIT is appropriate for families with children in the 2- to 8-year-old range. Although PCIT is primarily an individual treatment, a group format has also recently been introduced (Niec et al., 2005).

Similar to the HNC program, PCIT is divided into two phases. The first phase, child-directed interaction (CDI), is based on Hanf's Child's Game. During this phase, parents are encouraged to follow the child's lead using nondirective "PRIDE" skills including (1) praising the child, (2) reflecting child statements, (3) imitating the play, (4) describing child behavior, and (5) using enthusiasm in play with the child. As with the HNC program, the therapist coaches the parent in these skills, and criteria for mastery are met through behavioral observations of parent-child interactions. In the second phase of PCIT, parent-directed interaction (PDI), parents lead the play and are coached in giving appropriate commands and directives and enforcing consequences for compliance and noncompliance. Labeled praise is also introduced in this phase (whereas in the HNC program, labeled praise is introduced in the initial phase of the intervention). A primary component of PDI includes training parents in appropriate use of time out. "House rules" (equivalent to standing rules in HNC) are also introduced and implemented during PDI. Hembree-Kigin and McNeil (1995) have published a clinician's manual for PCIT.

Incredible Years—BASIC

A third PT program for young (3- to 8-year-old) children with OB, which includes some components of the Hanf and HNC programs, is the "Incredible Years" BASIC program developed by Webster-Stratton (2005). The core PT component of this program is a videotape modeling/group discussion intervention that consists of a standard package of videotape programs of modeled parenting skills shown by a therapist to groups of parents. The 250 video vignettes (each of which lasts approximately 2 minutes), presented during the 12–14-week program, include examples of parents interacting with their children in both appropriate and inappropriate ways. After each vignette, the therapist leads a discussion of the relevant interactions and solicits parental responses to the vignettes. In this program, the children do not attend the therapy sessions, although parents are given homework exercises to practice parenting skills with their children. The BASIC program has been implemented with both nonreferred (e.g., Webster-Stratton, 1981) and clinic-referred families (e.g., Webster-Stratton, 1984) and as a selective preventive intervention with Head Start mothers (e.g., Webster-Stratton, 1998).

In addition to these three Hanf-based PT programs, we review two additional widely recognized PT programs for OB: "Triple P-Positive Parenting Program" (Triple P; e.g., Sanders et al., 2003) and "Parent Management Training-Oregon" (PMTO; e.g., Patterson et al., 1975).

Triple P-Positive Parenting Program

The Triple P program developed by Sanders and colleagues (2003) in Australia consists of five levels of intervention, ranging from a universal prevention program to an intensive and individualized treatment targeting children with serious CP. This program combines PT strategies with a range of family support materials and services. The group of interventions was designed for use with parents of children from birth to age 16, although the majority of outcome research has focused on families with young (2 to 8 years) children.

The Level 1 intervention (Universal Triple P) is a universal prevention program designed to provide parents with easy access to parenting information using media sources (e.g., newspaper, radio, TV), a set of "tip sheets," and videotapes that demonstrate parenting strategies. Level 2 (Selected Triple P) is a brief (one- to two-session) intervention conducted by a primary health-care provider. This level is designed for parents of children with mild conduct problem behaviors (including OB) or for parents who have a specific behavioral concern. The Selected Triple P intervention includes the provision of problem-specific and developmental guidance and also incorporates tip sheets and videotapes demonstrating parenting strategies. Level 3 (Primary Care Triple P) is a four-session intervention, again conducted by a primary health-care provider. This level is appropriate for parents of children with mild to moderate CP behaviors and includes the provision of parenting advice and opportunities for parents to learn and practice skills to address problem behavior. Level 4 (Standard Triple P) is a more intensive intervention, including 8 to 10 sessions for parents of children with more severe CP. This level includes many components of traditional PT programs such as a focus on parent-child interaction and training in parenting skills designed to be applicable to a range of problem behavior. There are individual, group, and self-directed treatment options for Level 4 (Morawska et al., 2005). The Level 5 intervention (Enhanced Triple P) is appropriate when there is family dysfunction (e.g., parental depression, marital conflict) in addition to serious youth CP. At this level, a behavioral family intervention is individually tailored to families' needs, and treatment strategies often include home visits focused on parenting practices, training in coping skills, and management of mood problems, marital conflict, and/or family stress. Mental health practitioners typically administer Level 4 and Level 5 interventions.

Parent Management Training—Oregon

In addition to his seminal contributions regarding the theoretical and empirical knowledge base concerning conduct problems, Patterson has also been extremely influential with respect to the development and evaluation of family-based intervention strategies for children with CP. The PMTO program for preadolescent children (3 to 12 years of age) is delineated in the treatment manual by Patterson et al. (1975). Prior to beginning treatment, parents are given a copy of either *Living with Children* (Patterson, 1976) or *Families* (Patterson, 1975) to provide a conceptual background for the treatment sessions and to facilitate generalization and maintenance. After the reading assignment, the next step is to teach the parents to pinpoint problem behaviors of concern and to track the child's behavior. Once parents have mastered these skills, they are assisted in establishing a positive reinforcement system and using points, tangible reinforcers, and social reinforcement (i.e., praise). Over time, tangible reinforcers are faded. After the point system is well established, the parents are taught to use a five-minute time-out procedure for noncompliance or aggressive behavior. [Response cost (e.g., loss of privileges) and work chores are sometimes used with older children.] As treatment progresses, parents become increasingly responsible for designing and implementing behavior management programs. Parents are also taught to monitor or supervise their children, even when they are away from home. Then, problem-solving and negotiation strategies are taught to the parents. Patterson and Chamberlain (1988) also estimate that 30% of treatment time is devoted to dealing with problems such as marital difficulties, personal adjustment problems, and family crises.

Interventions for Oppositional Behavior in the School

For children who attend preschool or elementary school, the therapist also needs to consider whether intervention concerning the child's behavior in school is indicated. Assessment data can guide the therapist in choosing among three options (McMahon & Forehand, 2003). First, if there is no evidence of school behavior problems, a school intervention obviously is not necessary. However, even in this case, the child's behavior in the school setting should be monitored during and after intervention. This will allow detection of any behavioral difficulties that may arise and also provides the opportunity to see if the child's behavior improves with PT. Second, if behavioral difficulties exist in the school setting but they are not severe, the therapist may choose to implement PT and monitor the child's behavior in the school setting. However, the evidence for positive effects of PT in the school setting has been mixed (see below). Monitoring the child's behavior in the school setting will allow the therapist to determine whether intervention in school is necessary or not. Third, if severe behavioral difficulties exist in the school setting, the therapist will likely need to recommend intervention simultaneously in the home and school settings. When intervention in the school is necessary, the therapist may choose to implement an in-class intervention, a home-based reinforcement program, or both (e.g., McMahon et al., 2006; Walker & Walker, 1991).

ISSUES IN INTERVENTION EFFECTIVENESS

Generalization and Social Validity

The short-term efficacy of behavioral PT in producing changes in both parent and child behaviors has been demonstrated repeatedly (e.g., Serketich & Dumas, 1996), but generalization of these effects is also important to demonstrate. Forehand and Atkeson (1977) described four types of generalization of PT intervention effects: setting, temporal, sibling, and behavioral. A number of investigations assessing the various types of generalization have, for the most part, supported the efficacy of behavioral PT programs.

Each of the PT programs described earlier in the chapter has documented setting generalization from the clinic to the home for parent and child behavior and for parents' perception of child adjustment (e.g., Fleischman, 1981; Peed et al., 1977; Sanders et al., 2000; Schuhmann et al., 1998; Webster-Stratton, 1984). Temporal generalization has also been demonstrated over follow-up periods of one to six years (e.g., Baum

& Forehand, 1981; Bor et al., 2002; Hood & Eyberg, 2003; Patterson & Fleischman, 1979; Reid et al., 2003). Studies done 4.5 to 14 years after completion of the HNC program suggest that the children were functioning well compared to peers in terms of parent-, teacher-, and self-reported adjustment (Forehand & Long, 1988; Long et al., 1994).

Several investigators have now assessed setting generalization from the clinic or home setting to the school. In their meta-analytic study, Serketich and Dumas (1996) reported an effect size of 0.73 for PT when the outcome was based on teacher report, and McNeil et al. (1991) demonstrated generalization of PCIT to the classroom using both observational data and teacher ratings of conduct problem behavior. However, evidence of behavioral contrast effects (i.e., behavior worsens at school as it improves at home) has occasionally been found (e.g., Johnson et al., 1976; Wahler, 1975), and other investigators have failed to find evidence of generalization to school or a failure to maintain this generalization (e.g., Breiner & Forehand, 1981; Taylor et al., 1998).

Several parent training programs (HNC, PCIT, PMTO, BASIC) have demonstrated sibling generalization (e.g., Brestan et al., 1997; Gardner et al., 2006; Horne & Van Dyke, 1983; Humphreys et al., 1978), and this generalization has been maintained up to a one-year follow-up for PMTO (Horne & Van Dyke, 1983). Behavioral generalization from the treatment of child noncompliance to other behaviors (e.g., aggression, temper tantrums) has been demonstrated for the HNC (Wells et al., 1980a), BASIC (Webster-Stratton, 1984), and PMTO (e.g., Fleischman, 1981) programs.

The social validity of family-based interventions with children with CP has been assessed by various methods, including measures of consumer satisfaction completed by parents (see McMahon & Forehand, 1983) and treatment acceptability (e.g., Cross Calvert & McMahon, 1987), and by determining the clinical significance of improvements (Sheldrick et al., 2001). PT programs have provided strong evidence of consumer satisfaction at posttreatment and/or follow-up periods of a year or more (e.g., Baum & Forehand, 1981; Brestan et al., 1999; Leung et al., 2003; McMahon et al., 1984; Patterson et al., 1982; Taylor et al., 1998). They have also provided normative comparisons indicating that, by the end of treatment, child and/or parent behavior more closely resembles that in nonreferred families (e.g., Forehand et al., 1980; Sanders & Christensen, 1985; Sheldrick et al., 2001). In their meta-analytic review of PT, Serketich and Dumas (1996) reported that 17 of 19 intervention groups dropped below the clinical range after treatment on at least one measure, and 14 groups did so on all measures.

It is apparent that evidence for the generalization and social validity of family-based interventions with young children with OB is extensive and, for the most part, positive. A number of studies have examined the role of adjunctive treatments in facilitating generalization and/or social validity, over and above that obtained by standard PT programs. Adjunctive treatments have included components designed to facilitate maternal self-control/self-management (e.g., Sanders & Glynn, 1981; Wells et al., 1980b), child self-control (Baum et al., 1986), maternal depression

(Griest et al., 1982; Sanders & McFarland, 2000), parental knowledge of social learning principles (McMahon et al., 1981), generalization to specific settings in the home and community (e.g., Sanders & Christensen, 1985), marital/parental support, communication, and problem solving (e.g., Dadds et al., 1987; Griest et al., 1982; Webster-Stratton, 1994), discrimination training for mothers ("synthesis teaching"; Wahler et al., 1993), and parental stress (Kazdin & Whitley, 2003).

Comparison Studies

Each of the PT programs has been positively evaluated compared with no-treatment and waiting-list control conditions (e.g., Bor et al., 2002; Peed et al., 1977; Schuhmann et al., 1998; Scott et al., 2001; Wiltz & Patterson, 1974) or an attention-placebo condition (Walter & Gilmore, 1973). Furthermore, comparisons with groups of nonreferred "normal" samples have indicated greater similarity in parent/child behaviors and/or parental perceptions of children after treatment (e.g., Forehand et al., 1980; Patterson, 1974).

As evidence for the efficacy of various interventions with children with OB has accumulated, increased attention has been focused on the relative efficacy of these interventions compared to other forms of treatment. One or more of these PT programs have been shown to be relatively more efficacious than family systems therapies (e.g., Patterson & Chamberlain, 1988; Wells & Egan, 1988), the STEP program (Baum et al., 1986), and available community mental health services (e.g., Patterson et al., 1982; Taylor et al., 1998). In a subset of analyses with 6- to 12-year olds, McCart et al. (2006) demonstrated that the mean effect size for PT was higher than the mean effect size for youth cognitive-behavioral therapy in decreasing conduct problems (ES = 0.45 and 0.23, respectively) in their meta-analytic study.

Mechanisms and Moderation

Changes in parenting behavior have now been shown in several studies to mediate the effects of PT with young children with OB (e.g., Beauchaine et al., 2005; DeGarmo et al., 2004; Feinfield & Baker, 2004; Gardner et al., 2006). This is a critical finding that goes to the core of PT, as improvement in parenting behavior is hypothesized to be the central mechanism by which change in child behavior occurs.

In general, there has been a dearth of attention paid to the extent to which PT may be differentially efficacious with different subgroups of children, parents, and families, or as a function of different aspects of PT (e.g., treatment delivery mode). A recent meta-analytic study that examined moderators of PT found that more severe child conduct problems, single-parent status, economic disadvantage (i.e., low socioeconomic status), and group-administered (as opposed to individually administered) PT resulted in poorer child behavior outcomes in PT (Lundahl et al., 2006).

In addition, economic disadvantage and PT alone (as opposed to multicomponent interventions that included PT) were also associated with poorer parent behavior and parental perception outcomes. Child age was not a significant moderator, which others have also reported (e.g., McCart et al., 2006). Lundahl et al. (2006) found that among disadvantaged families, individual PT was associated with more positive child and parent behavioral outcomes than group PT.[1] Other researchers have identified adult attachment status (Routh et al., 1995) and marital distress (Dadds et al., 1987) as moderators of PT outcome. Child gender does not appear to moderate PT outcomes, although the research is limited. Beauchaine et al. (2005) reported that child comorbid anxiety/depression (but not ADHD or child gender), maternal depression, parental history of substance abuse, marital satisfaction, and single-parent status moderated the effects of the BASIC PT intervention (in contrast to interventions that did not include the BASIC component).

Effectiveness/Dissemination

Large-scale effectiveness trials as well as cross-cultural dissemination studies are becoming increasingly more common. These research efforts provide essential information on the feasibility of transporting interventions for OB to real-world settings and utilizing such interventions with diverse populations of children and families.

Currently, several effectiveness trials of PT programs have been conducted, and several have been evaluated in international settings. For example, cross-cultural replications of the BASIC program (Webster-Stratton, 2005) have been conducted in the UK (Gardner et al., 2006; Scott et al., 2001) and Canada (e.g., Taylor et al., 1998). Triple P has also been implemented and evaluated in a number of international locations (e.g., Hong Kong: Leung et al., 2003; China: Crisante & Ng, 2003; Germany: Cina et al., 2006). A cross-cultural implementation of PMTO is also currently underway in Norway (Ogden et al., 2005). Several of these international implementations have also served as effectiveness trials. For example, international implementations of the BASIC program were conducted in local community mental health centers (e.g., Scott et al., 2001; Taylor et al., 1998) and through volunteer organizations (Gardner et al., 2006). The PMTO implementation in Norway (Ogden et al., 2005) is currently being piloted in the elementary school system and the child welfare system, with the ultimate goal of nationwide implementation. Several other PT effectiveness trials have been conducted in the countries where the interventions were developed. For example, Group Triple P has been implemented in a high-risk health region in Australia with another high-risk region used as a control (Zubrick et al., 2005). Additionally, several trials of PMTO have been conducted by community clinicians, unsupervised by OSLC staff

---

[1] However, individual versus group administration of PT was not a significant moderator in the meta-analyses reported by McCart et al. (2006).

(e.g., Fleischman, 1981), and versions of PCIT have also been evaluated in community care settings (e.g., Franco et al., 2005; Pade et al., 2006).

CASE EXAMPLE[2]

We present two example sessions occurring during Phase I (Differential Attention) and Phase II (Compliance Training) of HNC. The mother, Mrs. M, and her 4-year-old son, John, sought help because of John's intense OB at home, including excessive noncompliance and aversive behavior.

In prior Phase I sessions, Mrs. M learned attending, rewarding, and ignoring skills. This session began with a five-minute observation of Mrs. M and John engaging in activities selected by the child (Child's Game). Recorded behaviors included Mrs. M's use of praise and attending statements, commands, questions, and criticisms. After discussing her use of positive attention during the observation, the therapist asked about Mrs. M's use of reinforcement at home. Mrs. M had noted daily practice of the Child's Game on her home recording sheet. Mrs. M also reported using attending and reward statements frequently in other situations and indicated that John seemed to be responding, as his behavior was becoming less aversive. She also reported ignoring most of John's whining and demanding attention.

At the previous session, Mrs. M identified three "OK" behaviors that she would like to increase. The therapist and Mrs. M focused on a single "OK" behavior in the current session: John remaining quietly in his room during a one-hour rest period. The therapist and Mrs. M discussed how she might accomplish this goal using attends, rewards, and ignoring. They decided that Mrs. M would initiate the period by taking John to his room and telling him that it is rest time. After he remained quietly in his room for five minutes, she should go to the room and provide positive attention. The therapist told Mrs. M to initially provide positive attention for each five-minute period that John stayed quietly in his room. During subsequent weeks, she could gradually lengthen the intervals between attending/rewarding statements but was never to fade out her attention entirely. She was instructed to ignore any of John's attempts to gain attention and calmly return him to his room if he left it. Mrs. M and the therapist then role-played the situation and then explained, demonstrated, and role-played the new plan with John.

Following completion of Phase I, Mrs. M and John began Phase II (Compliance Training). The following is an example of a Phase II session. In prior Phase II sessions, Mrs. M learned how to deliver clear instructions and had been introduced to the consequences for compliance and noncompliance, including the use of time out. This session initially consisted of a five-minute observation of Mrs. M and John engaging in activities selected by the mother (Parent's Game). Recorded behaviors included Mrs. M's use

---

[2]Adapted from McMahon and Forehand (2003).

of positive attention, commands, and warnings, and John's compliance. Following the observation, the therapist discussed Mrs. M's use of clear instructions and rewards and attends for compliance.

The therapist then asked Mrs. M about her use of time out at home. The homework assignment had been to use time out in one situation (for John not picking up his toys when told to do so before dinner). Mrs. M had kept a record of the number of instructions and warnings that were issued, the extent to which John complied, how often she had praised John for compliance, and the use of time out (including John's behavior during time out and her response). The therapist and Mrs. M discussed this record and how Mrs. M felt the use of time out had gone. She indicated that using time out was stressful because she "hated" confrontations with John. However, she stated that time out was effective and was less stressful than nagging or screaming. Mrs. M indicated that she felt she had used time out for noncompliance and positive attention for compliance effectively.

Based on Mrs. M's meeting criteria during the initial five-minute observation and her report of appropriately using the clear instructions sequence at home, the therapist decided Mrs. M was ready to use time out as needed throughout the day. The therapist encouraged Mrs. M to use time out but cautioned that it was only effective within the context of a positive environment created by positive attention for John's appropriate behavior. They then discussed other examples of noncompliance and the use of clear instructions, warnings, time out, and praise for compliance in these situations. The therapist requested that Mrs. M keep a record of each of these situations during the week. The rest of the session was spent practicing Parent's Game.

CONCLUSIONS

Summary

A PT approach to intervention for young children with OB is arguably the intervention of choice, given the substantial empirical support for efficacy, generalization, and social validity. In fact, a recent meta-analysis suggests that, even for school-aged children (aged 6–12 years; for whom individually focused interventions might also be appropriate), PT is superior to child-focused cognitive-behavioral approaches (McCart et al., 2006). There is also growing empirical support for the premise that change in parental behavior serves as a primary mechanism in producing child behavioral change. Meta-analytic research suggests that the efficacy of PT for child behavioral change is less for single-parent and economically disadvantaged families; greater when provided to children with more severe conduct problems; perhaps greater when administered to individual families rather than in groups; and comparable for boys and girls and for majority and minority samples. Large-scale effectiveness and dissemination trials are providing important information regarding the feasibility of implementing PT interventions in the real world.

Increasing the Clinical Utility of Parent Training Interventions for Oppositional Behavior

We have recently presented a number of suggestions for increasing the clinical utility of PT interventions for OB (McMahon, 2006). First, it is critical that policy makers select PT programs that have sufficient empirical support. Reference to reviews (e.g., Lundahl et al., 2006; McCart et al., 2006; McMahon et al., 2006) and lists of "best practices" (e.g., Metzler et al., 2002) can be helpful starting points for the identification of potential PT interventions.

With respect to mode of delivery, group-based PT can be a cost-effective alternative to individual family treatment in some instances, although PT conducted with individual families may be more efficacious, especially with economically disadvantaged families (Lundahl et al., 2006). In some cases, self-administered PT may also be sufficient (Morawska et al., 2005). Specific guidelines for the selection of particular modes of PT are needed.

Interest in interventions for the *prevention* of conduct problems has burgeoned over the past 15 years, stimulated in part by increased knowledge about the early-starter pathway of conduct problems. PT interventions for children's OB may have significant preventive effects (on the occurrence of later conduct problems), especially if applied during the preschool years (e.g., Reid, 1993). If that should prove to be the case, there will be significant implications for reducing the need for ongoing interventions throughout the developmental period and adulthood.

Perhaps the most compelling reason for the application of PT on a large scale is its potential cost-effectiveness. Specifically, the empirical support for PT, the availability of therapist manuals (which assist in standardization and dissemination) for many PT programs as well as multiple-level delivery systems, and the potential for preventive effects all contribute to cost-effectiveness. An economic analysis indicated that PT was more cost-effective in preventing later crime than home visiting plus day care or supervision of delinquents (Greenwood et al., 1996). Further, when analyzed as part of a cost-benefit study conducted by the Washington State Institute of Public Policy (Aos et al., 2004), PCIT was shown to save taxpayers approximately $3,427 per participant in the program, compared to the cost of one offense (including the crime itself, associated law enforcement costs, adjudication, and punishment/rehabilitation).

Despite this very positive evaluation of PT as an intervention for young children with OB, a number of areas warrant continued and increased attention. These include (1) development of treatment selection guidelines, (2) continued emphasis on both identification and elaboration of the processes of family engagement and change in PT (Nock & Ferriter, 2005), (3) examination of strategies for enhancing outcome and generalization of effects, especially with respect to underserved groups, such as the economically disadvantaged, (4) the role of PT as a preventive intervention, and (5) greater attention to the conceptual, empirical, and pragmatic issues that are involved in large-scale dissemination.

REFERENCES

American Psychiatric Association (2000). *Diagnostic and Statistical Manual of Mental Disorders,* 4th ed. (rev. ed.). Washington, DC.

Angold, A., & Costello, E. J. (2001). The epidemiology of disorders of conduct: Nosological issues and comorbidity. In J. Hill & B. Maughan (Eds.), *Conduct Disorders in Childhood and Adolescence* (pp. 126–168). Cambridge: Cambridge University Press.

Aos, S., Lieb, R., Mayfield, J., Miller, M., & Pennucci, A. (2004). *Benefits and Costs of Prevention and Early Intervention Programs for Youth* [online]. Available at: http://www.wsipp.wa.gov/rptfiles/04-07-3901.pdf.

Baum, C. G., & Forehand, R. (1981). Long-term follow-up assessment of parent training by use of multiple-outcome measures. *Behavior Therapy, 12,* 643–652.

Baum, C. G., Reyna McGlone, C. L., & Ollendick, T. H. (1986). *The efficacy of behavioral parent training: Behavioral parent training plus clinical self-control training, and a modified STEP program with children referred for noncompliance.* Paper presented at the meeting of the Association for Advancement of Behavior Therapy, Chicago.

Beauchaine, T. P., Webster-Stratton, C., & Reid, M. J. (2005). Mediators, moderators, and predictors of 1-year outcomes among children treated for early-onset conduct problems: A latent growth curve analysis. *Journal of Consulting and Clinical Psychology, 73,* 371–388.

Bor, W., Sanders, M. R., & Markie-Dadds, C. (2002). The effects of the Triple P-Positive Parenting Program on preschool children with co-occuring disruptive behavior and attentional/hyperactive difficulties. *Journal of Abnormal Child Psychology, 30,* 571–587.

Breiner, J. L., & Forehand, R. (1981). An assessment of the effects of parent training on clinic-referred children's school behavior. *Behavioral Assessment, 3,* 31–42.

Brestan, E. V., Eyberg, S. M., Boggs, S. R., & Algina, J. (1997). Parent-Child Interaction Therapy: Parents' perceptions of untreated siblings. *Child & Family Behavior Therapy, 19*(3), 13–28.

Brestan, E. V., Jacobs, J. R., Rayfield, A. D., & Eyberg, S. M. (1999). A consumer satisfaction measure for parent-child treatments and its relation to measures of child behavior change. *Behavior Therapy, 30,* 17–30.

Brinkmeyer, M., & Eyberg, S. M. (2003). Parent-Child Interaction Therapy for oppositional children. In A. E. Kazdin & J. R. Weisz (Eds.), *Evidence-Based Psychotherapies for Children and Adolescents* (pp. 204–223). New York: Guilford Press.

Campbell, S. B. (1995). Behavior problems in preschool children: A review of recent research. *Journal of Child Psychology and Psychiatry and Allied Disciplines, 36,* 113–149.

Chamberlain, P., & Patterson, G. R. (1995). Discipline and child compliance in parenting. In M. H. Bornstein (Ed.), *Handbook of Parenting: Vol. 4. Applied and Practical Parenting* (pp. 205–225). Hillsdale, NJ: Erlbaum.

Chamberlain, P., Reid, J. B., Ray, J., Capaldi, D. M., & Fisher, P. (1997). Parent inadequate discipline (PID). In T. A. Widiger, A. J. Frances, H. A. Pincus, R. Ross, M. B. First, & W. Davis (Eds.), *DSM-IV Sourcebook,* Vol. 3 (pp. 569–629). Washington, DC: American Psychiatric Association.

Cina, A., Bodenmann, G., Hahlweg, K., Dirscherl, T., & Sanders, M. R. (2006). Triple P (Positive Parenting Program): Theoretical and empirical background and first experiences in the German-speaking areas. *Journal of Family Research, 6,* 66–88.

Crisante, L., & Ng, S. (2003). Implementation and process issues in using Group Triple P with Chinese parents: Preliminary findings. *Australian eJournal for the Advancement of Mental Health, 2*(3), 1–10.

Cross Calvert, S., & McMahon, R. J. (1987). The treatment acceptability of a behavioral parent training program and its components. *Behavior Therapy, 18,* 165–179.

Dadds, M. R., Schwartz, S., & Sanders, M. R. (1987). Marital discord and treatment outcome in behavioral treatment of child conduct disorders. *Journal of Consulting and Clinical Psychology, 55,* 396–403.

DeGarmo, D. S., Patterson, G. R., & Forgatch, M. S. (2004). How do outcomes in a specified parent training intervention maintain or wane over time? *Prevention Science, 5,* 73–89.

Dumas, J. E. (1989). Treating antisocial behavior in children: Child and family approaches. *Clinical Psychology Review, 9,* 197–222.

Dumas, J. E. (1996). Why was this child referred? Interactional correlates of referral status in families of children with disruptive behavior problems. *Journal of Clinical Child Psychology, 25,* 106–115.

Essau, C. A. (2003). Epidemiology and comorbidity. In C. A. Essau (Ed.), *Conduct and Oppositional Defiant Disorders: Epidemiology, Risk Factors, and Treatment* (pp. 33–59). Mahwah, NJ: Erlbaum.

Feinfield, K. A., & Baker, B. L. (2004). Empirical support for a treatment program for families of young children with externalizing problems. *Journal of Clinical Child and Adolescent Psychology, 33,* 182–195.

Fleischman, M. J. (1981). A replication of Patterson's "Intervention for boys with conduct problems." *Journal of Consulting and Clinical Psychology, 49,* 342–351.

Forehand, R., & Atkeson, B. M. (1977). Generality of treatment effects with parents as therapists: A review of assessment and implementation procedures. *Behavior Therapy, 8,* 575–593.

Forehand, R., & Long, N. (1988). Outpatient treatment of the acting out child: Procedures, long term follow-up data, and clinical problems. *Advances in Behaviour Research and Therapy, 10,* 129–177.

Forehand, R., Wells, K. C., & Griest, D. L. (1980). An examination of the social validity of a parent training program. *Behavior Therapy, 11,* 488–502.

Franko, E., Soler, R. E., & McBride, M. (2005). Introducing and evaluating Parent-Child Interaction Therapy in a system of care. *Child and Adolescent Psychiatric Clinics of North America, 14,* 351–366.

Garcia, M. M., Shaw, D. S., Winslow, E. B., & Yaggi, K. E. (2000). Destructive sibling conflict and the development of conduct problems in young boys. *Developmental Psychology, 36,* 44–53.

Gardner, F., Burton, J., & Klimes, I. (2006). Randomised controlled trial of a parenting intervention in the voluntary sector for reducing child conduct problems: Outcomes and mechanisms of change. *Journal of Child Psychology and Psychiatry, 47,* 1123–1132.

Greenberg, M. T., Speltz, M. L., DeKlyen, M., & Jones, K. (2001). Correlates of clinic referral for early conduct problems: Variable- and person-oriented approaches. *Development and Psychopathology, 13,* 255–276.

Greene, R. W., Ablon, J. S., Goring, J. C., Fazio, V., & Morse, L. R. (2004). Treatment of oppositional defiant disorder in children and adolescents. In P. M. Barrett & T. H. Ollendick (Eds.), *Handbook of Interventions That Work with Children and Adolescents* (pp. 369–393). New York: Wiley.

Greenwood, P. W., Model, K. E., Rydell, C. P., & Chiesa, J. (1996). *Diverting Children from a Life of Crime: Measuring Costs and Benefits.* Santa Monica, CA: The RAND Corporation.

Griest, D. L., Forehand, R., Rogers, T., Breiner, J. L., Furey, W., & Williams, C. A. (1982). Effects of parent enhancement therapy on the treatment outcome and generalization of a parent training program. *Behaviour Research and Therapy, 20,* 429–436.

Hanf, C. (1969). *A two-stage program for modifying maternal controlling during mother-child (M-C) interaction.* Paper presented at the meeting of the Western Psychological Association, Vancouver, BC.

Hembree-Kigin, T. L., & McNeil, C. B. (1995). *Parent-Child Interaction Therapy.* New York: Plenum Press.

Hinshaw, S. P., & Lee, S. S. (2003). Conduct and oppositional defiant disorders. In E. J. Mash & R. A. Barkley (Eds.), *Child Psychopathology,* 2nd ed. (pp. 144–198). New York: Guilford Press.

Hood., K., & Eyberg, S. M. (2003). Outcomes of Parent-Child Interaction Therapy: Mothers' reports on maintenance three to six years after treatment. *Journal of Clinical Child and Adolescent Psychology, 32,* 419–429.

Horne, A. M., & Van Dyke, B. (1983). Treatment and maintenance of social learning family therapy. *Behavior Therapy, 14,* 606–613.

Humphreys, L., Forehand, R., McMahon, R., & Roberts, M. (1978). Parent behavioral training to modify child noncompliance: Effects on untreated siblings. *Journal of Behavior Therapy and Experimental Psychiatry, 9,* 235–238.

Johnson, S. M., Bolstad, O. D., & Lobitz, G. K. (1976). Generalization and contrast phenomena in behavior modification with children. In L.A. Hamerlynck, L.C. Handy, & E.J. Mash (Eds.), *Behavior Modification and Families* (pp. 160–188). New York: Brunner/Mazel.

Kazdin, A. E. (1995). *Conduct Disorders in Childhood and Adolescence*, 2nd ed. Thousand Oaks, CA: Sage Publications.

Kazdin, A. E., & Whitley, M. K. (2003). Treatment of parental stress to enhance therapeutic change among children referred for aggressive and antisocial behavior. *Journal of Consulting and Clinical Psychology, 71*, 504–515.

Leung, C., Sanders, M. R., Leung, S., Mak, R., & Lau, J. (2003). An outcome evaluation of the implementation of the Triple P-Positive Parenting Program in Hong Kong. *Family Process, 42*, 531–544.

Long, P., Forehand, R., Wierson, M., & Morgan, A. (1994). Does parent training with young noncompliant children have long-term effects? *Behaviour Research and Therapy, 32*, 101–107.

Lundahl, B., Risser, H. J., & Lovejoy, M. C. (2006). A meta-analysis of parent training: Moderators and follow-up effects. *Clinical Psychology Review, 26*, 86–104.

McCart, M. R., Priester, P. E., Davies, W. H., & Azen, R. (2006). Differential effectiveness of behavioral parent-training and cognitive-behavioral therapy for antisocial youth: A meta-analysis. *Journal of Abnormal Child Psychology, 34*, 527–543.

McMahon, R. J. (2006). Parent training interventions for preschool-age children. In R. E. Tremblay, R. G. Barr, & R. DeV. Peters (Eds.), *Encyclopedia on Early Childhood Development* [online]. Montreal, Quebec: Centre of Excellence for Early Childhood Development; 1–8. Retrieved May 23, 2006, from http://www.excellence-earlychildhood.ca/documents/McMahonRJANGxp.pdf.

McMahon, R. J., & Forehand, R. L. (1983). Consumer satisfaction in behavioral treatment of children: Types, issues, and recommendations. *Behavior Therapy, 14*, 209–225.

McMahon, R. J., & Forehand, R. L. (2003). *Helping the Noncompliant Child: Family-Based Treatment for Oppositional Behavior*, 2nd ed. New York: Guilford Press.

McMahon, R. J., Forehand, R., & Griest, D. L. (1981). Effects of knowledge of social learning principles on enhancing treatment outcome and generalization in a parent training program. *Journal of Consulting and Clinical Psychology, 49*, 526–532.

McMahon, R. J., Tiedemann, G. L., Forehand, R., & Griest, D. L. (1984). Parental satisfaction with parent training to modify child noncompliance. *Behavior Therapy, 15*, 295–303.

McMahon, R. J., Wells, K. C., & Kotler, J. S. (2006). Conduct problems. In E. J. Mash & R. A. Barkley (Eds.), *Treatment of Childhood Disorders*, 3rd ed. (pp. 137–268). New York: Guilford Press.

McNeil, C. B., Eyberg, S., Eisenstadt, T. H., Newcomb, K., & Funderburk, B. (1991). Parent-Child Interaction Therapy with behavior problem children: Generalization of treatment effects to the school setting. *Journal of Clinical Child Psychology, 20*, 140–151.

Metzler, C., Eddy, M., & Taylor, T. K. (2002). The evidence standards of ten "best practices" lists and the evidence base of the top family-focused programs. In C. Metzler (Chair), *Finding Common Ground Among "Best Practices" Lists: The Evidence Base and Program Elements of Top Family Focused and School-Based Programs.* Symposium conducted at the meeting of the Society for Prevention Research, Seattle, WA, May.

Miller, G. E., & Prinz, R. J. (1990). Enhancement of social learning family interventions for childhood conduct disorder. *Psychological Bulletin, 108*, 291–307.

Moffitt, T. E., Caspi, A., Harrington, H., & Milne, B. (2002). Males on the life-course persistent and adolescence-limited antisocial pathways: Follow-up at age 26. *Development and Psychopathology, 14*, 179–206.

Morawska, A., Stallman, H. M., Sanders, M. R., & Ralph, A. (2005). Self-directed behavioral family intervention: Do therapists matter? *Child & Family Behavior Therapy, 27*(4), 51–72.

Niec, L. N., Hemme, J., Yopp, J., & Brestan, E. (2005). Parent-Child Interaction Therapy: The rewards and challenges of a group format. *Cognitive and Behavioral Practice, 12*, 113–125.

Nock, M. K., & Ferriter, C. (2005). Parent management of attendance and adherence in child and adolescent therapy: A conceptual and empirical review. *Clinical Child and Family Psychology Review, 8*, 149–166.

Nock, M. K., Kazdin, A. E., Hiripi, E., & Kessler, R. C. (2007). Lifetime prevalence, correlates, and persistence of oppositional defiant disorder: Results from the National Comorbidity Survey replication. *Journal of Child Psychology and Psychiatry, 48*, 703–713.

Ogden, T., Forgatch, M. S., Askeland, E., Patterson, G. R., & Bullock, B. M. (2005). Implementation of parent management training at the national level: The case of Norway. *Journal of Social Work Practice, 19*, 317–329.

Pade, H., Taube, D. O., Aalborg, A. E., & Reiser, P. J. (2006). An immediate and long-term study of a temperament and Parent-Child Interaction Therapy based community program for preschoolers with behavior problems. *Child & Family Behavior Therapy, 28*(3), 1–28.

Patterson, G. R. (1974). Interventions for boys with conduct problems: Multiple settings, treatments, and criteria. *Journal of Consulting and Clinical Psychology, 42*, 471–481.

Patterson, G. R. (1975). *Families: Applications of Social Learning to Family Life* (rev. ed.). Champaign, IL: Research Press.

Patterson, G. R. (1976). *Living with Children: New Methods for Parents and Teachers* (rev. ed.). Champaign, IL: Research Press.

Patterson, G. R., & Chamberlain, P. (1988). Treatment process: A problem at three levels. In L. C. Wynne (Ed.), *The State of the Art in Family Therapy Research: Controversies and Recommendations* (pp. 189–223). New York: Family Process Press.

Patterson, G. R., Chamberlain, P., & Reid, J. B. (1982). A comparative evaluation of a parent training program. *Behavior Therapy, 13*, 638–650.

Patterson, G. R., & Fleischman, M. J. (1979). Maintenance of treatment effects: Some considerations concerning family systems and follow-up data. *Behavior Therapy, 10*, 168–185.

Patterson, G. R., Reid, J. B., & Dishion, T. J. (1992). *Antisocial Boys*. Eugene, OR: Castalia.

Patterson, G. R., Reid, J. B., Jones, R. R., & Conger, R. E. (1975). *A Social Learning Approach to Family Intervention: Vol. 1. Families with Aggressive Children*. Eugene, OR: Castalia.

Peed, S., Roberts, M., & Forehand, R. (1977). Evaluation of the effectiveness of a standardized parent training program in altering the interaction of mothers and their noncompliant children. *Behavior Modification, 1*, 323–350.

Reid, J. B. (1993). Prevention of conduct disorder before and after school entry: Relating interventions to developmental findings. *Development and Psychopathology, 5*, 243–262.

Reid, M. J., Webster-Stratton, C., & Hammond, M. (2003). Follow-up of children who received the Incredible Years intervention for oppositional defiant disorder: Maintenance and prediction of 2-year outcome. *Behavior Therapy, 34*, 471–491.

Routh, C. P., Hill, J. W., Steele, H., Elliott, C. E., & Dewey, M. E. (1995). Maternal attachment status, psychosocial stressors and problem behaviour: Follow-up after parent training courses for conduct disorder. *Journal of Child Psychology and Psychiatry, 36*, 1179–1198.

Sanders, M. R., & Christensen, A. P. (1985). A comparison of the effects of child management and planned activities training in five parenting environments. *Journal of Abnormal Child Psychology, 13*, 101–117.

Sanders, M. R., & Glynn, T. (1981). Training parents in behavioral self management: An analysis of generalization and maintenance. *Journal of Applied Behavior Analysis, 14*, 223–237.

Sanders, M. R., Markie-Dadds, C., Tully, L., & Bor, B. (2000). The Triple P-Positive Parenting Program: A comparison of enhanced, standard, and self-directed behavioral family intervention for parents of children with early onset conduct problems. *Journal of Consulting and Clinical Psychology, 68*, 624–640.

Sanders, M. R., Markie-Dadds, C., & Turner, K. M. T. (2003). Theoretical, scientific, and clinical foundations of the Triple P-Positive Parenting Program: A population approach to the promotion of parenting competence. *Parenting Research and Practice Monograph No. 1*, University of Queensland, Australia. Retrieved March 4, 2004, from http://www.triplep.net/01_about/pdf/Monograph1.pdf.

Sanders, M. R., & McFarland, M. (2000). Treatment of depressed mothers with disruptive children: A controlled evaluation of cognitive behavioral family intervention. *Behavior Therapy, 31*, 89–112.

Schuhmann, E. M., Foote, R., Eyberg, S. M., Boggs, S., & Algina, J. (1998). Parent-Child Interaction Therapy: Interim report of a randomized trial with short-term maintenance. *Journal of Clinical Child Psychology, 27*, 34–45.

Scott, S., Spender, Q., Doolan, M., Jacobs, B., & Aspland, H. (2001). Multicentre controlled trial of parenting groups for child antisocial behaviour in clinical practice. *British Medical Journal, 323,* 1–7.

Serketich, W. J., & Dumas, J. E. (1996). The effectiveness of behavioral parent training to modify antisocial behavior in children: A meta-analysis. *Behavior Therapy, 27,* 171–186.

Sheldrick, R. C., Kendall, P. C., & Heimberg, R. G. (2001). The clinical significance of treatments: A comparison of three treatments for conduct disordered children. *Clinical Psychology: Science and Practice, 8,* 418–430.

Speltz, M. L., McClellan, J., DeKlyen, M., & Jones, K. (1999). Preschool boys with oppositional defiant disorder: Clinical presentation and diagnostic change. *Journal of the American Academy of Child and Adolescent Psychiatry, 38,* 838–845.

Taylor, T. K., Schmidt, F., Pepler, D., & Hodgins, H. (1998). A comparison of eclectic treatment with Webster-Stratton's Parent and Children's Series in a children's mental health center: A randomized controlled trial. *Behavior Therapy, 29,* 221–240.

Wahler, R. G. (1975). Some structural aspects of deviant child behavior. *Journal of Applied Behavior Analysis, 8,* 27–42.

Wahler, R. G., Cartor, P. G., Fleischman, J., & Lambert, W. (1993). The impact of synthesis teaching and parent training with mothers of conduct-disordered children. *Journal of Abnormal Child Psychology, 21,* 425–440.

Walker, H. M., & Walker, J. E. (1991). *Coping with Noncompliance in the Classroom: A Positive Approach for Teachers.* Austin, TX: Pro-Ed.

Walter, H. I., & Gilmore, S. K. (1973). Placebo versus social learning effects in parent training procedures designed to alter the behavior of aggressive boys. *Behavior Therapy, 4,* 361–377.

Webster-Stratton, C. (1981). Modification of mothers' behaviors and attitudes through a videotape modeling group discussion program. *Behavior Therapy, 12,* 634–642.

Webster-Stratton, C. (1984). Randomized trial of two parent-training programs for families with conduct-disordered children. *Journal of Consulting and Clinical Psychology, 52,* 666–678.

Webster-Stratton, C. (1994). Advancing videotape parent training: A comparison study. *Journal of Consulting and Clinical Psychology, 62,* 583–593.

Webster-Stratton, C. (1998). Preventing conduct problems in Head Start children: Strengthening parent competencies. *Journal of Consulting and Clinical Psychology, 66,* 715–730.

Webster-Stratton, C. (2005). The Incredible Years: A training series for the prevention and treatment of conduct problems in young children. In E. D. Hibbs & P. S. Jensen (Eds.), *Psychosocial Treatments for Child and Adolescent Disorders,* 2nd ed. (pp. 507–555). Washington, DC: American Psychological Association.

Wells, K. C., & Egan, J. (1988). Social learning and systems family therapy for childhood oppositional disorder: Comparative treatment outcome. *Comprehensive Psychiatry, 29,* 138–146.

Wells, K. C., Forehand, R., & Griest, D. L. (1980a). Generality of treatment effects from treated to untreated behaviors resulting from a parent training program. *Journal of Clinical Child Psychology, 9,* 217–219.

Wells, K. C., Griest, D. L., & Forehand, R. (1980b). The use of a self-control package to enhance temporal generality of a parent training program. *Behaviour Research and Therapy, 18,* 347–358.

Wiltz, N. A., & Patterson, G. R. (1974). An evaluation of parent training procedures designed to alter inappropriate aggressive behavior of boys. *Behavior Therapy, 5,* 215–221.

Zubrick, S. R., Ward, K., Silburn, S. R., Lawrence, D., Williams, A. A., Blair, E., et al. (2005). Prevention of child behavioral problems through universal implementation of a group behavioral family intervention. *Prevention Science, 6,* 287–304.

14

Treating Conduct Problems, Aggression, and Antisocial Behavior in Children and Adolescents: An Integrated View

PAUL BOXER and PAUL J. FRICK

INTRODUCTION

Conduct disorder (CD) consists of persistent engagement in behavior that violates the rights of others and/or exhibits clear disregard for the law or for age-appropriate social norms (American Psychiatric Association, 2000). To qualify for the diagnosis of CD, a youth must, within the year preceding assessment, have engaged in at least three behaviors drawn from four categories—*aggression toward people or animals* (e.g., physical cruelty, intimidation, forced sexual activity), *property destruction* (fire-setting or otherwise), *deceitfulness or theft* (e.g., breaking and entering, lying for instrumental gain), or *serious developmentally based rule violations* (e.g., truancy, staying out all night without permission). Further, one of those behaviors must have been present within the six months leading up to the diagnostic assessment.

CD is associated with a variety of functional impairments or personal costs for the individual youth (e.g., academic failure, relationship disturbance, legal involvement, and comorbid psychopathology such as depression or attention deficit hyperactivity disorder; Frick, 1998). However, the greater cost of CD in many ways accrues through consequences to other individuals and society in general (cf. Frick, 2001). Youth

PAUL BOXER • Rutgers University and **PAUL J. FRICK** • University of New Orleans

who engage in behaviors consistent with the diagnosis of CD harm others directly and indirectly, causing reduced quality of life, emotional distress, and potential physical or psychological injury to their victims. These youth also exact high monetary costs through property destruction, vandalism, theft, and expenses associated with the juvenile justice system.

Children with CD are only a subset of children with problem behaviors that involve infringement on the well-being of others and society. Individuals meeting DSM criteria for CD are displaying forms of aggressive and antisocial behavior that become clinically salient (i.e., diagnosable) only through their aggregation. Even taken independently, though, each criterion symptom of CD can be a destructive and costly behavior, and youth who exhibit "subclinical" levels of CD problems certainly warrant concern.

To discuss adequately the range of potentially effective treatments for children with severe conduct problems, it is essential to assume a broader view of these youth than those who would be diagnosable with CD. In this chapter, we discuss not only effective treatments for CD but also effective strategies implemented to deal more broadly with aggression, violence, and delinquency in youth. Our belief is that evidence-based practice in treating CD and related problems will be most effective when these problems are understood within a developmental perspective. Our developmental view involves several basic assumptions. *First*, we assume that one must understand how children normally develop the capacity to inhibit problem behavior in order to understand adequately how these processes may go awry in the case of CD and related problem behavior. *Second*, we recognize that problem behaviors are multiply determined, often involving many different causal processes (Dodge & Pettit, 2003). *Third*, we recognize that these causal processes may vary across children who show severe problem behaviors. There may be many different pathways through which children develop problem behaviors (Frick, 2006).

In this chapter, we start with a review of research that helps to place CD and other problems behaviors within such a developmental framework. We then review current best-practice interventions for these problem behaviors. We consider how evidence-based best practices might translate into "real-world," everyday clinical practice and offer case material in support of our views. Finally, we offer suggestions to guide future applied research in this area.

DEVELOPMENTAL FOUNDATIONS OF HABITUAL AGGRESSIVE AND ANTISOCIAL BEHAVIOR

Once conduct problems have persisted beyond the very early childhood years—when some problem behavior is expected and thus is quite normative (e.g., kicking, biting, hitting; Tremblay, 2000)—they denote a fairly reliable individual-difference characteristic (Huesmann & Guerra, 1997). Across studies, time periods, and cultures, aggression has exhibited a high degree of intrapersonal continuity; that is, individuals who are more aggressive than their peers in childhood tend to remain in that relative position in adulthood (e.g., Huesmann et al., 2006). Similarly, severe conduct problems in childhood predict criminality and antisocial behavior in adulthood (see Frick & Loney, 1999, for a review).

Conduct problems are a prime example of what developmental psychopathologists describe as "equifinality" (Cicchetti & Rogosch, 1996) or "multicausality" (Cowen, 2000): problematic developmental outcomes (e.g., problem behavior) resulting from a variety of different risk factors that can operate on multiple levels of influence. Contemporary research on the development of conduct problems views these problems from a *developmental-ecological* perspective (also referred to as an individual-contextual or social-contextual perspective; e.g., Conger & Simons, 1997; Dodge & Pettit, 2003). This model posits generally that conduct problems emerge and become habitual through the interaction of individual and contextual factors. With respect to individually based factors, the risk for conduct problems is increased by temperamental predispositions toward impulsivity, thrill-seeking, irritability, and emotional lability (cf. Frick & Morris, 2004) as well as low intelligence and learning problems (e.g., Huesmann et al., 1987). Partly through genetic transmission of these characteristics, aggression and related problem behavior exhibit strong intergenerational continuity (Miles & Carey, 1997). Intergenerational continuity also likely accrues through social learning processes between parents and children. In terms of contextually based factors, then, the risk for conduct problems is increased not only by exposure to antisocial models in the family (e.g., Dubow et al., 2003) but also by exposure to deviant behavior in peers, in neighborhoods, and in the media (e.g., Boxer et al., 2003; Espelage et al., 2003; Huesmann et al., 2003).

In the general population of youth, individuals who exhibit habitual antisocial behavior tend to be those who possess a variety of dispositional and contextual risk factors. Of course, in any population there will be individuals at the extreme high end of the continuum. For example, studies have identified subgroups of youth who maintain persistently high levels of aggressive behavior over time (e.g., Broidy et al., 2003). Some typical risk factors (such as poor family interactions and socioeconomic adversity) can predict this trajectory pattern (NICHD Early Child Care Research Network, 2004). However, as Frick (2006) has noted, broad, cumulative risk models such as the general developmental-ecological view may not be able to account fully for conduct problems in such extreme groups. Rather, there may be several distinct patterns of individual and contextual risk that distinguish important subgroups within severely antisocial and aggressive youth. A *developmental pathways* approach attempts to define these subgroups.

One oft-noted pathway distinction drawn to describe serious antisocial behavior has been Moffitt's (1993) taxonomy of life-course persistent antisocial behavior versus adolescence-limited antisocial behavior. Individuals whose antisocial behavior began early in childhood (also referred to as the "early-starter" or "childhood-onset" group; e.g., Hinshaw et al., 1993) tend to be more severely aggressive and exhibit higher neurological or physiological risk with a greater likelihood of comorbid psychopathology (e.g., attention deficit hyperactivity disorder) compared to those who manifest temporary adolescent "flirtations" with antisocial behavior or whose antisocial pattern begins during adolescence. Recently, Frick and colleagues (e.g., 2000) have presented empirical evidence demonstrating that an additional distinction can be drawn within the early-starter group. That is, some children in this higher-risk group manifest even greater risk through the presence of callous and unemotional (CU) traits that are measurable fairly early in middle childhood. Children who score highly on measures of these traits are those who tend to lack guilt and remorse and who show a disregard for the feelings of others. These children also tend to change friends often and fail to attend to conventional obligations like schoolwork and promises (Frick et al., 2000). Antisocial youth high on CU traits tend to engage in more serious violent and nonviolent antisocial behaviors and to evince antisocial behavior earlier and more persistently than those low on CU traits (e.g., Frick et al., 2003).

As highlighted by McMahon and Frick (2005), understanding developmental research and theory on aggressive and antisocial behavior is critical to the assessment of conduct problems for proper diagnosis and intervention planning. Further, Boxer and colleagues (Boxer & Dubow, 2002; Boxer et al., 2005a; Guerra et al., 2005) have emphasized the importance of linking developmental theoretical propositions regarding aggression directly to intervention activities. Having described the current state of theory and research on the development of aggression and conduct problems, we now turn to a review of evidence-based interventions for those behaviors.

Because we recognize that many readers will be clinicians working in private practice, university or community-based clinics, or schools, we focus our review on evidence-based practices amenable to these sorts of settings. We focus on specific intervention programs that have met stringent objective criteria for designation as effective or efficacious. Generally, the more stringent criteria for designating a treatment as one that "works" include randomized assignment to conditions with adequate sample sizes in formal evaluations, independent replication of effects by a research team different from the progenitors of the treatment, replication of effects across diverse populations and settings, and statistically and clinically significant immediate as well as sustained effects.

We recognize that these well-established specific interventions rely on theoretical principles and models that have led to treatment effectiveness across a wide range of intervention strategies and modalities. For example, Frick (2001) noted the general effectiveness of treatments for conduct problems that rely upon contingency management strategies. This state of affairs supporting theoretically driven practice is fortunate given that everyday intervention work with aggressive, conduct-disordered youth typically does not permit the implementation of procedures necessary to mint empirically validated programs, such as highly controlled experimental conditions and intensive program supervision (Boxer & Butkus, 2005). We therefore discuss the empirically validated programs as top-notch *exemplars* of empirically and theoretically derived intervention strategies, and we will attend in particular to how the best-practice programs might be made more useful to the practicing clinician.

INTERVENTIONS FOR CD AND AGGRESSION

Our review of relevant developmental research on aggression and conduct problems indicates that habitual problem behavior emerges over time as the product of both individual (e.g., temperament) and ecological (e.g., exposure to violence) risk factors; that some youth show high levels of conduct problems fairly early and stay at that level across development; and that within this group of youth, some individuals show very high levels of serious conduct problems along with the presence of certain affective traits. What these conclusions suggest first of all is that clinicians should be prepared to administer interventions targeting a variety of personal and contextual risk factors to children and adolescents. Further, clinicians should recognize that habitual conduct problems can emerge fairly early in development in some children and, if left unchecked, may develop into quite serious problems. This implies that even young children might profit from interventions that address individual and ecological risk factors. Finally, for clinicians working with more serious and persistently antisocial youth, the added risk factor of callous and unemotional traits will require attention through intervention.

Our review is structured with respect to the general modalities in which the best-practice programs might be implemented. The practicing clinician may find this organization to be useful in matching a particular form of treatment to his or her typical client population.

TREATMENTS FOR PARENTS AND FAMILIES WITH YOUNG CHILDREN

The Incredible Years

Webster-Stratton and colleagues (e.g., Webster-Stratton & Hammond, 1997; Webster-Stratton et al., 1988, 2004) have produced a well-validated set of programs targeting the reduction and prevention of current and future conduct problems in young children (aged 2–8). The *Incredible Years* package of interventions for parents, teachers, and children has been recognized as a "model" program (highest designation) by the Blueprints for Violence Prevention program and as an effective or empirically supported treatment by, among others, the Society for Clinical Child and Adolescent Psychology (SCCAP), the Center for Substance Abuse Prevention (CSAP), and the Office of Juvenile Justice and Delinquency Prevention (OJJDP). These interventions have been evaluated as clinician-mediated treatments for individual parents and small groups of parents as well as self-instructional videotape-mediated treatments for individuals and groups.

The Incredible Years intervention has been shown to be efficacious (i.e., producing treatment effects under controlled laboratory conditions; e.g., Webster-Stratton & Hammond, 1997) as well as effective (i.e., producing effects under "real-world" practice conditions; e.g., Taylor et al., 1998). Importantly, Incredible Years has produced immediate reductions in conduct problems (Webster-Stratton & Hammond, 1997) as well as longer-term prevention of further problems and enhancement in social competence (Reid et al., 2003).

Incredible Years is a treatment package that relies upon the teaching, practice, and maintenance of behavioral strategies fundamental to reducing problem behavior and promoting positive behavior. For example, in the core parent training program, parents learn skills for noncorporal discipline strategies (e.g., redirection, ignoring, use of natural and logical consequences), anger management and problem solving, and collaborative communication with teachers and other caretakers. Supplemental programming for teachers focuses on classroom management skills in addition to instruction on teaching social skills and anger management techniques to students. Supplemental programming for students emphasizes social skills, self-control strategies, and the promotion of good study habits and techniques. All of these approaches use direct training techniques including videotape modeling, role-playing activities, guided practice, and live feedback from trainers and group members.

The Incredible Years package clearly appears to exert its effects through simple yet consistent and comprehensive training based upon well-established behavioral principles. Thus, it is important to recognize that although Incredible Years is probably the best-validated program of its kind, several other similar approaches or resources can produce success, such as Kazdin's Parent Management Training (Kazdin, 1997) or McMahon and Forehand's (2003) and Barkley's (1997) parent training manual approaches. As Frick (2001) has noted, behavioral approaches relying principally on contingency management or parent training strategies are useful for treating CD and are predicated on the empirically derived notion that children who develop conduct problems emerge from family environments that fail to socialize appropriate behaviors and/or to manage effectively children's existing temperamental vulnerabilities (e.g., Abramowitz & O'Leary, 1991). Incredible Years steps beyond just the parenting environment to modify children's skills and behavioral contingencies across settings, yielding a more powerful but no less theoretically grounded intervention into the development of conduct problems.

What should be taken from the consistent and longstanding success of Incredible Years and similar programs is the fact that behavioral approaches are likely to have the greatest utility in working with parents whose young children are beginning to exhibit the development of conduct problems. Although a comprehensive behavioral treatment strategy that includes work with parents, teachers, and children themselves might seem too intensive for a young child, research indicates clearly that such an approach is, in fact, necessary to prevent more severe behaviors in the future. Whereas these approaches clearly are most effective for young children, the principles have been extended for use in older youth (e.g., Barkley, 1997).

Further, it is important to acknowledge that with appropriate clinical training, supervision, and access to fairly inexpensive resources [e.g., the McMahon & Forehand (2003) manual], implementing behaviorally based parent training and school consultation is a very reasonable goal for practicing clinicians who might be unfamiliar with this therapeutic approach. It also is worth underscoring the fact that even the Incredible Years program, which was built on group-based instruction and skills training, also has shown clinical utility as an individual and/or self-administered treatment (Webster-Stratton, 1990). Therefore, other than having access to appropriate training and resources, there are essentially no treatment-oriented barriers to the implementation of parent training activities in everyday practice with children and families.

Functional Family Therapy

Alexander and colleagues (e.g., Alexander & Parsons, 1973; Morris et al., 1988; Sexton & Alexander, 2003) have developed a well-supported model of family therapy targeting the treatment of aggressive and antisocial behavior in adolescents (aged 11–18). *Functional Family Therapy* (FFT) has been designated a model intervention by the Blueprints program and recognized as effective by, among others, OJJDP, the Surgeon General, and the Centers for Disease Control (CDC). FFT is provided directly by clinicians and has been evaluated successfully in a variety of settings including mental health clinics, clients' homes, and juvenile court clinics (see Alexander et al., 1998).

Like the Incredible Years, FFT relies upon a solid foundation of established behavioral principles in the service of effecting behavioral change in youth clients. For example, FFT targets enhancements in communication and mutual problem-solving skills between parents and adolescents as well as improvements in parental contingency management. However, FFT also aims to modify structural and systemic family processes that maintain adolescent problem behaviors and/or that prevent the parent from implementing behavioral programs, such as persistent conflict and enmeshment or inappropriate power hierarchies between parents and adolescents. FFT proceeds through three general phases of treatment, beginning with *engagement and motivation* (i.e., altering family dynamics and individual cognitive and emotional factors that prevent engaging in behavioral change) and proceeding through *behavioral change* (i.e., training and supporting new parent-adolescent interactional styles and increasing positive parenting skills) and, finally, *generalization* (i.e., supporting the transfer of new skills to other settings such as school or the legal system).

A key feature of FFT is that it is an office-based, single-therapist-mediated treatment strategy that essentially can be adapted quite well to typical clinical practice across a variety of settings. In addition, its first-phase emphasis on encouraging families to engage in and commit to behavior change is highly consistent with a wealth of clinical research findings indicating that the initial steps of family contact and engagement with the therapist are critical to positive treatment outcomes (see, e.g., Szapocznik et al., 1990).

FFT and similar programs (e.g., Dishion & Kavanagh's *Adolescent Transitions Program*) utilize a number of interventions similar to those used in traditional parent training programs discussed in the context of the Incredible Years package. Thus, as Frick (2001) highlighted, contingency management and parent training approaches are critically important to the prevention and reduction of conduct programs. The key difference between Incredible Years (and similar programs) and FFT (and similar programs) is a focus on the process of engaging and motivating the family and a focus on the broader family system. The increased autonomy and parent-child conflict that often accompany adolescence necessitate the structural, systemic, and strategic approaches implemented in FFT and similar programs.

TREATMENTS FOR SMALL GROUPS OF YOUTH

Anger Coping Program and Coping Power Program

Lochman and colleagues (e.g., Lochman, 1992; Lochman & Wells, 2004) have designed two small-group programs targeting aggression and anger dysregulation in preadolescents (aged 8–12). The Anger Coping Program (ACP) typically has been implemented as a school-based, selected program for youth only. The Coping Power Program (CPP) represents an extended version of the ACP with more sessions for youth and the addition of a parent component. The ACP has been designated as effective by the Center for Mental Health Services and OJJDP, and the CPP has been labeled as effective by the Center for Substance Abuse Prevention and exemplary by OJJDP. In formal evaluations, both programs have been implemented by closely supervised doctoral students (Lochman, 1992) as well as masters- and doctoral-level clinicians (Lochman et al., 1998, cited in Lochman et al., 2003), primarily in school settings.

Both the ACP and the CPP are derived from social-cognitive theory on the development of aggression, which posits generally that aggression is maintained by crystallized cognitive structures (e.g., attitudes, beliefs) and online information processing skills (e.g., attention control, problem solving) that support the use of aggression as a habitual behavioral response (see Boxer et al., 2005a). In practice, ACP and CPP target social-cognitive processes through fairly standard cognitive-behavioral techniques such as self-control training, reframing, and perspective-taking, with an explicit focus on the problematic cognitive processes commonly associated with aggression (Boxer & Dubow, 2002). For example, ACP and CPP employ attribution retraining activities (e.g., Hudley & Graham, 1993) designed to mitigate the effects of aggressive children's hostile attributional biases—i.e., their automatic assumptions of hostility in the presence of otherwise ambiguous social stimuli.

Although the Centers for Disease Control has designated social-cognitive intervention as a best-practice strategy for reducing and preventing aggression (Thornton et al., 2000), the majority of well-researched programs deriving from this model are universal prevention programs not tested for use with small groups. However, it should be noted that in many ways the social-cognitive approach shares features with the more traditional small-group approach to dealing with youth conduct problems of anger management training (Feindler & Scalley, 1998) and that some researchers have observed effectiveness for programs relying on social-cognitive components in small-group interventions with highly aggressive and antisocial youth (Guerra & Slaby, 1990). Still, ACP and CPP represent exemplary applications of a general strategy for treating conduct problems via a small-group format in community-based settings.

It is worth noting with respect to small-group treatment for conduct problems that in recent years, much has been made of the potential for "peer contagion" processes occurring in such groups. Dishion et al.'s (1999) seminal review in this area advanced a compelling case that aggregating antisocial youth, particularly adolescents, in small-group therapy could produce the iatrogenic effect of increasing problem behaviors in those youth. Dishion et al. proposed that these effects would most likely accrue through "deviancy training processes" whereby youth provide mutual reinforcement for each other's antisocial behaviors and values in the context of service delivery. However, socialization of behavior in small groups can occur in both directions, with youth showing more or less aggression after treatment depending upon the interaction between pre-intervention level of aggression of others in their group and their own level of pre-intervention aggression (Boxer et al., 2005b). Further, a recent meta-analysis of youth psychotherapy outcome studies suggests that iatrogenic effects are generally quite unlikely in group treatments (Weiss et al., 2005). Thus, the evidence base at this time does not indicate that group treatment for conduct problems should be abandoned. However, such treatment does need to be done cautiously to ensure that inappropriate behavior is not encouraged by peers within the group. For example, group treatment should take place in relatively small groups, with close adult supervision and a behavioral management system designed to limit behavioral problems during the group.

TREATMENTS FOR INDIVIDUAL YOUTH ACROSS SYSTEMS

Multisystemic Therapy

Henggeler and colleagues (e.g., Henggeler et al., 1992, 1998) have developed a community-based, individual/family-focused, multiple-component intervention strategy for adolescents (aged 12–17). *Multisystemic Therapy* (MST) has been recognized as a "model" program by the Blueprints organization and as an effective treatment by CSAP, OJJDP, and the Surgeon General's office. MST is implemented as a multifaceted intervention bringing together a variety of individual practitioners representing numerous community-based agencies in the service of treating individual youth. MST has produced substantial short-term (Henggeler et al., 1986) as well as long-term (up to four years; Borduin et al., 1995) reductions in a host of conduct problems and related behaviors including behavioral problems (e.g., Henggeler et al., 1986) and substance use (Henggeler et al., 1991), in addition to marked reductions in out-of-home placements (Henggeler et al., 1992) and recidivism (Borduin et al., 1995).

MST, as its name suggests, is quite literally a multisystemic intervention approach. Youth and their families are engaged as the focus of home- and agency-based treatments from several different sources, including individual and family therapists as well as interventionists from a range of other potential service providers such as youth development agencies and neighborhood/family centers, schools, probation offices and diversion programs, and psychiatric clinics. MST is explicitly based on a developmental-ecological model of aggressive and antisocial behavior and thus attempts to modify as many risk-promoting processes as possible in the personal functioning and social ecology of the target youth. Thus, the full spectrum of treatment for an individual case might include treatments utilizing problem-solving and social skills training, family structural and strategic intervention, parenting skills training, psychopharmacological treatment, and involvement in prosocial community activities.

It might be more apt to describe MST as a family of evidence-based interventions united in a single principled approach. That is, within each class of intervention delivered in the MST framework, therapists and other service providers are expected to adhere not only to a best-practice strategy in selecting treatments for various issues, but also to a set of nine principles reflecting the broader ecological, strengths-oriented MST approach (see Henggeler et al., 1998). For example, MST providers are expected to focus explicitly on increasing or enhancing the positive aspects of a youth's individual or family functioning (principle #2) and to promote generalization of new skills and interaction sequences across settings and over time (principle #9). Individual therapists are relatively free to pick and choose among existing best-practice, evidence-based strategies for various individual and family concerns. Therefore, specific interventions within an MST case might include individual cognitive-behavioral therapy (CBT), behavioral parent training, and (primarily for comorbid psychopathologies such as ADHD) psychopharmacological therapy.

In MST, an individual case is essentially managed by a full-time therapist who maintains a fairly low caseload (i.e., about three to five cases at a time) along with frequent and (as needed) intensive supervision. This permits the therapist to spend as much time as necessary on individual cases and provides ongoing opportunities for expert consultation with respect to treatment selection and adherence to the MST model and principles. Relatedly, the primary treating therapist is expected to be available 24 hours a day, 7 days a week for crisis consultation. MST interventions are delivered in "real-world" settings—family homes, schools, and neighborhood centers. This works to reduce some of the typical barriers to successful treatment (e.g., transportation) while increasing ecological validity (generalizability). Although MST might be seen as taxing for the individual practicing clinician, the MST model and outcome evaluations certainly underscore the need for a multiple-component approach to intervening in serious conduct problems. Whereas the full implementation of MST might not be feasible for the typical clinician on account of limitations in financial as well as human resources, it certainly is possible for clinicians to adopt an MST-like approach to their work with youth exhibiting conduct problems. In fact, we address this issue directly in our case example.

CASE EXAMPLE OF AN OFFICE-BASED MULTICOMPONENT INTERVENTION

Broad meta-analytic reviews of youth psychotherapy outcomes have indicated generally that behaviorally based approaches are more effective than nonbehaviorally based approaches (Weisz et al., 1995b); behavioral approaches appear to be the stated treatment of choice for clinicians when dealing with aggression and conduct problems, particularly with young children (Weersing et al., 2002). Still, many therapists report fairly eclectic use of treatment techniques that are sensitive to variation in presenting problems across clients in typical child mental health practice (Weersing et al., 2002).

For the purposes of integrating best practices into everyday treatment, the tendency toward eclecticism might be viewed as a positive. As is evident from the approaches described above, the clinician treating conduct problems in children and adolescents should be prepared to implement a variety of specific intervention techniques. For example, behavioral parent training can require multiple modes of client interaction, such as direct skills training, cognitive restructuring, and psychoeducation. Any clinical contact, of course, requires the development of a therapeutic alliance along with the appropriate use of rapport building and other skills such as empathic listening (Karver et al., 2005). Therefore, clinicians with broadly based training are poised to provide the services necessary for evidence-based practice in the treatment of conduct problems, even with the typical limitations of clinical practice such as time, resources, and location. The key to implementing evidence-based strategies in typical clinical settings is to tailor empirically validated techniques as much as possible to those settings.

With that sort of tailoring in mind, our case example is based on clinical material presented in detail by Boxer and Butkus (2005). This case involved the successful treatment of an early adolescent (aged 11 years and attending sixth grade at start of treatment) African-American male diagnosed with Conduct Disorder, Childhood-Onset type (American Psychiatric Association, 2000) at initial evaluation. Psychological treatment in this case was provided in an outpatient mental health clinic through services funded by the county community mental health program via Medicaid. The client, Robert (pseudonym), was referred to the clinic in the early spring of his sixth-grade year by his legal guardian and maternal grandmother, Ms. Johnson.

Prior to the initial diagnostic evaluation, Robert had been suspended from school on four occasions due to behavioral misconduct and had been caught stealing an expensive portable compact disc player from his grandmother. Although this specific incident of theft prompted Ms. Johnson to seek mental health treatment, she had observed over the prior months that Robert had begun to lie to her frequently and to display a negative, callous, and "hard" attitude toward others. Robert acknowledged the validity of his grandmother's concerns and, during the individual interview portion of the evaluation, reported a more elaborated recent history of engagement in aggressive and antisocial behavior, including unprovoked aggression (i.e., "jumping" peers on the street with his currently incarcerated older brother, Jake) and shoplifting (also with his older brother). The persistence and intensity of Robert's conduct problems, and the extent to which he expressed a fondness for and identification with his delinquent older brother, were of serious concern. Along with the primary diagnosis of CD, Robert carried a preexisting diagnosis of ADHD for which he had been receiving pharmacotherapy through his pediatrician.

Robert had experienced a fairly extensive social history of family conflict, traumatic loss, and early deprivation. He was removed from his mother's custody at 18 months due to neglectful conditions accruing from his mother's substance abuse and had endured the murders of his father and uncle. At age 5, Robert was exhibiting very high levels of verbal and physical aggression in his kindergarten classroom, in addition to hyperactive behaviors, and consequently during that year was seen for 20 sessions of psychotherapy and psychiatric consultation in our clinic. He was discharged with diagnoses of ADHD and posttraumatic stress disorder in addition to a suspected reading disorder and an ongoing regimen of Ritalin. By the time Robert returned to our clinic at age 11, he clearly was beginning to fit the profile of the most severe trajectory of conduct problems; i.e., the early-starter and potentially callous type. Unchecked, it was quite likely that Robert's behavior would progress to far more serious manifestations, with significantly more deleterious consequences.

We conceptualized this case from the standpoint of the cognitive-ecological model (e.g., Guerra et al., 2005), a special case of the broader developmental-ecological model that places great emphasis on the role of social cognitions in maintaining aggressive behavior while retaining an important focus on the contexts in which those cognitions develop and are reinforced. Robert clearly presented with an array of biopsychosocial risk factors and acting-out behaviors consistent with this view, including what appeared to us as a strong identification with his aggressive, delinquent older brother Jake as an index of his cognitive orientation to the world.

In terms of formulating a general treatment approach, we focused heavily on two key factors. First, following best-practice strategies, we wanted to ensure as much involvement from Ms. Johnson as possible. Second, following the tenets of cognitive-ecological theory, we wanted to target Robert's beliefs and attitudes about aggressive and antisocial behavior that seemed to be driven by his identification with Jake. We assembled a treatment approach consisting of individual social-cognitive-behavioral psychotherapy with Robert (with activities targeting arousal control, problem solving, and attitude changes); parent management training with Ms. Johnson as well as Robert's mother, who had visitation with Robert on weekends, including psychoeducation on the development of aggression, the various concepts and skills being taught to Robert, and the use of praise in supporting desired behavior; and some limited contingency management with Robert's classroom teacher (with a daily checklist filled out and signed by the teacher, and brought home by Robert, to testify to Robert's classroom behavior). The therapist in this case (Boxer) served as the coordinator of all three of these separate strategies, linked formally in the treatment plan agreed upon by Robert and Ms. Johnson at the outset of treatment. Ongoing pharmacological treatment was handled separately by Robert's pediatrician.

Twelve sessions of psychotherapy, which included brief (5- to 10-minute) meetings with Ms. Johnson followed by 40-minute meetings with Robert, were conducted between the initial evaluation and the clinic-required three-month treatment review. Outcome assessment data, collected at the initial evaluation and about one month after the treatment review meeting, supported this conclusion, with clinically significant improvements noted in Ms. Johnson's ratings of Robert's externalizing behavior via Achenbach's (1991) Child Behavior Checklist as well as clinician ratings on Hodges' (1995) Child and Adolescent Functional Assessment Scale.

Robert's case illustrates the implementation of evidence-based strategies in the context of a "real-world" treatment setting. Although no empirically validated treatment package per se was utilized, all of the therapeutic techniques were derived from the general theoretical foundations supporting the best-practice intervention programs described above. Importantly, as described by Boxer and Butkus (2005), the procedures implemented would conform well to typical managed care considerations (e.g., limits on number of sessions; clear evidence of positive outcomes).

DIRECTIONS FOR APPLIED RESEARCH

As Weisz and colleagues (1995a) pointed out, there are striking differences between research therapies developed and evaluated under highly controlled research conditions and those implemented and fine-tuned in the actual world of everyday clinical practice. There is little evidence to suggest that this state of affairs has changed much since the time of Weisz et al.'s (1995) treatment of the subject. In fact, Weisz et al. (2005) recently reported the results of a comprehensive analysis of youth treatment outcome studies conducted between 1962 and 2002 and concluded that there is still a lack of real clinical representativeness with respect to therapist, client, and setting characteristics.

The ongoing divide between tightly controlled research-derived treatment and real-world clinical practice certainly is not desirable for any sort of psychosocial adjustment problem affecting children and adolescents. But given some of the high stakes (e.g., incarceration, violent victimization, school failure, juvenile justice expenses, etc.) attendant to conduct disorder and related problem behaviors, the issue seems particularly pressing in this arena. As illustrated by the multisytemic therapy framework, there is clear support for treatment approaches to conduct problems that rest on a behavioral and cognitive-behavioral foundation and that make explicit efforts to bring as many social contexts or systems as possible to bear on the problem. This seems to be the most important, basic premise to working with aggressive and antisocial youth.

As noted, internally valid and highly efficacious approaches already exist, and of course therapists with appropriate resources can be advised to adopt those approaches directly. However, it is important to be pragmatic in acknowledging that for the majority of clinicians working with youth, this may not be feasible. Certainly, scholars have acknowledged that there is something to be said for therapists with years of experience who make very skillful choices in their implementation of eclectic practices (Weisz et al., 1995a). Still, as is clear from this review, the evidence base is quite consistent with respect to the theories and principles that underlie efficacious treatment. Thus, we envision three important directions for future applied research.

First, designing, implementing, and evaluating new intervention packages through randomized controlled trials should be complemented or perhaps replaced by "second-level" evaluation studies to assess the effectiveness of *existing* best-practice approaches across different settings and for different client groups. For example, does MST or FFT work equally well for adolescents living in the inner city as well as in rural settings? Do outcomes vary depending upon whether services are provided by paraprofessionals, school counselors, social workers, or clinical psychologists? Do outcomes vary for youth who retain fairly positive social status among their peers as compared to those who are victimized or rejected by their peers? Certainly, these sorts of issues are being addressed by the developers of current best-practice programs. However, the important point here is that it will be fruitful for the field if other groups of clinical researchers take up the mantle of assessing ecological validity for best-practice interventions.

Second, given the theoretical consistency across best-practice strategies, and the clear implications of basic research on the development of aggression and conduct problems, it is worth considering whether clinical effectiveness can be promoted by disseminating broad treatment *models* rather than specific treatment *packages*. Rather than attempt to force practicing clinicians to adopt well-established intervention packages wholesale, it might be possible to enhance therapists' effectiveness across the board by disseminating more general treatment guidelines based on theory and research across multiple intervention packages, along the lines of the "Practice Parameters" offered by the American Academy of Child and Adolescent Psychiatry for a variety of specific psychiatric conditions.

Third, implementation of an individualized and multicomponent treatment for youth with severe aggression or conduct problems can be greatly enhanced by additional research investigating the various mechanisms that can play a role in the development of problem behaviors. For example, Frick (2006) has suggested that the different processes involved in the development of childhood and adolescent-onset patterns of conduct disorder, as well as differences between youth with and without callous-unemotional traits, could suggest that there may also be differences in the effectiveness of certain types of evidenced-based interventions for these distinct groups of antisocial youth. As a case in point, Hawes and Dadds (2005) recently reported that children with callous-unemotional traits showed a less overall positive response to a parenting intervention (similar to Incredible Years) than other children with conduct problems. Target children without callous traits showed greater improvement with a part of the intervention that focused on teaching parents more effective discipline strategies.

Enhancing the interplay between research investigating the developmental mechanisms involved in the etiology of conduct problems and research determining which interventions are most effective for different groups of children with conduct problems could be critical for improving future interventions (Frick, 2001). Further, research on the developmental mechanisms that can place a child at risk for displaying severe conduct problems could suggest interventions that attempt to enhance development (e.g., enhance the development of emotional regulation skills) to prevent the emergence of serious behavior problems (Frick, 2006). Given the serious consequences to the child and his or her family, school, and community that result from conduct problems and aggression, this possibility of effective early prevention may be one of the most important areas of promise for the future of evidence-based practice.

REFERENCES

Abramowitz, A. J., & O'Leary, S. G. (1991). Behavioral interventions for the classroom: Implications for students with ADHD. *School Psychology Review, 20,* 220–234.

Achenbach, T. M. (1991). *Manual for the Child Behavior Checklist/4-18 and 1991 Profile.* Burlington, VT: University of Vermont, Department of Psychiatry.

Alexander, J., Barton, C., Gordon, D., Grotpeter, J., Hansson, K., Harrison, R., et al. (1998). *Blueprints for Violence Prevention, Book Three: Functional Family Therapy.* Boulder, CO: Center for the Study and Prevention of Violence.

Alexander, J. F., & Parsons, B. V. (1973). Short-term behavioral intervention with delinquent families: Impact on family process and recidivism. *Journal of Abnormal Psychology, 81,* 219–225.

American Psychiatric Association (2000). *Diagnostic and Statistical Manual of Mental Disorders,* 4th ed. (rev. ed.). Washington, DC.

Barkley, R. A. (1997). *Defiant Children,* 2nd ed. New York: Guilford Press.

Borduin, C. M., Mann, B. J., Cone, L. T., Henggler, S. W., Fucci, B. R., Blaske, D. M., et al. (1995). Mutisystemic treatment of serious juvenile offenders: Long-term prevention of criminality and violence. *Journal of Consulting and Clinical Psychology, 63,* 569–578.

Boxer, P., & Butkus, M. (2005). Individual social-cognitive intervention for aggressive behavior in early adolescence: An application of the cognitive-ecological framework. *Clinical Case Studies, 4,* 277–294.

Boxer, P., & Dubow, E. F. (2002). A social-cognitive information-processing model for school-based aggression reduction and prevention programs: Issues for research and practice. *Applied & Preventive Psychology, 10,* 177–192.

Boxer, P., Edwards-Leeper, L., Goldstein, S.E., Musher-Eizenman, D., & Dubow, E. F. (2003). Exposure to "low-level" aggression in school: Associations with aggressive behavior, future expectations, and perceived safety. *Violence and Victims, 18,* 691–705.

Boxer, P., Goldstein, S .E., Musher-Eizenman, D., Dubow, E. F., & Heretick, D. (2005a). Developmental issues in the prevention of school aggression from the social-cognitive perspective. *Journal of Primary Prevention, 26,* 383–400.

Boxer, P., Guerra, N. G., Huesmann, L. R., & Morales, J. (2005b). Proximal effects of a small-group selected prevention program on aggression in elementary school children: An investigation of the peer contagion hypothesis. *Journal of Abnormal Child Psychology, 33,* 325–338.

Broidy, L. M., Nagin, D. S, Tremblay, R. E., Bates, J. E., Brame, B., Dodge, K. A., et al. (2003). Developmental trajectories of childhood disruptive behaviors and adolescent delinquency: A six-site, cross-national study. *Developmental Psychology, 39,* 222–245.

Cicchetti, D., & Rogosch, F. A. (1996). Equifinality and multifinality in developmental psychopathology. *Development and Psychopathology, 8,* 597–600.

Conduct Problems Prevention Research Group (1999). Initial impact of the Fast Track Prevention Trial for conduct problems: II. Classroom effects. *Journal of Consulting and Clinical Psychology, 67,* 648–657.

Conger, R. D., & Simons, R. L. (1997). Life-course contingencies in the development of adolescent antisocial behavior: A matching law approach. In T. P. Thornberry (Ed.), *Advances in Criminological Theory* (pp. 55–99). New Brunswick, NJ: Transactional.

Cowen, E. L. (2000). Now that we all know primary prevention in mental health is great, what is it? *Journal of Community Psychology, 28,* 5–16.

Dishion, T., & Kavanagh, K. (2003). *Intervening in Adolescent Problem Behavior.* New York: Guilford Press.

Dishion, T. J., McCord, J., & Poulin, F. (1999). When interventions harm: Peer groups and problem behavior. *American Psychologist, 54,* 755–764.

Dodge, K. A. (1991). The structure and function of reactive and proactive aggression. In D. Pepler & K. H. Rubin (Eds.), *The Development and Treatment of Childhood Aggression* (pp. 201–218). Hillsdale, NJ: Erlbaum.

Dodge, K. A., & Pettit, G. S. (2003). A biopsychosocial model of the development of chronic conduct problems in adolescence. *Developmental Psychology, 39,* 349–371.

Dubow, E. F., Huesmann, L. R., & Boxer, P. (2003). Theoretical and methodological considerations in cross-generational research on parenting and child aggressive behavior. *Journal of Abnormal Child Psychology, 31,* 185–192.

Espelage, D. L., Holt, M. K., & Henkel, R. R. (2003). Examination of peer-group contextual effects on aggression during early adolescence. *Child Development, 74,* 205–220.

Feindler, E., & Scalley, M. (1998). Adolescent anger-management groups for violence reduction. In K. C. Stoiber & T. R. Kratochwill (Eds.), *Handbook of Group Intervention for Children and Families* (pp. 100–119). Needham Heights, MA: Allyn & Bacon.

Frick, P. J. (1998). *Conduct Disorders and Severe Antisocial Behavior.* New York: Plenum.

Frick, P. J. (2001). Effective interventions for children and adolescents with conduct disorder. *Canadian Journal of Psychiatry, 46,* 597–608.

Frick, P. J. (2006). Developmental pathways to conduct disorder. *Child and Adolescent Psychiatric Clinics of North America.*

Frick, P. J., Bodin, S. D., & Barry, C. T. (2000). Psychopathic traits and conduct problems in community and clinic-referred samples of children: Further development of the Psychopathy Screening Device. *Psychological Assessment, 12,* 382–393.

Frick, P. J., Cornell, A. H., Bodin, S. D., Dane, H. A., Barry, C. T., & Loney, B. R. (2003). Callous-unemotional traits and developmental pathways to severe conduct problems. *Developmental Psychology, 39,* 246–260.

Frick, P. J., & Loney, B. R. (1999). Outcomes of children and adolescents with conduct disorder and oppositional defiant disorder. In H. C. Quay & A. Hogan (Eds.), *Handbook of Disruptive Behavior Disorders* (pp. 507–524). New York: Plenum.

Frick, P., Morris, A. S. (2004). Temperament and developmental pathways to severe conduct problems. *Journal of Clinical Child and Adolescent Psychology, 33,* 54–68.

Guerra, N. G., Boxer, P., & Kim, T. (2005). A cognitive-ecological approach to serving students with emotional and behavioral disorders: Application to aggressive behavior. *Behavioral Disorders, 30,* 277–288.

Guerra, N. G., & Slaby, R. G. (1990). Cognitive mediators of aggression in adolescent offenders: 2. Intervention. *Developmental Psychology, 26,* 269–277.

Hawes, D. J., & Dadds, M. R. (2005). The treatment of conduct problems in children with callous-unemotional traits. *Journal of Consulting and Clinical Psychology, 73,* 737–741.

Henggeler, S. W., Borduin, C. M., Melton, G. B., Mann, B. J., Smith, L., Hall, J. A., et al. (1991). Effects of multisystemic therapy on drug use and abuse in serious juvenile offenders: A progress report from two outcome studies. *Family Dynamics of Addiction Quarterly, 1,* 40–51.

Henggeler, S. W., Cunningham, B., Pickrel, S. G., Schoenwald, S. K., & Brondino, M. J. (1996). Multisystemic therapy: An effective violence prevention approach for serious offenders. *Journal of Adolescence, 19,* 47–61.

Henggeler, S. W., Melton, G. B., & Smith, L. A. (1992). Family preservation using multisystemic therapy: An effective alternative to incarcerating serious juvenile offenders. *Journal of Consulting and Clinical Psychology, 60,* 953–961.

Henggeler, S. W., Rodick, J. D., Borduin, C.M., Hanson, C. L., Watson, S. M., & Urey, J. R. (1986). Multisystemic treatment of juvenile offenders: Effects on adolescent behavior and family interactions. *Developmental Psychology, 22,* 132–141.

Henggeler, S. W., Schoenwald, S. K., Borduin, C. M., Roweland, M. D., & Cunningham, P. B. (1998). *Multisystemic Treatment of Antisocial Behavior in Children and Adolescents.* New York: Guilford Press.

Hinshaw, S. P., Lahey, B. B., & Hart, E. L. (1993). Issues of taxonomy and comorbidity in the development of conduct disorder. *Development and Psychopathology, 5 ,* 31–49.

Hodges, K. (1995). *The Child and Adolescent Functional Assessment Scale.* Ann Arbor, MI: Author.

Hudley, C., & Graham, S. (1993). An attributional intervention to reduce peer-directed aggression among African-American boys. *Child Development, 64,* 124–138.

Huesmann, L. R., Dubow, E. F., Eron, L. D., & Boxer, P. (2006). Middle childhood family-contextual and personal factors as predictors of adult outcomes. In A. C. Huston & M. Ripke (Eds.), *Developmental Contexts of Middle Childhood* (pp. 62–86). Cambridge: Cambridge University Press.

Huesmann, L. R., Eron, L. D., & Yarmel, P. W. (1987). Intellectual functioning and aggression. *Journal of Personality and Social Psychology, 52,* 232–240.

Huesmann, L. R., & Guerra, N. G. (1997). Children's normative beliefs about aggression and aggressive behavior. *Journal of Personality and Social Psychology, 72,* 408–419.

Huesmann, L. R., Moise-Titus, J., Podolski, C., & Eron, L. D. (2003). Longitudinal relations between children's exposure to television violence and their aggressive and violent behavior in young adulthood: 1977–1992. *Developmental Psychology, 39,* 201–222.

Karver, M. S., Handelsman, J. B., Fields, S., & Bickman, L. (2005). A theoretical model of common process factors in youth and family therapy. *Mental Health Services Research, 7,* 35–51.

Kazdin, A. E. (1997). Parent management training: Evidence, outcomes, and issues. *Journal of the American Academy of Child and Adolescent Psychiatry, 36,* 1349–1356.

Kazdin, A. E., & Weisz, J. R. (Eds.) (2003). *Evidence-Based Psychotherapies for Children and Adolescents.* New York: Guilford Press.

Lochman, J. E. (1992). Cognitive-behavioral interventions with aggressive boys: Three-year follow-up and preventive effects. *Journal of Consulting and Clinical Psychology, 60,* 426–432.

Lochman, J. E., Barry, T. D., & Pardini, D. A. (2003). Anger Control Training for aggressive youth. In A. E. Kazdin & J. R. Weisz (Eds.), *Evidence-Based Psychotherapies for Children and Adolescents* (pp. 263–281). New York: Guilford Press.

Lochman, J. E., Rahmani, C. H., Flagler, S. L., Nyko-Silva, I., Ross, J. J., & Johnson, J. L. (1998). *Dissemination of the Anger Coping Program.* Unpublished manuscript, University of Alabama-Tuscaloosa.

Lochman, J. E., & Wells, K. C. (2002). The Coping Power Program for preadolescent aggressive boys and their parents: Outcome effects at the one-year follow-up. *Journal of Consulting and Clinical Psychology, 72,* 571–578.

McMahon, R. J., & Forehand, R. L. (2003). *Helping the Noncompliant Child: Family-Based Treatment for Oppositional Behavior,* 2nd ed. New York: Guilford Press.

McMahon, R. J., & Frick, P. J. (2005). Evidence-based assessment of conduct problems in children and adolescents. *Journal of Clinical Child and Adolescent Psychology, 34,* 477–505.

Metropolitan Area Child Study Research Group (2002). A cognitive-ecological approach to preventing aggression in urban settings: Initial outcomes for high-risk children. *Journal of Consulting and Clinical Psychology, 70,* 179–194.

Miles, D. R., & Carey, G. (1997). Genetic and environmental architecture of human aggression. *Journal of Personality and Social Psychology, 72,* 207–217.

Moffitt, T. E. (1993). Adolescent-limited and life-course-persistent antisocial behavior: A developmental taxonomy. *Psychological Review, 100,* 674–701.

Morris, S. B., Alexander, J. F.. & Waldron, H. (1988). Functional family therapy. In I. R. H. Falloon (Ed.), *Handbook of Behavioral Family Therapy* (pp. 107–127). New York: Guilford Press.

MTA Cooperative Group (1999). A 14-month randomized clinical trial of treatment strategies for Attention Deficit-Hyperactivity Disorder. *Archives of General Psychiatry, 56,* 1073–1086.

Nagin, D. S., & Tremblay, R. E. (1999). Trajectories of boys' physical aggression, opposition, and hyperactivity on the path to physically violent and nonviolent juvenile delinquency. *Child Development, 70,* 1181–1196.

NICHD Early Child Care Research Network (2004). Trajectories of physical aggression from toddlerhood to middle childhood. *Monographs of the Society for Research in Child Development, 69*(4).

Reid, M. J., Webster-Stratton, C., & Hammond, M. (2003). Follow-up of children who received the Incredible Years intervention for oppositional-defiant disorder: Maintenance and prediction of 2-year outcome. *Behavior Therapy, 34,* 471–491.

Sexton, T. L., & Alexander, J. F. (2002). Functional Family Therapy: An empirically supported, family based intervention model for at-risk adolescents and their families. In T. Patterson (Ed.), *Comprehensive Handbook of Psychotherapy, Vol. 2: Cognitive Behavioral Approaches* (pp. 117–140). New York: Wiley.

Szapocznik, J., Perez-Vidal, A., Hervis, O. E., Brickman, A., & Kurtines, W. (1990). Innovations in family therapy: Strategies for overcoming resistance to treatment. In R. A. Wells & V. J. Giannetti (Eds.), *Handbook of Brief Psychotherapies* (pp. 93–114). New York: Plenum Press.

Taylor, T. K., Schmidt, F., Pepler, D., & Hodgins, H. (1998). A comparison of eclectic treatment with Webster-Stratton's Parents and Children Series in a children's mental health center: A randomized controlled trial. *Behavior Therapy, 12,* 634–642.

Thornton, T. N., Craft, C. A., Dahlberg, L. L., Lynch, B. S., & Baer, K. (2000). *Best Practices of Youth Violence Prevention: A Sourcebook for Community Action.* Atlanta: Centers for Disease Control and Prevention.

Tremblay, R. E. (2000). The development of aggressive behaviour during childhood: What have we learned in the past century? *International Journal of Behavioral Development, 24,* 129–141.

Webster-Stratton, C. (1990). Enhancing the effectiveness of self-administered videotape parent training for families with conduct-problem children. *Journal of Abnormal Child Psychology, 18,* 479–492.

Webster-Stratton, C., & Hammond, M. (1997). Treating children with early-onset conduct problems: A comparison of child and parent training interventions. *Journal of Consulting and Clinical Psychology, 65,* 93–109.

Webster-Stratton, C., Kolpacoff, M., & Hollinsworth, T. (1988). Self-administered videotape therapy for families with conduct-problem children: Comparison with two cost-effective treatments and a control group. *Journal of Clinical Child Psychology, 56,* 558–566.

Webster-Stratton, C., Reid, M. J., & Hammond, M. (2004). Treating children with early-onset conduct problems: Intervention outcomes for parent, child, and teacher training. *Journal of Clinical Child and Adolescent Psychology, 33,* 105–124.

Weersing, V. R., Weisz, J. R., & Donenberg, G. R. (2002). Development of the Therapy Procedures Checklist: A therapist-report measure of technique use in child and adolescent treatment. *Journal of Clinical Child and Adolescent Psychology, 31,* 168–180.

Weiss, B., Caron, A., Ball, S., Tapp, J., Johnson, M., & Weisz, J. R. (2005). Iatrogenic effects of group treatment for antisocial youth. *Journal of Consulting and Clinical Psychology, 73,* 1036–1044.

Weisz, J. R., Donenberg, G. R., Han, S. S., & Weiss, B. (1995a). Bridging the gap between laboratory and clinic in child and adolescent psychotherapy. *Journal of Consulting and Clinical Psychology, 63,* 688–701.

Weisz, J. R., Doss, A. J., & Hawley, K. M. (2005). Youth psychotherapy outcome research: A review and critique of the evidence base. *Annual Review of Psychology, 56,* 337–363.

Weisz, J. R., Weiss, B., Han, S. S., Granger, D. A., & Morton, T. (1995b). Effects of psychotherapy with children and adolescents: A meta-analysis of treatment outcome studies. *Psychological Bulletin, 117,* 450–468.

15

Components of Evidence-Based Interventions for Bullying and Peer Victimization

ANNE K. JACOBS

After several widely publicized school shootings, efforts to stem school-related violence have gained popularity and greater media exposure. Bullying, or peer victimization, is one specific form of repetitive violence common to schools that involves a real or perceived power imbalance between a bully and a victim. Bullying includes harassment, intimidation, social ostracism, and physical aggression. Bullying behavior can occur at a number of levels, including person to person, through notes, or through forms of electronic communication such as e-mail. Bullying is a common phenomenon, with over a quarter of students reporting frequent involvement in bullying (Limber et al., 1997; Nansel et al., 2001) and over 70% reporting being a victim at least once (Glover et al., 2000; Hoover et al., 1992).

There are at least four active roles that students can take during peer victimization. First, bullies are students who frequently dole out relational or physical aggression toward students perceived as being weaker. Second, victims seldom engage in aggression but are frequent targets of physical and or relational aggression. Third, students who both engage in bullying and are frequent victims themselves are classified as bully-victims or provocative victims. Finally, students can participate by being bystanders to acts of bullying. These bystanders can take steps to help the victim, join in on the bullying once it has begun, or reinforce the bully by providing an audience to the aggressive behavior (Olweus, 1993; Zerger, 1996). These roles tend to be stable over time, and the effects of each of these behaviors can reach into adulthood (Olweus, 1993).

ANNE K. JACOBS • University of Kansas

CONSEQUENCES ASSOCIATED WITH BULLYING

Several negative outcomes have been linked to the various roles students may take in bullying. In addition to low academic achievement (Glew et al., 2005), victims report having a number of physical and psychological difficulties in adulthood, including depression, low self-esteem (Limber & Nation, 1998; Olweus, 1993) and suicidal ideation (Rigby, 1996). Bullies generally have higher rates of other antisocial acts, are more likely to be truant or drop out of school, and are at a greater risk for being arrested as adults (Olweus, 1993). Compared to students who frequently bully and those who are frequently victimized, bully-victims have a higher rate of anxiety and psychosomatic symptoms (Kaltiala-Heino et al., 2000). Bully-victims also report higher rates of depression and suicidal ideation (Espelage & Swearer, 2003). Passively observing acts of bullying negatively affects students and is linked to increased fears of being bullied and decreased school attendance (Lee, 1993). Students even report that they refuse to use the restroom at school due to fears of being victimized there (Vernon et al., 2003). In an effort to prevent or ameliorate the negative outcomes linked to bullying, a growing body of research on factors related to peer victimization has been developed.

Traditionally, bullying has been seen as a problem behavior of individual students. Broadening this view to conceptualizing bullying as a social phenomenon that is best understood within the ecology in which it occurs is arguably the most important development in the understanding of bullying (Espelage & Swearer, 2003). Viewing peer victimization as a social or group phenomenon leads to the conclusion that interventions should be wide in scope to address the students' social climate (Salmivalli, 1999; Twemlow et al., 2001, 2003). It follows that interventions focused solely on individual roles in bullying have not been shown to be as effective in preventing bullying as comprehensive programs (Limber, 2004) that address the social dynamics, multiple roles, and environment in which bullying occurs. Anecdotal reports indicate that when an individual bully is removed from a particular school, another one emerges to take his or her place in the social arena. In addition to taking an ecological view of bullying, a number of factors consistently emerge in the research literature as likely being relevant to the prevention of bullying.

FACTORS RELATED TO BULLYING

Attitudes

Cognitive mechanisms, such as attitudes toward the use of aggression, have been explored in their relation to children victimizing peers. Studies have demonstrated that from middle childhood (Huesmann & Guerra, 1997) through adolescence (Vernberg et al., 1999), endorsing the attitude that aggression is a legitimate, acceptable means to an end has been clearly linked to bullying others. Likewise, negative attitudes toward victims, such as the belief that they deserve the victimization, have been linked to aggressive acting out toward peers (Slaby & Guerra, 1988). Although boys are more likely than girls to strongly endorse these attitudes, the relationship between these cognitive mechanisms and aggressive behavior holds true for both genders (Vernberg et al., 1999). Attitudes and beliefs concerning the acceptability of aggression have not been linked just to the behavior of bullies, but to that of bystanders as well. Increases in positive attitudes regarding the use of aggression predicted greater frequency of elementary school bystanders' joining in on bullying once it had begun; likewise, decreases in the endorsement of positive attitudes about aggression predicted increases in bystander helping behavior (Jacobs, 2001).

Empathy

Students' feelings of empathy have also been linked to their involvement in peer victimization. As expected, a lack of empathy for the victim or beliefs that the victim is somehow different or deserving of the bullying is linked to both participating in bullying and reinforcing peers when they bully (Hoover et al., 1992; Rigby & Slee, 1991). For bystanders, greater empathy for the victims was linked to greater helping behaviors in childhood (Boulton & Underwood, 1992) and early adolescence (Zerger, 1996). Bystanders who were more likely to join in bullying once it had begun reported lower levels of empathy (Zerger, 1996).

Adult Supervision and Sanctions

Research shows that levels of peer victimization are related to the presence of teachers and the actions that these adults take once they observe bullying. Student reports of bullying tend to be higher in locations that typically lack consistent adult supervision such as hallways, playgrounds, cafeterias, restrooms, and buses (Meraviglia et al., 2003; Vernon et al., 2003). Sadly, even when adults are present in these areas, they may not take appropriate action to stop aggression. According to social learning theories, teachers and other adults in the school have the potential to encourage students to help victims when they themselves intervene in bullying episodes (Barnett, 1987; Hampson, 1981); conversely, they have the potential to create a "norm of nonintervention" (Piliavin et al., 1982). Students are adept at picking up on these nonspoken norms (Newman-Carlson & Horne, 2004) and reflect these norms in their own behaviors. Accordingly, the frequency of observing adult sanctions for bullying has been linked to lower levels of aggressive bystander behavior (Vernberg et al., 2000). An increase in observed frequency of adult sanctions predicted more frequent female helping behaviors during bullying episodes, while a decrease in observed sanctions over time predicted greater joining in behavior for both boys and girls (Jacobs, 2001). Given the strong link

Table 1. Evidence-Based Components of Antibullying Programs

Program	Grades	Ed	Behav	Skills	Bystanders	Mentors	Teachers	Parents
					Components			
Bullying Prevention Program (BPP; Olweus, 1993)	4–7	X	X		X	X	X	X
Modified BPP (Orpinas et al., 2003)	K–5	X	X	X	X	X	X	X
Creating a Peaceful School Learning Environment (CAPSLE; Twemlow et al., 2001)	3–5	X	X	X	X	X	X	X
Steps to Respect (Frey et al., 2005)	3–6	X		X			X	X
Peer Supporters (Menesini et al., 2003)	6–8	X		X	X	X		
Social Skills Group Intervention (S.S.GRIN; DeRosier, 2004)	3	X	X	X				
Bulli & Pupe (Baldry & Farrington, 2004)	Ages 10–16	X		X				
Bully Busters (Newman-Carlson & Horne, 2004)	6–8	X	X	X			X	

Ed = psychoeducattion to decrease pro-bullying attitudes and increase empathy; *Behav* = increased supervision, positive reinforcement for prosocial behavior, consequences for bullying behavior; *Skills* = conflict resolution, anger management, communication skills; *Bystanders* = focus on bystander behavior; *Mentors* = peer mentors, befriending interventions; *Teachers* = teacher training & support; *Parents* = communication with parents.

between teacher and student behavior, it is discouraging that teachers typically intervene in only a small percentage of bullying episodes (Craig et al., 2000).

School Climate

Students' perceptions of the overall school climate and sense of connectedness to their school have been found to be related to academic and social behavior. Positive ratings of school climate have been linked to higher grades (Barber & Olsen, 1997) and lower levels of delinquency (Neumark-Sztainer et al., 1997). Less favorable ratings of school climate and lower levels of student connectedness correlated with more frequent bullying and violence perpetrated at school (Bosworth et al., 1999; Elliott & Voss, 1974; Gilbert, 1995). For bystanders of bullying, greater connectedness to school predicted increased helping behavior in girls, while decreases in positive school perceptions related to greater joining in behavior for girls (Jacobs, 2001).

The number and type of antibullying programs are vast and varied, but common threads can be found between programs. Many programs use education to alter students' attitudes toward aggression and increase empathy for victims. Teacher training and behavioral interventions are used to enhance adult supervision and create clear sanctions for aggressive behavior and reinforcement of prosocial behavior. The involvement of other resources such as parents, bystanders, and peer mentors focuses on improving the overall school climate. It is not surprising that the antibullying programs that demonstrate positive outcomes comprise many of these interventions to target the factors linked in the research literature to bullying (Table 1).

EVIDENCE-BASED ANTIBULLYING PROGRAMS

The emergence of antibullying state laws includes several state statutes that address the implementation of bullying prevention programs (Limber & Small, 2003). The fact that schools continue to use counterproductive strategies to reduce bullying (Limber, 2004) highlights the importance of increasing awareness of evidence-based interventions for peer victimization. Numerous bullying and prevention and intervention school-based programs exist, and the number increases substantially when one includes programs targeting violence at school in general. Identifying all of the individual programs marketed to schools is a daunting task. Some programs comprise only manuals, while others include videos, music, online games, and guest speakers. Because many schools tend to create their own bullying programs or modify existing ones, a review of evidence-based and counterproductive components is important in helping consumers determine whether a program is likely to be effective in reducing peer victimization. In the following section, the components of eight antibullying programs with promising results are discussed. When available, information regarding the number of schools implementing the programs is reported.

Olweus Bullying Prevention Program

Several promising school-based programs exist that target a large number of risky student behaviors, of which bullying is just one component (e.g., Cunningham & Henggeler, 2001), but among programs specifically targeting bullying, the Olweus Bullying Prevention Program (BPP; Olweus, 1993) has emerged as the "gold standard." The BPP has been evaluated numerous times using age-cohort designs and a comparison to a control group. When implemented in primary and secondary schools, the Olweus program demonstrated a reduction in bullying by approximately 50% (Olweus, 1993), with the effects being maintained at a two-year follow-up (1997). The program also resulted in decreases in truancy, vandalism, and theft; improvement in overall school climate; and increased student satisfaction (Olweus, 1993). Despite varying results in replications across different countries thought to be related to differing levels of program implementation (for review, see Smith & Ananiadou, 2003), the BPP remains the model antibullying program to date. This program was selected as a Blueprints for Violence Prevention Model Program by the University of Colorado's Center for the Study and Prevention of Violence based on its evidence of deterring childhood aggression using a strong research design, positive effects that endure one year postintervention, and success in multiple site replications (Center for the Study and Prevention of Violence, 2002). The BPP is also a "model program" identified by the Substance Abuse and Mental Health Services Administration and has been named as a "promising program" by the Surgeon General's report on youth violence.

As reflected in the body of research on bullying, the BPP addresses the ecology of bullying by providing a comprehensive approach to reducing peer victimization with interventions at the school, classroom, and individual levels (Olweus, 1993). The school-level interventions include administration and evaluation of a student questionnaire to inform staff about the nature and level of bullying behavior, school conference day, teacher training and teacher groups to raise the awareness of bullying and counteract passive acceptance of bullying behaviors, the creation of a Bullying Prevention Coordinating Committee, Parent Teacher Association meetings, parent circles to discuss bullying issues, and increased adult supervision of areas in the school where bullying is most likely to occur. Class meetings, creation and enforcement of classroom rules targeting bullying and bystander behavior, praise for prosocial behavior, and cooperative learning activities are all interventions at the classroom level, while individual discussions with frequent bullies and victims along with their parents and changing classes to separate bullies and victims occur at the student level of intervention. The BPP is being used in at least 18 states and in hundreds of schools worldwide (USDHHS, n.d.). In addition, many bullying intervention and prevention programs evaluated in the research literature are based, at least in part, on the BPP.

Modified BPP

One antibullying program implemented in an elementary school supplemented the Olweus BPP with other components such as positive incentives for appropriate student behavior and student education in conflict resolution, anger management, respect, and communication skills. Orpinas and colleagues found in a pre-posttest design that self-reported aggression decreased for the younger students by 40% and self-reported victimization decreased for students in all grades (Orpinas et al., 2003). The results indicated that not only might the added educational and skills components be useful in reducing bullying, but the level of effectiveness varies by age.

Creating a Peaceful School Learning Environment (CAPSLE)

The CAPSLE program, also known as the Peaceful Schools Program, is another comprehensive schoolwide antibullying program for elementary schools that comprises three core and two support components (Twemlow et al., 1999, 2003). The first core component is a positive climate campaign to emphasize positive social skills not just between students, but also between students and adults in the school. The second core component, a classroom management plan, is a method of discipline that raises students' awareness of bullying dynamics and changes their behavior accordingly. The Gentle Warriors Program, the third core component, is a unique physical education program influenced by defensive martial arts that helps students focus on self-regulation skills. The support components of the CAPSLE program are mentoring programs for teachers and students to help them avoid taking a negative role in bullying.

An initial evaluation comparing a school receiving the intervention to a control school showed significant decreases in discipline referrals, lower student suspension rates, and significantly increased achievement scores in the CAPSLE school (Twemlow et al., 2001). A larger RCT study of the program using random assignment of schools to one of three conditions (CAPSLE, school psychiatric consultant comparison intervention, control group) was recently completed (Fonagy et al., 2005). Outcome measures were comprehensive and included self-report, peer report, and direct observation. Compared to control schools, CAPSLE moderated the developmental trend of increasing peer-reported victimization, aggression, and aggressive bystanding in the intervention schools. These effects were maintained at the one-year follow-up. CAPSLE also moderated a decline in empathy compared to the school psychiatric consultant and control conditions. Direct observations indicated that CAPSLE produced a significant decrease in off-task and disruptive classroom behaviors. Approximately 200 schools have ordered the CAPSLE manual and materials. The CAPSLE program is being implemented in 20 schools across three states, and current projects include implementation in a fourth state and in two Jamaican schools.

Steps to Respect

The Steps to Respect program utilizes a schoolwide program for grades 3–6 including staff training to increase their awareness of and intervention in bullying (Frey et al., 2005). This program also added a classroom curriculum teaching social-emotional skills and engaged parents in the program through communications such as take-home letters. An experimental trial of this program showed relative declines in bullying based on observations of playground behavior, a positive change in attitudes toward aggression, and a trend for decreased bystander reinforcement of bullying (Frey et al., 2005). Unfortunately, no significant differences in self-reported aggression emerged between experimental and control groups. Additional positive findings included decreased argumentative behavior, increased prosocial interactions, and greater reports of adult responsiveness to bullying. The Steps to Respect program is being used across the United States and Canada in approximately 3,300 schools (USDHHS, n.d.).

Peer Supporters

One study looked at interventions at the classroom and individual levels. Menesini and colleagues (2003) examined the effects of providing peer supporters for victims of bullying and providing education and awareness exercises in Italian middle-school classrooms. When comparing experimental and control classes using peer nominations and student questionnaires, the researchers found that these interventions countered the developmental increase in bullying behavior in middle schools and prevented the developmental increase in attitudes supporting aggression. Although there was no random assignment of classrooms to conditions, the study shows promising results. Decreasing the incidents of bullying is considered a sign of success, but it is important to note that countering the developmental trend for increasing bullying and attitudes supporting the use of aggression is also the mark of a promising program.

Social Skills Group Intervention (S.S.GRIN)

DeRosier (2004) examined the effects of a general social skills intervention, S.S.GRIN, on bullying behavior among third-grade students. Third graders were randomly assigned to a treatment or control group, and the outcome was evaluated using peer nominations and questionnaires. There were no significant changes in reports of peer disliking; however, positive changes were found in reports of student behavior. Aggressive students who received the social skills training showed greater declines in bullying behavior and fewer antisocial affiliations than did aggressive students in the control group. Other positive results included increased peer liking, enhanced self-esteem and self-efficacy, and decreased social anxiety. Also impressive were the maintenance of the positive effects and additional gains were found in a one-year follow-up study (DeRosier & Marcus, 2005).

Bulli & Pupe (Bullies and Dolls)

A short-term intervention using a three-hour session once a week for three weeks, presented to middle- and high school students in Italy, showed mixed results in reducing bullying (Baldry & Farrington, 2004). The Bulli & Pupe intervention included three videos with a booklet, inter-active classroom lessons, role-plays, group discussions, and focus groups designed to develop social cognitive skills related to the negative effects of bullying. Classrooms were randomly assigned to either the treatment or control group, and a student survey was given four months after the inter-vention. Older students, those in their third year of middle school and those in their first year of high school, reported a decrease in self-victimization while younger students reported an increase in being victimized. The researchers theorized that the cognitive skills presented in the intervention might be more appropriate for the older students' developmental level.

Bully Busters

Newman-Carlson and Horne (2004) evaluated the effects of a psychoed-ucational intervention for teachers in reducing bullying among middle-school students. The intervention relied on a teacher training manual, *Bully Busters: A Teacher's Manual for Helping Bullies, Victims, and Bystanders* (Newman et al., 2000), that included education about bullying and victimization, intervention and prevention techniques, stress-management information, classroom activities, and a classroom curriculum resource. Teachers were also assigned to teacher support groups focused on the bullying prevention program. The researchers used a quasi-experimental, pre-posttest design with a control group to evaluate Bully Busters. This teacher-based intervention resulted in increased teacher knowledge and use of the intervention skills and a greater sense of personal self-efficacy for participating teachers. The treatment group showed a significant decrease in disciplinary referrals, which were used to measure bullying behavior. Bully Busters has been implemented in four states, and at least 2,000 manuals have been sold (USDHHS, n.d.).

COUNTERPRODUCTIVE INTERVENTIONS

While it is important to understand what works to decrease bullying, it is equally important to be aware of what does not work. School staff members need to use their limited time and resources in the most effective manner possible. Implementing ineffective programs not only wastes resources but can increase the staff's sense of hopelessness, decrease morale, and make it less likely that the school would or could invest in a different, more effective program. In some cases, ineffective programs may actually increase the problem of bullying. Given the social dynamics of bullying, it is unlikely that quick, easy interventions are likely to have any effect. Having a well-known speaker at an assembly, promoting a simple motto, or showing a video on bullying may be good ways to initially raise awareness, but they are insufficient by themselves to change behavior (e.g., Okayasu & Takayama, 2004). As demonstrated in the study by Baldry and Farrington (2004), brief interventions can show mixed results and care should be taken to determine whether the adverse outcomes for younger students are due to the sensitization effect or a true increase in bullying.

Discipline methods that gained popularity after the Columbine school shooting in 1999 such as sending the bully to an alternative school or other zero-tolerance policies remove the bully from much-needed positive models of behavior and do not stem the problem of bullying at school (Limber & Small, 2003). Harsh, punitive responses to bullying run the risk of decreasing students' willingness to report aggressive or dangerous behaviors of their peers (Jacobs, 2001), and merely removing a bullying student from a school does not address the social climate or the behaviors of bystanders who contribute to peer victimization. Furthermore, zero-tolerance policies have not been shown to be effective in increasing overall student safety (Skiba, 2000).

Peer mediation and conflict-resolution strategies are popular and may be effective in addressing certain issues between students. These techniques, however, are not appropriate to the problem of bullying given the nature of this social behavior (Limber, 2004; Limber & Nation, 1998). Bullying is defined by the imbalance of power between the two parties, while mediation and conflict resolution are used in situations where parties are assumed to have equal power. Interventions relying on conflict resolution as an agent of change have shown mixed results in decreasing bullying (Smith et al., 2003). In some cases, peer mediation has been shown to be ineffective and possibly harmful when used with students to address aggressive behaviors (Gottfredson, 1987; U.S. Department of Health and Human Services, 2001).

Finally, interventions focused on only one group of students involved in bullying are unlikely to adequately address the social dynamics of the problem. For example, interventions designed to increase social skills of the victims sound promising but have not been shown to be effective in combating the problem of peer victimization when used alone (Fox & Boulton, 2003). It is also noteworthy that group treatment of bullies is ill-advised (Limber, 2004). Much in the same way that group therapy for antisocial youth may result in unintended negative effects (Dishion et al., 1994), group meetings with bullies would likely be counterproductive. Ultimately, such interventions might serve to increase the bullies' negative social network and serve as a breeding ground for new and creative ways to torment their peers.

CASE EXAMPLE OF IMPLEMENTATION PROBLEMS OF AN EVIDENCE-BASED ANTIBULLYING PROGRAM

A junior high school principal contacted a professor of clinical child psychology at a local university in a Midwestern city in response to a teacher request for consultation related to concerns with the level of bullying behavior between students. An additional teacher concern was the perception that incidents of students disrespecting and bullying teachers were increasing. The consulting university personnel administered and scored a student survey regarding levels of bullying, victimization, adult sanctions for bullying, bystander behavior, empathy, and attitudes toward aggression. Not only did the students report frequent episodes of bullying, but when visiting the school, the professor and graduate student observed fistfights between students, students using inappropriate language toward teachers, and an apparent lack of effective sanctions for such behaviors. Teachers reported feeling frustrated and even scared as student behaviors escalated to include a sexually threatening note left with a used condom addressed to a specific female teacher. As a result of the survey, the teachers wrote recommendations for the Olweus BPP to be included in the five-year school improvement plan. One experienced teacher emerged as a strong proponent and leader of the intervention program, but teacher support overall varied. Some teachers were enthusiastic about the interventions, while other teachers voiced the opinion that younger teachers did not know how to handle student behavior and that a schoolwide intervention was not necessary.

The modified BPP was implemented during the second year of contact with the junior high school. School-level interventions included a school conference and Parent Teacher Organization meetings where the student survey results were presented. In contrast to the Olweus BPP, the implementation did not include the creation of a Bullying Prevention Coordinating Committee or parent circles to discuss bullying. Great emphasis was placed on increasing adult supervision, and teacher meetings were organized for each section of the hallway on both floors of the school. In these meetings, teachers discussed increasing supervision in the hallways and bathrooms in their sections of the school and helping their classes create rules regarding student social behaviors. One particularly enthusiastic teacher group provided awards for good hallway behavior, thereby adding positive reinforcement for appropriate behavior to the increased sanctions for bullying. The classroom-level interventions implemented included class meetings, creation of class rules regarding bullying, and praise for prosocial behavior. Some teachers had already implemented cooperative learning opportunities. Other interventions included a bullying "hotline" staffed by a graduate student, and the student council created an antibullying video that it presented at a school assembly. Teacher groups provided reports on incidents of bullying observed in the hallways and bathrooms.

What Worked

A teacher group on a first-floor hallway was cohesive in its support for the BPP. All members attended regular weekly meetings and were united in creating classroom rules targeting bullying behavior, providing increased supervision of their hallway and bathroom, tracking down students to ensure that appropriate consequences were applied for bullying behavior, and rewarding students verbally and with candy for positive hallway behaviors. These teachers utilized discussions with the consulting university personnel and shared effective interventions and social support with each other during their weekly meetings. Initially, teacher reports of bullying in this hallway increased from baseline. The teachers interpreted this increase as being due to a sensitization effect. As the weeks went by, teacher reports of aggressive student behavior in their hallway decreased dramatically and teachers openly voiced satisfaction with their interventions.

What Did Not Work

Throughout the junior high school, there were varying levels of teacher buy-in to the BPP and correspondingly mixed results. While the active teachers' group on the first floor reported great satisfaction with the interventions as well as decreases in bullying between classes, results were less positive on the second floor of the school. The group of teachers on the second floor who voiced their opinion that a schoolwide intervention was not warranted and, thus, did not meet together or engage in the interventions reported increases in the frequency of bullying in their hallway. They did not see the first floor as being successful in their efforts, but rather blamed the program for merely "shifting the problem" up to their floor. With the school divided on the program, it was important for someone in a leadership position to take a stand. The school's principal retired at the end of the program's second year and his replacement did not provide many follow-up efforts. The first-floor teachers' group continued its efforts as the program in the rest of the school gradually ended with active opposition to the program from one teacher and indifference from many. In implementing schoolwide programs, it is important to attend to teacher and administrative buy-in. Clearly, in this case many teachers and certainly the new principal did not feel a sense of ownership of the program and thus felt that it was a burden rather than a help.

EVALUATING BULLYING PREVENTION PROGRAMS

Measures

Evaluations of bullying prevention program generally use a variety of measures. The most commonly used form of measurement appears to be questionnaires completed by the students. These questionnaires usually contain a variety of items to measure factors such as students' attitudes toward aggression, empathy for victims, reports of observed adult sanctions, frequency of victimization of self, victimization of others, and bystander behaviors such as helping the victim, joining in, or watching passively (Olweus, 1993; Rigby & Slee, 1991; Vernberg et al., 1999). Peer nominations are another source of useful information on student behaviors in regards to bully, victim, and bystander behaviors. Some studies gather teacher reports on levels of bullying, although peer victimization generally occurs in places that lack adult supervision (Meraviglia et al., 2003; Olweus, 1993). As several programs strive to increase teacher awareness of bullying, some studies include teacher reports of their attitudes and perceptions of peer victimization. Direct observation seems to be an ideal, yet expensive, measure of bullying behavior. Observations are free of the specific reporter biases that may encumber student and teacher questionnaires and seem to overcome the sensitization issue whereby reports of bullying initially increase after a school's awareness of such behaviors has been raised (Smith et al., 2003). While several programs have included direct observation in their evaluations, this method is time-consuming and expensive, which makes it prohibitive for some evaluations. More recently, the idea of using real-time reporting of bullying behaviors has been put forth (Espelage & Swearer, 2003). Using this method, students would be paged or otherwise prompted at specific times to complete questions related to bullying.

EVALUATIONS OF ANTIBULLYING PROGRAMS

The relatively young body of research on outcomes of antibullying programs is quite small compared to the outcome literature on the treatment of specific childhood psychological disorders. For example, a literature search on peer-reviewed journals through PsycINFO (1806–2005) using the terms "bullying," "children or adolescents," "intervention," and "outcome or evaluation" returned only 12 articles. A similar search using the terms "depression," "children or adolescents," "treatment," and "outcome or evaluation" resulted in a return of 407 articles. Numerous antibullying programs are marketed to schools; the official Web site for the U.S. Department of Health and Human Services' "Stop Bullying Now!" National Bullying Prevention Campaign (http://www.stopbullyingnow. hrsa.gov/index.asp) lists 29 such programs. Only a handful, however, have been scientifically evaluated in peer-reviewed journals. The manner in which these programs are evaluated ranges from simple pre-posttest designs to randomized trials comparing a program to an alternative intervention and a control group.

Evaluation of schoolwide programs is fraught with challenges and unique obstacles. Approval for such evaluations involves satisfying the requirements of the researchers' institutional review board, the school district, and the concerns of individual principals, teachers, and parents. In addition to the expense and coordination of providing an intervention and gathering data at the school and student levels, parents understandably pressure schools to avoid being in the control group for a study. Schools that agree to provide data while not receiving an intervention will sometimes choose to implement a different intervention program for their students during the course of the study, thus confounding the experimental comparisons. These considerations, as well as the recent increase in awareness of the long-term problems associated with bullying, explain the relatively small number of extant evaluation studies. Nonetheless, several programs have demonstrated promising results in decreasing peer victimization.

MOVING FORWARD TOWARD GREATER CLINICAL UTILITY

Increase Program Buy-In

While the literature base on bullying prevention is not large, it is clear that several interventions have been shown successful in decreasing bullying. The promise of effective programs spurs researchers to the next level of studies. The previous case example not only reflects the dose-response aspect of the BPP program documented by Olweus (1999) but also illustrates an important area of research needed in order to move effective bullying interventions into greater use. Understanding teacher buy-in and other potential barriers to implementation is a crucial next step in bullying research (Forgatch, 2003). Various levels of buy-in have been proposed for examination, including factors at the level of the individual, school, community, and overall culture (Vernberg & Gamm, 2003). Kallestad and Olweus (2003) have already begun investigations into factors related to teacher implementation. The case example given typifies the lack of shared vision (Vernberg & Gamm, 2003) that can prevent successful implementation of an effective program.

Identify Critical Components

The second area for researchers to tackle, which may also help improve program buy-in and implementation, is to identify the critical components of bullying prevention programs. It is important for an intervention program to fit into a school's ethos in order to have a chance at maximum implementation and success, but deciding which component to modify or eliminate from a manualized treatment must be guided by research as opposed to personal tastes. A complicating factor is the difficulty of measuring a "clean" intervention. Schools generally have several educational or intervention programs that may overlap with some of the factors related to bullying, such as programs targeting gang violence, sexual harassment, or racial- or sexual orientation-based aggression. There have not been many efforts to dismantle the Olweus BPP and determine the effects of the individual components; however, the evaluation of Bully Busters suggests that the teacher training and support elements of a schoolwide antibullying program can be effective as standalone interventions (Newman-Carlson & Horne, 2004). Thus, school-level components are likely to be active ingredients in larger antibullying programs.

Have Simple Standardized Measures

A third area of research helpful in expanding the clinical utility of bullying programs relates to the way in which these programs are evaluated. Having some standardization of measures would allow for comparison across schools and studies. Although it may be useful to have a questionnaire tailored to a school's particular need, administering a standardized section of a questionnaire consistently would not only greatly add to the research literature but would also help schools make meaningful comparisons to schools in other states and countries. Even ensuring that schools are using the same definition of bullying would aid in this effort (Rigby, 2003). In order for schools to realistically evaluate bullying programs when their resources are already stretched thin, such information must be presented in a brief, easy-to-administer format or be available in data routinely collected by schools. Information gleaned from office referrals for inappropriate behavior, suspension records, and even nursing records can provide insight into how well a program is or is not working.

Tailor to Students' Developmental Levels

A fourth step to increase the clinical utility of antibullying programs is to further investigate how the factors linked to bullying change in their relationship to this behavior at different ages. Several promising programs had results that varied with the age or grade level of the students involved (e.g., Baldry & Farrington, 2004; Orpinas et al., 2003). Greater investigation into which factors have the greatest influence on bullying at different ages and the manner in which interventions are presented to students will help program developers gain positive results for a larger range of school grades. Bullying behaviors decrease in the high school years, but they certainly do not disappear completely. Very few programs, however, target bullying in high school. Tailoring effective antibullying programs to reach this age range would be an important advancement.

The current state of the literature on antibullying programs is at an exciting stage. Researchers have generated much information on diverse factors related to bullying behavior and expanded the view of bullying to include various roles of all students involved. This research has increased the understanding of students' social experiences, their feelings about themselves in relation to their school, and the interplay between student and teacher behaviors. Comparing the research on antibullying programs to the criteria for *well-established* and *probably efficacious* psychosocial interventions (Lonigan et al., 1998) is somewhat challenging. In many cases, random assignment and comparing the intervention to a no-treatment control group or to an alternative treatment are undesirable, if not impossible, within most school systems. Following the criteria summarized by Lonigan and colleagues (1998), the antibullying programs seem to fall short, and even the Olweus BPP, with all of its accolades, only meets the criteria for *probably efficacious* interventions. This is not to say that antibullying program evaluations should not be held to high standards, and developers and researchers of these programs are trying to address evaluation issues by using methods such as age-cohort designs. The CAPSLE program evaluation is one example of success in designing and carrying out a true randomized controlled trial for a schoolwide program. In light of the challenges of implementing and evaluating schoolwide programs as opposed to individual therapeutic interventions, several programs targeting peer victimization have shown promising results in changing student behavior.

Increasing the research literature on effective bullying interventions is not enough. The information about effectiveness will be almost useless if it is not disseminated effectively so that school consumers can make informed choices. Through public health campaigns, such as the "Stop Bullying Now!" campaign by the U.S. Department of Health and Human Services (http://www.stopbullyingnow.hrsa.gov/index.asp), the message about effective antibullying programs is being disseminated to the general public. While some states are requiring schools to put such programs in place, schools now have easy-to-access online information about the components of effective programs (e.g., http://www.colorado.edu/cspv/blueprints/). The literature on antibullying programs has demonstrated not just how to evaluate programs but also how to educate potential consumers about the results.

REFERENCES

Baldry, A. C., & Farrington, D. P. (2004). Evaluation of an intervention program for the reduction of bullying and victimization in schools. *Aggressive Behavior, 30,* 1–15.

Barber, B. K., & Olsen, J. A. (1997). Socialization in context: Connection, regulation, and autonomy in the family, school, and neighborhood, and with peers. *Journal of Adolescent Research, 12,* 287–315.

Barnett, M. A. (1987). Empathy and related responses in children. In N. Eisenberg & J. Strayer (Eds.), *Empathy and Its Development* (pp. 146–162). New York: Cambridge University Press.

Bosworth, K., Espelage, D. L., & Simon, T. R. (1999). Factors associated with bullying behavior in middle school students. *Journal of Early Adolescence, 19,* 341–362.

Boulton, M. J., & Underwood, K. (1992). Bully/victim problems among middle school children. *British Journal of Educational Psychology, 62,* 73–87.

Center for the Study and Prevention of Violence (2002). Blueprints model program selection criteria. Retrieved September 12, 2006, from http://www.colorado.edu/cspv/blueprints/model/criteria.html.

Craig, W. M., Pepler, D., & Atlas, R. (2000). Observations of bullying in the playground and in the classroom. *School Psychology International, 21,* 22–36.

Cunningham, P. B., & Henggeler, S. W. (2001). Implementation of an empirically based drug and violence prevention and intervention program in public school settings. *Journal of Clinical Child Psychology, 30,* 221–232.

DeRosier, M. E. (2004). Building friendships and combating bullying: Effectiveness of a school-based social skills group intervention. *Journal of Clinical Child and Adolescent Psychology, 33,* 196–201.

DeRosier, M. E., & Marcus, S. R. (2005).Building friendships and combating bullying: Effectiveness of S.S.GRIN at one-year follow-up. *Journal of Clinical Child and Adolescent Psychology, 34,* 140–150.

Dishion, T. J., Patterson, G. R., & Griesler, P. C. (1994). Peer adaptation in the development of antisocial behavior: A confluence model. In L. R. Huesmann (Ed.), *Aggressive Behavior: Current Perspectives* (pp. 61–95). New York: Plenum Press.

Elliott, D. S., & Voss, H. L. (1974). *Delinquency and Dropout.* Lexington, MA: Lexington Books.

Espelage, D. L., & Swearer, S. M. (2003). Research on school bullying and victimization: What have we learned and where do we go from here? *School Psychology Review, 32,* 365–383.

Fonagy, P., Twemlow, S. W., Vernberg, E. V., Mize, J. A., Dill, E. J., Little, T. D., et al. (2005). *A Randomized Controlled Trial of a Child-Focused Psychiatric Consultation and a School Systems-Focused Intervention to Reduce Aggression.* Manuscript in preparation.

Forgatch, M. S. (2003). Implementation as a second stage in prevention research. Prevention and Treatment, 6, Article 24. Retrieved on November 29, 2005, from http://journals.apa.org/ prevention/volume6/pre0060021a.html.

Fox, C. L., & Boulton, M. J. (2003). Evaluating the effectiveness of a social skills training (SST) programme for victims of bullying. *Educational Research, 45,* 231–247.

Frey, K. S., & Hirschstein, M. K., Snell, J. L., Edstrom, L. V., MacKenzie, E. P., & Broderick, C. J. (2005). Reducing playground bullying and supporting beliefs: An experimental trial of the Steps to Respect program. *Developmental Psychology, 41,* 479–491.

Gilbert, S. E. (1995). Violence in schools: Why—and what can we do about it? *Journal of Health Care for the Poor and Underserved, 6,* 205–208.

Glew, G. M., Fan, M. Y., Katon, W., Rivara, F. P., & Kernick, M. A. (2005). Bullying, psychosocial adjustment, and academic performance in elementary school. *Archives of Pediatric and Adolescent Medicine, 159,* 1026–1031.

Glover, D., Gough, G., Johnson, M., & Cartwright, N. (2000). Bullying in 25 secondary schools: Incidence, impact and intervention. *Educational Research, 42,* 141–156.

Gottfredson, D. C. (1987). An evaluation of an organization development approach to reducing school disorder. *Education Review, 11,* 739–763.

Hampson, R. B. (1981). Helping behavior in children: Addressing the interaction of a person-situation model. *Developmental Review, 1,* 93–112.

Hoover, J. H., Oliver, R., & Hazler, R. J. (1992). Bullying: Perceptions of adolescent victims in the Midwestern USA. *School Psychology International, 13,* 5–16.

Huesmann, L. R., & Guerra, N. G. (1997). Children's normative beliefs about aggression and aggressive behavior. *Journal of Personality and Social Psychology, 72,* 408–419.

Jacobs, A. K. (2001). Predicting change in bystander behavior during middle childhood: An examination of contextual factors and cognitive mechanisms. Unpublished doctoral dissertation, University of Kansas, Lawrence.

Kallestad, J. H., & Olweus, D. (2003). Predicting teachers' and schools' implementation of the Olweus Bullying Prevention Program: A multilevel study. *Prevention and Treatment, 6,* Article 21. Retrieved on November 29, 2005, from http://journals.apa.org/prevention/volume6/pre0060021a.html.

Kaltiala-Heino, R., Rimpela, M., Rantanen, P., & Rimpela, A. (2000). Bullying at school: An indicator of adolescents at risk for mental disorders. *Journal of Adolescence, 23,* 661–674.

Lee, F. (1993). Disrespect rules. *The New York Times Educational Supplement,* 16.

Limber, S. P. (2004). Reflections on bullying prevention in a post-Columbine era. In G. Melton (Chair), 2004 Distinguished Contributions to Psychology in the Public Interest (Early Career) Award. Invited address conducted at the annual convention of the American Psychological Association, Hawaii.

Limber, S. P., Cummingham, P., Florx, V., Ivey, J., Nation, M., Chai, S., & Melton, G. (1997). Bullying among school children: Preliminary findings from a school-based intervention program. Paper presented at the Fifth International Family Violence Research Conference, Durham, NH.

Limber, S. P., & Nation, M. M. (1998). Bullying among children and youth. In J. L. Arnette & M. C. Walsleben (Eds.), *Combating Fear and Restoring Safety in Schools* (p. 5). Washington, DC: Department of Justice, Office of Juvenile Justice and Delinquency Prevention.

Limber, S. P., & Small, M. A. (2003). State laws and policies to address bullying in schools. *School Psychology Review, 32,* 445–455.

Lonigan, C. J., Elbert, J. C., & Johnson, S. B. (1998). Empirically supported psychosocial interventions for children: An overview. *Journal of Clinical Child Psychology, 27,* 138–145.

Menesini, E., Codecasa, E., Benelli, B., & Cowie, H. (2003). Enhancing children's responsibility to take action against bullying: Evaluation of a befriending intervention in Italian middle schools. *Aggressive Behavior, 29,* 1–14.

Meraviglia, M. G., Becker, H., Rosenbluth, B., Sanchez, E., & Robertson, T. (2003). The Expect Respect Project: Creating a positive elementary school climate. *Journal of Interpersonal Violence, 18,* 1347–1360.

Nansel, T. R., Overpeck, M., Pilla, R. S., Ruan, W. J., Simons-Morton, B., & Scheidt, P. (2001). Bullying behaviors among US youth: Prevalence and association with psychosocial adjustment. *JAMA, 285*, 2094–2100.

Newman, D. A., Horne, A. M., & Bartolomucci, L. (2000). *Bully Busters: A Teacher's Manual for Helping Bullies, Victims, and Bystanders.* Champaign, IL: Research Press.

Newman-Carlson, D., & Horne, A. M. (2004). Bully Busters: A psychoeducational intervention for reducing bullying behavior in middle school students. *Journal of Counseling and Development, 82*, 259–267.

Neumark-Sztainer, D., Story, M., French, S. A., & Resnick, M. D. (1997). Psychosocial correlates of health compromising behaviors among adolescents. *Health Education Research, 12*, 37–52.

Okayasu, T., & Takayama, I. (2004). Implementation and evaluation of a bullying prevention program focused on educational movements in junior high school. *Japanese Journal of Counseling Science, 37*, 155–167.

Olweus, D. (1993). *Bullying at School: What We Know and What We Can Do.* Cambridge, MA: Blackwell Publishers.

Olweus, D. (1997). Tackling peer victimization with a school-based intervention program. In D. P. Fry & K. Bjorkqvist (Eds.), *Cultural Variation in Conflict Resolution: Alternatives to Violence* (pp. 215–231). Hillsdale, NJ: Lawrence Erlbaum Associates.

Olweus, D. (1999). Norway. In P. K. Smith, Y. Morita, J. Junger-Tas, D. Olweus, R. Catalano, & P. Slee (Eds.), *The Nature of School Bullying: A Cross-National Perspective* (pp. 28–48). New York: Routledge.

Orpinas, P., Horne, A. M., & Staniszewski, D. (2003). School bullying: Changing the problem by changing the school. *School Psychology Review, 32*, 431–444.

Piliavin, J. A., Dovidio, J. F., Gaertner, S. L., & Clark, R. D. (1982). Responsive bystanders: The process of intervention. In V. J. Derlega & J. Grzelak (Eds.), *Cooperation and Helping Behavior: Theories and Research* (pp. 279–304). New York: Academic Press.

Rigby, K. (1996). *Bullying in Schools: And What to Do About It.* Bristol, PA: Jessica Kingsley Publishers.

Rigby, K. (2003). Consequences of bullying in schools. *Canadian Journal of Psychiatry, 48*, 583–590.

Rigby, K., & Slee, P. T. (1991). Bullying among Australian school children: Reported behavior and attitudes towards victims. *Journal of Social Psychology, 131*, 615–627.

Salmivalli, C. (1999). Participant role approach to school bullying: Implications for intervention. *Journal of Adolescence, 22*, 453–459.

Skiba, R. J. (2000). Zero tolerance, zero evidence: An analysis of school disciplinary practice (Rep. No. SRS2). Indiana Education Policy Center. Retrieved on November 29, 2005, from http://www.indiana.edu/~safeschl/ztze.pdf.

Slaby, R. G., & Guerra, N. G. (1988). Cognitive mediators of aggression in adolescent offenders: 1. Assessment. *Developmental Psychology, 24*, 580–588.

Smith, P. K., & Ananiadou, K. (2003). The nature of school bullying and effectiveness of school-based interventions. *Journal of Applied Psychoanalytic Studies, 5*, 189–209.

Smith, P. K., Ananiadou, K., & Cowie, H. (2003). Interventions to reduce school bullying. *Canadian Journal of Psychiatry, 48*, 591–599.

Twemlow, S. W., Fonagy, P., Sacco, F. C., Gies, M., Evans, R., & Ewbank, R. (2001). Creating a Peaceful School Learning Environment: A controlled study of an elementary school intervention to reduce violence. *American Journal Psychiatry, 158*, 808–810.

Twemlow, S. W., Fonagy, P., & Sacco, F. C. (2003). Modifying social aggression in schools. *Journal of Applied Psychoanalytic Studies, 5*, 211–222.

Twemlow, S. W., Sacco, F. C., & Twemlow, S. W. (1999). *Creating a Peaceful School Learning Environment: A Training Program for Elementary Schools.* Agawam, MA: T & S Publishing Group.

U.S. Department of Health and Human Services (2001). Youth violence: A report of the Surgeon General. Retrieved on November 29, 2005, from http://www.surgeongeneral. gov/library/youthviolence.

U.S. Department of Health and Human Services (n.d.). *Stop Bullying Now! What Adults Can Do: Additional Resources.* Retrieved on September 12, 2006, from http://www. bullyingresources.org/stopbullyingnow/indexAdult.asp?Area=ProgramResources.

Vernberg, E. M., & Gamm, B. K. (2003). Resistance to violence prevention interventions in schools: Barriers and solutions. *Journal of Applied Psychoanalytic Studies*, 5, 125–138.

Vernberg, E. M., Jacobs, A. K., & Hershberger, S. L. (1999). Peer victimization and attitudes about violence during early adolescence. *Journal of Clinical Child Psychology*, 28, 386–395.

Vernberg. E. M., Jacobs, A. K., Twemlow, S. W., Sacco, F., & Fonagy, P. (2000). Developmental patterns in aggression, victimization, and violence-related cognitions. In E. M. Vernberg (Chair), *Violence Against Peers: Developmental Inevitability or Unacceptable Risk?* Symposium conducted at the annual meeting of the American Psychological Association, Washington, DC.

Vernon, S., Lundblad, B., & Hellstrom, A. L. (2003). Children's experiences of school toilets present a risk to their physical and psychological health. *Child: Care, Health and Development*, 29, 47–53.

Zerger, A. K. (1996). Bystanders and attitudes about violence during early adolescence. Unpublished master's thesis, University of Kansas, Lawrence, Kansas.

Pediatric/Medically Related Disorders

16

Pain and Pain Management

LINDSEY L. COHEN, JILL E. MACLAREN, and CRYSTAL S. LIM

THE NATURE OF PEDIATRIC PAIN

Pain is the most common reason people seek out health care, pain costs to society are exorbitant, and pain is detrimental to quality of life (e.g., Stewart et al., 2003). The importance of attending to pain is highlighted by directives that it be considered the "fifth vital sign" (along with core temperature, heart rate, respiration, and blood pressure) and monitored in routine medical care (American Pain Society Quality of Care Committee, 1995). Recently, the International Association for the Study of Pain (IASP) and the World Health Organization (WHO) posited that "the relief of pain should be a human right" (for more information, see http://www.painreliefhumanright.com/). Despite growing recognition of the importance of pain, it is undertreated such that it is arguably a critical public health issue (Bond & Breivik, 2004; Brennan & Cousins, 2004), and this is especially the case in pain in children (Finley et al., 2005; Schechter et al., 1993).

There are various potential explanations for the relative lack of attention to children's pain. For instance, there are inaccurate but long-held myths that children do not experience pain as intensely as adults, that children are more resilient from pain than adults, and that children do not experience long-term repercussions from untreated pain (for a review, see Kenny, 2001). These misconceptions continue to be problematic despite a growing body of research refuting each of these claims (for review, see Young, 2005). Unfortunately, children are at unique risk for the under-treatment of pain because they lack the verbal ability and personal power to demand adequate pain management. Further, children often do not understand the reason for their suffering, and they experience frequent pain as part of their routine health care (McGrath, 2005). As a result,

LINDSEY L. COHEN • Georgia State University, **JILL E. MACLAREN** • Yale University and **CRYSTAL S. LIM** • Georgia State University

pain is a frequent and vivid part of childhood, and research is accumulating to suggest that early pain might have long-term negative repercussions on pain sensitivity, immune functioning, neurophysiology, attitudes, and health-care behavior (for review, see Young, 2005).

ASSESSMENT OF PEDIATRIC PAIN

Accurate assessment is critical in determining whether pain is present, making diagnostic decisions, deciding whether and what type of intervention is necessary for treatment, and knowing when to modify or terminate treatment. Given that pain is an internal and subjective experience (Merskey & Bogduk, 1994), self-report is considered the "gold standard" of pain assessment. Unfortunately, children often do not possess the cognitive and verbal abilities to clearly articulate their pain, and their reports are often viewed with skepticism. This issue has led professionals to develop and validate a host of tools to measure children's pain. These instruments include self-reports (e.g., faces scales), observer ratings, and behavior observational scales. For a review of pediatric pain assessment, see Finley and McGrath (1998).

MODELS OF PEDIATRIC PAIN

Models of pain are important to guide research and the development of interventions. Descartes proposed the specificity theory in the 1700s, which posited a direct link between pain receptors and a pain center in the brain. Melzack and Wall refuted the specificity theory with the Gate Control Theory (1965), which identified a central mechanism that modulates pain experiences. The Gate Control Theory opened the door for the psychological study of pain by proposing active influences of attention, prior experience, beliefs, thoughts, and emotions on pain experience. Psychological research has extended our understanding of pediatric pain and introduced a number of empirically supported interventions for both acute and chronic pain. Stimulus-response (Figure 1) and ecological (Figure 2) models extend the

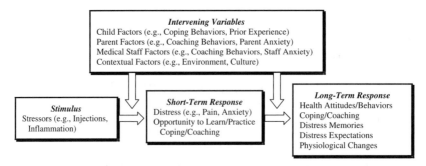

Figure 1. Stimulus Response Model of Pain

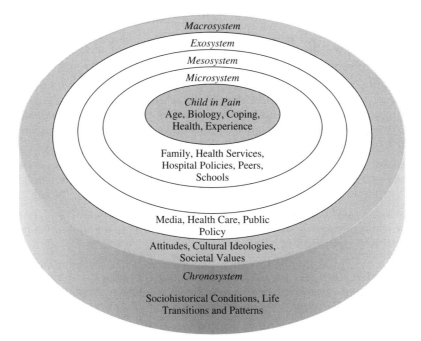

Figure 2. Ecological Model of Pediatric Pain

gate control theory by specifying individual and contextual variables that can influence the pain experience (see Kazak & Kunin-Batson, 1998; and Figures 1 and 2).

ACUTE PEDIATRIC PAIN MANAGEMENT

Acute pain is typically short, fast, and sharp, often with an identifiable cause. Acute pain is a relatively specific group; however, there are qualitatively different pain experiences within this category. For example, children undergoing routine immunizations likely have a very different experience of medical procedures than children undergoing port-a-cath access or bone marrow aspiration as part of cancer treatment. Further, procedural pain is qualitatively different from postoperative pain. Thus, it is helpful to organize pain management interventions by pain associated with specific procedures for medical conditions as well as by type of procedure.

Burn Treatment

Burn injuries are painful, and this pain is further compounded by the requirement of invasive procedures as part of injury treatment such as debridement (removal of dead skin) and physical therapy. Multiple behavioral component strategies including distraction, relaxation, imagery, and reinterpretation of pain have been effective for management of pain from debridement (Elliot and Olson, 1983).

Single-component strategies have also been evaluated for the treatment of pain during burn debridement. Hypnosis has shown promise in the treatment of debridement pain in adults (Patterson et al., 1992), although the literature is not as extensive in children. Martin-Herz et al. (2000) provide rationale and support for the use of thought stopping and positive self-statements, relaxation techniques (including deep breathing and muscle relaxation), and operant techniques (nonreinforcement of escape behaviors) for burn treatment. Although there are few randomized trials evaluating the efficacies of these strategies in burn patients specifically, these interventions have demonstrated efficacy in other procedures, and the authors argue that they are also applicable in the context of pediatric burn debridement.

One of the most recent advances in behavioral interventions for burn debridement is the use of virtual-reality distraction. In one study, Das (2005) evaluated an age-appropriate virtual-reality videogame and found a decrease in pain when children used virtual reality compared to when they did not. Virtual reality has also been evaluated for the management of pain during burn rehabilitation. Hoffman et al. (2001) demonstrated that a virtual "Snow World" decreased pain reports during physical therapy in children and adults.

The issue of who performs burn treatment procedures has also been a topic of investigation. For example, Tarnowski et al. (1987) found that child involvement in debridement procedures resulted in less pain and distress than therapist-only debridement. Overall, multicomponent interventions and virtual reality show promise for pain management related to burn debridement. However, more research systematically evaluating interventions for this procedure are warranted.

Cancer Treatment

Cancer treatments include venipuncture, port access procedures, and bone marrow aspirations and lumbar punctures (BMA/LPs). Each of these procedures is associated with high anxiety and pain. Cognitive-behavioral packages (e.g., distraction, deep breathing, imagery) have proven helpful at reducing distress across these procedures (e.g., Jay et al., 1985) and have been shown to be an effective adjuvant to (Kazak et al., 1996) or even comparable to general anesthesia for BMA/LPs (Jay et al., 1985).

Virtual-reality distraction has also been used for children's cancer procedural pain. For example, Wint et al. (2002) demonstrated that virtual-reality skiing was somewhat helpful to adolescents undergoing LPs. Gershon et al. (2004) found virtual reality was beneficial to children undergoing port access procedures. An interactive toy distraction was also shown to lower port access distress in oncology patients (Dahlquist et al., 2002).

Immunizations

The most common painful events during infancy are immunizations (Reis et al., 2003). In contrast to multicomponent interventions for other procedures, most interventions for immunization pain have been single-component in nature, with distraction as the most commonly evaluated intervention (Blount et al., 2003). A variety of distraction strategies have received empirical attention (e.g., party blowers, cartoon movies, music), and outcomes have been assessed on multiple dimensions (e.g., parent-report, self-report, observational distress). Despite the variability in strategies, results of most studies in preschoolers demonstrate the efficacy of distraction as an intervention for pediatric pain and distress (for reviews, see Kleiber & Harper, 1999; Piira et al.,2002). Further, distraction has been supported as both time- and cost-efficient (DeMore & Cohen, 2005). Notably, those strategies that required an overt response from the child and those that involved multiple sensory modalities were the most effective (DeMore & Cohen, 2005). In terms of the efficacy of behavioral interventions for infants, Cohen and colleagues (2002, 2006) found that distraction lowered children's behavioral distress during the preinjection anticipatory phase (2006) and postinjection recovery phase (2002, 2006), but not during the anticipatory or procedural phase (2002, 2006). In contrast, Cramer-Berness and Friedman (2005) found that encouraging parents to use techniques that were commonly effective at comforting their infants was superior to distraction and control for infant immunization distress. The inconsistent results with regards to the effectiveness of distraction for infants suggest that continuing examination of this intervention is warranted.

Venipuncture

Venipuncture (drawing blood from a vein) is another procedure that children commonly undergo for routine health care. As with immunizations, distraction has received a good deal of empirical evidence for venipuncture. Manne et al. (1990) found that party-blower distraction/paced breathing reinforced with prizes was an effective avenue at reducing venipuncture distress.

As with immunizations, although distraction has demonstrated efficacy in these procedures, there is little consensus on the *type* of distractor that is most effective. In an effort to address this question, MacLaren and Cohen (2005) compared an interactive toy report with a cartoon movie for children's venipuncture distress. Results indicated that those children who received a more passive distraction strategy (movie) were less distressed. The authors suggested that children's anticipatory distress may have interfered with their ability to interact with the distractor, highlighting the importance of considering children's previous experience and preprocedural distress when selecting a distraction strategy. In sum, distraction appears to be the greatest empirical support for managing children's pain during venipuncture procedures.

Postoperative Pain

There is a wealth of literature in support of preparation programs for children's surgery distress (for review, see O'Conner-Von, 2000). However, most of the outcomes in these studies have been children's behavior and adjustment to hospitalization, rather than pain. Those studies that have evaluated pain outcomes have generally implemented specific pain management techniques rather than general preparation strategies. For example, Huth et al. (2004) evaluated an audiotaped imagery intervention provided a week in advance and also while children were recovering from pediatric tonsillectomy. Results indicated that children in the imagery condition reported significantly less pain in recovery than children in the control group. Jaw relaxation and music distraction have also demonstrated efficacy for postoperative pain (Good et al., 1999).

Consistent with conclusions drawn by Powers (1999) across acute painful procedures, cognitive-behavioral packages (e.g., distraction, relaxation) appear to have strong empirical support. Future research examining promising interventions for acute pain (e.g., virtual reality) is needed.

CHRONIC AND RECURRENT PEDIATRIC PAIN MANAGEMENT

Chronic pain has been defined as pain that lasts for longer than six months; however, some recognize that pediatric chronic pain might be of shorter durations (Task Force on Taxonomy, 1994). Chronic and recurrent pain in children is common, with conservative prevalence rates estimated at 15% to 20% of community samples (Goodman & McGrath, 1991). The most common types of pediatric chronic and recurrent pain are headache, recurrent abdominal pain, and musculoskeletal pain. As with acute pain, chronic and recurrent pain is a broad and diverse category. It is important to distinguish between chronic pain conditions and diseases that are associated with pain in children. Specifically, chronic pain conditions are illnesses where the cause of pain is dysfunctional pain signaling (e.g., fibromyalgia), whereas in diseases associated with pain, pain is a secondary complication of an identified illness (e.g., cancer; Zeltzer & Schlank, 2005).

Recurrent Headache

Recurrent pediatric headaches are typically subdivided into unspecified tension-type headaches and migraines (Larsson, 1999). Psychological interventions for these conditions have typically included relaxation, biofeedback, and multicomponent cognitive-behavioral interventions (for a review, see Holden et al., 1999).

Relaxation interventions have included muscle relaxation, self-hypnosis, autogenic training, and guided imagery and appear to be one of the most common clinical approaches to treating pediatric recurrent headache. In fact, in a review of the literature, Holden et al. (1999) deemed relaxation as a "well-established and efficacious treatment" for recurrent headaches in children and adolescents. Since the review by Holden et al. (1999), additional research has supported this conclusion. For example, Andrasik et al. (2003) found that a group relaxation intervention and relaxation tapes used at home reduced headache days, anxiety, and depression in 6- to 16-year-old children with recurrent tension-type headaches.

Biofeedback has also received empirical support in the treatment of pediatric recurrent headache. This intervention uses electronic equipment to monitor and display physiological indices associated with tension headaches (e.g., heart rate, forehead muscle tension, temperature) (Spirito & Kazak, 2006). Small sample studies have supported biofeedback as an intervention for tension-type headache (Arndorfer and Allen, 2001) and migraines (Allen et al., 2002). Balancing the limitations (e.g., small sample size, treatment confounds) and positive results, biofeedback has been considered a "probably efficacious" treatment for children with recurrent headaches (Holden et al., 1999; Spirito & Kazak, 2006). Multiple-component cognitive-behavioral treatments (CBT) for headache (e.g., relaxation, imagery, problem solving, cognitive restructuring) have also received some empirical support (e.g., Kroener-Herwig & Denecke, 2002; McGrath et al., 1992), as have group interventions (Kroener-Herwig & Denecke, 2002).

For children and adolescents with recurrent headache, research suggests that relaxation techniques may the most effective at reducing symptoms. Although research biofeedback and multicomponent CBT interventions are limited by small sample sizes and other confounds to date, these interventions are promising and warrant further investigation.

Recurrent Abdominal Pain

Recurrent abdominal pain (RAP) is the most common gastrointestinal disorder in children, with prevalence rates of about 10 to 15% in school-aged children (Janicke & Finney, 1999). Most of the psychological interventions examined to treat pain in children with RAP have been cognitive-behavioral. An eight-session family-based intervention including topics such as pain monitoring, reinforcement of nonpain behavior, engagement in competing activities, relaxation, and imagery was effective in decreasing pain reported by children, their mothers, and their teachers (Sanders et al., 1989). However, a subsequent study (Sanders et al., 1994) with added intervention components (parent training in contingency management) found no differences at the end of intervention in self-reported or observed pain when compared to standard medical care. The treatment effect may have been delayed in this study, however, as there were promising results for the CBT intervention at 6- and 12-month follow-ups. More recently, a brief intervention (five sessions) including active management of pain episodes, modeling and practicing pain management techniques, and parent training demonstrated efficacy with significantly less pain evidenced immediately and at 6- and 12-month follow-up (Robins et al., 2005). Overall, CBTs for children with RAP have been considered "probably efficacious" (Janicke & Finney, 1999).

Sickle Cell Disease

Sickle cell disease (SCD) is a group of genetic disorders characterized by abnormal hemoglobin, causing red blood cells to become rigid and crescent-shaped (Graumlich et al., 2001; Thompson & Gustafson, 1996). For children with SCD, the most common and most debilitating symptom of the disease is recurrent, painful, vaso-occlusive episodes (Shapiro, 1993). In addition to recurrent pain, children with SCD may also experience chronic pain. Therefore, many of the psychological interventions that have been examined in children with SCD have focused on teaching pain management skills for recurrent episodes as well as for general chronic pain associated with the disease.

Thomas and colleagues (Thomas et al., 1998, 1999) created a six-month weekly group-session CBT package (e.g., relaxation) for adolescents and adults with SCD. In the pilot study (Thomas et al., 1998), the intervention revealed no significant group differences in psychological functioning when compared to controls; however, they did observe a trend in reduced anxiety and depression in the CBT group. In a later larger study, Thomas et al. (1999) found that patients receiving CBT used more positive and less negative cognitive coping styles, had higher levels of behavioral activity, felt more able to control and decrease their pain, and experienced less affective pain compared to the waiting list and attentional control groups. An additional evaluation also revealed that the cognitive-behavioral intervention was cost-effective, especially during the first six months following the intervention (Thomas et al., 2001). However, the inclusion of adolescents and adults limits this intervention's generalizability to children.

Family-based interventions have also been examined in children with SCD. Kaslow et al. (2000) designed a six-session intervention consisting of various components (e.g., describing the stress-coping-adjustment model; presenting preventative health-care strategies; teaching age-appropriate pain management techniques, such as relaxation and guided imagery; developing active problem-focused coping strategies; and focusing on interpersonal relationships). When compared to children receiving standard medical treatment, children and parents in the family-based intervention demonstrated higher disease knowledge. However, children's pain was not directly examined. In addition, Powers et al. (2002) studied the effects of a six-session CBT package (e.g., deep breathing, modeling, behavioral rehearsal) for families with a child with SCD. Results from three children, ranging in age from 9 to 12, who completed the training indicated decreases in negative thinking and the use of coping skills on most days pain occurred. In addition, children reported that using coping skills was moderately effective for reducing pain.

The effectiveness of biofeedback training has also been examined in children with SCD. Cozzi et al. (1987) examined the effectiveness of six biofeedback sessions in eight children and adolescents with SCD. Significant reductions were found in the frequency of headaches, analgesic use, perceived pain intensity, frequency of self-treated crises, and anxiety.

In addition, after six months, significant reductions in the number of headaches were maintained.

For managing pain associated with SCD, CBT interventions that are family-based may be the most helpful at reducing pain. However, many of the studies reviewed utilized small sample sizes. Future research should evaluate these interventions with larger samples to determine whether the interventions are efficacious.

Juvenile Rheumatoid Arthritis

Juvenile rheumatoid arthritis (JRA) is a musculoskeletal autoimmune disorder that is characterized by inflammation in organs, joints, and other body parts that causes intense pain episodes (Jaworski, 1993). To date, only two studies have systematically examined psychological interventions designed for children with JRA.

Lavigne et al. (1992) examined a six-session psychological treatment package (relaxation, biofeedback training, operant strategies), and Walco et al. (1992) evaluated an eight-session CBT intervention (e.g., relaxation, imagery, problem solving). Both of these interventions resulted in significant decreases in pain. However, both enrolled small samples, had relatively high attrition rates, and lacked control groups. Although there are no other experimental evaluations of psychological interventions for children with JRA, recent research suggests that more than one-third of parents utilize complementary and alternative pain management techniques, such as naturopathy and acupuncture, to treat their child's JRA-related pain (Feldman et al., 2003). Continuing to evaluate the effectiveness of CBT interventions for reducing pain associated with JRA is warranted.

CONCLUSIONS

There is strong evidence that children's acute and chronic pain can be managed via psychological approaches. To further research clinical avenues in pediatric pain management, several specific recommendations are in order. First, interventions have predominately targeted the individual child or proximal factors (e.g., parents, staff) but have largely ignored the important distal factors (e.g., culture, environment). It is important to recognize that changes are necessary on various levels to make a significant impact on children's pain. Second, treatment research has largely conceptualized pediatric pain as negative and to be diminished however possible. There might be value in viewing children's pain, especially predictable pain (e.g., needle injections), as an opportunity for the child and parent to master a stressor. Families might be able to achieve self-efficacy over a stressor, which may generalize to other stressful life events. Third, translational research is necessary to ensure that evidence-based approaches are being put into actual clinical practice (Scott-Finley & Estabrooks, 2006). A bridge is needed to connect research endeavors to the everyday care of pediatric patients. Along these lines, pain management researchers should consider the feasibility of their interventions in terms of cost, time, ease, acceptance, and other factors to ensure that the treatments are reasonable given the particulars of the patient population and the health-care environment. Taking this view one step further, it is important to educate the public in terms of children's pain and methods of pain control. The greater the transparency across science, practice, and the public, the increased likelihood of changing our culture to one embracing child pain relief. Fourth, a developmental framework is essential. The unique developmental characteristics of children and their environments result in adult interventions not being directly applicable in this population (McGrath, 2005). Unlike adult pain management strategies, pediatric treatment is often targeted at the *other* individuals who are important and proximate to the pediatric patient rather than the actual patient. In addition, knowledge of children's cognitive, emotional, and social changes should guide the development and implementation of pain management strategies. Fifth, socio-cultural factors have been largely unexplored but might prove valuable in understanding children's pain (for a review, see Craig & Riddel, 2003). Findings regarding socio-cultural influences on pain would help health-care professionals effectively understand, diagnose, and treat children's pain. Sixth, examination of contextual factors and patient individual differences that influence the effectiveness of treatments is in order. Research is accumulating to support interventions for pediatric pain, but how best to tailor these treatments to individual patients is in order. Seventh, the long-term gains of pain management are largely unexplored. Investigations documenting that pediatric pain relief benefits the individual child and society as a whole, both in the short and long term, would go far to further the cause of pediatric pain management. Finally, multidisciplinary efforts are in order. Psychology, pharmacology, nursing, physical therapy, and other health-care fields have each made great strides in pediatric pain control; however, joint efforts would prove synergistic in the efforts to alleviate child suffering. In conclusion, psychology's efforts in pediatric pain management are promising; however, there continues to be much work to do to truly relieve the unnecessary pain children face every day.

REFERENCES

Allen, K. D., Elliott, A. J., & Arndorfer, R. E. (2002). Behavioral pain management for pediatric headache in primary care. *Children's Health Care, 31,* 175–189.

American Pain Society Quality of Care Committee (1995). Quality improvement guidelines for the treatment of acute pain and cancer pain. *Journal of the American Medical Association, 274,* 1874–1880.

Andrasik, F., Grazzi, L., Usai, S., D'Amico, D., Leone, M., & Bussone, G. (2003). Brief neurologist-administered behavioral treatment of pediatric episodic tension-type headache. *Neurology, 60,* 1215–1216.

Arndorfer, R. E., & Allen, K. D. (2001). Extending the efficacy of a thermal biofeedback treatment package to the management of tension-type headaches in children. *Headache, 41,* 183–192.

Blount, R. L., Piira, T., & Cohen, L. L. (2003). Management of pediatric pain and distress due to painful medical procedures. In M. C. Roberts (Ed.), *Handbook of Pediatric Psychology*, 3rd ed. (pp. 216–233). New York: Guilford Press.

Bond, M., & Breivik, H. (2004). Why pain control matters in a world full of killer diseases. *Pain: Clinical Updates*, *12* (4), 1–4.

Brennan, F., & Cousins, M. J. (2004). Pain relief as a human right. *Pain: Clinical Updates*, *12*(5), 1–4.

Cohen, L. L. (2002). Reducing infant immunization distress through distraction. *Health Psychology*, *21*, 207–211.

Cohen, L. L., Bernard, R. S., Greco, L. R., & McClellan, C. B. (2002). A child-focused intervention for coping with procedural pain: Are parent and nurse coaches necessary? *Journal of Pediatric Psychology*, *27*, 749–757.

Craig, K., & Riddel, R. (2003). Social influences, culture, and ethnicity. In G. A. Finley & P. J. McGrath (Eds.), *Pediatric Pain: Biological and Social Context, Progress in Pain Research and Management*, Vol. 26 (pp. 159–182). Seattle: IASP Press.

Cramer-Berness, L. J., & Friedman, A. G. (2005). Behavioral interventions for infant immunizations. *Children's Health Care*, *34*, 95–111.

Cozzi, L., Tryon, W. W., & Sedlacek, K. (1987). The effectiveness of biofeedback-assisted relaxation in modifying sickle cell crises. *Biofeedback & Self Regulation*, *12*, 51–61.

Dahlquist, L. M., Pendley, J. S., Landtrip, D. S., Jones, C. L., & Steuber, C. P. (2002). Distraction interventions for preschoolers undergoing intramuscular injections and subcutaneous port access. *Health Psychology*, *21*, 94–99.

Das, D., Grimmer, K., Sparnon, A., McRae, S., & Thomas, B. (2005). The efficacy of playing a virtual reality game in modulating pain for children with acute burn injuries: A randomized controlled trial. *BMC Pediatrics*, *5*, 1–10.

DeMore, M., & Cohen, L. L. (2005). Distraction for pediatric immunization pain: A critical review. *Journal of Clinical Psychology in Medical Settings*, *12*, 281–291.

Elliot, C. H., & Olson, R. A. (1983). The management of children's distress in response to painful medical treatment for burn injuries. *Behavior Research and Therapy*, *21*, 675–683.

Feldman, D. E., Duffy, C., De Civita, M., Malleson, P., Philibert, L., Gibbon, M., et al. (2003). Factors associated with the use of complementary and alternative medicine in juvenile idiopathic arthritis. *Arthritis & Rheumatism*, *51*, 527–532.

Finley, G. A., Franck, L. S., Grunau, R . E., & von Baeyer, C. L. (2005). Why children's pain matters. *Pain: Clinical Updates*, *13*(5), 1–6.

Finley, G. A., & McGrath, P. J. (1998). Introduction: The roles of measurement in pain management and research. In G. A. Finley & P. J. McGrath (Eds.), *Measurement of Pain in Infants and Children*, Vol. 10 (pp. 1–4). Seattle: IASP Press.

Gershon, J., Zimand, E., Pickering, M., Rothbaum, B. O., & Hodges, L. (2004). A pilot and feasibility study of virtual reality as a distraction for children with cancer. *Journal of the American Academy of Child and Adolescent Psychiatry*, *43*, 1243–1249.

Good, M., Stanton-Hicks, M., Grass, J. A., Anderson, G. C., Choi, C., Schoolmeesters, L. J., et al. (1999). Relief of postoperative pain with jaw relaxation, music, and their combination. *Pain*, *81*, 163–172.

Goodman, J. E., & McGrath, P. J. (1991). The epidemiology of pain in children and adolescents: A review. *Pain*, *46*, 247–264.

Graumlich, S. E., Powers, S. W., Byars, K. C., Schwarber, L. A., Mitchell, M. J., & Kalinyak, K. A. (2001). Multidimensional assessment of pain in pediatric sickle cell disease. *Journal of Pediatric Psychology*, *26*, 203–214.

Hoffman, H. G., Patterson, D. R., Carrougher, G. J., & Sharar, S. R. (2001). Effectiveness of virtual reality-based pain control with multiple treatments. *The Clinical Journal of Pain*, *17*, 229–235.

Holden, E. W., Deichmann, M. M., & Levy, J. D. (1999). Empirically supported treatments in pediatric psychology: Recurrent pediatric headache. *Journal of Pediatric Psychology*, *24*, 91–109.

Huth, M. M., Broome, M. E., & Good, M. (2004). Imagery reduces children's post-operative pain. *Pain*, *110*, 439–448.

Janicke, D. M., & Finney, J. W. (1999). Empirically supported treatments in pediatric psychology: Recurrent abdominal pain. *Journal of Pediatric Psychology*, 24, 115–127.

Jaworski, T. M. (1993). Juvenile rheumatoid arthritis: Pain-related and psychosocial aspects and their relevance for assessment and treatment. *Arthritis Care and Research*, 6, 187–196.

Jay, S. M., Elliot, C. H., Ozolins, M., Olson, R. A., & Pruitt, S. D. (1985). Behavioral management of children's distress during painful medical procedures. *Behavior Research and Therapy*, 23, 513–520.

Jay, S. M., Elliot, C. H., Fitzgibbons, I., Woody, P., & Seigel, S. E. (1995). A comparative study of cognitive behavioral therapy versus general anesthesia for painful medical procedures in children. *Pain*, 62, 3–9.

Kaslow, N. J., Collins, M. H., Rashid, F. L., Baskin, M. L., Griffith, J. R., Hollins, L., et al. (2000). The efficacy of a pilot family psychoeducational intervention for pediatric sickle cell disease (SCD). *Families, Systems & Health*, 18, 381–404.

Kazak, A. E., Penati, B., Boyer, B. A., Himelstein, B., Brophy, P., Waibel, M. K., et al. (1996). A randomized controlled prospective outcome study of a psychological and pharmacological intervention protocol for procedural distress in pediatric leukemia. *Journal of Pediatric Psychology*, 21, 615–631.

Kenny, N.P. (2001). The politics of pediatric pain. In G. A. Finley & P. J. McGrath (Eds.), *Acute and Procedure Pain in Infants and Children, Progress in Pain Research and Management*, Vol. 20 (pp. 147–158). Seattle: IASP Press.

Kleiber, C., & Harper, D. C. (1999). Effects of distraction on children's pain and distress during medical procedures: A meta-analysis. *Nursing Research*, 48, 44–49.

Kroener-Herwig, B., & Denecke, H. (2002). Cognitive-behavioral therapy of pediatric headache: Are there differences in efficacy between a therapist-administered group training and a self-help format? *Journal of Psychosomatic Research*, 53, 1107–1114.

Larsson, B. (1999). Recurrent headaches in children and adolescents. In P. J. McGrath & G. A. Finley (Eds.), *Chronic and Recurrent Pain in Children and Adolescents, Progress in Pain Research and Management*, Vol. 13 (pp. 115–140). Seattle: IASP Press.

Lavigne, J. V., Ross, C. K., Berry, S. L., Hayford, J. R., & Pachman, L. M. (1992). Evaluation of a psychological treatment package for treating pain in juvenile rheumatoid arthritis. *Arthritis Care and Research*, 5, 101–110.

MacLaren, J. E., & Cohen, L. L. (2005). A comparison of distraction strategies for venipuncture distress in children. *Journal of Pediatric Psychology*, 30, 387–396.

Manne, S. L., Redd, W. H., Jacobsen, P. B., Gorfinkle, K., Schorr, O., & Rapkin, B. (1990). Behavioral intervention to reduce child and parent distress during venipuncture. *Journal of Consulting and Clinical Psychology*, 58, 565–572.

Martin-Herz, S. P., Thurber, C. A., & Patterson, D. R. (2000). Psychological principles of burn wound pain in children. II: Treatment applications. *Journal of Burn Care and Rehabilitation*, 21, 458–472.

McGrath, P. A. (2005). Children—Not simply "little adults." In E. Merskeuy, J. D. Loeser, & R. Dubner (Eds.), *The Paths of Pain 1975–2005*. Seattle: IASP Press.

McGrath, P. J., Humphreys, P., Keene, D., Goodman, J. T., Lascelles, M. A., Cunningham, S. J. et al. (1992). The efficacy and efficiency of a self-administered treatment for adolescent migraine. *Pain*, 49, 321–324.

Melzack, R., & Wall, P. D. (1965). Pain mechanisms: A new theory. *Science*, 150, 971–979.

Merskey, H., & Bogduk, N. (Eds.) (1994). *Classification of Chronic Pain: Descriptions of Chronic Pain Syndromes and Definitions of Pain Terms*, 2nd ed. Seattle: IASP Press.

O'Conner-Von, S. (2000). Preparing children for surgery: An integrative research review. *AORN Journal*, 71, 334–343.

Patterson, D. R., Everett, J. J., Burns, G. L., & Marvin, J. A. (1992). Hypnosis for the treatment of burn pain. *Journal of Consulting and Clinical Psychology*, 60, 713–717.

Piira, T., Hayes, B., & Goodenough, B. (2002). Distraction methods in the management of children's pain: An approach based on evidence or intuition? *The Suffering Child*, 1, 1–10.

Powers, S. W. (1999). Empirically supported treatments in pediatric psychology: Procedure related pain. *Journal of Pediatric Psychology*, 24, 131–145.

Powers, S. W., Mitchell, M. J., Graumlich, S. E., Byars, K. C., & Kalinyak, K. A. (2002). Longitudinal assessment of pain, coping, and daily functioning, in children with sickle cell disease receiving pain management skills training. *Journal of Clinical Psychology in Medical Settings, 9,* 109–119.

Reis, E. C., Roth, E. K., Syphan, J. L., Tarbell, S. E., & Holubkov, R. (2003). Effective pain reduction for multiple immunization injections in young infants. *Archives of Pediatrics and Adolescent Medicine, 157,* 1115–1120.

Robins, P. M., Smith, S. M., Glutting, J. J., & Bishop, C. T. (2005). A randomized controlled trial of cognitive-behavioral family intervention for pediatric recurrent abdominal pain. *Journal of Pediatric Psychology, 30,* 397–408.

Sanders, M. R., Rebgetz, M., Morrison, M., Bor, W., Gordon, A., Dadds, M., et al. (1989). Cognitive-behavioral treatment of recurrent nonspecific abdominal pain in children: An analysis of generalization, maintenance, and side effects. *Journal of Consulting and Clinical Psychology, 57,* 294–300.

Sanders, M. R., Shepherd, R. W., Cleghorn, G., & Woolford, H. (1994). The treatment of recurrent abdominal pain in children: A controlled comparison of cognitive-behavioral family intervention and standard pediatric care. *Journal of Consulting and Clinical Psychology, 62,* 306–314.

Schechter, N. L., Berde, C. B., & Yaster, M. (1993). Pain in infants, children, and adolescents: An overview. In N. L. Schechter, C. B. Berde, & M. Yaster (Eds.), *Pain in Infants, Children, and Adolescents* (pp. 3–9). Baltimore: Williams & Wilkins.

Scott-Findlay, S., & Estabrooks, C. A. (2006). Knowledge translation and pain management. In G. A. Finley, P. J. McGrath, & C. T. Chambers (Eds.), *Bringing Pain Relief to Children: Treatment Approaches* (pp. 199–228). Totowa, NJ: Humana Press.

Shapiro, B. S., Dinges, D. F., Orne, E. C., Bauer, N., Reilly, L. B., Whitehouse, W. G., et al. (1995). Home management of sickle cell-related pain in children and adolescents: Natural history and impact on school attendance. *Pain, 61,* 139–144.

Spirito, A., & Kazak, A. E. (2006). *Effective & Emerging Treatments in Pediatric Psychology.* New York: Oxford University Press.

Stewart, W. F., Ricci, J. A., Chee, E., Morganstein, D., & Lipton, R. (2003). Lost productive time and cost due to common pain conditions in the US workforce. *JAMA, 290,* 2443–2454.

Tarnowski, K. J., McGrath, M. L., Calhoun, M. B., & Drabman, R. S. (1987). Pediatric burn injury: Self- versus therapist-mediated debridement. *Journal of Pediatric Psychology, 12,* 567–579.

Task Force on Taxonomy (1994). *Classification of Chronic Pain: Descriptions of Chronic Pain Syndromes and Definitions of Pain Terms.* Seattle: IASP Press.

Thomas, V. J., Dixon, A. L., & Milligan, P. (1999). Cognitive-behaviour therapy for the management of sickle cell disease pain: An evaluation of a community-based intervention. *British Journal of Health Psychology, 4,* 209–229.

Thomas, V. J., Greun, R., & Shu, S. (2001). Cognitive-behavioural therapy for the management of sickle cell disease pain: Identification and assessment of costs. *Ethnicity & Health, 6,* 59–67.

Thomas, V. J., Wilson-Barnett, J., & Goodhart, F. (1998). The role of cognitive-behavioural therapy in the management of pain in patients with sickle cell disease. *Journal of Advanced Nursing, 27,* 1002–1009.

Thompson, R. J. & Gustafson, K. E. (1996). *Adaptation to Childhood Chronic Illness.* Washington, DC: American Psychological Association.

Walco, G. & Ilowite, N. (1992). Cognitive-behavioral intervention for juvenile primary fibromyalgia syndrome. *Journal of Rheumatology, 22,* 525–528.

Walco, G. A., Varni, J. W., & Ilowite, N. T. (1992). Cognitive-behavioral pain management in children with juvenile rheumatoid arthritis. *Pediatrics, 89,* 1075–1079.

Wint, S., Eshelman, D., Steele, J., & Guzzetta, C. (2002). Effects of distraction using virtual reality glasses during lumbar punctures in adolescents with cancer. *ONF, 29,* 8–15.

Young, K. (2005). Pediatric procedural pain. *Annals of Emergency Medicine, 45,* 160–171.

Zeltzer, L. K., & Schlank, C. B. (2005). *Conquering Your Child's Pain: A Pediatrician's Guide for Reclaiming a Normal Childhood.* New York: HarperCollins Publishers.

17

Evidence-Based Treatments for Children with Chronic Illnesses

T. DAVID ELKIN and LAURA STOPPELBEIN

A discussion of the use of evidence-based treatments (EBTs) in children with chronic illnesses presents a problematic but well-known dilemma. Many of the treatments for psychological distress in these children have historically been modified from better-known and validated treatments in children without chronic illness. In other words, what works in children who are not ill has been taken and modified to work with children who are ill. Any discussion of EBTs in children with chronic illness must take into consideration the work that has been done in the non-ill population.

We will discuss the general themes, assessments, and interventions that have been discussed in the literature. One of the main overarching themes in pediatric psychology (in which psychological applications are made with children with chronic illnesses) is that psychological difficulties are similar, regardless of setting. When dealing with food refusal, the mental health worker will use similar interventions in children who are healthy and those who have a specific gastrointestinal disorder, such as Crohn's disease. Modifications may have to be made, given the unique medical history and care these ill children receive; but overall, the interventions will appear similar. In taking EBTs that have been demonstrated in healthy populations, researchers have had to adapt and modify these interventions. Thus, the literature has only recently begun to report EBTs in children who have chronic illnesses.

In order to address the use of EBTs in this population, we will discuss the use of psychological interventions in several broad illness categories, with a view toward the application of these interventions across a range of illnesses.

T. DAVID ELKIN and LAURA STOPPELBEIN • University of Mississippi Medical Center

DIABETES

Type 1 diabetes is among the most common pediatric chronic illnesses, occurring in 1.7 per 1,000 school-aged youths (Centers for Disease Control, 2005). Type 1 diabetes occurs because of pancreatic failure, which subsequently results in an absence of usable insulin in the body. Because type 1 diabetes is typically diagnosed during childhood or adolescence, type 2 diabetes has historically been thought of as a disease that did not affect children and adolescents. However, over the past decade there has been a sharp rise in the number of children and adolescents who are diagnosed with type 2 diabetes, and recent studies suggest that as many as 10–20% of new cases of diabetes in youths are type 2 (American Diabetes Association, 2000). The recent increase in type 2 diabetes among children and adolescents is thought to be related to increases in sedentary lifestyles and the subsequent increases in obesity among youths. Unlike type 1 diabetes, in which there is a lack of usable insulin, type 2 diabetes results from insulin resistance, in which the body's ability to use insulin that is being secreted by the pancreas is reduced. Oftentimes, type 2 diabetes can be controlled simply by diet and exercise alone or with the addition of oral medications, but many individuals with type 2 diabetes eventually develop insulin deficiency similar to that seen in type 1 diabetes, thus resulting in the need to complete a more complicated and restricted regimen of adherence behaviors.

Treatment for youths with type 1 diabetes is often complex and includes insulin administration via multiple insulin injections or subcutaneous insulin pump, frequent blood glucose monitoring, adherence to a strict diet that includes counting carbohydrates or calories, as well as frequent exercise. The consequences of not adhering to all four components (e.g., insulin injection, monitoring, diet, and exercise) of disease management can have both long- and short-term health consequences, many of which are severe and would significantly shorten one's life span or significantly impact quality of life. The most immediate consequences of nonadherence include the risk of hypo- or hyperglycemia. Left untreated, these conditions can result in headache, nausea, coma, retinopathy, renal failure, heart disease, and even death.

Psychological treatment for youths diagnosed with type 1 diabetes can be divided into two broad categories. First, there are interventions that address behaviors thought to directly influence metabolic control such as diet or blood glucose monitoring (e.g., adherence behaviors). The second category includes interventions that target distal factors that indirectly affect adherence and metabolic control (e.g., family functioning, stress, social skills). Many of the interventions targeting adherence behaviors or metabolic control as the primary outcome variable are behaviorally oriented. While behavioral interventions delivered in a group setting (e.g., Anderson et al., 1989; Mendez & Belendez, 1997) appear to be effective in increasing adherence behaviors and management of diabetes-related tasks, interventions that are disseminated in an individual format appear to have greater promise in influencing not only adherence behaviors but also measures of metabolic control (e.g., Epstein et al., 1981). In particular, behavioral programs that include direct reinforcement for specific adherence behaviors seem to be effective in improving regimen adherence. For example, Wysocki et al. (1989) found that behavioral contracting for blood glucose monitoring significantly improved adherence and that those in the treatment group had better metabolic control than those in the conventional therapy group.

Other intervention programs have attempted to influence variables that are indirectly related to adherence and metabolic control. For example, there is some evidence to suggest that individuals with diabetes may be susceptible to stress-related hyperglycemia (Gilbert et al., 1989); despite the fact that experimental manipulations of stress have shown an equivocal relation between stress and metabolic control in children (Gilbert et al., 1989), there appears to be a significant relation between self-report of stress and poorer metabolic control (Hanson et al., 1987). Consequently, interventions specifically addressing coping skills and stress/anxiety reduction have been developed and evaluated among children and adolescents with type 1 diabetes. Grey et al. (2000) assessed a coping skills program for adolescents (aged 12–20) with type 1 diabetes that emphasized social problem solving, social skills training, conflict resolution, and cognitive behavior modification in situations specifically related to diabetes (e.g., managing food choices with friends) and in situations faced by all adolescents (e.g., drug/alcohol use). The results suggest that the adolescents in the coping skills program had lower HbA1c levels than those in the comparison groups at 3, 6, and 12 months after treatment initiation. Additionally, those in the intervention group reported increases in self-efficacy and reported that diabetes had less of an impact on their quality of life during the follow-up periods.

Other studies have attempted to decrease stress through behavioral interventions known to decrease anxiety such as stress management and problem-solving training (Boardway et al., 1993). While many of these studies have reported improvements in subjective experiences of stress or anxiety, they do not appear to have significantly impacted metabolic control. For example, Silverman and his colleagues (2003) found some improvement in self-care behaviors following an intervention that included training in cognitive restructuring and effective problem-solving techniques, but they did not provide information about the impact of the intervention on metabolic control. While many studies focus on increasing coping skills or reducing stress, there have been a few interventions aimed specifically at decreasing the social stress associated with treatment of type 1 diabetes. For example, Gross and his colleagues (1985) conducted a series of studies examining the effectiveness of a social skills training program to improve interpersonal functioning by teaching diabetes-specific assertiveness skills. Overall, the results of the studies suggest that the program was effective in improving the targeted social skills but did not have as much of an impact on metabolic control. Others such as Kaplan et al. (1985) compared a social skills program for children with diabetes to an educational program and found that those in the social skills training group had lower HbA1c values at four months' posttreatment than those in the education group.

While intrapersonal factors such as perceived stress or coping style influence adherence behaviors, the importance of the environment in maintaining good metabolic control is undeniable. For example, family conflict has been found to negatively impact metabolic control in both cross-sectional and longitudinal studies with youths (Anderson et al., 2002; Wysocki, 1993), while parental involvement, parental warmth, and diabetes-specific support provided by parents may serve as protective factors against regimen nonadherence (La Greca et al., 1995; Lewin et al., in press; Ott et al., 2000). Consequently, researchers have attempted to evaluate programs that specifically address parent-child conflict, family problem-solving skills, and family communication. Wysocki and his colleagues (2000) evaluated the effectiveness of a behavioral family systems therapy (BFST) compared to standard diabetes treatment among a group of adolescents diagnosed with type 1 diabetes and their families. The results suggest marked improvement in parent-adolescent relations and diabetes-specific conflict. However, improvements in treatment adherence were not significant and the relation between treatment and glycated hemoglobin was variable, with some adolescents showing improvements (e.g., younger children or boys in the treatment group) in metabolic control while others seemed to have a worsening of metabolic control (e.g., older girls in the treatment group). In an attempt to further evaluate the usefulness of BFST, Harris et al. (2005) completed home-based BSFT treatment for adolescents with poorly controlled type 1 diabetes. While the initial posttreatment evaluation suggested improvements in maternal-reported family conflict and overall behavior problems, these effects were not maintained at the six-month follow-up. Additionally, no changes were observed in metabolic control for the adolescents.

It may be that the focus of interventions such as BFST is too narrow or that other factors may moderate the relation between familial factors and regimen adherence. Therefore, to successfully treat youths with type 1 diabetes, attention should be given to both intrapersonal as well as familial variables. A model that incorporates individual and familial influences on regimen adherence and may provide some guidance for clinicians treating youths with type 1 diabetes was recently proposed by Greening and her colleagues (in press). This model suggests that intrapersonal variables such as coping style and health locus of control may moderate the relation between parental involvement in diabetes care and a child's adherence behaviors. This model suggests that when treating families of children with diabetes, clinicians should address not only parental involvement in diabetes care but also provide treatment that increases self-efficacy and adaptive coping in the child/adolescent while simultaneously reducing the response costs associated with regimen adherence.

While BFST has focused primarily on the family environment, other treatment programs have attempted to take an ecological approach to treatment and include strategies that can be implemented in the larger social and community context of the child as a means of increasing adherence behaviors or improving metabolic control. Recently, the efficacy of programs such as multisystemic therapy (MST; Henggeller, et al., 1999), an intervention originally designed for use with adolescents who were engaging in antisocial behaviors, has been evaluated with youths who are diagnosed with type 1 diabetes. MST takes a socio-ecological and family systems approach to treatment. In a multiple-baseline study of MST, Ellis and her colleagues (2003) found that among a small sample of adolescents with poorly controlled diabetes, MST was effective in improving the overall health status of the participants and resulted in fewer hospitalizations and emergency room visits. More recently, the results from a randomized controlled trial of MST with youths in poor metabolic control found that those in the MST group had fewer hospital admissions during treatment, and the costs associated with their treatment were significantly less when compared with youths in the standard care condition (Ellis et al., 2005).

While many studies have examined the efficacy of treatment programs for youths with type 1 diabetes, very few interventions qualify as empirically supported treatments. Based on the recommendations made by the Division of Clinical Psychology Task Force (Chambless, 1996) and then later modified by the Society for Pediatric Psychology (Spirito, 1999), only a handful of interventions would fall into the "well-established treatment," "probably efficacious treatment," or the "promising interventions" categories. Lemanek and her colleagues (2001) attempted to use the criteria set forth by the Chambless task force (1996) and Spirito (1999) to identify empirically supported treatments for improving behavioral adherence or metabolic control. Of the 11 studies that met their initial inclusion criteria for the study (i.e., included youths younger than 18 years of age, directly measured adherence, the intervention specifically targeted nonadherence and obtained significant improvement in adherence rates), none met the highest standard of support (i.e., the well-established treatment), and only two types of treatments fell into the probably efficacious category. The programs included in this category were operant learning procedures such as those employed by Wysocki et al. (1989), in which direct reinforcement was used to increase adherence behaviors and multicomponent treatment, which emphasizes training in self-management skills. An additional intervention strategy that included cognitive and behavioral self-regulation strategies such as those employed by Schafer et al. (1982) was included in the promising intervention category (Lemanek et al., 2001). In another attempt to determine the overall efficacy of psychological interventions for children with diabetes, Beale (2006) found an overall medium effect size (ES; $d = 0.67$) for psychological treatments of type 1 diabetes to be comparable to the ES reported for psychological treatment with other chronic illness populations (Beale, 2006). However, the ES reported by Beale (2006) is based on outcome data that not only included metabolic control and adherence behaviors but also other psychological variables such as social support or self-efficacy; when calculated for only adherence behaviors, the ES may differ significantly from this estimate.

Needless to say, clinicians working with children and families diagnosed with type 1 diabetes have a wide variety of treatment programs from which to draw. However, when the Chambless (1996) criteria for EST are applied, only a few of these intervention programs meet the necessary criteria. Therefore, regardless of the targeted outcome (e.g., adherence behavior, stress reduction, family conflict), additional studies that include prospective randomized clinical trials of youths with diabetes are needed.

CANCER

The past two decades have seen significant improvements in the medical treatment of pediatric cancer, and 5-year survival rates for pediatric cancer patients are approaching 80% (Ries et al., 2005). However, treatment for cancer continues to involve the use of invasive medical procedures as well as aggressive chemotherapy regimens, which can have adverse long-term physical and mental health consequences. In general, psychological treatment for pediatric cancer patients falls into three broad categories: interventions that address the medical needs of the child, interventions that address the psychosocial needs of the child, and interventions that address the psychosocial needs of the parents/family of the identified patient.

Research examining interventions that target the medical needs of the child/patient tend to address either the side effects of chemotherapy treatment or procedural pain management. We will focus on treatments for the side effects of chemotherapy because chemotherapy regimens are often associated with a number of undesirable side effects but most notably anticipatory and postchemotherapy nausea and vomiting. It is estimated that more than one-fourth of children and adolescents develop anticipatory nausea over the course of treatment, with rates being higher among adolescents than children. Additionally, nearly 80% of adolescents experience postchemotherapy nausea and vomiting (Dolgin et al., 1989). Since anticipatory nausea is thought to be the result of classical conditioning, the use of cognitive-behavioral techniques that disrupt the conditioning process can be effective in alleviating anticipatory nausea. A number of studies have examined the effectiveness of using relaxation, imagery, distraction, or some combination of these three techniques to treat anticipatory nausea in pediatric cancer patients. For example, in a small sample of adolescents, Zeltzer et al. (1983) found that using a relatively short (one- to three-session) imagery-based intervention was effective in reducing the frequency and intensity of vomiting. Additionally, a six-month follow-up assessment revealed a significant decrease in anxiety symptoms from pretreatment levels. Others have reported single-case studies of imagery-based interventions for nausea and found decreases in the frequency of both anticipatory and postchemotherapy nausea (Ellenberg et al., 1980; Kaufman et al., 1989). In one of the few controlled studies of chemotherapy-related nausea reduction, Cotanch et al. (1985) found imagery-based interventions to be superior to interventions that included a combination of relaxation and distraction in reducing the intensity, frequency, amount, and duration of vomiting. More recently, Zeltzer et al. (1991) completed a randomized control study in which children were assigned to either treatment using imagery-based techniques, treatment using distraction and relaxation, or an attention-control group. Their findings suggest that either treatment was superior to the attention-control condition in duration of nausea; however, those who received the imagery treatment also reported less anticipatory emesis than those in the relaxation/distraction group. Therefore, the findings suggest that imagery-based interventions are an effective way to treat the nausea and vomiting associated with chemotherapy and are considered a well-established treatment based on the criteria set forth by the Chambless task force (1996).

While it appears that cognitive-behavioral interventions for nausea and vomiting have been somewhat successful in reducing the physiological side effects of chemotherapy, the findings regarding the effectiveness of cognitive-behavioral techniques for addressing other psychosocial issues faced by children and adolescents diagnosed with cancer have been equivocal. Although childhood cancer survivors tend to be well adjusted and do not typically show elevated levels of depression or anxiety (Recklitis et al., 2003; Stoppelbein et al., 2006), some may experience low self-esteem and decreased hopefulness about the future. Hinds and her colleagues (2002) examined the effectiveness of a behavioral psychoeducational program for increasing self-efficacy, hopefulness, and self-esteem among newly diagnosed adolescents. The program was brief, consisting of three sessions, and focused on teaching self-care coping skills. Although there were no differences between the treatment group and the control group on the measures of interest, those in the treatment group tended to show an increase in hopefulness during the follow-up assessments. Others have attempted to use behavioral techniques to address the long-term consequences of cancer such as peer difficulties (Barakat et al., 2003; Varni et al., 1993).

Because children and adolescents diagnosed with cancer do not typically exhibit significant psychological sequelae or distress, some have suggested that the current measures of psychopathology fail to adequately assess the specific psychological distress experienced for pediatric cancer survivors and their parents (Kazak, 2005). For example, while many now acknowledge the risk of posttraumatic stress symptoms (PTSS) following the diagnosis of cancer, it was not until the most recent revision of the *Diagnostic and Statistical Manual of Mental Disorders—Fourth Edition* (DSM-IV; American Psychiatric Association, 1994) that being diagnosed with or having a loved one diagnosed with a life-threatening illness such as cancer was recognized as a traumatic event. A diagnosis of a life-threatening illness such as cancer is an unpredictable event that elicits distress and feelings of helplessness from patients and loved ones, and while pediatric cancer patients do not exhibit symptoms traditionally associated with depression or anxiety (Recklitis et al., 2003; Stoppelbein et al., 2006), there is research to suggest that they may be at risk for developing posttraumatic stress symptoms (PTSS; Kazak et al., 2001; Stoppelbein et al., 2006).

Epidemiological research suggests that 2–20% of children diagnosed with cancer meet criteria for posttraumatic stress disorder (PTSD; Kazak et al., 1997, 2001;Pelcovitiz et al., 1998). In addition to the obvious impact that a cancer diagnosis has on the patient, parents of children diagnosed with cancer may be at greater risk for PTSS than the child/patient. Parents of childhood cancer survivors may display no significant depression and anxiety but still have marked symptomatology (Stoppelbein et al., 2006). Consequently, interventions that address PTSS within the family or the child's caretaker have been designed and evaluated empirically.

Kazak and her colleagues (1999, 2004) recently completed a series of studies evaluating the efficacy of a family-based cognitive-behavioral intervention program for reducing PTSS, the Surviving Cancer Compe- tently Intervention Program (SCCIP; Kazak et al., 1999). The program consists of four group sessions that are completed in a single day and is designed for use with adolescent long-term cancer survivors (e.g., 1–10 years' posttreatment) and their families. The initial findings suggested that the program was effective in decreasing PTSS and anxiety among the adolescents, their parents, and their siblings. Additionally, there was some support for the effectiveness of the intervention on parental perceptions of family cohesion as well. More recently, Kazak and her colleagues (2004) conducted a randomized clinical trial comparing the effectiveness of SCCIP to a waitlist control group. The results indicated a significant treatment effect for adolescents PTSS and a marginal effect for father's PTSS, but the effect for mothers was not statistically significant.

Recently, Kazak and her colleagues (2005) evaluated a shorter version of SCCIP with caregivers of children newly diagnosed with cancer. Although the sample size was small, the results were promising and suggested the program was effective in reducing general anxiety and PTSS within the caregivers. Since women are particularly vulnerable to developing stress- related disorders and for experiencing depression, anxiety, and PTSS (Kessler et al., 2005), many of the interventions have focused on allevi- ating this distress and increasing adaptive coping skills among mothers of newly diagnosed pediatric cancer patients. Sahler et al. (2002) completed a randomized clinical trail assessing the efficacy of a problem-solving skills training program with mothers of children newly diagnosed with cancer. The program consisted of one-hour individual sessions conducted over eight weeks. The intervention appeared to be effective in increasing constructive problem-solving skills but was not as effective in decreasing dysfunctional problem solving. Additionally, those in the intervention program had significantly less negative affectivity, and these effects were maintained at the three-month follow-up assessment. In a follow-up study, Sahler et al. (2005) replicated these findings in another sample of mothers with children who were newly diagnosed with cancer. A Spanish-language version of the program was also tested among a sample of monolingual Spanish-speaking mothers, and the results were similar to those found for the English version of the program. However, in contrast to the success of these programs, other psychoeducational programs have not been as effective in alleviating the distress of parents. For example, Hoekstra-Weebers et al. (1998) compared the efficacy of a psychoeducational program for parents of children newly diagnosed with cancer to a standard care condition. Although the evaluation of the intervention by participants was positive, the treatment was no more effective than the standard care received by the parents in alleviating general distress or anxiety or in increasing the parent's perception of social support.

Again, it seems that while many of the interventions for children with cancer are promising, only a few meet the Chambless (1996) criteria for ESTs. Imagery-based interventions for nausea and vomiting and family-based interventions for long-term coping with cancer appear to be effective interventions. The psychological care for children with cancer is currently moving from description to intervention, and more prospective randomized trials of other targeted interventions are needed.

SICKLE CELL DISEASE

Sickle cell disease (SCD) is a chronic condition that affects individuals of African and Mediterranean origins. In the United States, this results in approximately 1 in 500 African Americans being affected by the disease (Lemanek et al., 1995). SCD is characterized by abnormal shaping of red blood cells, often referred to as "sickling." This abnormality can result in the formation of masses that block vessels, leading to a variety of problems such as vaso-occlusive crises ("pain crises"), splenic sequestration syndrome, growth retardation, and cerebrovascular accidents (Ris & Gruenich, 2000).

The focus of most psychological interventions in children and adolescents with SCD has been on alleviating pain crises. Other areas are being investigated, such as feeding disorders (Lemanek et al., 2002), enuresis (Barakat et al., 2001), and adherence (Jensen et al., 2005). However, the literature in these other areas is still relatively undeveloped and thus does not qualify for a thorough discussion in the context of empirically supported treatments.

Prior to 1999, there was little evidence for empirically supported treatments in pediatric SCD and pain management (Walco et al., 1999). Since that time, researchers in pain management in pediatric SCD have reported evidence of promising and emerging results for cognitive coping skills (Gil et al., 2000, 2001). Karen Gil and her colleagues have reported that cognitive coping skills training in this population resulted in a reduced number of medical contacts as well as reduced self-report of pain compared to no intervention. It would appear that this line of research offers evidence of promising efficacy in managing pain in children and adolescents with SCD. Further randomized controlled trials would be necessary to confirm this as an EBT for this particular population.

Likewise, Powers and his colleagues (2002) have reported findings from pilot studies in which pain management skills are taught in a family setting, using a cognitive-behavioral framework. Patients and their families are trained to manage pain crises and use behavioral techniques such as distraction and breathing in order to reduce pain sensitivity and increase pain coping abilities. These findings indicate that this type of intervention may be useful as well. However, these studies need to be replicated in order to meet criteria for EBTs.

Clearly, more research is needed in this historically understudied population. We expect that over the next decade, more evidence of empirically supported treatments will emerge, which will greatly improve the overall well-being and quality of life for these children, adolescents, and their families.

CONCLUSION

Children with chronic illnesses represent a small but significant population. While many of the diseases they and their families must cope with are relatively rare, these diseases can produce sizable psychological distress. Over the past decade, a growing number of researchers have developed and tested interventions that are specifically targeted. This has resulted in a burgeoning, if somewhat immature, literature. In this chapter, we have attempted to highlight some of these targeted interventions in three of the most prominent disease categories in children: diabetes, cancer, and sickle cell. Overall, cognitive-behavioral interventions have shown the most promise, but what has become obvious is that targeted interventions are needed to address specific problems, especially when those problem areas are in the context of certain diseases. Future research will continue to refine this effort of identifying specific strategies for specific diseases in children.

REFERENCES

American Diabetes Association (2000). *American Diabetes Association Complete Guide to Diabetes*. Alexandria, VA.

American Psychiatric Association (1994). *Diagnostic and Statistical Manual of Mental Disorders*, 4th ed. Washington, DC.

Anderson, B. J., Vangsness, L., Connell, A., Butler, D., Goebel-Fabbri, A., & Laffel, L. M. B. (2002). Family conflict, adherence, and glycemic control in youth with short duration type I diabetes. *Diabetic Medicine, 19*, 635–642.

Anderson, B. J., Wolf, F. M., Burkhart, M. T., Cornell, R. G., & Bacon, G. E. (1989). Effects of peer-group intervention on metabolic control of adolescents with IDDM. *Diabetes Care, 12*, 179–183.

Barakat, L. P., Hetzke, J. D., Foley, B., Carey, M. E., Gyato, K., & Phillips, P. C. (2003). Evaluation of a social skills training group intervention with children treated for brain tumors: A pilot study. *Journal of Pediatric Psychology, 28*, 299–307.

Barakat, L. P., Smith-Whitley, K., Schulman, S. (2001). Nocturnal enuresis in pediatric sickle cell disease. *Journal of Developmental and Behavioral Pediatrics, 22*,300–305.

Beale, I. L. (2006). Scholarly literature review: Efficacy of psychological interventions for pediatric chronic illnesses. *Journal of Pediatric Psychology, 31*(5), 437–451.

Boardway, R. H., Delamater, A. M., Tomakowsky, J., & Gutai, J. P. (1993). Stress management training for adolescents with diabetes. *Journal of Pediatric Psychology, 18,* 29–45.

Centers for Disease Control. *Diabetes Projects.* Retrieved February 7, 2006, from http://www.cdc.gov/diabetes/projects/cda2.htm.

Chambless, D. L., Baker, M. J., Baucom, D. H., Beutler, L. E., Calhoun, K. S., Crits-Christophe, P., et al. (1996). An update on empirically validated therapies. *Clinical Psychologist, 49,* 5–18.

Cotanch, P., Hockenberry, M., & Herman, S. (1985). Self-hypnosis as antiemetic therapy in children receiving chemotherapy. *Oncology Nursing Forum, 12,* 41–46.

Dolgin, M. J., Katz, E. R., Zeltzer, L. K., & Landsverk, J. (1989). Behavioral distress in pediatric patients with cancer receiving chemotherapy. *Pediatrics, 84,* 103–110.

Ellenberg, L., Kellerman, J., Dash, J., Higgins, G., & Zeltzer, L., (1980). Use of hypnosis for multiple symptoms in an adolescent girl with leukemia. *Journal of Adolescent Health Care, 1,* 132–136.

Ellis, D. A., Naar-King, S., Frey, M., Rowland, M., & Greger, N. (2003). Case study: Feasibility of multisystemic therapy as a treatment for urban adolescents with poorly controlled type I diabetes. *Journal of Pediatric Psychology, 28,* 287–293.

Ellis, D. A., Naar-King, S., Frey, M., Templin, T., Rowland, M., & Cakan, N. (2005). Multisystemic treatment of poorly controlled type I diabetes: Effects on medical resource utilization. *Journal of Pediatric Psychology, 30,* 656–666.

Epstein, L. H., Beck, S., Figueroa, J., Farkas, G., Kazdin, A. E., Daneman, D., et al. (1981). The effects of targeting improvements in urine glucose on metabolic control in children with insulin dependent diabetes. *Journal of Applied Behavior Analysis, 14,* 365–375.

Frederick, C. J. (1985). Selected foci in the spectrum of posttraumatic stress disorders. In J. Laube & S. A. Murphy (Eds.), *Perspectives on Disaster Recovery* (pp. 110–130). Norwalk, CT: Appleton-Century-Crofts.

Gil, K. M., Anthony, K., Carson, J., Redding-Lallinger, R., Daeschner, C., & Ware, R. (2001). Daily coping practice predicts treatment effects in children with sickle cell disease. *Journal of Pediatric Psychology, 26,* 163–173.

Gil, K. M., Carson, J., Sedway, J. W., Porter, L., Schaeffer, J., & Orringer, E. (2000). Follow-up of coping skills training in adults with sickle cell disease: Analysis of daily pain and coping practice diaries. *Health Psychology, 19,* 85–90.

Gilbert, B. O., Johnson, S. B., Silverstein, J., & Malone, J. (1989). Psychological and physiological responses to acute laboratory stressors in insulin-dependent diabetes mellitus adolescents and nondiabetic controls. *Journal of Pediatric Psychology, 14,* 577–591.

Greening, L., Stoppelbein, L., & Reeves, C. (in press). A model for promoting adolescents adherence to treatment for type I diabetes mellitus. *Children's Health Care.*

Grey, M., Boland, E. A., Davidson, M., Li, J., & Tamborlane, W. V. (2000). Coping skills training for youth with diabetes mellitus has long-lasting effects on metabolic control and quality of life. *Journal of Pediatrics, 137,* 107–113.

Gross, A. M., Magalnick, L. J., & Richardson, P. (1985). Self-management training with families of insulin-dependent diabetic children: A controlled long-term investigation. *Child and Family Behavior Therapy, 7,* 35–50.

Hanson, C. L., Henggeler, S. W., & Burghen, G. A. (1987). Social competence and parental support as mediators of the link between stress and metabolic control in adolescents with insulin-dependent diabetes mellitus. *Journal of Consulting and Clinical Psychology, 55,* 529–533.

Harris, M. A., Harris, B. S., & Mertlich, D. (2005). Brief report: In-home family therapy for adolescents with poorly controlled diabetes: Failure to maintain benefits at 6-month follow-up. *Journal of Pediatric Psychology, 30,* 683–688.

Henggeler, S. W., Rowland, M. D., Randall, J., Ward, D. M., Pickrel, S. G., Cunningham, P. B., et al. (1999). Home-based multisystemic therapy as an alternative to the hospitalization of youths in psychiatric crisis: Clinical outcomes. *Journal of American Academy of Child and Adolescent Psychiatry, 38,* 1331–1339.

Hinds, P. S., Quargnenti, A., Bush, A. J., Pratt, C., Fairclough, D., Rissmiller, G., et al. (2000). An evaluation of the impact of a self-care coping intervention on psychological and clinical outcomes in adolescents with newly diagnosed cancer. *European Journal of Oncology Nursing, 4,* 6–17.

Hoekstra-Weebers, J. E. H. M., Heuvel, F., Jaspers, J. P. C., Kamps, W. A., & Klip, E. C. (1998). Brief report: An intervention program for parents of pediatric cancer patients: A randomized controlled trial. *Journal of Pediatric Psychology, 23,* 207–214.

Jensen, S. A., Elkin, T. D., Hilker, K., Jordan, S., Iyer, R., & Smith, M. G. (2005). Caregiver knowledge and adherence in children with sickle cell disease: Knowing is not doing. *Journal of Clinical Psychology in Medical Settings, 12*(4), 333–337.

Kaplan, R. M., Chadwick, M. W., & Schimmel, L. E. (1985). Social learning intervention to promote metabolic control in type I diabetes mellitus: Pilot experiment results. *Diabetes Care, 8,* 152–155.

Kaufman, K. L., Tarnowski, K. J., & Olson, R. (1989). Self-regulation treatment to reduce the aversiveness of cancer chemotherapy. *Journal of Adolescent Health Care, 10,* 323–327.

Kazak, A. E. (2005). Evidence-based interventions for survivors of childhood cancer and their families. *Journal of Pediatric Psychology, 30,* 29–39.

Kazak, A. E., Alderfer, M. A., Streisand, R., Simms, S., Rourke, M. T., Barakat, L. P., et al. (2004). Treatment of posttraumatic stress symptoms in adolescent survivors of childhood cancer and their families: A randomized clinical trial. *Journal of Family Psychology, 18,* 493–504.

Kazak, A. E., Barakat, L., Alderfer, M., Rourke, M., Meeske, K., Gallagher, P., et al. (2001). Posttraumatic stress in survivors of childhood cancer and mothers: Development and validation of the Impact of Traumatic Stressors Interview Schedule (ITSIS). *Journal of Clinical Psychology in Medical Settings, 8,* 307–323.

Kazak, A. E., Barakat, L. P., Meeske, K., Christakis, D., Meadows, A. T., Casey, R., et al. (1997). Posttraumatic stress, family functioning, and social support in survivors of childhood leukemia and their mothers and fathers. *Journal of Consulting and Clinical Psychology, 65,* 120–129.

Kazak, A. E., Simms, S., Alderfer, M. A., Rourke, M. T., Crump, T., McClure, K., et al. (2005). Feasibility and preliminary outcomes from a pilot study of a brief psychological intervention for families of children newly diagnosed with cancer. *Journal of Pediatric Psychology, 30,* 644–655.

Kazak, A. E., Simms, S., Barakat, L., Hobbie, W., Foley, B., Golomb, V., et al. (1999). Surviving Cancer Competently Intervention Program (SCCIP): A cognitive-behavioral and family therapy intervention for adolescent survivors of childhood cancer and their families. *Family Process, 38,* 175–191.

Kessler, R. C., Chiu, W. T., Demler, O., & Walters, E. E. (2005). Prevalence, severity, and comorbidity of 12-month DSM-IV disorders in the national comorbidity survey replication. *Archives of General Psychiatry, 62,* 617–627.

La Greca, A. M., Auslander, W. F., Greco, P., Spetter, D., Fisher, E. B., & Santiago, J. V. (1995). I get by with a little help from my family and friends: Adolescents' support for diabetes care. *Journal of Pediatric Psychology, 20,* 449–476.

Lemanek, K. L., Brown, R. T., Armstrong, F. D., Hood, C., Pegelow, C., & Woods, G. (2002). Dysfunctional eating patterns and symptoms of pica in children and adolescents with sickle cell disease. *Clinical Pediatrics, 41,* 493–500.

Lemanek, K. L., Buckloh, L. M., Woods, G., & Butler, R. (1995). Diseases of the circulatory system: Sickle cell and hemophilia. In M. Roberts (Ed.), *Handbook of Pediatric Psychology,* 2nd ed. (pp. 286–309). New York: Guilford Press.

Lemanek, K. L., Kamps, J., & Chung, N. B. (2001). Empirically supported treatments in pediatric psychology: Regimen adherence. *Journal of Pediatric Psychology, 26,* 253–275.

Lewin, A. B., Heidgerken, A. D., Geffken, G. R., Williams, L. B., Storch, E. A., Gelfand, K. M., et al. (in press). The relation between family factors and metabolic control: The role of diabetes adherence. *Journal of Pediatric Psychology.*

McQuaid, E. L., & Nassau, J. H. (1999). Empirically supported treatments of disease-related symptoms in pediatric psychology: Asthma, diabetes, and cancer. *Journal of Pediatric Psychology, 24,* 305–328.

Mendez, F. J., & Belendez, M. (1997). Effects of a behavioral intervention on treatment adherence and stress management in adolescents with IDDM. *Diabetes Care, 20,* 1370–1375.

Noll, R. B., Bukowski, W. M., Davies, W. H., Koontz, K., & Kulkarni, R. (1993). Adjustment in the peer system of adolescents with cancer: A two-year study. *Journal of Pediatric Psychology, 18,* 351–364.

Noll, R. B., Garstein, M. A., Vannatta, K., Correll, J., Bukowski, W. M., & Davies, W. H. (1999). Social, emotional, and behavioral functioning of children with cancer. *Pediatrics, 103,* 71–78.

Ott, J., Greening, L., Palardy, N., Holderby, A., & DeBell, W. K. (2000). Self-efficacy as a mediator variable for adolescents' adherence to treatment for insulin-dependent diabetes mellitus. Children's Health Care, 29, 47–63.

Pelcovitz, D., Libov, B. G., Mandel, F., Kaplan, S., Weinblatt, M., & Septimus, A. (1998). Posttraumatic stress disorder and family functioning in adolescent cancer. *Journal of Traumatic Stress, 11,* 205–221.

Powers, S., Mitchell, M., Graumlich, S., Byars, K., & Kalinyak, K. (2002). Longitudinal assessment of pain, coping, and daily functioning in children with sickle cell disease receiving pain management skills training. *Journal of Clinical Psychology in Medical Settings, 9,* 109–119.

Recklitis, C., O'Leary, T., & Diller, L. (2003). Utility of routine psychological screening in the childhood cancer survivor clinic. *Journal of Clinical Oncology, 21,* 787–792.

Ries, L., Eisner, M., Kosary, C., Hankey, B., Miller, B., Clegg, L., et al. (Eds). *SEER Cancer Statistics Review, 1975–2002,* National Cancer Institute. Bethesda, MD; http://seer.cancer.gov/csr/1975_2002/, based on November 2004 SEER data submission, posted to the SEER Web site 2005.

Ris, M. D., & Gruenich, R. (2000). Sickle cell disease. In K. Yeates, M. Ris, & H. Taylor (Eds.), *Pediatric Neuropsychology: Research, Theory, and Practice* (pp. 320–335). New York: Guilford Press.

Sahler, O. J. Z., Fairclough, D. L., Phipps, S., Mulhern, R. K., Dolgin, M. J., Noll, R. B., et al. (2005). Using problem-solving skills training to reduce negative affectivity in mothers of children with newly diagnosed cancer: Report of a multisite randomized trial. *Journal of Consulting and Clinical Psychology, 73,* 272–283.

Sahler, O. J. Z., Varni, J. W., Fairclough, D. L., Butler, R. W., Noll, R. B., Dolgin, M. J., et al. (2002). Problem-solving skills training for mothers of children with newly diagnosed cancer: A randomized trial. *Journal of Developmental and Behavioral Pediatrics, 23,* 77–87.

Silverman, A. H., Hains, A. A., Davies, W. H., & Parton, E. (2003). A cognitive behavioral adherence intervention for adolescents with type I diabetes. *Journal of Clinical Psychology in Medical Settings, 10,* 119–127.

Spirito, A. (1999). Introduction to the special series on empirically supported treatments in pediatric psychology. *Journal of Pediatric Psychology, 24,* 87–90.

Stoppelbein, L. A., Greening, L., & Elkin, T. D. (2006). Risk of posttraumatic stress symptoms: A comparison of child survivors of pediatric cancer and parental bereavement. *Journal of Pediatric Psychology, 31*(4), 367–376.

Varni, J. W., Katz, E. R., Colegrove, R., & Dolgin, M. (1993). The impact of social skills training on the adjustment of children with newly diagnosed cancer. *Journal of Pediatric Psychology, 18,* 751–767.

Walco, G., Sterling, C., Conte, P., & Engel, R. (1999). Empirically supported treatments in pediatric psychology: Disease-related pain. *Journal of Pediatric Psychology, 24,* 155–167.

Wysocki, T. (1993). Associations among teen-parent relationships, metabolic control and adjustment to diabetes in adolescents. *Journal of Pediatric Psychology, 18,* 441–452.

Wysocki, T., Green, L., & Huxtable, K. (1989). Blood glucose monitoring by diabetic adolescents: Compliance and metabolic control. *Health Psychology, 8,* 267–284.

Wysocki, T., Harris, M. A., Greco, P., Bubb, J., Danda, C. E., Harvey, L. M., et al. (2000). Randomized, controlled trial of behavior therapy for families of adolescents with insulin-dependent diabetes mellitus. *Journal of Pediatric Psychology, 25,* 23–33.

Zeltzer, L. K., Dolgin, M. J., LeBaron, S., & LeBaron, C. (1991). A randomized, controlled study of behavioral intervention for chemotherapy distress in children with cancer. *Pediatrics, 88,* 34–42.

Zeltzer, L. K., Kellerman, J., Ellenberg, L., Dash, J., & Rigler, D. (1983). Hypnosis for reduction of vomiting associated with chemotherapy and disease in adolescents with cancer. *Journal of Adolescent Health Care, 4,* 77–84.

18

Evidence-Based Therapies for Enuresis and Encopresis

PATRICK C. FRIMAN

The alimentary process terminates with the elimination of waste, specifically urine and feces. Among the most common, persistent, and stressful presenting complaints in primary medical care for children are two disorders involving developmentally inappropriate elimination of waste—enuresis (urine) and encopresis (feces). Evidence is found for their commonality and persistence in prevalence and age-range estimates. Prevalence estimates range as high as 2% of 5-year-old children for encopresis and 25% of 6-year-old children for enuresis and, although both are much less prevalent by the teenage years, they are not rare. For example, as many as 8% of boys and 4% of girls are still enuretic at age 12 (Byrd et al., 1996; Gross & Dornbusch, 1983; Foxman et al., 1986; Friman & Jones, 1998). Evidence of their stress-inducing properties is found in their relationship with child abuse; incontinence is one of its leading causes (Finn, 2005; Helfer & Kempe, 1976). Evidence is also found in surveys of child-reported stressors; it is exceeded only by divorce and parental fights (Van Tijen et al., 1998). Nocturnal enuresis (NE) and encopresis usually occur independently but can co-occur. This chapter will briefly describe both disorders in terms of their diagnosis, etiology, and evaluation and then more fully describe evidence-based treatments used for them.

ENURESIS

Diagnosis

"Enuresis" is the technical term used for the regular passage of urine into locations other than those specifically designed for that purpose. The diagnostic criteria in the fourth edition of the *Diagnostic and Statistical*

PATRICK C. FRIMAN • Girls and Boys Town, The University of Nebraska School of Medicine

Manual for Mental Disorders (DSM-IV; American Psychiatric Association, 1994) include repeated voiding of urine into clothing or bed at least twice a week for at least three months. If the frequency is smaller than that but the voiding is a cause of significant distress or impairment to social, academic, or occupational functioning, it satisfies diagnostic criteria. The child must be at least 5 years of age or exhibit that level of developmental ability if developmental delays are present. The condition cannot be directly due to the physiological effects of a substance (e.g., diuretics) or a general medical condition. The DSM further classifies NE into primary (in which the person has never achieved urinary continence) and secondary (in which incontinence develops after a period of continence) cases. Additionally, the DSM subdivides NE into three subtypes—nocturnal, diurnal, and combined nocturnal and diurnal. This chapter will focus solely on nocturnal enuresis (NE) because it is, by a very wide margin, the most frequently presenting type.

Etiology

Multiple variables have been identified as partial causes for NE, and these will be only briefly described here. Fuller discussions are widely available (e.g., Christophersen & Friman, 2004; Friman, 1986, 1995; Friman & Jones, 1998, 2005; Houts, 1991; Levine, 1982). Perhaps the most salient etiological variable is family history. The probability of NE increases as function of closeness and number of blood relations with a positive history (Kaffman & Elizur, 1977). Delayed physiological maturation, especially in the areas of bone growth, secondary sexual characteristics, and stature, is correlated with NE (Fergusson et al., 1986). A strong association between functional bladder capacity and NE has been established (Troup & Hodgson, 1971). Although the abundant research on sleep dynamics and NE has been marred by design flaws (cf. Friman, 1986, 1995), a recent study appears to support what parents have long suspected, specifically, that deep sleep and slowness to arouse may increase the likelihood of NE (Gellis, 1994). Although there is a long history of attributing NE to psychological (e.g., psychopathology) and/or characterological (e.g., laziness) variables, there appears to be no relationship in the vast majority of cases (Friman et al., 1998; Friman, 2002). There was initial enthusiasm for a finding of reduced antidiuretic hormone (ADH) in a small sample of enuretic children (Norgaard et al., 1985), but the findings have not been replicated across large numbers of children, and treatments that increase ADH have had limited success (Moffat et al., 1993; see also Houts, 1991; Houts et al., 1994). Finally, there are numerous and well-known potential physiopathological (i.e., medical) causes (e.g., urinary tract infection, diabetes, bladder instability).

Evaluation

The treatment of NE should not proceed until a medical examination has been conducted, because medical causes need to be either ruled out medically or diagnosed and treated (Christophersen & Friman, 2004; Friman, 1986, 1995; Friman & Jones, 1998, 2005). The evaluation should also include a history with questions derived from diagnostic criteria (e.g., primary vs. secondary) and the etiological factors mentioned above. Some screening for mental health problems should be included (e.g., behavior checklists, related inquiry); if clinically significant problems are detected, they should be targeted in the ultimate treatment plan. In addition to addressing medical and psychological complications, the evaluation should address three other very important topics. First, all sources of punishment for urinary accidents should be identified and eliminated. Second, the motivational level and availability of social resources for the parents should be assessed because these will influence the number of components included in treatment. For example, if the parent is minimally motivated and/or has few social resources (e.g., single working parent), the number will be lower. Third, the motivational level and likely cooperation of the child should be assessed. Optimal treatment plans involve multiple components and require compliance from the child for completion of most steps. An unmotivated or noncompliant child would be difficult to treat with any method known to cure NE. Fortunately, NE itself usually contributes to the afflicted child's motivation. As the quantity of pleasant experiences missed (e.g., sleepovers, camp) and unpleasant experiences encountered (e.g., wetness, social detection, embarrassment) accumulates, motivation naturally increases.

Treatment

The need for treatment of NE predates modern civilization, and the variety of techniques used in antiquity appear to have been limited only by the imagination of the ancient therapists and their tolerance for inflicting unpleasantness on young children in order to possibly secure therapeutic gain. Penile binding, buttock and sacrum burning, and forced urine-soaked pajama wearing are among the many highly aversive treatments reported in a review of ancient approaches to NE (Glicklich, 1951). In fairness to the ancient therapists, the health-based consequences of prolonged NE during their time were severe, due to the limited means for cleaning bedding and the ineffective methods for managing infection. The evolution of treatment for NE that began in earnest early in the 20th century abandoned the physically harsh treatments in favor of approaches that were more humane from a physical perspective but still problematic from a psychological one. Specifically, with the rise of Freudian psychodynamics came psychopathological characterizations of common childhood problems such as NE (Friman, 2002). Although more protected from harsh physical treatment than their ancestral peers, early 20th-century enuretic children were often subject to stigma, isolation, and other negative social consequences.

The advent of behavioral theory, and the conditioning type treatments derived from it, inaugurated a virtual paradigmatic shift in treatment. Specifically, behavioral theory rendered psychopathological interpretations obsolete and aversive physical treatments unnecessary (e.g., Christophersen & Friman, 2004; Friman, 1986, 1995; Friman & Jones, 1998, 2005). The cardinal conditioning-type treatment for NE has been the urine alarm; if not the first, certainly the foremost early user of it was Herbert Mower (Mower & Mower, 1938). Since the mid-1970s, psychological research on medically uncomplicated NE in children has been dominated by either the development of alternative behavioral procedures based on operant conditioning or improving urine alarm treatments (Houts, 2000; Mellon & McGrath, 2000). Controlled evaluations of the urine alarm indicate that this relatively simple device is 65–75% effective, with a duration of treatment around 5 to 12 weeks and a 6-month relapse rate of 15–30% (e.g., Butler, 2004; Doleys, 1977; Houts et al., 1994; Mellon & McGrath, 2000). Most of this research has been conducted using the bed device and, less frequently, the pajama device. Treatment involving the alarm used alone, or in strategic combinations with other treatment components, has been established as "effective treatments" according to the "Chambless criteria" (Mellon & McGrath, 2000). Thus, the urine alarm is a core treatment component that can be augmented by a range of other strategies. The sections below will describe alarm-based treatments in terms of method, process, and outcome and will then describe the augmentive components with the most empirical support because they have been shown to be effective when used either in isolation or as part of a treatment package.

Bed Devices

The urine alarm uses a moisture-sensitive switching system that, when closed by contact with urine seeped into pajamas or bedding, completes a small-voltage electrical circuit and activates a stimulus that is theoretically strong enough to cause waking (e.g., buzzer, bell, light, or vibrator). The device is placed on the bed or sewn into the pajamas. The bed device typically involves two aluminum foil pads, one of which is perforated, with a cloth pad between them. The bed pads are placed under the sheets of the target enuretic child's bed with the perforated pad on top. A urinary accident results in urine seeping through perforations in the top pad, collecting in the cloth pad, and causing contact with the bottom sufficient to complete an electrical circuit and activate a sound-based alarm mechanism. In principle, the awakened child turns off the alarm and completes a series of responsibility-training steps associated with their accidents, such as completing urination in the bathroom, changing pajamas and sheets, and returning to bed. In practice, the alarm often alerts parents first, who then waken the child and guide him through the training steps (Friman & Jones, 1998, 2005).

Pajama Devices

Pajama devices are similar in function, yet simpler in design. The alarm itself is either placed into a pocket sewn into the child's pajamas or pinned to them. Two wire leads extending from the alarm are attached (e.g., by small alligator clamps) on or near the pajama bottoms. When the child wets during the night, absorption of urine by the pajamas completes an electrical circuit between the two wire leads and activates the alarm. A range of stimuli is available for use with the pajama devices and includes buzzing, ringing, vibrating, and lighting.

Child- and Parent-Focused Methods

Actual alarm use can be divided into different methods, depending on the primary management role of the child and parent. In the child-focused method, the alarm awakens the child, who independently completes the responsibility-training procedure. The most recent example of child-focused methods involves the use of a vibrating (rather than sound-producing) urine alarm (Ruckstuhl & Friman, 2003). In the parent-focused method, the alarm awakens or alerts the parent, who awakens the child and guides her through the training procedure. The training procedures vary across published accounts and guides but generally include full arousal, going to the bathroom to complete (or attempt) urination, changing bedding and pajamas, resetting the alarm, and going back to bed. Parent-focused methods are obviously dependent on the saliency of the alarm stimulus and, with the bed device wire leads, can be extended to the parent's auditory range (e.g., in the parent's bedroom). For the pajama device, either a very loud alarm or periodic checking is necessary to allow parents to readily attend to accidents. Although it seems logical that no matter what method or device is used, reduced latency between onset of urination and awakening is best, but no data are available to support this position.

Underlying Process

The mechanism of action in alarm treatment was initially described as classical conditioning, with the alarm as the unconditioned stimulus, bladder distention as the conditioned stimulus, and waking as the conditioned response (Mowrer & Mowrer, 1938). More recent literature emphasizes a negative reinforcement or avoidance paradigm (Friman, 1995; Friman & Jones, 1998, 2005; Ruckstuhl & Friman, 2003) in which the child increases sensory awareness of urinary need and exercises anatomical responses (e.g., contraction of the pelvic floor muscles) that effectively avoid setting off the alarm (Mellon et al., 1997). Cures are obtained slowly, however, and during the first few weeks of alarm use the child often awakens only after voiding completely. The aversive properties of the alarm, however, inexorably strengthen those responses necessary to avoid it.

Evidence of Effectiveness

Reports of controlled comparative trials show the alarm-based treatment is superior to drug treatment and other nondrug methods such as retention control training. In fact, numerous reviews of the literature show its success rate is higher and its relapse rate lower than any other method—ranging as high as 80% for success and as low as 17% for relapse (Butler, 2004; Christophersen & Friman, 2004; Friman & Jones, 1998; Doleys, 1977; Houts et al., 1994; Mellon & McGrath, 2000). One problem with interpreting the review literature on alarm treatment is that adjunctive components are often added to improve effectiveness, resulting in treatment "packages" to be described below. Additionally, there is very little research on child-based methods and apparently only one available study on the vibrating urine alarm. In that study, the use of the alarm produced an approximately 50% success rate (Ruckstuhl & Friman, 2003).

Treatment Packages

The oldest, best-known and empirically supported treatment package is Dry Bed Training (DBT; Azrin et al., 1974). Initially evaluated for use with a group of adults with profound mental retardation, it has been systematically replicated numerous times across child populations. In addition to the bed alarm, its initial composition included overlearning, intensive cleanliness (responsibility) training, intensive positive practice (of alternatives to wetting), hourly awakenings, close monitoring, and rewards for success. In subsequent iterations, the stringency of the waking schedule was reduced and retention control training was added (e.g., Bollard & Nettlebeck, 1982). Other similar programs were also developed, the best-known and empirically supported of which is Full Spectrum Home Training (FSHT; Houts & Liebert, 1985; Houts et al., 1984a). It includes the alarm, cleanliness training, retention control training, and overlearning. Multiple variations are now available (e.g., Christophersen & Friman, 2004; Friman, 1986, 1995; Friman & Jones, 1998; 2005). Component analyses have been conducted on both major programs, and the findings show that the alarm is the critical element and that the probability of success increases as the number of additional components are added (Bollard & Nettlebeck, 1982; Houts et al., 1986). Therefore, the following section will describe a broad range of additional components, starting with those that either have independent empirical support or have been part of programs that have empirical support. The section will then describe a series of components that have yet to be evaluated alone or as part of a treatment program but are frequently prescribed, and the logic of their inclusion is consistent with the learning and physiological dynamics of learning and urination.

Empirically Supported Components of Conventional Programs

Retention Control Training (RCT)

The emergence of RCT followed the observation that many enuretic children had reduced functional bladder capacity (Muellner, 1960, 1961; Starfield, 1967). RCT expands functional bladder capacity by requiring children to drink extra fluids (e.g., 16 oz of water or juice) and delay urination as long as possible and thus increase the volume of their diurnal urinations and expand the interval between urges to urinate at night (Muellner, 1960, 1961; Starfield, 1967; Starfield & Mellits, 1968). Parents are instructed to establish a regular time for RCT each day and conclude the training at least a few hours before bedtime. Progress can be assessed by monitoring the amount of time the child is able to delay urination and/or the volume of urine he is able to produce in a single urination (Christophersen & Friman, 2004; Friman, 1986, 1995; Friman & Jones, 1998, 2005). Either or both can be incorporated into a game context wherein children earn rewards for progress. RCT is successful in as many as 50% of cases (Doleys, 1977; Starfield & Mellits, 1968).

Kegel/Stream Interruption Exercises

Kegel exercises involve purposeful manipulation of the muscles necessary to prematurely terminate urination or contraction of the muscles of the pelvic floor (Kegel, 1951; Muellner, 1960). Originally developed for stress incontinence in women (Kegel), a version of these exercises—stream interruption—has been used in NE treatment packages for years (Christophersen & Friman, 2004; Friman, 1986, 1995; Jones & Friman, 1998, 2005). For children, stream interruption requires initiating and terminating urine flow at least once a day during a urinary episode. The use of stream interruption exercises in the treatment of NE is logical from a physiological perspective, because terminating an actual or impending urinary episode involves the same muscle systems. A major study of Kegel exercises showed that their regular practice eliminated accidents in 47 of 79 children with diurnal enuresis. Stream interruption was used to train the appropriate muscle contractions, but dry contraction composed the exercise and it was held for 5 to 10 seconds, followed by a 5-second rest, 10 times, on 3 separate occasions a day (Schneider et al.,1994). Of the 52 children who also wet at night, nocturnal episodes were eliminated in 18 and improved in 9 children.

Waking Schedule

This treatment component involves waking enuretic children and guiding them to the bathroom for urination. Results obtained are attributed to a change in arousal, increased access to the reinforcing properties of dry nights (Bollard & Nettlebeck, 1982), and urinary urge in lighter stages of sleep (Scharf & Jennings, 1988). In a representative study using a staggered waking schedule, four of nine children reduced their accidents to less than twice a week, suggesting a waking schedule may improve, but is unlikely to cure, NE (Creer & Davis, 1975). The early use of waking schedules typically required full awakening, often with sessions that occurred in the middle of the night (e.g., Creer & Davis, 1975; Azrin et al., 1974). But subsequent research showed partial awakening (e.g., Rolider & Van Houten, 1986; Rolider et al., 1984) or conducting waking ns just before the parent's normal bedtime (Bollard & Nettlebeck, was just as effective. Thus, these less stringent methods are now a ational component of multicomponent treatment plans (e.g., Friman, 1986, 1995; Friman & Jones, 1998, 2005; Houts & Liebert, 1985). In fact, a component analysis of Dry Bed Training showed that a combination of the reduced effort waking schedule and the urine alarm produced results that were close to those produced by the full program (Bollard & Nettlebeck, 1982).

Overlearning

An adjunct related to RCT involves overlearning. Like the RCT procedure, this method requires that children drink extra fluids—but just prior to bedtime. Overlearning is an adjunctive strategy only and is used primarily to enhance the maintenance of treatment effects established by alarm-based means. Thus, it should not be initiated until a dryness criterion has been reached (e.g., seven dry nights; Houts & Liebert, 1985).

Cleanliness Training

Some form of consequential effort directed toward returning soiled beds, bed clothing, and pajamas to a presoiled state is a standard part of DBT (Azrin et al., 1974), FSHT (Houts et al., 1984a, 1985; Houts & Liebert, 1985), and other variations (e.g., Luciano et al., 1993). It has not been evaluated independently of other components and, thus, the extent of its contribution to outcome is unknown. Its contribution to the logic of treatment, however, suggests its status as a treatment component is probably permanent.

Reward Systems

Contingent rewards alone are unlikely to cure NE but are a component of Dry Bed Training (Azrin et al., 1974), have been included in many multiple-component treatment programs since then (e.g., Luciano et al., 1993), and are routinely recommended in papers describing effective treatment (e.g., Chrisophersen & Friman, 2004; Friman, 1986, 1995; Friman & Jones, 1998, 2005). With the current state of the literature, it is impossible to determine their independent role in treatment. A plausible possibility is that they sustain the enuretic child's motivation to participate in treatment, especially when the system reinforces success in small steps. If dry nights are initially infrequent and motivation begins to wane, decreases in the size of the urine stain can be used as the criteria for earning a reward. In the initial report of this method, tracing paper was laid over the spot and the number of 1-inch squares contained within the spot was counted (Ruckstuhl & Friman, 2003).

Additional Components with Less Empirical Support and/or Conventional Usage

Self-Monitoring

Self-monitoring provides data that can be used to evaluate progress and, when used for that purpose, does not appear to involve treatment. One simple method for monitoring NE merely requires the child to record on a calendar whether the previous night was wet or dry. A more complex and more sensitive method involves the size of spot measure described above (Ruckstuhl & Friman, 2003). In addition to supplying data, however, the literature on self-monitoring shows it has reactive properties and thus can actually be considered a treatment component. The direction of the change self-monitoring brings about is determined by the valence of the behaviors that are monitored (e.g., Nelson, 1977). Because nocturnal wetting is view negatively by afflicted children, their self-monitoring of it could produce decreases.

Hypnotism

A major obstacle to appraising hypnotism from an evidence-based perspective is the difficulty in operationally defining what it actually is. Here it will be considered hyper-relaxation brought about by an arousal reducing verbal interaction between child and therapist, the end result of which is an increase in instructional control or susceptibility to suggestion. Once the relaxed state is achieved, the therapist makes a number of suggestions pertaining to continence. In the best-known study using hypnosis for treatment of enuresis, 31 of 40 subjects became fully continent (Olness, 1975). A subsequent independent study reported full continence in 20 of 28 bedwetting participants (Stanton, 1979). The results of the two studies, although remarkable, were reported more than 25 years ago, and full independent replications have not been reported. Additionally, studies attempting to determine the additive role of hypnosis to treatment packages have produced inconsistent results (e.g., Edwards & Van Der Spuy, 1985; Banerjee et al., 1993). Therefore, the evidence-based picture of hypnosis is unclear from two perspectives: clear operationalized descriptions of the independent variable and outcome data.

Paired Associations

Paired association involves pairing Kegel exercises (stream interruption) with the urine alarm in a reward-based program. In a typical scenario, a tape recording of the urine alarm sounding at strategically placed temporal intervals is taken into the bathroom by the child and played as urination proceeds. At each sounding of the alarm on the tape, the child stops urine flow. The number of starts and stops are then included in part of a reward-based interaction between child and parent. The paired-association procedure has not yet been evaluated, but some basic literature supports its potential effectiveness. For example, sleeping persons can make discriminations between stimuli on the basis of meaningfulness and prior training (Oswald et al., 1960), and the probability of a correct discrimination is significantly improved through contingent reinforcement (Zung & Wilson, 1961). Thus, reinforcing a relationship between stream interruption and the alarm while the child is awake may increase the probability the child will interrupt urination in response to the alarm while asleep.

Cognitive Therapy

Cognitive therapy, a version of psychotherapy, competed favorably with conditioning treatment in a comparative trial more than a decade ago (Ronen et al., 1992). Although two other papers describing successful cognitive therapy have been published by the same group (Ronen et al., 1995; Ronen & Wozner, 1995), they essentially report the same findings. From an evidence-based perspective, these findings should be viewed with caution, for several reasons. After more than a decade, the findings still have not been independently replicated, despite the ease of their application. Second, the findings are dramatically inconsistent, with over 50 years of research showing the routine success of behavioral approaches and routine failure of purely psychological (e.g., cognitive) approaches to treatment of NE (Friman, 1986, 1995; Friman & Jones, 1998; Houts, 1991, 2000; Mellon & McGrath, 2000). Third, the authors made no attempt to explain how a purely cognitive approach could so powerfully influence a problem that has such a fundamentally biological basis. Fourth and finally, the original study is flawed methodologically in several ways (see Houts, 2000, for a thorough critique).

Medication

Although the primary purpose of this chapter is to survey evidence-based psychological approaches to NE, the literature indicates that physicians prescribe drug therapy for NE more frequently than they do any other treatment (Blackwell & Currah, 1973; Cohen, 1975; Fergusson et al., 1986; Rauber & Maroncelli, 1984; Vogel et al., 1996). Because of the necessity of physician involvement in NE, the widespread use of drug therapy by physicians, and the dominating influence of the biobehavioral model of NE, it is likely that medication will often be part of treatment (e.g., Christophersen & Friman, 2004; Friman 1995; Friman & Jones, 1998, 2005; Houts, 1991; Mellon & McGrath, 2000). Therefore, the two most commonly prescribed types of medications—antidepressants and antidiuretics—will be briefly discussed here.

Tricyclic Antidepressants

Historically, tricyclic antidepressants were the drugs of choice for treatment of NE, and imipramine was the most frequently prescribed drug treatment (Blackwell & Currah, 1973; Foxman et al., 1986; Rauber & Maroncelli, 1984; Stephenson, 1979). The mechanism by which imipramine reduces bed wetting is still, for the most part, unknown (Stephenson, 1979). In doses between 25 and 75 mg given at bedtime, imipramine has produced initial reductions in wetting in substantial numbers of enuretic children, often within the first week of treatment (Blackwell & Currah, 1973). Reviews of both short- and long-term studies show NE usually recurs when tricyclic therapeutic agents are withdrawn (Ambrosini, 1984). The permanent cure produced with imipramine is reported to be 25% (ranging from 5–40%) (Blackwell & Currah, 1973; Houts et al., 1994). There are some concerns with the use of imipramine for NE, ranging from a potential detrimental effect on behavioral treatment (Houts et al., 1984b) to a large number of unpleasant and sometimes unhealthful side effects (e.g., Cohen, 1975; Friman, 1986; Herson et al., 1979).

Antidiuretics

As described in the section on etiology, Norgaard and colleagues reported on a small number of enuretic children who had abnormal circadian patterns of ADH (Norgaard et al., 1985; Rittig et al., 1989). As a result of these reports, desmopressin (DDAVP), an analogue of ADH, has rapidly became a popular treatment for NE, and it appears to have displaced the tricyclics as the most prescribed treatment. DDAVP concentrates urine, thereby decreasing urine volume and intravesical pressure, which makes the physiological dynamics that precede urination less probable and nocturnal continence more probable. DDAVP also has far fewer side effects than imipramine (Dimson, 1986; Ferrie et al., 1984; Norgaard et al., 1985; Novello & Novello, 1987; Pedersen et al., 1985; Post et al., 1983). Recommended dosages are 10 to 20 ug taken at bedtime.

Research on DDAVP has yielded mixed results, with success in some studies (Dimson, 1986; Pederson et al., 1985; Post et al., 1983) but not in others (Ferrie et al., 1984; Scharf & Jennings, 1988). A recent review indicated that fewer than 25% of children become dry on the drug (a much larger percentage show some improvement) and, similar to tricyclics, its effects appear to last only as long as the drug is taken and are less likely to occur in younger children or children who have frequent accidents (Moffat et al., 1993; see also Houts et al., 1994; Pederson et al., 1985; Post et al., 1983). Additionally, DDAVP is very expensive. Nonetheless, its treatment effects, when they occur, are as immediate as imipramine but with fewer side effects. Thus, DDAVP may be preferable to imipramine as an adjunct to treatment, and a review of the relevant literature suggested including it with alarm-based treatment has the potential to boost the already high success obtained by the alarm to 100% (Mellon & McGrath, 2000).

FUNCTIONAL ENCOPRESIS (FE)

Diagnosis

FE is a common, undertreated, and often overinterpreted form of fecal incontinence. The definition of FE has remained relatively consistent across versions of the DSM, and the current version (DSM-IV; American Psychiatric Association, 1994) lists four criteria: (1) repeated passage of feces into inappropriate places whether involuntary or intentional; (2) at least one such event a month for at least three months; (3) chronological age is at least 4 years (or equivalent developmental level); and (4) the behavior is not due exclusively to the direct physiological effects of a substance or a general medical condition except through a mechanism involving constipation. The DSM also describes two types: primary, in which the child has never had fecal continence, and secondary, in which incontinence returns after at least six months of continence. Because research on treatment typically does not distinguish between the two, they will be collapsed here.

Although all forms of incontinence require evaluation and treatment, FE, when left untreated, is more likely than other forms (such as NE) to lead to serious and potentially life-threatening medical sequelae and seriously impaired social acceptance, relations, and development. The reasons for the medical sequelae will be summarized briefly in the Etiology and Evaluation sections below. The primary reason for the social impairment is that soiling evokes more revulsion from peers, parents, and important others than other forms of incontinence (and most other behavioral problems). As an example, severe corporal punishment for fecal accidents was still recommended by professionals in the late 19th century (Henoch, 1889).

Etiology

Successful treatment for FE targets the processes that cause the condition, and 90–95% of cases occur as a function of, or in conjunction with, reduced colonic motility, constipation, and fecal retention, and the various behavioral/dietary factors contributing to these conditions. These factors include (1) insufficient roughage or bulk in the diet; (2) irregular diet; (3) insufficient oral intake of fluids; (4) medications that may have a side effect of constipation; (5) unstructured, inconsistent, and/or punitive approaches to toilet training; and (6) toileting avoidance by the child. Any of these factors, singly or in combination, increases the risk of reduced colonic motility, actual constipation, and corresponding uncomfortable or painful bowel movements. Uncomfortable or painful bowel movements, in turn, negatively reinforce fecal retention, and retention leads to a regressive reciprocal cycle often resulting in regular fecal accidents. When the constipation is severe or the cycle is chronic, fecal impaction, a large blockage caused by the collection of hard, dry stool, may develop. Not infrequently, liquid fecal matter will seep around the fecal mass, producing "paradoxical diarrhea." Although the child is actually constipated, he or she appears to have diarrhea. Some parents will attempt to treat this type of "diarrhea" with over-the-counter antidiarrheal agents, which only worsen the problem.

Of note is that a small minority of cases do not involve any problems with colonic motility or constipation; they involve regular, well-formed, soft bowel movements that occur somewhere other than the toilet. The process underlying these cases is not well understood except that they tend to be treatment-resistant (Christophersen & Friman, 2004; Friman & Jones, 1998; also see Landman & Rappaport, 1985).

Evaluation

As with NE, treatment for encopresis should not proceed until the afflicted child has received a medical evaluation, for two fundamental reasons. First, encopresis can be the result of organic diseases (e.g., Hirschsprung's disease, hypothyroidism) and, although rare, these are real and need to be ruled out or identified and treated before a behavioral approach to treatment is pursued. The second reason involves the medical risk posed by fecal matter inexorably accumulating in an organ with a limited amount of space. An unfortunately all-too-frequent presenting problem in medical clinics is an encopretic child who has been in extended therapy with a nonmedical professional and whose initial evaluation did not include referral for a medical evaluation and whose treatment did not address the etiology of FE. As a result, the children's colonic systems can become painfully and dangerously distended, sometimes to the point of being life-threatening (e.g., McGuire et al., 1983). The medical evaluation will typically involve a thorough medical, dietary, and bowel history. In addition, abdominal palpitation and rectal examination are used to check for large amounts of fecal matter, very dry fecal matter in the rectal vault, and poor sphincter tone. Approximately 70% of constipation can be determined on physical exam, and detection can be increased to above 90% with a KUB (X-ray of kidneys, ureter, and bladder) (Barr et al., 1979).

Following the medical evaluation, a full fecal elimination history should be obtained, including toilet training, dietary habits, parent and child responses to accidents and successful bowel movements, parent-child interactional style, level of instructional control, and emotional and psychological functioning. Regarding the latter, although the primary causes of encopresis are biological and not psychological (see also Friman et al., 1988), in some cases it is secondary to extraordinary emotional disturbance and thus resistant to behavioral/medical treatment focused only on toileting (e.g., Landman & Rappaport, 1985). In such cases, the emotional condition may be a treatment priority, especially when there is no evidence of constipation or fecal retention.

Treatment-Retentive FE

There are multiple parallels between evidence-supported treatment for NE and FE. For example, as with NE, the best-supported treatments for encopresis include multiple components and are typically delivered in a "package"-type format. Additionally, there are core components, which can be augmented by additional approaches to treatment. Distinct from NE, the core components of treatment for FE are primarily medical and include full bowel evacuation, facilitating medication, dietary recommendations, and scheduled toilet sitting. Early research on the medical approach to treatment produced successful outcomes (e.g., Davidson,

1958; Davidson et al., 1963; Levine, 1982), but more recent research has achieved somewhat lower levels of success. As a result, the primarily medical approach for encopresis does not meet the Chambless criteria for any category of efficacy (e.g., McGrath et al., 2000). However, there is mounting evidence showing that augmenting medical treatment with biofeedback and/or behavioral components improves success rates sufficiently well for various combinations to earn efficacious or probably efficacious ratings (Cox et al., 1998, 2003; Christophersen & Friman, 2004; McGrath et al., 2000; Stark et al., 1990, 1997). The greater success of augmented approaches notwithstanding, the medical approach to FE remains the dominant method of treatment prescribed in the medical community (the primary source of treatment for the vast majority of cases), has its own rather extensive supportive literature, is closely linked to causal mechanisms, and represents a significant departure from the failed psychodynamic approach to FE (e.g., Christophersen & Friman, 2004; Friman, 2002, 2003; Friman & Jones, 1998, 2005; Levine, 1982). For these reasons, the primary components of the medical approach will be described below and will be followed by a description of some of the biofeedback and behavioral approaches to treatment of FE.

Medical Treatment

Bowel Evacuation

The primary goal of FE treatment is the establishment of regular bowel movements in the toilet, and the first step is to cleanse the bowel completely of resident fecal matter (Christophersen & Friman, 2004; Friman, 2003; Levine, 1982). A variety of methods are used, the most common of which involve enemas and/or laxatives. Although any properly trained professional can assist with the recommendations of these (e.g., with suggestions about timing, interactional style, behavioral management, etc.), the evacuation procedure must be prescribed and overseen by the child's physician. Typically, evacuation procedures are conducted in the child's home, but severe resistance can necessitate medical assistance, in which case they must be completed in a medical setting. The ultimate goal, however, is complete parent management of evacuation procedures because they are to be used whenever the child's eliminational pattern suggests excessive fecal retention.

Facilitating Medication

Successful treatment for FE will almost always require inclusion of medications that soften fecal matter, ease its migration through the colon, and/or aid its expulsion from the rectum. The discovery of the therapeutic benefits of facilitating medication represents the advent of the medical approach to FE and the departure from the historically psychodynamic approach (Davidson, 1958; Davidson et al., 1963; Levine, 1982). The decision to use medication as well as the type of medication is the consulting physician's to make but, as with bowel evacuation, any trained professional can inform the decision and educate the parent about its use. Generally, it is best to avoid interfering with the sensitive biochemistry of the alimentary system (the colonic portion of it in particular) and, thus, inert or only mildly noninert substances are preferred. Formerly, the most frequently used substance was mineral oil, used either alone or in combination with other ingredients such as magnesium. As indicated, prescription of the substance is the physician's prerogative, but ensuring compliance with the prescription is typically a psychological task. Children will often resist ingesting substances with odd tastes and textures. Therefore, to gain their cooperation, it is often necessary to mix the substances with a preferred liquid (e.g., orange juice) and follow ingestion with praise and appreciation. A recent development, however, makes this task even easier while also improving outcomes for children with FE. Polyethylene glycol (trade name, Miralax) is an odorless, tasteless powdered laxative that can be mixed with food or liquid with limited possibility of child detection, it has produced excellent results in treatment of childhood constipation and FE, and it is increasingly becoming the preferred medical treatment option (e.g., Tucker, 2003).

Dietary Changes

As indicated in the section on etiology, diet often plays a causal role in FE, and dietary changes are often part of treatment. Increased dietary fiber increases colonic motility and the moisture in colonic contents and facilitates easier and more regular bowel movements. Although some evaluative trials have not included fiber-based recommendations in the treatment protocol, there is no medical reason for this nor did the research yield results that would contribute substantively to established etiological theory (e.g., Houts & Peterson, 1986; see also McGrath et al., 2000).

Dietary changes can also be enhanced with over-the-counter preparations with dense fiber content (e.g., *Metamucil, Perdiem*). In addition to recommendations about increases in fiber, some investigators have also included recommendations about increased fluid intake. The reason for this is ensuring that a child with FE is sufficiently hydrated to maintain soft stools.

Scheduling Toilet Sits

Regularity is the goal of treatment; therefore, regular toilet sits are an important part of it. The time should not be during school hours because unpleasant social responses to bowel movements in the school setting can cause regressive responses to treatment (e.g., stool retention; see Levine, 1982). Choosing among the times that remain (morning, afternoon, or evening) is guided by the child's typical habits and child-parent time constraints. Establishing a time shortly after food intake can increase chances of success through the influence of the gastrocolonic reflex. In the early stages of treatment, or in difficult cases, two scheduled attempts a day (e.g., after breakfast and dinner) are often necessary. The time the child is required to sit on the toilet should be limited to 10 or fewer minutes in order to avoid unnecessarily increasing the aversive properties of the toileting experience. The child's feet should be supported by a flat surface (e.g., floor or a small stool) to increase comfort, maintain circulation in the extremities, and facilitate the abdominal push necessary to expel fecal matter from the body. The time should also be unhurried and free from distraction or observation by anyone other than the managing parent. Allowing children to listen to music, read, or talk with the parent may improve child attitude toward toileting requirements. Generally, toileting should be a relaxed, pleasant, and ultimately private affair.

Supplements to Medical Treatment: Biofeedback and Behavioral Treatments

Biofeedback

The best-known and most specific supplemental approach to treatment of FE is biofeedback. Briefly, biofeedback uses sensors attached to strategic parts of the body to amplify physiological responses (e.g., heart rate, skin temperature, muscle tension), allowing the person to perceive them more vividly than would otherwise be possible. Typically, the responses are "fed" back to the subject using enhanced auditory, tactile, or visual display (Friman, in press). The earliest biofeedback study on FE showed that afflicted children often do not detect a full bowel until their intracolonic pressure exceeds extraordinary levels, sometimes more than 10 times the pressure needed to establish detection in nonencopretic children (Meunier et al., 1976). As a result, these children often fail to detect peristalsis, have grossly delayed urges to defecate, exhibit infrequent and very large bowel movements, and have chronic fecal accidents. There is also a subsample of children with FE who paradoxically contract their external anal sphincter as they "bear down" for a bowel movement, thus attempting and preventing a successful movement with the same action (e.g., Loening-Baucke, 1990).

Generally, biofeedback treatment for FE involves training the voluntary contraction of the external anal sphincter and functionally related muscle systems in response to rectal filling. The training improves rectal sensory perception, strength, coordination, or some combination of these three components. The sensory training is achieved by inducing intrarectal pressure using a balloon feedback device inserted into the rectum. The balloon is then filled with air to produce a sensation of rectal filling. The children are subsequently trained to detect the stimulation resulting from the distension and to respond either with contraction of the external sphincter if they are not on the toilet or with relaxation if they are. The overarching purpose of the training (typical of all biofeedback programs; Friman, in press) is to increase awareness of a subtle sensation (fecal material in the rectum) and train appropriate responses. Biofeedback can be used in isolation, but it is often combined with other components. There was initial evidence of its success (e.g., Loening-Baucke, 1990);

however, several large studies, one by the author of the first major study to recommend biofeedback, have provided data that call into question the additive value of biofeedback for medical treatment (e.g., Loening-Baucke, 1995; Nolan et al., 2001; van der Plas et al., 1996) and for medical plus behavioral treatment (Cox et al., 1996).

Behavioral Treatment

A broad range of components loosely grouped under the term "behavioral treatments" have been combined with medical treatments as well as medical plus biofeedback treatments. The primary component includes two types of consequential events. The first involves requiring that children participate in their own cleaning, including wiping and caring for soiled clothing. Although this component has not been independently evaluated, it is a routine component in most treatment programs, and there is no apparent logical basis to exclude it. The second consequential event involves rewards for efforts or success. These have been included in multiple evaluations involving successful treatment of single subjects (e.g., Houts & Peterson, 1986; O'Brien et al., 1986) and groups of subjects (see McGrath et al., 2000). Additional behavioral components include stimulus control procedures, enhanced scheduling, enhanced health education, relaxation techniques, and various types of monitoring. Behavioral components have been included in almost all empirically supported approaches to treatment of FE.

Evidence of Effectiveness

Over the past 20 years, several descriptive and controlled experimental studies have supplemented variations on the medical treatments described above with behavioral approaches, which has led to several comprehensive biobehavioral treatment packages for FE (e.g., Christophersen & Friman, 2004; Friman 2003; Friman & Jones, 1998; McGrath et al., 2000). The research suggests that effective treatment for FE, as with effective treatment for NE, depends upon core treatment components (i.e., medical treatment), and the probability of success mounts with the inclusion of other components, especially those composing the behavioral approach to treatment.

The literature on this "comprehensive approach" includes multiple single-subject evaluations (e.g., O'Brien et al., 1986) and group trials (e.g., Lowery et al., 1985). For example, in a study of 58 children with encopresis, 60% were completely continent after five months, and those who did not achieve full continence averaged a 90% decrease in accidents (Lowery et al., 1985). A more recent study reported on a comparison of three treatment conditions: (1) medical care (including enemas for disimpaction and laxatives to promote frequent bowel movements); (2) Enhanced Toilet Training—a comprehensive approach very similar to the one described above (using reinforcement and scheduling to promote response to defecation urges and instruction and modeling to promote appropriate straining, along with laxatives and enemas); and (3) biofeedback (directed at relaxing the external anal sphincter during attempted defection, along with toilet training, laxatives, and enemas). At three months after treatment, the Enhanced Toilet Training group significantly benefited more children than the other two treatments, with fewer treatment sessions and lower costs (Cox et al., 1998).

The multiple successes of the single-subject and group evaluations of the comprehensive approach to treatment have led to evaluation of group treatment. In the initial evaluation, 18 encopretic children between the ages of 4 and 11 years and their parents were seen in groups of three to five families for six sessions. Noteworthy is that all of these children had previously failed a medical regimen. The sessions in this trial focused on a much-expanded regimen very similar to that described above. Soiling accidents decreased by 84% across the groups, and these results were maintained or improved at six months' follow-up (Stark et al., 1990). Additionally, the results were subsequently replicated in a much larger group (Stark et al., 1997). The successes of the comprehensive approach to treatment in small N and large N studies (focused on treating individuals) and large N studies treating groups have led treatment to be supplied entirely by an interactive Internet-based program that has shown to be highly effective (Ritterbrand et al., 2003).

FE (Without Constipation)

Treatment of nonretentive FE has been the focus of far less research than treatment of the retentive type; therefore, it would be premature to argue that any known approach is empirically supported. From the small available literature, it appears that treatment of these children should be preceded by a comprehensive psychological evaluation. Virtually all investigators who have described this subsample of children report emotional and behavioral problems and treatment resistance (e.g., Landman & Rappaport, 1985), and it is possible that some of these children's soiling is related to modifiable aspects of their social ecology. Some investigators have employed versions of the approach outlined above and included supportive verbal therapy (Landman & Rappaport, 1985), or they have specifically taught parents how to manage their children's misbehavior (Stark et al., 1990). Thus, it appears that effective treatment of this subsample would involve only some components of the comprehensive approach to treatment (e.g., facilitating medication may not be needed) combined with some form of treatment for psychological and behavioral problems.

CONCLUSION

NE and FE have been misunderstood, misinterpreted, and mistreated for centuries. During the last half of the 20th century, however, and particularly toward its end, a fuller, biobehavioral understanding of their causal conditions and an empirically supported approach to their treatment emerged. The biobehavioral understanding and approach to NE and FE are dramatically different than the psychogenic understanding and approach of history. The biobehavioral approach addresses the physiology of elimination primarily and addresses the psychology of the child as a set of variables that are not causal but can be critical to active participation in treatment. The psychogenic approach, however, addressed the psychology of the child primarily, especially insofar as causal variables were of interest, and gave minimal attention to the physiology of elimination. Although evaluation and treatment of NE and FE absolutely require the direct involvement of a physician, ideal management involves a partnership among the physician, therapist, and family. This united, empirically supported, biobehavioral approach can alleviate incontinence and eliminate or at least minimize the possibility of the damaging overinterpretation and dangerous forms of treatment that blemished the approach to NE and FE from antiquity throughout large portions of the 20th century.

REFERENCES

Ambrosini, P. J. (1984). A pharmacological paradigm for urinary continence and enuresis. *Journal of Clinical Psychopharmacology, 4,* 247–253.

American Psychiatric Association (1994). *Diagnostic and Statistical Manual of Mental Disorders,* 4th ed. Washington, DC.

Azrin, N. H., Sneed, T. J., & Foxx, R. M. (1974). Dry-bed training: Rapid elimination of childhood enuresis. *Behavior Research & Therapy, 12,* 147–156.

Banerjee, S., Srivastav, A., & Palan, B. (1993). Hypnosis and self-hypnosis in the management of nocturnal enuresis: A comparative study with imipramine therapy. *American Journal of Clinical Hypnosis, 36,* 113–119.

Barr, R. G., Levine, M. D., Wilkinson, R. H., & Mulvihill, D. (1979). Chronic and occult stool retention: A clinical tool for its evaluation in school aged children. *Clinical Pediatrics, 18,* 674–686.

Blackwell, B., & Currah, J. (1973). The psychopharmacology of nocturnal enuresis. In I. Kolvin, R. C. MacKeith, & S. R. Meadow (Eds.), *Bladder Control and Enuresis* (pp. 231–257). Philadelphia: Lippincott.

Bollard, J., & Nettlebeck, T. (1982). A component analysis of dry-bed training for treatment of bed-wetting. *Behavior Research & Therapy, 20,* 383–390.

Butler, R. J. (2004). Childhood nocturnal enuresis: Developing a conceptual framework. *Clinical Psychology Review, 24,* 909–931.

Byrd, R. S., Weitzman, M., Lanphear, N. E., & Auinger, P. (1996). Bed-wetting in US children: Epidemiology and related behavior problems, *Pediatrics, 98,* 414–419.

Christophersen, E. R., & Friman, P. C. (2004). Elimination disorders. In R. Brown (Ed.), *Handbook of Pediatric Psychology in School Settings* (pp. 467–488). Mahwah, NJ: Lawrence Erlbaum.

Cohen, M. W. (1975). Enuresis. *Pediatric Clinics of North America, 22,* 545–560.

Cox, D. J., Sutphen, J., Borowitz, S., Kovatchev, B., & Ling, W. (1998). Contribution of behavior therapy and biofeedback to laxative therapy in the treatment of pediatric encopresis. *Annals of Behavioral Medicine, 20*(2), 70–76.

Cox, D. J., Sutphen, J., Ling, W., Quillian, W., & Borowitz, S. (1996). Additive benefits of laxative, toilet training, and biofeedback therapies in the treatment of pediatric encopresis. *Journal of Pediatric Psychology, 21,* 659–670.

Creer, T. L., & Davis, M. H. (1975). Using a staggered waking procedure with enuretic children in an institutional setting. *Journal of Behavior Therapy & Experimental Psychiatry, 6,* 23–25.

Davidson, M. (1958). Constipation and fecal incontinence. *Pediatric Clinics of North America, 5,* 749–757.

Davidson, M., Kugler, M. M., & Bauer, C. H. (1963). Diagnosis and management in children with severe and protracted constipation and obstipation. *Journal of Pediatrics, 62,* 261–275.

Dimson, S. B. (1977). Desmopressin as a treatment for enuresis. *Lancet, 1,* 1260.

Dimson, S. B. (1986). DDAVP and urine osmolality in refractory enuresis. *Archives of Diseases in Children, 61,* 1104–1107.

Doleys, D. M. (1977). Behavioral treatments for nocturnal enuresis in children: A review of the literature. *Psychological Bulletin, 84,* 30–54.

Edwards, S., & Van Der Spuy, H. (1985). Hypnotherapy as a treatment for enuresis. *Journal of Child Psychology and Psychiatry, 26,* 161–170.

Fergusson, D. M., Horwood, L. J., & Sannon, F. T. (1986). Factors related to the age of attainment of nocturnal bladder control: An 8-year longitudinal study. *Pediatrics, 78,* 884–890.

Ferrie, B. G., MacFarlane, J., & Glen, E. S. (1984). DDAVP in young enuretic patients: A double-blind trial. *British Journal of Urology, 56,* 376–378.

Finn, R. (2005). Clinic rounds. *Pediatric News, 39*(11), 43.

Foxman, B., Valdez, R. B., & Brook, R. H. (1986). Childhood enuresis: Prevalence, perceived impact, and prescribed treatments. *Pediatrics, 77,* 482–487.

Friman, P. C. (in press). Behavior assessment. In D. Barlow, F. Andrasik, & M. Hersen. *Single Case Experimental Designs.* Boston: Allyn & Bacon.

Friman, P. C. (1986). A preventive context for enuresis. *Pediatric Clinics of North America, 33,* 871–886.

Friman, P. C. (1995). Nocturnal enuresis in the child. In R. Ferber & M. H. Kryger (Eds.), *Principles and Practice of Sleep Medicine in the Child* (pp. 107–114). Philadelphia: Saunders.

Friman, P.C. (2002). The Psychopathological Interpretation of Common Child Behavior Problems: A Critique and Related Opportunity for Behavior Analysis. Invited address at the 28th annual convention of the Association for Behavior Analysis, Toronto, Canada.

Friman, P. C. (2003). A biobehavioral bowel and toilet training treatment for functional encopresis. In W. O'Donohue, S. Hayes, and J. Fisher. Cognitive Behaviour Therapy: Empirically supported Techniques in Your Practice (pp.51–58). New York: Wiley.

Friman, P. C., Handwerk, M. L., Swearer, S. M., McGinnis, C., & Warzak, W. J. (1998). Do children with primary nocturnal enuresis have clinically significant behavior problems? *Archives of Pediatrics and Adolescent Medicine, 152,* 537–539.

Friman, P. C., & Jones, K. M. (1998). Elimination disorders in children. In S. Watson & F. Gresham (Eds.), *Handbook of Child Behavior Therapy* (pp. 239–260). New York: Plenum Press.

Friman, P. C., & Jones, K. M. (2005). Behavioral treatment for nocturnal enuresis. *Journal of Early and Intensive Behavioral Intervention, 2,* 259–267.

Gellis, S. S. (1994). Are enuretics truly hard to arouse? *Pediatric Notes, 18,* 113.

Glicklich, L. B. (1951). An historical account of enuresis. *Pediatrics, 8,* 859–876.

Gross, R. T., & Dornbusch, S. M. (1983). Enuresis. In M. D. Levine, W. B. Carey, A. C. Crocker, & R. T. Gross (Eds.), *Developmental-Behavioral Pediatrics* (pp. 575–586). Philadelphia: Saunders.

Helfer, R. & Kempe, C. H. (1976). *Child Abuse and Neglect.* Cambridge, MA: Ballinger.

Henoch, E. H. (1889). *Lectures on Children's Diseases,* Vol. 2. London: New Syndenham Society.

Herson, V. C., Schmitt, B. D., & Rumack, B. H. (1979). Magical thinking and imipramine poisoning in two school-aged children. *Journal of the American Medical Association, 241,* 1926–1927.

Houts, A. C. (1991). Nocturnal enuresis as a biobehavioral problem. *Behavior Therapy, 22,* 133–151.

Houts, A. C. (2000). Commentary: Treatments for enuresis: Criteria, mechanisms, and health care policy. *Journal of Pediatric Psychology, 25,* 219–224.

Houts, A. C., Berman, J. S., & Abramson, H. (1994). Effectiveness of psychological and pharmacological treatments for nocturnal enuresis. *Journal of Consulting and Clinical Psychology, 62,* 737–745.

Houts, A. C., & Liebert, R. M. (1985). *Bedwetting: A Guide for Parents.* Springfield, IL: Thomas.

Houts, A. C., & Liebert, R. M., & Padawer, W. (1984a). A delivery system for the treatment of primary enuresis. *Journal of Abnormal Child Psychology, 11,* 513–519.

Houts, A. C., & Peterson, J. K. (1986). Treatment of a retentive encopretic child using contingency management and diet modification with stimulus control. *Journal of Pediatric Psychology, 11,* 375–383.

Houts, A. C., Peterson, J. K., & Liebert, R. M. (1984b). The effects of prior imipramine treatment on the results of conditioning therapy with NE. *Journal of Pediatric Psychology, 9,* 505–508.

Houts, A. C., Peterson, J. K., & Whelan, J. P. (1986). Prevention of relapse in Full-Spectrum Home Training for primary NE: A component analysis. *Behavior Therapy, 17,* 462–469.

Jenson, W. R., & Sloane, H. N. (1979). Chart moves and grab bags: A simple contingency management. *Journal of Applied Behavior Analysis, 12,* 334.

Kaffman, M., & Elizur, E. (1977). Infants who become enuretics: A longitudinal study of 161 Kibbutz children. *Monographs of the Society for Research on Child Development, 42,* 2–12.

Kegel, A. H. (1951). Physiologic therapy for urinary stress incontinence. *Journal of the American Medical Association, 146,* 915–917.

Landman, G. B., & Rappaport, L. (1985). Pediatric management of severe treatment-resistant encopresis. *Development and Behavioral Pediatrics, 6,* 349–351.

Levine, M. D. (1982). Encopresis: Its potentiation, evaluation, and alleviation. *Pediatric Clinics of North America, 29,* 315–330.

Loening-Baucke, V. A. (1990). Modulation of abnormal defecation dynamics by biofeedback treatment in chronically constipated children with encopresis. *Journal of Pediatrics, 116,* 214–221.

Loening-Baucke, V. A. (1995). Biofeedback treatment for chronic constipation and encopresis in childhood: Long term outcome. *Pediatrics, 96,* 105–110.

Lowery, S., Srour, J., Whitehead, W. E., & Schuster, M. M. (1985). Habit training as treatment of encopresis secondary to chronic constipation. *Journal of Pediatric Gastroenterology and Nutrition, 4,* 397–401.

Luciano, M., Molina, F., Gomez, I., & Herruzo, J. (1993). Response prevention and contingency management in the treatment of nocturnal enuresis: A report of two cases. *Child and Family Behavior Therapy, 15,* 613–615.

McGrath, M. L., Mellon, M. W., & Murphy, L. (2000). Empirically supported treatments in pediatric psychology: Constipation and encopresis. *Journal of Pediatric Psychology, 25,* 225–254.

McGuire, T., Rothenberg, M B., & Tyler, D. C. (1983). Profound shock following intervention for chronic untreated stool retention. *Clinical Pediatrics, 23,* 459–461.

Mellon, M. W., & McGrath, M. L. (2000). Empirically supported treatments in pediatric psychology: Nocturnal enuresis. *Journal of Pediatric Psychology, 25,* 193–214.

Mellon, M. W., Scott, M. A., Haynes, K. B., Schmidt, D. F., & Houts, A. C. (1997). EMG recording of pelvic floor conditioning in nocturnal enuresis during urine alarm treatment: A preliminary study. Paper presentation at the Sixth Florida Conference on Child Health Psychology, University of Florida, Gainesville, FL.

Meunier, P., Marechal, J. M., & De Beaujeu, M. J. (1979). Rectoanal pressures and rectal sensitivity in chronic childhood constipation. *Gastroenterology, 77,* 330–336.

Moffatt, M. E. K., Harlos, S., Kirshen, A. J., & Burd, L. (1993). Desmopressin acetate and nocturnal enuresis: How much do we know? *Pediatrics, 92,* 420–425.

Mowrer, O. H., & Mowrer, W. M. (1938). Enuresis: A method for its study and treatment. *AmericanJournal of Orthopsychiatry, 8,* 436–459.

Muellner, R. S. (1960). Development of urinary control in children. *Journal of the American Medical Association, 172,* 1256–1261.

Muellner, R. S. (1961). Obstacles to the successful treatment of primary enuresis. *Journal of the American Medical Association, 178,* 147–148.

Nelson, R. (1977). Methodological issues in assessment via self-monitoring. In J. D. Cone & R. P. Hawkins (Eds.), *Behavioral Assessment: New Directions in Clinical Psychology*. New York: Bruner/Mazel.

Nolan, T., Debelle, G., Oberklaid, F., & Coffey, C. (1991). Randomized controlled trial of biofeedback training in persistent encopresis with anismus. *Archives of Diseases in Childhood, 79*, 131–135.

Norgaard, J. P., Pedersen, E. B., & Djurhuus, J. C. (1985). Diurnal antidiuretic hormone levels in enuretics. *Journal of Urology, 134*, 1029–1031.

Novello, A. C., & Novello, R. (1987). Enuresis. *Pediatric Clinics of North America, 34*, 719–733.

O'Brien, S., Ross, L., & Christophersen, E. R. (1986). Primary encopresis: Evaluation and treatment. *Journal of Applied Behavior Analysis, 19*, 137–145.

Olness, K. (1975). The use of self hypnosis in the treatment of childhood nocturnal enuresis. *Clinical Pediatrics, 14*, 273–279.

Oswald, K., Taylor, A. M., & Treisman, M. (1960). Discriminative responses to stimulation during human sleep. *Brain, 83*, 440–445.

Pedersen, P. S., Hejl, M., & Kjoller, S. S. (1985). Desamino-D-arginine vasopressin in childhood nocturnal enuresis. *Journal of Urology, 133*, 65–66.

Post, E. M., Richman, R. A., & Blackett, P. R. (1983). Desmopressin response of enuretic children. *American Journal of Diseases in Children, 137*, 962–963.

Rauber A., & Maroncelli, R. (1984). Prescribing practices and knowledge of tricyclic antidepressants among physicians caring for children. *Pediatrics, 73*, 107–109.

Ritterband, L. M., Cox, D. J., Walker, L. S., Kovatchev, B., McKnight, L., Patel, K., et al. (2003). An internet intervention as adjunctive therapy for pediatric encopresis. *Journal of Consulting and Clinical Psychology, 71*, 910–917.

Rittig, S., Knudsen, U. B., Norgaard, J. P., Pedersen, E. B., & Djurhuus, J. C. (1989). Abnormal diurnal rhythm of plasma vasopressin and urinary output in patients with enuresis. *American Journal of Physiology, 252*, F664–F671.

Rolider, A., & Van Houten, R. (1986). Effects of degree of awakening and the criterion for advancing awakening on the treatment of bedwetting. *Education and Treatment of Children, 9*, 135–141.

Rolider, A., Van Houten, R., & Chlebowski, I. (1984). Effects of a stringent versus lenient awakening procedure on the efficacy of the dry bed procedure. *Child and Family Behavior Therapy, 14*, 1–14.

Ronen, T., Rahav, G., & Wozner, Y. (1995). Self-control and enuresis. *Journal of Cognitive Psychotherapy, 9*, 249–258.

Ronen, T., & Wozner, Y. (1995). A self-control intervention package for the treatment of primary nocturnal enuresis. *Child and Family Behavior Therapy, 17*, 1–17.

Ronen, T., Wozner, Y., & Rahav, G. (1992). Cognitive intervention in enuresis. *Child and Family Behavior Therapy, 14*, 1–14.

Ruckstuhl, L. E., & Friman, P. C. (2003). Evaluating the effectiveness of the vibrating urine alarm: A study of effectiveness and social validity. Paper presented at the 29th annual convention of the Association for Advancement of Behavior Theraphy, San Francisco, CA.

Scharf, M. B., & Jennings, S. W. (1988). Childhood enuresis: Relationship to sleep, etiology, evaluation, and treatment. *Annals of Behavioral Medicine, 10*, 113–120.

Schmitt, B. D. (1984). Nocturnal enuresis. *Primary Care, 11*, 485–495.

Schneider, M. S., King, L. R., & Surwitt, R. S. (1994). Kegel exercises and childhood incontinence: A new role for an old treatment. *Journal of Pediatrics, 124*, 91–92.

Stanton, H. (1979). Short term treatment of enuresis. *American Journal of Clinical Hypnosis, 22*, 103–107.

Starfield, B. (1967). Functional bladder capacity in enuretic and nonenuretic children. *Journal of Pediatrics, 70*, 777–782.

Starfield, B., & Mellits, E. D. (1968). Increases in functional bladder capacity and improvements in enuresis. *Journal of Pediatrics, 72*, 483–487.

Stark, L. J., Opipari, L. C., Donaldson, D. L., Danovsky, M. R., Rasile, D. A., & DelSanto, A. F. (1997). Evaluation of a standard protocol for rententive encopresis: A replication. *Journal of Pediatric Psychology, 22*, 619–633.

Stark, L., Owens-Stively, J., Spirito, A., Lewis, A., & Guevremont, D. (1990). Group behavioral treatment of retentive encopresis. *Journal of Pediatric Psychology, 15*, 659–671.

Stephenson, J. D. (1979). Physiological and pharmacological basis for the chemotherapy of enuresis. *Psychological Medicine, 9*, 249–263.

Troup, C. W., & Hodgson, N. B. (1971). Nocturnal functional bladder capacity in enuretic children. *Journal of Urology, 105*, 129–132.

Tucker, N. T. (2003). Managing defecation disorders in children. Special supplement to *Pediatric News*. New York: International Medical News Group.

van der Plas, R. N. Benninga, M. A., Buller, H. A., Bossuyt, P. M., Akkermans, I. M., Redekop, W. K., et al. (1996). Biofeedback training in treatment of childhood constipation: A randomised clinical trial. *Lancet, 348*(9030), 776–780.

Van Tijen, N. M., Messer, A. P., & Namdar, Z. (1998). Perceived stress of nocturnal enuresis in childhood. *British Journal of Urology, 81* (Suppl 3), 98–99.

Vogel, W., Young, M., & Primack W. (1996). A survey of physician use of treatment methods for functional enuresis. *Journal of Developmental Behavioral Pediatrics, 17*, 90–93.

Zung, W. W., & Wilson, W. P. (1961). Responses to auditory stimulation during sleep. *Archives of General Psychiatry, 4*, 548–552.

19

Evidence-Based Therapies for Children and Adolescents with Eating Disorders

DAVID H. GLEAVES and JANET D. LATNER

"'Is evidence-based treatment of anorexia nervosa possible?',
the answer must be 'Barely'."

(Fairburn, 2005, p. S29)

The principal eating disorders in the current *Diagnostic and Statistical Manual of Mental Disorders* (American Psychiatric Association, 2000) are anorexia nervosa (AN), bulimia nervosa (BN), and eating disorder not otherwise specified (EDNOS), which may designate binge eating disorder (BED) or atypical variants of AN or BN. As with adults, the atypical variants of eating disorders appear to be more common than the specified disorders (Kjelsås et al., 2004). In earlier versions of the DSM (up to the 3rd edition, revised), the eating disorders were listed within the *Disorders usually first evident in infancy, childhood, or adolescence* section. Given their prominence among adults, they were moved to their own section in the most recent edition. However, their common origin in childhood should not be forgotten and is the focus of this chapter.

Obesity is also a common eating-related problem among children and adolescents, and there are also several eating-/feeding-related problems that are usually first diagnosed in infancy or early childhood and are thus included in that section of the DSM-IV. These are pica, rumination disorder, and feeding disorder of infancy or early childhood (sometimes referred to as failure to thrive). In this chapter, we will focus on AN and BN and somewhat on BED. Pediatric obesity is covered by Johnston and Tyler (Chapter 20). Given that we will focus largely on treatment rather than

---

DAVID H. GLEAVES • University of Canterbury and **JANET D. LATNER** • University of Hawaii

DAVID H. GLEAVES • University of Canterbury and **JANET D. LATNER** • University of Hawaii

assessment, readers may want to consult Netemeyer and Williamson (2001) for an overview of the assessment of eating disorders among children and adolescents.

Anorexia Nervosa

AN involves a refusal to maintain a minimally normal body weight, an intense fear of gaining weight, and some form of body image disturbance. In postmenarcheal females, there is also amenorrhea. Within the current DSM scheme, there are restricting and binge eating/purging subtypes of AN. There is also commonly a wealth of additional psychopathology including mood disorders, substance use, and personality disorders (Gleaves & Eberenz, 1993), although the presence of such additional psychopathology is not as well established among children and adolescents as among adults. Among the former, what may be more often seen is oppositional and defiant behaviors that may lead to confusion as to whether or not the disordered eating is a manifestation of oppositional defiant disorder (Netemeyer & Williamson, 2001).

For adolescents, the prevalence rate of AN is not completely clear. However, Kjelsås et al. (2004) reported a lifetime prevalence of 0.7% and 0.2% among a sample of 14- to 15-year-old girls and boys, respectively. There are no clear data on the prevalence of AN among younger children, although cases have been reported in the literature. Of the psychiatric disorders, AN appears to have the highest mortality rate (Agras, 2001) (due to both physical complications and suicide) and may pose particular risks for the developing child or adolescent, such as impaired linear growth and osteoporosis (Katzman, 2005). Although some effects may be reversible if caught in time, others may be permanent.

Recognizing the disorder in children and adolescents presents many challenges. First, in a prepubescent female (or a male), the amenorrhea criterion is not applicable. Second, there may not be a noticeable weight loss but rather a failure to achieve normal weight or gain weight at a normal rate. Related to this challenge, normal weight is also sometimes a challenge to determine and quantify. Cutoffs based on body mass index [weight (in kg)/height (in meters)^2] are often used with adults, but BMIs are interpreted differently with children. Percent of expected weight (based on weight and age) is most meaningful (Fisher et al., 1995), with 15% below expected weight being the cutoff typically used (and is so designated in the DSM-IV). A related concern is that severe anorexia may inhibit normal skeletal development; thus, height may be affected. A third general challenge is that some children may not yet have the cognitive capacity to understand and express an abstract concept such as body image disturbance and may express only more concrete fears or exhibit a refusal to eat.

With AN, the primary targets for treatment are the low weight (and associated health concerns), the fear of gaining weight, and the body image concerns. The associated psychological problems noted above (e.g. depression, self-injury, or substance use) may also be the focus of treatment, as is family conflict. At times, there may be specific areas of family conflict, such as a history of incest, that appear related to the eating disorder.

Bulimia Nervosa

BN is characterized by recurrent episodes of binge eating (eating a large amount of food in a short period of time and feeling out of control) followed by some sort of compensatory behavior such as self-induced vomiting, use of laxatives, or excessive exercise. According to the current DSM classification, there are purging (vomiting or use of laxatives) and nonpurging (exercisers or dieters) subtypes. As with AN, there may also be a wealth of additional psychopathology (Gleaves et al., 1993), although its presence in adolescents or children is also less common than among adults.

Kjelsås et al. (2004) reported a prevalence of 1.2% of girls and 0.4% of boys aged 14 to 15. The exact prevalence among younger children is unknown, although young children do frequently report binge eating (Marcus & Kalarchian, 2003). As with AN, subclinical manifestations are much more common than full-blown disorders, with as many as half of high school students reporting some instances of binge eating or self-induced vomiting (Fisher et al., 1995). There also appears to be some individuals who engage in vomiting in the absence of binge eating (Binford & Le Grange, 2005). Recognizing and detecting the disorder may often be difficult due to the secrecy associated with the behaviors of binge eating and purging. Some researchers have also hypothesized that the reason why the prevalence of BN among children and adolescents is not higher is logistical rather than psychological. That is, most children do not have the money and privacy to allow for binge eating (Netemeyer & Williamson, 2001).

For BN, the primary targets for treatment are the out-of-control binge eating and purging, the excessive dietary restraint, and the weight- and appearance-related fears and cognitions. As with AN, when there is additional psychopathology or family dysfunction, these may also need to be targets for treatment.

Binge Eating Disorder

BED [currently listed in the "Criteria sets and axes provided for further study" (p. 759) section of the DSM-IV] is characterized by recurrent episodes of binge eating but in the absence of the regular use of compensatory behaviors. Such individuals are typically overweight. Although the exact prevalence of BED among the general child and adolescent population has yet to be determined, Decaluwé and Braet (2003) found that 9% of a sample of obese children and adolescents seeking weight loss treatment had objective bulimic episodes and 1% met criteria for BED. Binge eating was more common among girls than boys. Kjelsås et al. (2004) reported similar results (1.5% prevalence for girls and 0.9% for boys) among a sample of 14- to 15-year-olds. The experience of out-of-control eating may be more problematic for children than the consumption of large amounts of food is. Children aged 6–13 who had experienced episodes involving a loss of control over eating, regardless of the size of these episodes, were more likely to have disordered cognitions than children without such eating episodes (Tanofsky-Kraff et al., 2004). Similarly, 6–10-year-old children who reported loss-of-control eating were heavier and had greater body dissatisfaction, anxiety, and depression (Morgan et al., 2002).

With BED, the main target for treatment is the binge eating; however, the obesity may also be a focus. Body image concerns may be present, but to a lesser degree than with AN and BN. In contrast with those two disorders, the excessive dietary restraint is not as often present with BED.

INTERVENTIONS AND EMPIRICAL SUPPORT

Inpatient Treatment

Although most children and adolescents with eating disorders are treated on an outpatient basis, a minority need inpatient care, on either psychiatric or pediatric units. The admission criteria, goals, treatment strategies, and length of stay in such treatments vary widely across settings and countries, and there is little research evidence to guide these treatment decisions. However, Fisher et al. (1995) suggested a set of circumstances when hospitalization is justified: (1) Malnutrition is severe (under 75% of expected body weight), or medical complications of malnutrition are acute or severe (e.g., seizures, cardiac dysrhythmia, arrested growth); (2) psychiatric emergencies are acute (e.g., suicidal ideation or psychosis); or (3) the likelihood of outpatient treatment efficacy is low (e.g., failed prior treatment attempts, acute food refusal, severe psychiatric comorbidity, severe family dysfunction).

The primary goals of inpatient treatment include medical and nutritional stabilization, typically until patients have reached 85% to 90% of ideal body weight and are regularly eating and gaining weight (Robin et al., 1998). The National Institute for Clinical Excellence (NICE, 2004) in the UK recently issued a set of evidence-based guidelines for the treatment of eating disorders based on an exhaustive review of the available literature and rigorous consultation with mental health professionals, academics, and other experts. All guidelines were graded according to a coding scheme from A (strong empirical support from well-conducted trials) to C (expert opinion without strong empirical data). In describing the aim of inpatient treatment, NICE recommended refeeding and physical monitoring in combination with psychosocial interventions. However, this recommendation carried a grade of the lowest level (C), indicating expert opinion in the absence of empirical data. The most comparable guidelines in the United States are those recently issued by the APA (2006), which contain recommendations that are graded based on levels of clinical confidence (I, substantial confidence; II, moderate confidence; or III, may be recommended on an individual basis).

Guidelines for inpatient treatment primarily pertain to AN, as most patients with BN can be treated on an outpatient basis (Fairburn et al., 1993). However, reasons for the hospitalization of children or adolescents with BN may include (1) severe cardiac or physiological disturbances caused by binge eating and purging, (2) persistent suicidal ideation/attempts, self-harm, or psychosis, (3) intractable binge eating and purging that have not responded to outpatient treatment or partial hospitalization, or (4) serious comorbid conditions that interfere with treatment (Robin et al., 1998). The primary goal of treatment is to establish normal nutritional intake without purging, binge eating, or restricting (Fisher et al., 1995).

Only uncontrolled investigations have examined the outcome of inpatient treatment for adolescents with AN. In a naturalistic comparison of 21 adolescents with AN treated as inpatients and 51 treated as outpatients, the outpatients showed a better outcome two to seven years after initial presentation. The primary predictor of poorer outcome was admission to inpatient care (Gowers et al., 2000). Although this study was not randomized, it suggests that caution is necessary in prescribing inpatient care (Gowers & Bryant-Waugh, 2004). A number of other naturalistic outcome studies have documented the prognosis of adolescents treated as inpatients. Among 113 patients assessed at an average of 4.5 years after treatment, 72 were considered "healthy," 25 still had an eating disorder, 11 refused contact, and 5 had died (Steinhausen & Boyadjieva, 1996). The outcome was similar in a subsequent replication by the same group (Steinhausen et al., 2000). Among adolescents, long-term outcome is often good; 70% of women with adolescent-onset AN had a good outcome eight years after being hospitalized (Casper & Jabine, 1996), compared to the 42% of adult-onset patients who had a good outcome. However, these data may be more reflective of the natural course of the illness than of the efficacy of inpatient care. (For a review of the course and outcome of eating disorders in adolescents and adults, see Fisher, 2003.)

One study has attempted to randomize patients to different treatment settings. Crisp et al. (1991) directly compared inpatient treatment to two types of outpatient psychotherapy or no treatment in 90 adults with AN. The two types of outpatient treatment were (1) individual and family psychotherapy plus dietary counseling or (2) group psychotherapy plus dietary counseling. Not surprisingly, many patients randomized to inpatient care refused this form of treatment. Many of those assigned to the no-treatment condition also refused to "comply" with this condition. At one-year follow-up, the weight and eating disorder symptoms of all three treatment groups improved relative to the no-treatment group. The authors concluded that all three treatments were powerful in their effect. The methodological problems of this study highlight the difficulties in conducting randomized trials of this type.

Partial Hospitalization

Managed care restrictions have led to the development of treatments less costly than inpatient care. Partial hospitalization programs, also known as day hospitalization programs, are an increasingly common venue for providing treatment that is more intensive than outpatient care but less intensive (and therefore less costly) than inpatient. Day treatment programs also have the theoretical advantage of allowing patients to remain in their natural environments. This may permit a more rapid generalization of therapeutic skills to home and school settings, allow the continuation of social roles, and facilitate greater family contact and support (Zipfel et al., 2002).

By reviewing the charts of 59 patients transferred from inpatient to day program treatment, Howard et al. (1999) identified several prognostic indicators of the likelihood of treatment failure and inpatient readmission in patients with AN. These included long duration of illness (>2.5 years), amenorrhea, and low BMI (<19). This study was conducted with adults, so it did not take into account additional factors that may potentially affect treatment success in day programs for children and adolescents, such as level of development and family conflict.

The treatment goals and strategies of partial hospitalization programs are generally the same as those of inpatient programs. The primary difference is the amount of time spent on the unit. A detailed description of three day programs (for patients of all ages) reported the regular use of group meals, nutrition and cooking education groups, body image and counseling groups, and groups focused on social skills, assertiveness, family issues, and relationships (Zipfel et al., 2002).

A pediatric day treatment program that involved parents as participants and providers in the therapy followed up 32 girls with AN, nine months after treatment (Danziger et al., 1988). A healthy restoration of weight, menses, body image, eating and exercise habits, and social functioning was reported in the majority of cases. Uncontrolled studies on two of the day programs described by Zipfel and colleagues (2002) showed preliminary evidence of efficacy in a range of age groups. Williamson et al. (2001) compared treatment outcomes and direct costs associated with inpatient and partial day hospitalization treatment in 51 adult women with AN, BN, or subthreshold variants of each. Patients were nonrandomly assigned to treatment conditions based on disorder severity. Treatment outcomes were similar between the two types of treatment, and the cost savings with treatment initiated at the day hospital were $9,645, or 43% of the cost of inpatient cases. Across both conditions, 63% of cases were classified as recovered. Gerlinghoff et al. (1998) followed 65 patients out of 106 who had begun day treatment between 6 and 33 months earlier. Patients were primarily adults, diagnosed at baseline with AN, BN, and EDNOS. Statistically significant improvements were reported on weight (for those with AN), eating disorder symptoms, and general psychopathology. Although these initial findings suggest the utility and cost savings of partial hospitalization programs, randomized controlled studies are needed to compare the efficacy of day treatment with inpatient and outpatient treatments.

Outpatient Treatment

Family-Based Treatment

The NICE (2004) guidelines recommended that most patients with AN should be treated on an outpatient basis. This recommendation received a grading of C (expert opinion). In discussing the treatment of AN, these guidelines gave only one recommendation a grade higher than C: Family interventions that directly address the eating disorder for children and adolescents with AN were given a grade of B indicating support from well-conducted clinical studies. The APA (2006) guidelines called family treatment the most effective treatment for child and adolescent AN and gave this recommendation its highest grade (I).

Family therapy, as developed by clinical researchers at the Maudsley Hospital in the UK, is based on a model of mobilizing family resources to help the family refeed the patient (Lock et al., 2001). The therapist carefully emphasizes that the family should not be blamed for the illness but must take responsibility together for helping to overcome it. The first phase of treatment focuses on refeeding the patient, and the therapist reinforces strong alliances between the parents in their refeeding effort, and between the patient and any siblings available to provide support. The second phase focuses on family issues that may be interfering with refeeding. The third phase, initiated when healthy weight and eating patterns are achieved, focuses on establishing a relationship between the adolescent and the family that is not centered on the eating disorder (Le Grange, 1999). A number of controlled trials have investigated family therapy, but a limitation of this body of work is that the majority of studies have come from one setting, possibly limiting its generalizability. The research has also not yet identified the effective components of family therapy (Lock & Le Grange, 2005).

In AN patients whose weight had been restored by inpatient treatment, Russell et al. (1987) administered either individual supportive psychotherapy or family therapy focused on eating and weight. In a subgroup of 21 adolescents with a short duration of illness (<3 years), those receiving family therapy had greater weight gains and better psychological outcomes than those receiving individual treatment. The advantage of family therapy over individual therapy persisted in this subset of patients at a five-year follow-up, despite the natural trend toward improvement over time (Eisler et al., 1997). Robin and colleagues (1999) compared a similar form of family therapy, behavioral systems family therapy (BSFT), with a form of individual therapy, ego-oriented individual treatment (EOIT, described below under psychodynamic treatment), among 37 adolescents with AN. Eleven BSFT patients and 5 EOIT patients required concurrent hospitalization. After treatment and at a 12-month follow-up, two-thirds of all patients reached their target weight, but patients in the BSFT group had gained more weight. More BSFT patients than EOIT patients resumed menstruation (94% vs. 64%) after treatment, though the difference was no longer significant at follow-up. The results suggest that family therapy was faster-acting than individual treatment.

Several studies have compared different forms of family therapy. Family group psychoeducation, involving education classes and professionally led discussion groups on eating disorders, was compared with family therapy, both administered in eight sessions over four months, among 25 adolescent girls with AN and their families (Geist et al., 2000). All patients required concurrent hospitalization (for an average of eight weeks). Both groups achieved similar improvements in body weight, eating disorder psychopathology, and general psychopathology. In another study examining varying forms of family therapy, Eisler et al. (2000) compared conjoint family therapy (CFT), where 19 adolescents with AN were seen together with their parents, and separated family therapy (SFT), where 21 adolescents with AN were seen separately from their parents, but their parents had regular sessions with the same therapist. Four patients required concurrent hospitalization. Therapy goals and strategies were otherwise similar between the groups. Small but nonsignificant differences in eating disorder symptomatology were found in favor of SFT, whereas clearer differences in general psychopathology (mood, obsessionality, and psychosexual adjustment) were found in favor of CFT. In cases where high maternal criticism was directed at the patient, SFT was significantly superior.

In a study designed to determine the ideal dose of family therapy, Lock et al. (2005) compared the more standard therapy length of 20 sessions over 12 months to a short form offering 10 sessions over 6 months. The shorter therapy covered the first and second phases of family therapy but had less time to deal with general adolescent concerns. Eighty-six adolescents with AN were randomized to the two conditions. Similar gains in BMI, eating disorder psychopathology, and general psychopathology were achieved in both treatments at 12 months. Nineteen patients needed to be hospitalized after starting treatment; these were evenly distributed across treatment conditions. However, those with more severe eating-related obsessional thinking gained more weight, and those from nonintact families improved more on eating psychopathology, in the longer treatment. Overall, 96% of the sample no longer met criteria for AN, and 67% achieved a healthy BMI (>20) at one year. These findings suggest that for AN patients from intact families who are not exceptionally high on eating-related obsessionality, a shorter form of family therapy is likely to be effective.

The Lock et al. (2005) investigation had adequate power to have detected differences had they existed. However, other studies on AN that have found no differences between groups frequently have had small sample sizes, due in large part to the rarity of the disorder. In these studies, it is important not to mistake a lack of significant differences across conditions for treatment equivalence (Fairburn, 2005).

No controlled studies have examined family therapy for adolescents with BN, but Russell et al. (1987) did include a subgroup of 23 adults with BN of low weight randomly assigned to individual or family therapy. This subgroup generally did quite poorly, with only 3 of 19 achieving a good outcome (using the Morgan–Russell definition: having a healthy body weight, menstruating, and having no bulimic symptoms; Morgan & Russell, 1975) at five years. Individual therapy did not differ from family therapy in its efficacy with these BN patients. A case series described family therapy provided to eight adolescents with BN (Dodge et al., 1995). The Maudsley Hospital method of family therapy was modified slightly to address compensatory behaviors and shift the focus from weight gain to regular eating. (Le Grange et al., 2003, have also described the techniques of family therapy for adolescent BN.) One year after treatment initiation, significant reductions were found in eating pathology and in the level of deliberate self-harm, initially present in four of the cases. However, only one patient had a good outcome (based on the Morgan–Russell definition). Further research is needed before family therapy can be recommended for children or adolescents with BN.

Cognitive-Behavioral Therapy

Cognitive-behavioral therapy (CBT) involves identifying dysfunctional thoughts related to eating, weight, and body shape and challenging these thoughts through cognitive restructuring and behavioral experiments (Garner et al., 1997). It also aims to establish regular eating patterns through self-monitoring and dietary planning. No randomized controlled trials of CBT for children or adolescents with AN or BN have been conducted, so cautious speculation about its efficacy can be based only on studies with adults.

A handful of studies have examined CBT for AN. Channon et al. (1989) compared CBT to behavior therapy (BT) and a low-contact treatment by psychiatrists in 24 adults with AN. All patients improved significantly on nutritional and menstrual functioning and weight. The three treatments did not differ from each other on outcome, but CBT produced better compliance with treatment attendance than BT. Serfaty et al. (1999) also found a much lower dropout rate in CBT than in a comparison treatment group receiving dietary counseling—in fact, all patients had dropped out of dietary counseling by three months. All of these patients also refused to provide data for a six-month follow-up. Another study compared a 12-month course of CBT and nutritional counseling in adult AN patients following hospitalization (Pike et al., 2003). CBT recipients stayed in treatment significantly longer without relapsing (44 vs. 27 sessions on average); 22% vs. 53% of patients relapsed in CBT and nutritional counseling, respectively. Again, CBT was less likely to result in early dropouts. However, many of the patients in this trial were on antidepressant medication, and 88% of those showing a good response to CBT were taking medication compared to 40% of those who did not show a good response to CBT. This was a significant difference that was not found for nutritional counseling, suggesting a possible synergistic relationship between CBT and medication. However, nutritional counseling without concurrent psychotherapy may not provide a rigorous comparison group for CBT (Fairburn, 2005).

Complicating matters further, a recent study compared CBT to interpersonal therapy (IPT) and to a nonspecific clinical management condition providing supportive psychotherapy, in 55 women (aged 17–40) diagnosed with AN using a lenient weight criterion (BMI <19; McIntosh et al., 2005). Overall, only 30% of patients were considered much improved or as having minimal symptoms after the 20-week treatment. Contrary to the authors' predictions, on global measures of eating disorder symptoms, the nonspecific control treatment was superior to CBT and IPT. Thus, there is not yet strong support for the use of any specific individual psychotherapy for AN.

On the other hand, the efficacy of CBT for BN has been well established. CBT was recommended as the leading evidence-based treatment for BN by NICE (2004) and by the APA (2006). This was the first time that NICE has endorsed a specific psychotherapy as a treatment of choice. This recommendation was given a grade of "A," indicating strong evidence from randomized controlled trials.

CBT treatment typically has three stages. In the first, the cognitive-behavioral model of bulimia and other psychoeducational material is presented, and behavioral techniques (e.g., self-monitoring, meal planning, and stimulus control) are used to normalize eating behavior. In the second stage, additional attempts are made to establish healthy eating habits and to eliminate dieting. Cognitive interventions are used more in this stage, with the therapist helping the client examine his or her thoughts, beliefs, and values that maintain the eating problem. The final stage is concerned with preventing relapse. Treatment typically involves weekly sessions for four to five months and results in complete remission in about 40% of cases (Wilson & Fairburn, 2002). On average, patients' body weight does not change during treatment. CBT is quick-acting; most of the changes occur in the first few treatment sessions, significantly sooner than in comparison treatments (Wilson et al., 1999). For example, in comparison to IPT, more patients in CBT achieved remission by the end of treatment, although this difference leveled off by a one-year follow-up (Agras et al., 2000). This result was similar to that found in a previous comparison of CBT and IPT (Fairburn et al., 1995).

CBT has also been well established as a treatment for BED. Although inferences can only be made from research with adults, CBT is efficacious in reducing binge eating and associated psychopathology. These changes are also maintained in the longer term (Agras et al., 1997). However, CBT (and specialized psychotherapy more generally) is ineffective in reducing the obesity associated with BED. Two recommendations related to BED received a grade of A from NICE (2004): that CBT should be offered as a first-line treatment for adults with BED, and that psychological treatment has a limited effect on weight. The fact that descriptive studies with children documented the presence of BED among children about to receive treatment for obesity (Decaluwé & Braet, 2003) suggests that a research priority should be evaluating the effect of weight loss therapy on childhood BED.

In the absence of controlled trials for adolescents with BN, NICE (2004) recommended that CBT be used for this group, with age-related modifications to suit the patient's level of development and circumstances and including the family as appropriate (grade: C). However, Robin et al. (1998) cautioned that patients must have developed certain requisite cognitive abilities to engage in this treatment: (1) the ability to think abstractly about beliefs and attitudes regarding weight, shape, and appearance, and (2) the ability to consider alternative possibilities to presently held beliefs and to test alternative hypotheses. Robin and colleagues suggested that these cognitive skills are usually present by the age of 14 to 15. For children who do not yet have these skills, they suggest modifying CBT techniques to make them less abstract: simple behavioral experiments to disconfirm distorted beliefs, or concrete cognitive coping strategies such as overt self-statements or self-instruction.

Psychodynamic Therapy

Two studies have examined time-limited and standardized versions of psychodynamic treatment for AN in adults. In a controlled trial comparing four treatments lasting one year, 84 women with AN were randomly assigned to one of three specialized treatments, or to a low-contact control treatment with trainee psychiatrists who were replaced every six months (Dare et al., 2001). The first specialized treatment was focal psychoanalytic therapy, which addresses the meaning of the AN symptoms in light of the patient's history and family relationships, the effect of the symptoms on the patient's relationships, and the manifestation of these effects in the relationship with the therapist (transference). The second specialized treatment was cognitive analytic treatment (CAT), which combines elements of cognitive therapy with elements of psychodynamic therapy and focuses on interpersonal and transference issues. It aims to give patients a multifaceted understanding of themselves, which in turn would enable them to manage their emotions and relationships and eliminate the need for the eating disorder. The third treatment was family therapy. At the end of one year, the three specialized treatments did not differ from each other on outcome, but they were superior to control treatment (except CAT, which was not statistically different from control treatment). Overall, patients did poorly across all conditions: Thirty percent of patients in specialized treatment no longer met criteria for AN, compared to 5% of patients in the control treatment. The study may have had insufficient power to detect differences among the specialized treatments, and patients had a long history of illness (6.3 years on average), indicating poor prognosis. However, the results are consistent with an earlier study finding no differences between CAT and behavior therapy (with a substantial psychoeducation component), administered in 20 weekly sessions to adult AN patients (Treasure et al., 1995).

The Robin et al. (1999) trial of adolescents with AN compared family therapy to ego-oriented individual treatment (EOIT), focused on developing ego strength, coping skills, individuation from the family, and identifying and changing the dynamics blocking eating. Although EOIT was less immediately effective than family therapy, it led to a similar decrease in eating-related conflict during family interactions even though no conjoint family sessions took place. Based on the existing literature, psychodynamic therapy does not appear to be more effective than alternative specialized treatments for AN with adolescents or adults.

Interpersonal Therapy

Interpersonal therapy (IPT) aims to resolve interpersonal difficulties that contribute to the onset or maintenance of the eating disorder. Treatment focuses on problems in four areas: grief, interpersonal disputes, role transitions, and interpersonal deficits. The trial comparing CBT, IPT, and nonspecific clinical management in adult women with AN found IPT to be the least effective of the three treatments (McIntosh et al., 2005). In adults with BN, IPT is similar in efficacy to CBT in the long term, but its delayed benefits make it the less preferred treatment of the two. There is also evidence for the efficacy of IPT for BED in adults (Wilfley et al., 2002).

SUMMARY OF EVIDENCE-BASED TREATMENTS

The sentiment expressed by Fairburn (2005) in our opening quote does not suggest much optimism in terms of treatment for AN. However, the more positive side of the picture is that Fairburn's quote is based on the outcome with adults and that the outcome with children and adolescents appears to be more positive, as does the outcome with eating disorders other than AN. Thus, overall, the state of the research base varies depending on which disorder and which age group are being considered.

In a recent systematic review of randomized controlled trials of psychosocial interventions for adolescents with AN, Tierney and Wyatt (2005) concluded that only limited conclusions could be drawn from this small body of research. Many of the trials have been small and thus possibly underpowered to detect differences between interventions. No published trials have included a no-treatment control arm. Furthermore, most studies lacked a follow-up assessment. Thus, there is not yet strong support for the use of any specific individual psychotherapy for AN.

For BN, there is almost no published research with adolescents or children to inform treatment decisions, although two randomized trials of family therapy for BN are underway (Gowers & Bryant-Waugh, 2004). However, the efficacy of CBT for BN among adults has been well established, and CBT was recommended by NICE (2004) as the leading evidence-based treatment for BN. It recommended that CBT be used for this group, but with age-related modifications to suit the patient's level of development and circumstances, and including the family as appropriate (grade: C). Robin et al. (1998) made similar recommendations regarding how treatments may need to be modified to match the cognitive capacities of children and adolescents.

AN ILLUSTRATIVE CASE EXAMPLE

Natalie was a 12-year-old sixth grader at the time she was referred to an eating disorder treatment service by her family physician because of concerns that she was not eating enough (having passed out in school twice) and was "possibly vomiting." Data from a variety of assessment procedures (as recommended by Netemeyer & Williamson, 2001) including physical exam, nutritional assessment, interviews with both Natalie and her parents, self-report questionnaires and direct behavioral assessment were collected during the intake procedure.

In terms of her history (some gathered from her and some from her mother), Natalie had been slightly overweight as a child through elementary school. Although not initially a concern for Natalie, her mother (who was also weight-preoccupied) had insisted that the school cafeteria prepare special "diet" meals for her. Natalie herself began to become preoccupied after she unsuccessfully tried out for the middle-school cheerleading team. During the process, she was teased by some peers about looking "fat" in the uniform, and she reached the conclusion that she had failed to make the team for that reason. She began dieting excessively (fasting as her primary method) over the next several months. She lost 10 pounds initially and then maintained the new weight over the next several months even though she also grew two inches in height over the course of the year. She had not yet begun menstruating, and menarche may or may not have been delayed by her failure to gain weight. Her behaviors were socially reinforced by (among other things) her successfully making the cheerleading squad for the following year. However, after several months of restraint, she had her first binge eating episode. She felt extremely guilty but recommitted herself to her diet. After a subsequent period of fasting, she had her first fainting episode. Furthermore, the binge eating began to increase in frequency and, following a large binge on Halloween candy, she first tried self-induced vomiting (which she reported having read about in a magazine). She was not concerned about the vomiting except that she viewed it as "gross." For that reason, she had reportedly only done so "4 or 5 times" in total, although there were doubts about the accuracy of her self-report. At intake, Natalie also reported a long list of forbidden foods (those on which she would potentially binge).

Based on all the intake data and using DSM-IV criteria, Natalie fell into the category of EDNOS because she did not meet the weight criterion for AN but did not yet meet the frequency of binging and purging criterion for BN (assuming that her self-report was accurate). It was the treatment team's opinion that, if left untreated, her problems would progress into a more extreme disorder, and this concern was shared with Natalie and her parents. Outpatient treatment was recommended (both individual and group treatment) but with the condition that progress needed to occur or else inpatient treatment might be required.

Treatment was based on CBT for BN supplemented with work with her family (to address her mother's encouragement of unhealthy eating). As is common with adolescents (or persons with AN), treatment initially had to focus on Natalie's low motivation for change (Gowers & Smyth, 2004). Although she was unhappy with her developing binging problem, she was very reluctant to reduce her dieting. She argued that her weight loss was the best thing that had ever happened to her, that her eating was no different from her friends, and that no one would like her if she gained back any weight. She actually wanted to lose more weight and asked if she could lose 10 more pounds and *then* start the eating disorder treatment. However, when an older cheerleader at her school was hospitalized for AN, the seriousness of her state became clearer, with Natalie able to verbalize that she did not want to end up like the other girl.

Through initial meal planning with a dietitian and cooperation with the family (e.g., helping them learn to support Natalie without modeling or reinforcing pathological behavior), Natalie was able to normalize her eating (i.e., eating three meals a day of sufficient variety) and test her beliefs that she would gain excessive amounts of weight if she ate normally. She was gradually exposed to foods on her "forbidden" list without being allowed to either binge or purge. Natalie's therapist also helped Natalie better identify her emotions and situations that seemed to trigger feeling "fat." For her, although some of these were related to eating (e.g., having eaten a previously forbidden food), others had to do with interpersonal difficulties at school or conflict at home. Cognitive interventions in the form of positive self-statements and learning to challenge her own cognitions targeted Natalie's problematic attitudes regarding appearance and thinness and provided her with better skills for coping with stress at school and home. Behavioral tests were devised to test new hypotheses about her shape and weight, such as having Natalie wear an avoided short skirt to a party and observe whether her friends treated her with their usual friendliness or with scorn. To challenge Natalie's belief that she had made the cheerleading squad only because she had lost weight, her therapist asked Natalie to determine how many of the squad were fifth graders and how many were in the sixth. Natalie reported that only one came from the fifth grade, suggesting that it was most likely age and practice rather than appearance that determined who had made the team.

Within four months, Natalie's eating had normalized and without instances of binging or purging. She did gain some weight but remained in the normal range. She continued to be self-conscious about her appearance, but her therapist encouraged Natalie to make life decisions that challenged rather than maintained her schema. For example, among other decisions, she decided to go out for the basketball team instead of the cheerleading squad in junior high.

The case is typical of child or adolescent eating disorders in several ways. First, the majority fall into the EDNOS category rather than being prototypical diagnostic cases. Although this fact actually applies to adult cases of eating disorders as well (Fairburn & Bohn, 2005), it may be more of an issue for children and adolescents (Gowers & Bryant-Waugh, 2004). Second, changes in weight status are complicated by the fact that maturation is occurring, which may mask weight loss. Thus, documenting weight *loss* may not be as important as weight relative to what is expected at a particular height. However, in severe cases, height may also be affected. Third, low motivation is common in the early phases of treatment. That is, patients may not view their behaviors as problematic or recognize the seriousness. In some cases, they may use the eating behavior as a way of controlling their environment. However (fourth), if caught early, the problem may be relatively responsive to treatment that prevents such individuals from going down a path of self-destructive behaviors. Finally, effective treatments are modified, with caution, from those used with adults (see Bowers et al., 2003). That is, the bulk of the empirical research has been with adults. Furthermore, the vast majority has also been with BN; so treatments for AN are also modified from treatments of BN.

RECOMMENDATIONS FOR MOVING THE LITERATURE TOWARD GREATER CLINICAL UTILITY

At least one principal limitation with the current literature on the treatment of child and adolescent eating disorders is quite obvious. That is, the majority of it has been based on adults rather than children and/or adolescents. Extrapolating from the adult literature should not be viewed as completely inappropriate. In fact, Gowers and Bryant-Waugh (2004) recently listed four arguments in favor of such extrapolation. First, it can be argued that many young adults with eating disorders (such as those studied in the treatment research) are still struggling with adolescent issues and, in fact, that such issues underlie eating disorders. Second, the core and secondary psychopathology of eating disorders seems consistent across different age groups. Third, much of the "adult" treatment research actually included adolescents in the samples. Fourth, some of the treatments found to be effective for adult eating disorders (e.g., CBT) have also been found to be effective for children or adolescents with other disorders (e.g., depression). Additionally, there are data suggesting that cognitive-behavioral models, upon which many interventions are based, may be applicable to children and adolescents (Decaluwé & Braet, 2005).

However, there are also numerous reasons why such extrapolation may *not* be warranted (and Gowers & Bryant-Waugh, 2004, also went on to list five such reasons). First, as discussed above, atypical presentations may be more common among children and adolescents, and the adult literature is not based on such atypical cases. Second, particularly for AN, the treatment goals in children and adolescents may be different than with adults. That is, adult treatment may focus on a return to normal weight, whereas treatments with children and adolescents need to aim for a return to normal trajectory and development. Their third argument referred to pharmacological interventions and the fact that drugs may have different pharmacodynamics and pharmacokinetics in children. Fourth, parents will need to be involved in the treatment of children and most adolescents, another difference from the adult treatment literature. Fifth, particularly when treatment occurs in a hospital setting, there is a need to attend to children's social and educational needs. At the very least, there is a need for research to test the extrapolations that have been made from the adult literature. Thus, a primary recommendation for moving the literature forward is to do more treatment research with children and adolescents. This recommendation is particularly relevant for AN. As Fairburn (2005) noted, we do not yet know if family-based interventions really have a specific therapeutic effect or if their apparent effectiveness is simply a function of the good prognosis of AN in adolescence. Also, interventions designed to improve motivation and adherence to treatment are needed, as the vast majority of children and adolescents are brought to treatment by others rather than seeking it themselves. As there is virtually no research on the problem of BED and this disorder does seem to occur among this population (particularly among those seeking treatment for obesity), there is clearly a need for more research on that problem. Also needed are maintenance and effectiveness studies (Strober, 2005).

CONCLUSIONS

The eating disorders are, at the same time, potentially life-threatening and potentially very treatable. A key seems to be catching them early enough, which is a mandate for those working with children and adolescents. Much more research needs to be done with children and adolescents before we can make firm extrapolations from the adult literature. In the meantime, "clinical judgment is decisive when evidence is lacking on what treatment to use" (Wilson & Shafran, 2005, p. 81). Furthermore, the clinician should not forget that the most important *evidence* is that related to the client being treated. That is, treatment outcome evidence can and should be collected from work with individual clients. Although the methodology has been called "a neglected alternative" (Blampied, 2000, p. 960), single-case research designs are excellent ways of examining the efficacy of a treatment with the individual client as well as potentially contributing to and enriching the published evidence base.

REFERENCES

Agras, W. S. (2001). The consequences and costs of the eating disorders. *Psychiatric Clinics of North America, 24,* 371–379.

Agras, W. S., Telch, C. F., Arnow, B., Eldredge, K., & Marnell, M. (1997). One-year follow-up of cognitive-behavioral therapy for obese individuals with binge eating disorder. *Journal of Consulting and Clinical Psychology, 65,* 343–347.

Agras, W. S., Walsh, B. T., Fairburn, C. G., Wilson, G. T., & Kraemer, H. C. (2000). A multi-center comparison of cognitive-behavioral therapy and interpersonal psychotherapy for bulimia nervosa. *Archives of General Psychiatry, 57,* 459–466.

American Psychiatric Association (2000). *Diagnostic and Statistical Manual of Mental Disorders IV-TR* (4th ed., text rev.). Washington, DC.

American Psychiatric Association (2006). *Practice Guidelines for the Treatment of Patients with Eating Disorders,* 3rd ed. Retrieved September 27, 2006, from http://www.psych.org/psych_pract/treatg/pg/EatingDisorders3ePG_04-28-06.pdf.

Binford, R. B., & Le Grange, D. (2005). Adolescents with bulimia nervosa and eating disorder not otherwise specified-purging only. *International Journal of Eating Disorders, 38,* 157–161.

Blampied, N. M. (2000). Single-case research designs: A neglected alternative. *American Psychologist, 55,* 960.

Bowers, W. A., Evans, K., Le Grange, D., & Andersen, A. E. (2003). Treatment of adolescent eating disorders. In M. A. Reinecke, F. M. Dattilio, & A. Freeman (Eds.), *Cognitive Therapy with Children and Adolescents: A Casebook for Clinical Practice,* 2nd ed. (pp. 247–280). New York: Guilford Press.

Casper, R. C., & Jabine, L. N. (1996). An eight-year follow-up: Outcome from adolescent compared to adult onset anorexia nervosa. *Journal of Youth and Adolescence, 25,* 499–517.

Channon, S., de Silva, P., Hemsley, D., & Perkins, R. E. (1989). A controlled trial of cognitive-behavioural and behavioural treatment of anorexia nervosa. *Behaviour Research and Therapy, 27,* 529–535.

Crisp, A. H., Norton, K., Gowers, S., Halek, C., Bowyer, C., Yeldham, D., et al. (1991). A controlled study of the effect of therapies aimed at adolescent and family psychopathology in anorexia nervosa. *British Journal of Psychiatry, 159,* 325–333.

Danziger, Y., Carel, C. A., Varsano, I., Tyano, S., & Mimouni, M. (1988). Parental involvement in treatment of patients with anorexia nervosa in a pediatric day-care unit. *Pediatrics, 81,* 159–162.

Dare, C., Eisler, I., Russell, G., Treasure, J., & Dodge, E. (2001). Psychological therapies for adults with anorexia nervosa: Randomised controlled trial of out-patient treatments. *British Journal of Psychiatry, 178,* 216–221.

Decaluwé, V., & Braet, C. (2003). Prevalence of binge-eating disorder in obese children and adolescents seeking weight-loss treatment. *International Journal of Obesity, 27,* 404–409.

Decaluwé, V., & Braet, C. (2005). The cognitive behavioural model for eating disorders: A direct evaluation in children and adolescents with obesity. *Eating Behaviors, 6,* 211–220.

Dodge, E., Hodes, M., Eisler, I., & Dare, C. (1995). Family therapy for bulimia nervosa in adolescents: An exploratory study. *Journal of Family Therapy, 17,* 59–77.

Eisler, I., Dare, C., Hodes, M., Russell, G., Dodge, E., & Le Grange, D. (2000). Family therapy for adolescent anorexia nervosa: The results of a controlled comparison of two family interventions. *Journal of Child Psychology and Psychiatry, 41,* 727–736.

Eisler, I., Dare, C., Russell, G., Szmukler, G., Le Grange, D., & Dodge, E. (1997). Family and individual therapy in anorexia nervosa: A 5-year follow-up. *Archives of General Psychiatry, 54,* 1025–1030.

Fairburn, C. G. (2005). Evidence-based treatment of anorexia nervosa. *International Journal of Eating Disorders, 37* (Suppl), S26–S30.

Fairburn, C. G., & Bohn, K. (2005). Eating disorder NOS (EDNOS): An example of the troublesome "not otherwise specified" (NOS) category in DSM-IV. *Behaviour Research and Therapy, 43,* 691–701.

Fairburn, C. G., Marcus, M. D., & Wilson, G. T. (1993). Cognitive-behavioral therapy for bulimia nervosa and binge eating: A comprehensive manual. In C. G. Fairburn & G. T. Wilson (Eds.), *Binge Eating: Nature, Assessment, and Treatment* (pp. 361–404). New York: Guilford Press.

Fairburn, C. G., Norman, P. A., Welch, S. L., O'Connor, M. E., Doll, H. A., & Peveler, R. C. (1995). A prospective study of outcome in bulimia nervosa and the long-term effects of three psychological treatments. *Archives of General Psychiatry, 52,* 304–312.

Fisher, M. (2003). The course and outcome of eating disorders in adults and adolescents: A review. *Adolescent Medicine, 14,* 149–158.

Fisher, M., Golden, N. H., Katzman, D. K., Kreipe, R. E., Rees, J., Schebendach, J., et al. (1995). Eating disorders in adolescents: A background paper. *Journal of Adolescent Health, 16,* 420–437.

Garner, D. M., Vitousek, K. M., & Pike, K. M. (1997). Cognitive-behavioral therapy for anorexia nervosa. In D. M. Garner & P. E. Garfinkel (Eds.), *Handbook of Treatment for Eating Disorders,* 2nd ed. (pp. 94–144). New York: Guilford Press.

Geist, R., Heinmaa, M., Stephens, D., Davis, R., & Katzman, D. K. (2000). Comparison of family therapy and family group psychoeducation in adolescents with anorexia nervosa. *Canadian Journal of Psychiatry, 45*, 173–178.

Gerlinghoff, M., Backmund, H., & Franzen, U. (1998). Evaluation of a day treatment programme for eating disorders. *European Eating Disorders Review, 6*, 96–106.

Gleaves, D. H., & Eberenz, K. P. (1993). The psychopathology of anorexia nervosa: A factor analytic investigation. *Journal of Psychopathology and Behavioral Assessment, 15*, 141–152.

Gleaves, D. H., Williamson, D. A., & Barker, S. E. (1993). Confirmatory factor analysis of a multidimensional model of bulimia nervosa. *Journal of Abnormal Psychology, 102*, 173–176.

Gowers, S., & Bryant-Waugh, R. (2004). Management of child and adolescent eating disorders: The current evidence base and future directions. *Journal of Child Psychology and Psychiatry, 45*, 63–83.

Gowers, S. G., & Smyth, B. (2004). The impact of a motivational assessment interview on initial response to treatment in adolescent anorexia nervosa. *European Eating Disorders Review, 12*, 87–93.

Gowers, S. G., Weetman, J., Shore, A., Hossain, F., & Elvins, R. (2000). Impact of hospitalisation on the outcome of adolescent anorexia nervosa. *British Journal of Psychiatry, 176*, 138–141.

Howard, W. T., Evans, K. K., Quintero-Howard, C. V., Bowers, W. A., & Andersen, A. E. (1999). Predictors of success or failure of transition to day hospital treatment for inpatients with anorexia nervosa. *American Journal of Psychiatry, 156*, 1697–1702.

Katzman, D. K. (2005). Medical complications in adolescents with anorexia nervosa: A review of the literature. *International Journal of Eating Disorders, 37*, S52–S59.

Kjelsås, E., Bjornstrom, C., & Götestam, K. G. (2004). Prevalence of eating disorders in female and male adolescents (14–15 years). *Eating Behaviors, 5*, 13–25.

Le Grange, D. (1999). Family therapy for adolescent anorexia nervosa. *Journal of Clinical Psychology, 55*, 727–739.

Le Grange, D., Lock, J., & Dymek, M. (2003). Family-based therapy for adolescents with bulimia nervosa. *American Journal of Psychotherapy, 57*, 237–251.

Lock, J., Agras, W. S., Bryson, S., & Kraemer, H. C. (2005). A comparison of short- and long-term family therapy for adolescent anorexia nervosa. *Journal of the American Academy of Child & Adolescent Psychiatry, 44*, 632–639.

Lock, J., & Le Grange, D. (2005). Family-based treatment of eating disorders. *International Journal of Eating Disorders, 37* (Suppl), S64–S67.

Lock, J., Le Grange, D., Agras, W. S., & Dare, C. (2001). *Treatment Manual for Anorexia Nervosa: A Family-Based Approach.* New York: Guilford Press.

Marcus, M. D., & Kalarchian, M. A. (2003). Binge eating in children and adolescents. *International Journal of Eating Disorders, 34*, S47–S57.

McIntosh, V. V. W., Jordan, J., Carter, F. A., Luty, S. E., McKenzie, J. M., Bulik, C. et al. (2005). Three psychotherapies for anorexia nervosa: A randomized, controlled trial. *American Journal of Psychiatry, 162* (April), 741–747.

Morgan, C. M., Yanovski, S. Z., Nguyen, T. T., McDuffie, N. G. S., Jorge, M. R., Keil, M., et al. (2002). Loss of control over eating, adiposity, and psychopathology in overweight children. *International Journal of Eating Disorders, 31*, 430–441.

Morgan, H. G., & Russell, G. F. M. (1975). Value of family background and clinical features as predictors of long-term outcome in anorexia nervosa: Four-year follow-up study of 41 patients. *Psychological Medicine, 5*, 335–371.

National Institute for Clinical Excellence (2004). *Eating Disorders: Core Interventions in the Treatment and Management of Anorexia Nervosa, Bulimia Nervosa, and Related Eating Disorders.* London: National Institute for Clinical Excellence.

Netemeyer, S. B., & Williamson, D. A. (2001). Assessment of eating disturbance in children and adolescents with eating disorders and obesity. In J. K. Thompson & L. Smolak (Eds.), *Body Image, Eating Disorders, and Obesity in Youth: Assessment, Prevention, and Treatment* (pp. 215–233). Washington, DC: American Psychological Association.

Pike, K. M., Walsh, B. T., Vitousek, K., Wilson, G. T., & Bauer, J. (2003). Cognitive behavior therapy in the posthospitalization treatment of anorexia nervosa. *American Journal of Psychiatry, 160*, 2046–2049.

Roberts, M. C., Lazicki-Puddy, T. A., Puddy, R. W., & Johnson, R. J. (2003). The outcomes of psychotherapy with adolescents: A practitioner-friendly research review. *Journal of Clinical Psychology/In Session, 59*, 1177–1191.

Robin, A. L., Gilroy, M., & Dennis, A. B. (1998). Treatment of eating disorders in children and adolescents. *Clinical Psychology Review, 18*, 421–446.

Robin, A. L., Siegel, P. T., Moye, A. W., Gilroy, M., & Dennis, A. B., & Sikand, A. (1999). A controlled comparison of family versus individual therapy for adolescents with anorexia nervosa. *Journal of the American Academy of Child & Adolescent Psychiatry, 38*, 1482–1489.

Russell, G. F., Szmukler, G. I., Dare, C., & Eisler, I. (1987). An evaluation of family therapy in anorexia nervosa and bulimia nervosa. *Archives of General Psychiatry, 44*, 1047–1056.

Serfaty, M. A., Turkington, D., Heap, M., Ledsham, L., & Jolley, E. (1999). Cognitive therapy versus dietary counselling in the outpatient treatment of anorexia nervosa: Effects of the treatment phase. *European Eating Disorders Review, 7*, 334–350.

Steinhausen, H.-C., & Boyadjieva, S. (1996). The outcome of adolescent anorexia nervosa: Findings from Berlin and Sofia. *Journal of Youth and Adolescence, 25*, 473–481.

Steinhausen, H.-C., Seidel, R., & Metzke, C. W. (2000). Evaluation of treatment and intermediate and long-term outcome of adolescent eating disorders. *Psychological Medicine, 30*, 1089–1098.

Strober, M. (2005). The future of treatment research in anorexia nervosa. *International Journal of Eating Disorders, 37*, S90–S94.

Tanofsky-Kraff, M., Yanovski, S. Z., Wilfley, D. E., Marmarosh, C., Morgan, C. M., & Yanovski, J. A. (2004). Eating-disordered behaviours, body fat, and psychopathology in overweight and normal-weight children. *Journal of Consulting and Clinical Psychology, 72*, 1, 53–61.

Tierney, S., & Wyatt, K. (2005). What works for adolescents with AN? A systematic review of psychosocial interventions. *Eating and Weight Disorders, 10*, 66–75.

Treasure, J., Todd, G., Brolly, M., Tiller, J., Nehmed, A., & Denmen, F. (1995). A pilot study of a randomised trial of cognitive analytical therapy vs. educational behavioral therapy for adult anorexia nervosa. *Behaviour Research and Therapy, 33*, 363–367.

Wilfley, D. E., Welch, R. R., Stein, R. I., Spurrell, E. B., Cohen, L. R., Saelens, B. E., et al.. (2002). A randomized comparison of group cognitive-behavioral therapy and group interpersonal psychotherapy for the treatment of overweight individuals with binge-eating disorder. *Archives of General Psychiatry, 59*, 713–721.

Williamson, D. A., Thaw, J. M., & Varnado-Sullivan, P. J. (2001). Cost-effectiveness analysis of a hospital-based cognitive-behavioral treatment program for eating disorders. *Behavior Therapy, 32*, 459–477.

Wilson, G. T., & Fairburn, C. G. (2002). Treatments for eating disorders. In P. E. Nathan & J. M. Gorman (Eds.), *A Guide to Treatments That Work*, 2nd ed. (pp. 559–592). New York: Oxford University Press.

Wilson, G. T., Loeb, K. L., Walsh, B. T., Labouvie, E., Petkova, E., Liu, X., et al. (1999). Psychological versus pharmacological treatments of bulimia nervosa: Predictors and processes of change. *Journal of Consulting and Clinical Psychology, 67*, 451–459.

Wilson, G. T., & Shafran, R. (2005). Eating disorder guidelines from NICE. *Lancet, 365*, 79–81.

Zipfel, S., Reas, D. L., Thornton, C., Olmsted, M. P., Williamson, D. A., Gerlinghoff, M., et al. (2002). Day hospitalization programs for eating disorders: A systematic review of the literature. *International Journal of Eating Disorders, 31*, 105–117.

20

Evidence-Based Therapies for Pediatric Overweight

CRAIG A. JOHNSTON and CHERMAINE TYLER

In the United States, slightly over 17% of all children are classified as overweight, and the prevalence of overweight has significantly increased over the past four decades (Ogden et al., 2006). An additional 16.5% of U.S. children are considered at risk for overweight (Ogden et al., 2006). These prevalence rates reflect a 95% increase in extreme obesity that has been noted in children between 6 and 11 years of age (Klesges et al., 1993). Based on this alarming increase, the U.S. National Institutes of Health has identified the reduction of obesity in children as a primary goal under its current health initiative, Healthy People 2010 (2000). The most common determination of obesity for the United States is provided by the Centers for Disease Control (CDC; Ogden et al., 2000). The CDC uses body mass index (BMI) percentiles for weight classification and classifies children as *at risk* for overweight ($\leq$85th to 95th) or overweight ($\leq$95th). Further, overweight in children is not a serious health issue only in the United States, as it has reached epidemic proportions in Western and Western-izing countries as well (e.g., Finer, 2003; James, 2004). For example, it is estimated that over 22 million children under the age of 5 are overweight worldwide (Deckelbaum & Williams, 2001).

This increased prevalence and incidence are particularly concerning because overweight children are at risk for significant physical and emotional difficulties. Specifically, type 2 diabetes, sleep apnea, arthritis, gallstones, and some types of cancer have been associated with obesity (Must & Anderson, 2003; Wang & Dietz, 2002). The increased incidence of obesity in children has actually led to drastic increases in rates of childhood hyperinsulimia and type 2 diabetes (Sinha et al., 2002). Although the health consequences of obesity are severe in childhood and adolescence, overweight children will additionally suffer health problems later

---

CRAIG A. JOHNSTON and CHERMAINE TYLER • Department of Pediatrics-Nutrition, Baylor College of Medicine

in life given their increased risk of being an overweight adult (Erickson et al., 2003). While health risks increase substantially if obesity persists from childhood to adulthood (Kawachi, 1999; Rossner, 1998), even more alarming is the fact that obesity in adolescence, independent of adult obesity status, has been associated with the above-mentioned health consequences (Must & Anderson, 2003).

In addition to the physical consequences, multiple psychological consequences are associated with obesity. These problems include having a lowered self-concept, being less liked by peers, and having a negative self-image that impacts decision making and interactions with peers (Erickson et al., 2000; Thompson & Tantleff-Dunn, 1998; Whitaker et al., 1997; Zametkin et al., 2004). Further, overweight children and adolescents self-report having a quality of life that is similar to that of children who have cancer (Schwimmer et al., 2003). Fortunately, receiving treatment for overweight may attenuate some of the negative health and psychological consequences of obesity (Boreham & Riddoch, 2001; Holtz et al., 1999).

In light of the incidence of overweight in children and the impact it can have on their lives, the need for prevention and treatment of this condition is clear. However, prevention programs have yet to show promising results (e.g., CDC, 2005: Summerbell et al., 2005). Furthermore, the incidence and prevalence of this condition are expected to continue to increase throughout the next generation in the United States and worldwide. In fact, a report from the Surgeon General's office estimated that, left unabated, more preventable deaths will be associated with obesity than with cigarette smoking and that deaths related to obesity could replace those prevented by improved treatment for cancer, heart disease, and diabetes (DHHS, 2001).

In terms of treatment, an abundance of studies examining childhood overweight exist in the literature (Jelalian & Saelens, 1999). Most of these treatments take a multidisciplinary approach and include strategies for improving eating habits, increasing physical activity, and decreasing sedentary behavior. The greatest empirical support has been found for those therapies that are behaviorally based (e.g., Summerbell et al., 2003). In fact, Israel (1999) suggested that such treatments should be designated as "empirically supported," particularly for children between the ages of 8 and 12. If one applies the standards set forth by Chambless and Hollon (1998) for empirically supported therapies, behaviorally based treatments for obesity appear to meet criteria for "possibly efficacious."

This chapter will present three specific treatments that have obtained significant support in the literature. Although this chapter is by no means exhaustive in terms of treatments present in the literature, the following treatments have been subjected to randomized controlled trials with a follow-up of at least one year posttreatment. An overview of each treatment and an explanation of specific cognitive-behavioral treatment components are provided. Additionally, specific information about the multiple behaviors and persons targeted for change will be discussed. However, the main focus is on the approaches aimed at changing behaviors.

THE TRAFFIC LIGHT PROGRAM (TLP)

Epstein's (1996) TLP provides perhaps the best example of an evidence-based therapy for overweight children (Kazdin & Weisz, 1998). Specifically, multiple investigations have found the TLP to be superior to control conditions in randomized studies. For example, Epstein and colleagues demonstrated that receiving the TLP is superior to no treatment (Epstein et al., 1984a) and to an attention placebo control condition (Epstein et al., 1980, 1985a). Additionally, multiple components have been identified that add to the efficacy of the TLP. For example, including parents as participants in treatment (Epstein et al., 1981), providing exercise in addition to diet (Epstein et al., 1985a), and reinforcing the reduction of sedentary behavior (Epstein et al., 1995) have all been shown to increase either initial or follow-up outcomes. Perhaps the most impressive finding is that children who received the TLP demonstrated maintenance of effects in 10-year follow-up studies (i.e., Epstein et al., 1990, 1994). For a brief summary of literature regarding the TLP, the reader is directed to Table 1.

Overview

The TLP is a family-based behavioral treatment designed for a child who is considered either at risk for overweight (<85th percentile to 95th percentile for BMI) or overweight (<95th percentile for BMI) as defined by the Centers for Disease Control (CDC, 2000). Although the child is the target, parents are viewed as an integral part of treatment, and at least one parent must consent to attend and participate in weekly sessions. The importance of concurrent treatment of parents and children (Epstein et al., 1990) and of children and parents attending separate group treatment meetings (Brownell et al., 1983) has been established in the literature.

Sessions are held on a weekly basis and range in duration from 8 (Epstein et al., 1990) to 16 weeks (Epstein et al., 1995) with follow-up sessions (typically monthly) for the remainder of the year. During a treatment meeting, children and parents are first weighed and counseled together and are then separated for child and parent group meetings (Epstein et al., 1995). Both children and parents receive instruction in the use of various behavioral strategies during meetings. Therapists play an integral role in these interactions, reviewing and helping to calculate participants' self-monitored targeted behaviors (e.g., physical activity, television viewing), determining if weekly goals have been met, providing performance feedback, and ensuring that both parents and children have received contracted rewards.

The Traffic Light Diet itself (Epstein et al., 1985a) is used to decrease energy intake and promote healthy eating habits. Foods are categorized into the three colors of a traffic light based on their calorie and nutrient content. "Green" foods are low in calorie and high in nutrient content. These foods are primarily vegetables. "Yellow" foods are higher in calories but include nutrients necessary for a balanced diet. Examples of these foods include skim milk, lean meats, and fruits. "Red" foods are high in

Table 1. Studies Addressing the TLP

Citation	Purpose	Result
1. Epstein et al. (1980)	Compared behavior modification to nutrition education for weight loss	Behavior modification > nutrition education
2. Epstein et al. (1981)	Compared family-based behavior modification: 1. Parent/child target 2. Child target 3. Nonspecific target	Tentatively, 1>2 Children in 1, 2 & 3 were equal in weight changes; parents in 1 had greater losses
3. Epstein et al. (1984)	Compared effects of: 1. Diet 2. Diet and exercise 3. No treatment control	1-year outcomes: 1 & 2>3 2>3
4. Epstein et al. (1985b)	Compared effects of: 1. Parent managed program 2. Nutrition/exercise education	8–12-month outcomes: 1>2 Child intervention effective with parental involvement
5. Epstein et al. (1985a)	Compared effects of: 1. Lifestyle exercise 2. Aerobic exercise 3. Calisthenic exercise	1-year outcomes: 1>2 & 3 2 & 3 gained weight
6. Epstein et al. (1990)	Compared types of family-based treatment: 1. Parent and child 2. Child alone 3. Nonspecific control	10-year outcomes: 1>3 2 = 1 & 3
7. Epstein et al. (1994)	Examined maintenance effects (10 years)	TLP > nontargeted controls, calisthenics control
8. Epstein et al. (1995)	Compared types of active lifestyle reinforcement: 1. Reduce sedentary 2. Increase exercise 3. Combined	1>2 & 3 All groups reduced weight during treatment and follow-up
9. Epstein (1996)	Developed interventions targeting obese children and provided support for factors useful in treatment	Involvement of ≥ 1 parent is better than no involvement

calorie and low in nutrient content. Examples of these foods include potato chips, soda, and candy. Although the daily total caloric intake goal has varied across studies, parents and children are instructed to consume a restricted amount of calories (typically ranging from 900 to 1,300 kcal). In addition to this caloric goal, participants are instructed to eat seven or fewer "red" foods per week.

The physical activity instruction given to children and parents is disseminated through written manuals focused on the advantages of increased physical activity and the disadvantages of sedentary behaviors (Epstein et al., 1995). Physical activity is defined in terms of caloric expenditure and translated into activity points using number of calories burned in a 10-minute period of the activity according to weight. Children and parents are taught to calculate the caloric expenditure of each activity in which they participate. Sedentary behaviors are defined as behaviors that compete for being active (e.g., watching television, playing videogames, talking on the phone). Sedentary behaviors, such as listening to music or completing homework, are not specifically targeted for reduction. However, participants are rewarded for a gradual increase in physical activity and a gradual reduction in sedentary behaviors. Once the participant reaches the goal of 15 or fewer hours of sedentary behavior a week or 150 activity points, they are expected to maintain this change.

Specific Behavioral Components

Self-Monitoring

Participants are taught to record dietary and caloric intake, number of "red" foods consumed, and amount of time spent in physical and sedentary activities. A "habit book" is provided for maintaining the records so the therapist can monitor participant progress. Furthermore, participants are instructed to weigh themselves daily at home and chart their weights.

Stimulus Control

Parents and children are encouraged to change their environments to maximize the likelihood of behavior change. Specifically, families are taught to remove "red" foods from the home. Additionally, they are encouraged to decrease cues for sedentary behaviors, such as turning the television toward the wall. Finally, families are instructed to keep items associated with physical activity (e.g., exercise clothing, bikes) readily accessible.

Reinforcement (Contingency Management) and Modeling

Parents and children are taught how to establish contracts that specify rewards received when specific behaviors are displayed. Reciprocal contracting is also used (Epstein et al., 1990), teaching the child and parent to provide mutually agreed-upon reinforcers/rewards for each other when specified behavioral criteria are met. Parents are additionally trained to be role models for healthy behaviors and for reinforcement (e.g., praise, rewards) when children are successful in adapting target actions.

THE CAIR PROGRAM

Israel's CAIR program (Israel et al., 1984) has obtained considerable support in the child weight loss literature. This program has been compared to several control conditions in randomized studies. For example, two studies have been conducted that demonstrated the CAIR program is superior to a waitlist control condition (Israel et al., 1985, 1984). Program components such as directing more attention to child self-regulation (Israel et al., 1994) and having parents perform a helper role instead of a collaborative role in achieving concordant weight loss (Israel et al., 1990) have been identified as improving program results. Maintenance of these outcomes has been shown for as long as one year (Israel et al., 1984, 1985). For a brief summary of literature regarding CAIR, the reader is directed to Table 2.

Overview

The CAIR program is a family-based behavioral treatment designed for children who are either at risk for overweight or overweight. CAIR uses a "four-prong" format in which stimulus control cues, activity (exercise), food intake, and rewards are presented at each session and individualized for each family. Parents' participation in this program is viewed as essential. Parents are expected to help influence the child's behavior, monitor the child's food and caloric intake, and monitor the child's energy expenditure throughout the program.

Parents and children attend an orientation, eight weekly 90-minute sessions, and nine biweekly sessions. Prior to the official start of the weight reduction program, parents attend two classes to improve behavioral child management skills with a basis from *Living with Children* (Patterson, 1976). At each meeting, parents and children bring completed homework for discussion. Generally, they are instructed to complete self-monitoring of food intake and physical activity. Though there is variance, participants are

Table 2. Studies Addressing the CAIR Program

Citation	Purpose	Result
1. Israel et al. (1984)	Compared effects of 1. Helper parents 2. Weight loss parents	1 = 2
2. Israel et al. (1985)	Compared effects of 1. Weight reduction only (WRO) 2. Weight reduction + parent training 3. Waiting-list control	Parents and children in 1 & 2 lost weight; children in 1 & 2 improved eating habits. Families in 3 had weight gain.
3. Israel et al. (1987)	Examined relation between 1. baseline adherence of overweight children 2. attrition among families	Useful index for detecting high-risk subjects.
4. Israel et al. (1988)	Examined parent involved child weight control by 1. overall adherence 2. meeting goals	Overall adherence = % overweight loss. Meeting the goals ≠ weight loss.
5. Israel et al. (1990)	Examined parental help in weight loss of children	Overall rate of success > with parental help.
6. Israel et al. (1994)	Examined self-regulation intervention in children	Providing self-regulation = additional weight loss.

also expected to record specific efforts for behavior change. Children are encouraged to participate as much as possible in completing homework, but the primary responsibility for finishing assignments rests on the parents, with parents additionally being expected to reward treatment success (e.g., staying within the calorie intake level).

Specific Behavioral Components

Self-Monitoring

Similar to the TLP discussed above, participants are taught to monitor and record dietary and caloric intake, energy expenditure, and adherences to other behaviors associated with weight loss. The CAIR program relies on the parent being ultimately responsible for completing these records; however, depending on each child's ability, children are given self-monitoring tasks to encourage active participation.

Stimulus Control

Although stimulus cue control is an integral part of this program, the specifics that families are taught are unclear. However, the CAIR program appears to focus on using stimulus control to increase physical activity and to decrease caloric intake. Specifically, parents are to make healthy fruit and vegetable snacks more visible in the home and to have children engaged in eating in the absence of other competing activities (e.g., television watching).

Rewards

Rewards are based solely on progress in the program and are individualized for each family. Although the specific use and implementation of rewards is not provided, an important factor to note is the individualization of treatment for each family. Therapists meet independently with families, make phone calls between sessions, and have access to information provided in both the parent and child groups. Based on this information, therapists assess factors such as motivation (Israel et al., 1985) and provide an individualized reward system for each family. It appears that only the children are being rewarded, as there is no specific mention of parental rewards.

PARENTS AS EXCLUSIVE AGENTS OF CHANGE (PEAC) PROGRAM

Golan and colleagues (1998b) developed a program using parents as exclusive agents of change. Their PEAC program has also been examined in the context of a randomized control trial. Specifically, the PEAC program has demonstrated greater weight loss when parents are targeted as the primary agent of change compared to children alone being the primary target (Golan et al., 1998a, b). The PEAC program has identified additional factors impacted by treatment. For example, the PEAC parent-targeted program compared to a child-focused program resulted in lower attrition (Golan, et al., 1998b), decreased exposure to food stimuli, and healthy changes in eating habits (Golan et al., 1998a). Maintenance of these outcomes has been shown for as long as seven years (Golan & Crow, 2004a). For a brief summary of literature regarding PEAC, the reader is directed to Table 3.

Overview

The PEAC program is a family-based behavioral treatment designed for children who are overweight or at risk for overweight. Unlike the TLP or CAIR program, PEAC includes parents only in the treatment of pediatric overweight. This strategy is based on recommendations by Lerner (1982), who suggests that children will resist change and will rebel when subjected to change. Parents serve as sources of authority and role models for their children. Parents are taught strategies for providing an environment that promotes a healthy lifestyle (e.g., improved food choices; Golan et al., 1998a) and are encouraged to make family-based changes.

Parents attend four weekly sessions and then four biweekly sessions followed by six additional maintenance sessions that are spaced six weeks apart. Each session is one hour in duration, during which time parents learn how to change the family eating environment, to decrease sedentary lifestyle and exposure to food stimuli, to use behavior modification, and to implement relevant parenting skills. During the last seven months of intervention, an additional five sessions (15 minutes in duration) are conducted that include the entire family. This is the time when each family member is measured (i.e., height and weight) without a targeted child being identified.

Table 3. Studies Addressing theParent's as Exclusive Agents of Change Program

Citation	Purpose	Result
1. Golan et al. (1998a)	Compare effects of 1. family-based approach targeted parents 2. conventional approach targeted children	1 > 2 in reduction of weight and changes in eating habits
2. Golan et al. (1998b)	Compare effects of 1. family-based approach targeted parents 2. conventional approach targeted children	1 > 2
3. Golan & Crow (2004a)	Long-term study that compared effects of 1. targeted parents 2. targeted children (control intervention)	1 > 2

Specific Cognitive-Behavioral Components

Self-Monitoring

Parents are instructed to keep a seven-day food diary and to track changes in physical activity. However, it is unclear if this is done throughout the program. Children are not reported as participating in self-monitoring. In fact, it is unclear if the parents are instructed to teach their children these behavioral techniques.

Stimulus Control

Parents are instructed to reduce the presence and visibility of snacks. Furthermore, sweets and other types of less nutritious foods (e.g., ice cream) are to be removed from the home. The overall role of the parent is to establish a healthy food environment but not to restrict the amount of food eaten.

Beyond these two components, the cognitive-behavioral components used in the PEAC program are not discussed in detail in the literature; however, an overview is available (Golan et al., 1998a). Issues such as limits of responsibility, parental modeling, cognitive restructuring, and coping with resistance are listed. Several specific behaviors are also identified for change. For example, the activity level of the family is expected to increase, eating outside meal times is expected to decrease, and eating while watching television is expected to decrease. It may also be important to note that parents are encouraged to use an authoritative parenting style (Golan & Crow, 2004b) as they implement this program.

SUMMARY OF FAMILY-BASED BEHAVIORAL INTERVENTIONS

The importance of the inclusion of both parents and children is apparent, as each of the three programs demonstrates. However, unlike the TLP and CAIR programs, the PEAC program does not include children directly in the intervention. PEAC actually used a child-focused intervention as a control group and found that the parent-centered program resulted in better child weight loss than did the child as the agent of change control. The program has not, however, been compared to programs such as the TLP or CAIR in which both children and parents are included in treatment. Currently, however, the preponderance of empirical support for the treatment of pediatric overweight is for family-based (including both the child and parent) behavioral interventions (e.g., Epstein et al., 1981; Israel, 1999; McLean et al., 2003; Summerbell et al., 2003).

Additionally, the behavioral components used in each of these programs are, for the most part, consistent. For example, each program uses self-monitoring and stimulus control. Additionally, contingency management (i.e., reinforcement) appears to be used in each of the programs. However, the independent contribution of behavioral techniques is currently unknown. More specifically, dismantling studies have not been conducted to determine the relative impact that each strategy has on weight loss or weight maintenance in children. Two studies are noted that identify components that may have little additional effect in the treatment of childhood overweight. Problem solving does not appear to add to the effectiveness of treatment beyond standard family-based treatment (Epstein et al., 2000). Cognitive interventions also do not appear to improve outcomes compared to behavioral interventions (Herrera et al., 2004).

CASE EXAMPLE

Leah, a 12-year-old girl, presented for overweight treatment with her mother, Sharon. Sharon reported that although Leah did not appear overweight, she was concerned about her daughter's recent weight increase, especially given that she and her husband had always struggled with being significantly overweight and had recently been told by their physicians that they were at high risk for type 2 diabetes. Additionally, Sharon indicated that even her 16-year-old son, David, needed to lose weight as well. Sharon was encouraged to bring her entire family in for the next meeting before treatment began.

After some discussion on the importance of family involvement and environmental change, the entire family agreed to participate in a 12-week family-based weight management program. On the first day of treatment, all family members had their heights and weights taken and were given an introduction to the program, which included weekly nutrition meetings as well as a training session focusing on physical activity. During the 1.5-hour meetings, parents and children separately participated in 40-minute nutrition and physical activity training sessions. The nutrition classes focused on classifying foods into categories according to their nutritional and caloric content as well as identifying appropriate serving sizes. Lessons also focused on changing the eating environment for the family, including guidelines for eating out, for making fresh fruits and vegetables readily available, and for removing unhealthy foods from the home. The physical activity included pre- and poststretching with leisure- (e.g., walking, playing catch, and jumping rope) and training- (e.g., treadmill, stationary bike, elliptical machine) focused cardiovascular activities. Family members were encouraged to adopt their preferred physical activities as substitutes for sedentary activities.

All family members were weighed weekly at the beginning of the meeting, and weight changes were charted and discussed. A facilitator helped them to determine diet/activity changes that contributed to weight change and ways to improve their weights in the coming weeks. The family was taught to conduct a similar type of meeting at home each week to build an ongoing means of accountability for making changes beyond the termination of the program. During the weekly training hour, family members engaged in preferred activities in the workout facility with the trainer available for questions or assistance. The first month of the program the family made a number of changes, removing processed sweets, high-fat snacks, and nondiet sodas from the home. They increased fruit consumption and began engaging in leisure-time activity as a family, and they steadily lost weight each week.

The father, however, complained about the decreased amount of food served at meals, expressing annoyance at the types of food he was being asked to eat. On one occasion, Sharon left town for a few days for a business trip and returned to find her husband had taken the kids to buffet breakfasts each day she was away. At the following meeting, the father refused to attend or to chart his weight at home, and both children gained weight. The father did, however, encourage increased physical activity and engaged in basketball games with his children on a regular basis. Meanwhile, Sharon struggled to maintain a healthy eating environment at home given her husband's sabotage of her efforts and insistence that increased exercise would account for his eating patterns. Though the father never returned to the program, the other family members continued, monitoring their food and activity patterns and losing weight on a steady basis. Sharon reported that after a doctor visit when her husband was told his weight had increased since his previous visit, he began slowly to make changes, mostly decreasing visits to all-you-can-eat restaurants. He continued, however, to struggle with incorporating healthy options into his diet.

Monthly follow-up visits were conducted after the 12-week program ended, and Sharon and David demonstrated further weight loss during this time. Leah's weight was sustained, which indicated a significant change given that her height had increased from the beginning of their treatment. Sharon and the children also attended a follow-up a year following their beginning the program, and she had lost additional weight, for a total weight loss that exceeded 15% of her total initial weight. David and Leah had also significantly decreased their BMI percentile, having decreased in weight and increased in height.

FUTURE DIRECTIONS

With few empirically supported treatments for child overweight, a great deal of work remains to be done in this area. Actually, many of the children who have been successful in terms of weight loss continue to be overweight, and some significantly so (e.g., Epstein et al., 1990; Israel et al., 1985). Even though studies examining the TLP have produced robust effects, 70% remained overweight or obese at 10-year follow-up (Epstein et al., 1994). The other identified programs have not reported results beyond a one-year follow-up. Thus, programs that address maintenance of treatment effects are needed. Additionally, none of the available literature supporting the previously mentioned programs utilizes diverse participants. To date, no empirically supported programs have successfully been used with significantly overweight children, minorities, adolescents, or children from low-income families. Given the rates of overweight in children from these communities and their health problems, programs targeting these groups must be developed. Johnston and Steele (2007) began to address this issue by providing families with a modified version of the TLP in an applied setting. Results from this study showed a significant decrease in standardized body mass index for children who were provided the TLP. Although the results are encouraging, suggesting that this treatment may generalize to applied settings, results on long-term follow-up are lacking. Some work is being done to address a number of these issues, and brief explanations in each area as well as ideas for continued research are presented.

Internet-based programs may be useful in terms of sustaining healthy changes made during the course of an intense intervention. A study that examined the use of the Internet as an adjunct to a summer day camp for decreasing BMI, increasing fruit and vegetable consumption, and increasing physical activity showed there was a trend in the expected direction for each of these variables (Baranowski et al., 2003). However, no statistical differences were found between the control and treatment groups in terms of BMI. Another study focused specifically on using the Internet for weight loss in African-American girls showed a reduction in percent body fat but not BMI (Williamson et al., 2005). Overall, little evidence exists for Internet-only interventions resulting in weight loss, although there is a trend toward positive health outcomes. This mode of delivery may be used to bolster effects in standard treatments or to assist with maintenance upon completion of a treatment.

Another area of needed research is with very overweight children whose BMIs are at least 30 or greater than the 95th percentile for their age and gender. A modified version of the TLP has been used to determine the efficacy of this program for these children (Levine et al., 2001). Those who completed the program significantly reduced their weight and improved on several psychosocial variables (e.g., depression, anxiety); however, approximately one-third of the families did not complete the treatment. Furthermore, these children remained significantly overweight. Currently, treatments using weight loss medications (e.g., Chanoine et al., 2005; McDuffie et al., 2002), bariatric surgery (e.g., Davis et al., 2006), and meal replacements (Ball et al., 2003) are being assessed for use with this population. Although these therapies are beyond the scope of this chapter, the importance of addressing the specific needs of very overweight children is clear.

Research is also needed to determine effective treatments for children in low-income families. Given the increased risk of overweight and obesity in lower socioeconomic SES populations (e.g., Gordon-Larsen et al., 2003), interventions that specifically address the needs of these families need to be developed. A paucity of information is available on this topic. A major critique of family-based behavioral treatments for pediatric overweight is their lack of inclusion of lower-income groups. One recommendation for addressing this area was provided by Berkel et al. (2005). They suggest that although nutritious home-prepared meals are ideal for children, consumer demand for convenience may mean the most viable research option is to use meal replacements that meet the nutritional demands of children. These types of foods may also serve as a helpful adjunct to standard treatments.

Similar to the area of economic diversity, the impact of cultural diversity should be further explored. Ethnic minorities experience some of the highest rates of overweight in the United States (Hedley et al., 2004), and few studies have been conducted that address the specific treatment concerns for these groups. Issues such as recruitment, adherence, and retention need to be better understood to increase the efficacy of interventions (e.g., Keller et al., 2005). Overall, culturally appropriate interventions are needed that meet the unique needs of these populations.

Finally, weight management studies for adolescents are lacking. The most support for treatment of pediatric overweight is provided for children between the ages of 8 and 12 (e.g., Israel, 1999). However, treatments targeting adolescents have resulted in modest weight loss, with a trend toward weight regain at follow-up (e.g., Mellin et al., 1987; Rocchini et al., 1988). One study attempted to address overweight treatment in adolescents by including a peer-based "adventure therapy" component (Jelalian et al., 2006). In this study, a trend was found for this intervention to be most effective with older adolescents. Although the results appear promising and the inclusion of social support for change in adolescent weight loss is rather innovative, results remain inconclusive about the use of this as an adjunct to behavioral weight control interventions.

SUMMARY

A firm foundation of empirically supported treatments for pediatric overweight has been established. As this condition in children reaches epidemic proportions, the need for effective programs to treat the problem is clear. However, few studies have been conducted to determine the "effectiveness" of these interventions in applied settings (e.g., Kazdin & Weisz, 1998). Furthermore, these interventions have yet to demonstrate positive results with very overweight children, economically and culturally diverse families, or adolescents. Despite these critiques, the evidence for the benefits of these interventions is substantial, with one intervention demonstrating 10-year improvements in weight for children (Epstein et al., 1990). In order to advance this field, practitioners and researchers are encouraged to use the wealth of information obtained from the above-mentioned research groups as a basis for providing treatment. Furthermore, modifications and adjuncts to these programs are needed to better serve specific populations and to better combat this growing epidemic.

ACKNOWLEGEMENT.   Preparation of this paper was supported, in part, by USDA ARS 2533759358.

References

Ball, S. D., Keller, K. R., Moyer-Mileur, L. J., Ding, Y., Donaldson, D., & Jackson, W. D. (2003). Prolongation of satiety after low versus moderately high glycemic index meals in obese adolescents. *Pediatrics, 111,* 488–494.

Baranowski, T., Baranowski, J. C., Cullen, K. W., Thompson, D. I., Nicklas, T., Zakeri, I. E., et al. (2003). The Fun, Food, and Fitness Project (FFFP): The Baylor GEMS pilot study. *Ethnicity and Disease, 13*, S30–S39.

Berkel, L. A., Poston, W. S. C., Reeves, R. S., & Foreyt, J. P. (2005). Behavioral interventions for obesity. *Journal of the American Dietetic Association, 105*, S35–S43.

Boreham, C., & Riddoch, C. (2001). The physical activity, fitness and health of children. *Journal of Sports Science, 19*, 915–929.

Brownell, K. D., Kelman, J. H., & Stunkard, A. J. (1983). Treatment of obese children with and without their mothers: Changes in weight and blood pressure. *Pediatrics, 71*, 515–523.

Centers for Disease Control (2005). *Public Health Strategies for Preventing and Controlling Overweight and Obesity in School and Worksite Settings: A Report on the Recommendations of the Task Force on Community Preventive Services* (Morbidity and Mortality Weekly Report, 54, RR-10). Washington, DC: Government Printing Office.

Chambless, D. L., & Hollon, S. D. (1998). Defining empirically supported therapies. *Journal of Consulting and Clinical Psychology, 66*, 7–18.

Chanoine, J., Hampl, S., Jensen, C., Boldrin, M., & Hauptman, J. (2005). Effect of Orlistat on weight and body composition in obese adolescents: A randomized controlled trial. *Journal of the American Medical Association, 293*, 2873–2883.

Davis, M. M., Slish, K., Chao, C., & Cabana, M. D. (2006). National trends in bariatric surgery, 1996–2002. *Archives of Surgery, 141*, 71–74.

Deckelbaum, R. J., & Williams, C. L. (2001). Childhood obesity: The health issue. *Obesity Research, 9*, 239s–243s.

Department of Health and Human Services (2001). *The Surgeon General's Call to Action to Prevent and Decrease Overweight and Obesity* (Office of the Surgeon General). Washington, DC: Government Printing Office.

Epstein, L. H. (1996). Family-based behavioural intervention for obese children. *International Journal of Obesity, 20*, 14–21.

Epstein, L. H., Paluch, R. A., Gordy, C. C., Saelens, B. E., & Ernst, M. M. (2002). Problem solving in the treatment of childhood obesity. *Journal of Consulting and Clinical Psychology, 68*, 717–721.

Epstein, L. H., Valoski, A., Vara, L. S., McCurley, J., Wisniewski, L., Kalarchian, M. A., et al. (1995). Effects of decreasing sedentary behavior and increasing activity on weight change in obese children. *Health Psychology, 14*, 109–115.

Epstein, L. H., Valoski, A., Wing, R. R., & McCurley, J. (1990). Ten-year follow-up of behavioral, family-based treatment for obese children. *Journal of the American Medical Association, 264*, 2519–2523.

Epstein, L. H., Valoski, A., Wing, R. R., & McCurley, J. (1994). Ten-year outcomes of behavioral family-based treatment of childhood obesity. *Health Psychology, 13*, 371–372.

Epstein, L. H., Wing, R. R., Koeske, R. R., Andrasik, F. & Ossip, D. (1981). Child and parent weight loss in family-based behavior modification programs. *Journal of Consulting and Clinical Psychology, 49*, 674–685.

Epstein, L. H., Wing, R. R., Koeske, R. R., & Valoski, A. (1984). Effects of diet plus exercise on weight change in parents and children. *Journal of Consulting and Clinical Psychology, 52*, 429–437.

Epstein, L. H., Wing, R. R., Koeske, R. R., & Valoski, A. (1985a). A comparison of lifestyle exercise, aerobic exercise, and calisthenics on weight loss in obese children. *Behavior Therapy, 16*, 345–356.

Epstein, L. H., Wing, R. R., Steranchak, L., Dickson, B., & Michelson, J. (1980). Comparison of family-based behavior modification and nutrition education for childhood obesity. *Journal of Pediatric Psychology, 5*, 25–37.

Epstein, L. H., Wing, R. R., Woodall, K., Penner, B. C., Kress, M. J., & Koeske, R. (1985b). Effects of family-based behavioral treatment on obese 5- to 8-year-old children. *Behavior Therapy, 16*, 205–212.

Erickson, J., Forsen, T., Osmond, C., & Barker, D. (2003). Obesity from cradle to grave. *International Journal of Obesity and Related Metabolic Disorders, 27*, 722–727.

Erickson, S. J., Robinson, T. N., Haydel, K. F., & Killen, J. D. (2000). Are overweight children unhappy?: Body mass index, depressive symptoms, and overweight concerns in elementary school children. *Archives of Pediatric and Adolescent Medicine, 154*, 931–935.

Finer, N. (2003). Obesity. *Clinical Medicine, 3*, 23–27.

Golan, M., & Crow, S. (2004a). Targeting parents exclusively in the treatment of childhood obesity: Long-term results. *Obesity Research, 12*, 357–361.

Golan, M., & Crow, S. (2004b). Parents are key players in the prevention and treatment of weight-related problems. *Nutrition Reviews, 62*, 39–50.

Golan, M., Fainaru, M., & Weizman, A. (1998a). Role of behavior modification in the treatment of childhood obesity with the parents as the exclusive agents of change. *International Journal of Obesity, 22*, 1217–1224.

Golan, M., Weizman, A., Apter, A., & Fainaru, M. (1998b). Parents as the exclusive agent of change in the treatment of childhood obesity. *American Journal of Nutrition, 67*, 1130–1135.

Gordon-Larsen, P., Adair, L. S., & Popkin, B. M. (2003). The relationship of ethnicity, socioeconomic factors, and overweight in U.S. adolescents. *Obesity Research, 11*, 121–129.

Hedley, A. A., Ogden, C. L., Johnson, C. L., Carroll, M. D., Curtin, L. R., & Flegal, K. M. (2004). Prevalence of overweight and obesity among U.S. children, adolescents, and adults, 1999–2002. *Journal of the American Medical Association, 291*, 2847–2850.

Herrera, E. A., Johnston, C. A., & Steele, R. G. (2004). A comparison of cognitive and behavioral treatments for pediatric obesity. *Children's Health Care, 33*, 151–167.

Holtz, C., Smith, T. M., & Winters, F. D. (1999). Childhood obesity. *Journal of the American Osteopathic Association, 99*, 366–371.

Israel, A. C. (1999). Commentary: Empirically supported treatments for pediatric obesity: Goals, outcome criteria, and the societal context. *Journal of Pediatric Psychology, 24*, 249–250.

Israel, A. C., Guile, C. A., Baker, J. E., & Silverman, W. K. (1994). An evaluation of enhanced self-regulation training in the treatment of childhood obesity. *Journal of Pediatric Psychology, 19*, 737–749.

Israel, A. C., Silverman, W. K., & Solotar, L. C. (1987). Baseline adherence as a predictor of dropout in a children's weight-reduction program. *Journal of Consulting and Clinical Psychology, 55*, 791–793.

Israel, A. C., Silverman, W. K., & Solotar, L. C. (1988). The relationship between adherence and weight loss in a behavioral treatment program for overweight children. *Behavior Therapy, 19*, 25–33.

Israel, A. C., Solotar, L. C., & Zimand, E. (1990). An investigation of two parental roles in the treatment of obese children. *International Journal of Eating Disorders, 9*, 557–564.

Israel, A. C., Stolmaker, L., & Andrian, C. A. (1985). Thoughts about food and their relationship to obesity and weight control. *International Journal of Eating Disorders, 4*, 549–558.

Israel, A. C., Stolmaker, L., Sharp, J. P., Silverman, W. K., & Simon, L. G. (1984). An evaluation of two methods of parental involvement in treating obese children. *Behavior Therapy, 15*, 266–272.

James, P. (2004). Obesity: The worldwide epidemic. *Clinics in Dermatology, 22*, 276–280.

Jelalian, E., Mehlenbeck, R., Lloyd-Richardson, E. E., Birmaher, V., & Wing, R. R. (2006). "Adventure therapy" combined with cognitive-behavioral treatment for overweight adolescents. *International Journal of Obesity, 30*, 31–39.

Jelalian, E., & Saelens, B. E. (1999). Empirically supported treatments in pediatric psychology: Pediatric obesity. *Journal of Pediatric Psychology, 24*, 223–248.

Johnston, C. A., & Steele, R. G. (2007). Treatment of pediatric overweight: An examination of feasibility and effectiveness in an applied clinical setting. *Journal of Pediatric Psychology, 32*, 106–110.

Kawachi, I. (1999). Physical and psychological consequences of weight gain. *Journal of Clinical Psychiatry, 60*, 5–9.

Kazdin, A. E., & Weisz, J. R. (1998). Identifying and developing empirically supported child and adolescent treatments. *Journal of Consulting and Clinical Psychology, 66*, 19–36.

Keller, C. S., Gonzales, A., & Fleuriet, K. J. (2005). Retention of minority participants in clinical research studies. *Western Journal of Nursing Research, 27*, 292–306.

Klesges, R. C., Shelton, M. L., & Klesges, L. M. (1993). Effects of television on metabolic rate: Potential implications for childhood obesity. *Pediatrics, 91*, 281–286.

Lerner, R. M. (1982). Child development: Life-span perspectives. *Human Development, 25*, 38–41.

Levine, M. D., Ringham, R. M., Kalarchian, M. A., Wisniewski, L., & Marcus, M. D. (2001). Is family-based behavioral weight control appropriate for severe pediatric obesity? *International Journal of Eating Disorders, 30,* 318–328.

McDuffie, J. R., Calis, K. A., Uwaifo, G. I., Sebring, N. G., Fallon, E. M., Hubbard, V. S., & Yanovski, J. A. (2002). Three-month tolerability of Orlistat in adolescents with obesity-related comorbid conditions. *Obesity Research, 10,* 642–650.

McLean, N., Griffin, S., Toney, K., & Hardeman, W. (2003). Family involvement in weight control, weight maintenance and weight loss interventions: A systematic review of randomized trials. *International Journal of Obesity, 27,* 987–1005.

Mellin, L. M., Slinkard, L. A., & Irwin, C. E. (1987). Adolescent obesity intervention: Validation of the SHAPEDOWN program. *Journal of the American Dietetic Association, 87,* 333–338.

Must, A., & Anderson, S. E. (2003). Effects of obesity in children and adolescents. *Nutrition in Clinical Care, 6,* 4–12.

Ogden, C. L., Carroll, M. D., Curtin, L. R., McDowell, M. A., Tabak, C. J., & Flegal, K. M. (2006). Prevalence of overweight and obesity in the United States, 1999–2004. *Journal of the American Medical Association, 288,* 1549–1555.

Ogden, C. L., Kuczmarski, R. J., Flegal, K. M., Mei, Z., Guo, S., Wei, R., et al. (2000). Centers for Disease Control and Prevention 2000 growth charts for the United States: Improvements to the 1977 National Center for Health Statistics version. *Pediatrics, 109,* 45–60.

Patterson, G. R. (1976). *Living with Children: New Methods for Parents and Teachers,* 3rd ed. Champaign, IL: Research Press.

Rocchini, A. P., Katch, V., Anderson, J., Hinderlite, J., Becque, D., Martin, M., et al. (1988). Blood pressure in obese adolescents: Effects on weight loss. *Journal of the American Medical Association, 82,* 16–23.

Rossner, S. (1998). Childhood obesity and adulthood consequences. *Acta Peadiatrica, 87,* 1–5.

Schwimmer, J. B., Burwinkle, T. M., & Varni, J. M. (2003). Health-related quality of life of severely overweight children and adolescents. *Journal of the American Medical Association, 289,* 1813–1819.

Sinha, R., Fisch, G., Teague, B., Tamborlane, W. V., Banyas, B., Allen, K., et al. (2002). Prevalence of impaired glucose tolerance among children and adolescents with marked obesity. *New England Journal of Medicine, 346,* 802–810.

Summerbell, C. D., Ashton, V., Campbell, K. J., Edmunds, L. D., Kelly, S., & Waters, E. Interventions for treating obesity in children. *The Cochrane Review Database of Systematic Reviews* 2003, Issue 3, Art. No.: CD001872. DOI: 10.1002/14651858.CD001872.

Summerbell, C. D., Waters, E., Edmunds, L. D., Kelly, S., Brown, T., & Campbell, K. J. Interventions for preventing obesity in children. *The Cochrane Review Database of Systematic Reviews* 2005, Issue 3, Art. No.: CD001871.pub2. DOI: 10.1002/14651858.CD001871.pub2.

Thompson, J. K., & Tantleff-Dunn, S. (1998). Assessment of body image disturbance in obesity. *Obesity Research, 6,* 375–377.

U.S. Department of Health and Human Services (2000). *Healthy People 2010: Understanding and Improving Health,* 2nd ed. Washington, DC: Government Printing Office.

Wang, G., & Dietz, W. H. (2002). Economic burden of obesity in youths aged 6 to 17 years: 1979–1999. *Pediatrics, 109,* E81-1.

Whitaker, R. C., Wright, J. A., Pepe, M. S., Seidel, K. D., & Dietz, W. H. (1997). Predicting obesity in young adulthood from childhood and parental obesity. *New England Journal of Medicine, 337,* 869–873.

Williamson, D. A., Martin, P. D., White, M. A., Newton, R., Walden, H., York-Crowe, E., et al. (2005). Efficacy of an Internet-based behavioral weight loss program for overweight adolescent African-American girls. *Eating and Weight Disorders, 10,* 193–203.

Zametkin, A. J., Zoon, C. K., Klein, H. W., & Munson, S. (2004). Psychiatric aspects of child and adolescent obesity: A review of the past 10 years. *Journal of the American Academy of Child and Adolescent Psychiatry, 43,* 134–150.

Others Disorders and Problems

21

Evidence-Based Therapies for Autistic Disorder and Pervasive Developmental Disorders

JONATHAN M. CAMPBELL, CAITLIN V. HERZINGER, and CARRAH L. JAMES

The core features of autism were first described in Leo Kanner's (1943) remarkable description of 11 children who showed a cluster of social, communicative, and behavioral features unique from other diagnostic entities, such as mental retardation or childhood schizophrenia. One year after Kanner, Austrian physician Hans Asperger's initial report was published describing a group of four children who also showed unusual social and behavioral impairments. Although Asperger's disorder shares considerable symptom overlap with autism, the disorder has only recently become recognized in the United States as a distinct entity. In addition to autism ("autistic disorder") and Asperger's disorder, the DSM-IV-TR describes two additional subtypes of pervasive developmental disorders (PDD): Rett's disorder and childhood disintegrative disorder. Individuals who show social impairment and associated symptoms of autism but fail to meet diagnostic criteria for another PDD are diagnosed with pervasive developmental disorder, not otherwise specified (PDD-NOS). Regardless of diagnosis, all children with PDD show severe impairments, typically in communication and social interactions emerging in early childhood and deviating from overall developmental level. Children across the PDD spectrum usually engage in repetitious, stereotyped behaviors, interests, and activities, often similar to those described for children with autism. Most children with PDD, except for those with Asperger's disorder, function within the range of mental retardation.

JONATHAN M. CAMPBELL, CAITLIN V. HERZINGER, and CARRAH L. JAMES • University of Georgia

THE COMPLEX LANDSCAPE OF PDD SYMPTOMATOLOGY AND TREATMENT SERVICES

Prior to reviewing the evidence base for treatments for PDDs, several important points warrant discussion that necessitate tempering any conclusions reached about "what treatments work" for children with PDDs. First, children with PDDs are widely heterogeneous. By definition, children with PDDs exhibit a range of impairments and frequently exhibit a complex array of social, language, behavioral, and cognitive difficulties. For example, the range of intellectual functioning for children with autism can extend from mental retardation (MR) to superior cognitive ability. Furthermore, children with PDDs can show a remarkable combination of well-preserved or age-appropriate abilities in the presence of severe disability. The discrepancies between areas of functioning are perhaps best exemplified by prodigious savants, who may demonstrate memory, math, calendar-calculation, or musical talents in the presence of profound cognitive impairment.

Second, most children with PDDs present with comorbid neurocognitive, affective, or medical disorders. In the domain of neurocognitive functioning, MR frequently co-occurs with autism, with traditionally reported estimates ranging between 70–80%. As classification has included higher-functioning individuals on the PDD spectrum, such as those with Asperger's syndrome, the historical data most certainly overestimate the presence of MR for the entire PDD spectrum. Children across the PDD spectrum frequently show problems with various aspects of attention and executive functioning, such as sustaining attention and organizing academic tasks. Medical disorders most frequently reported for children with autism consist of epilepsy (20–30%); neurocutaneous syndromes, such as tuberous sclerosis and neurofibromatosis (1–4%); and chromosomal disorders, such as fragile X (1–8.1%; Fombonne, 2005). Internalizing disorders also frequently co-occur with PDDs, with estimates reported as high as 56% for the presence of either a depressive or anxiety disorder (Howlin, 2005).

Third, treatments for children with PDD may consist of *focal* (or *skills-based*) or *comprehensive* treatments (Rogers, 1998). Focal treatments are interventions designed to target specific core symptoms of PDD, such as increasing appropriate eye contact, or to target associated features of PDDs, such as reducing self-injurious behaviors. Examples of focal treatments are the use of differential reinforcement of alternative behavior (DRA) to decrease self-injury or prescribing a selective-serotonin reuptake inhibitor (SSRI) to improve mood. In contrast to focal interventions, comprehensive treatments are interventions designed to target a wide range of autistic symptomatology and improve the long-term outcomes of children with PDDs. Comprehensive treatment approaches for autism and PDDs are implemented typically via treatment teams, with high intensity (e.g., 20–40 hours per week), and over long periods of time (e.g., 2 to 3 years). Arguably the most well-known comprehensive treatment program is Lovaas' Young Autism Project (YAP), where preschool-aged children with autism received

40 or more hours of discrete trial training over a period of two or more years (Lovaas, 1987). Other comprehensive treatment programs include (1) the Treatment and Education of Autistic and Related Communication Handicapped Children (TEACCH) program, (2) the Learning Experiences...an Alternative Program (LEAP), and (3) the University of Colorado Health Sciences Center (UCHSC).

Fourth, due to the complex presentation of problems that overlap domains of professional expertise, such as speech-language pathology, psychology, special education, and psychiatry, the involvement of a range of professionals is the norm for intervention with children with PDDs. Indeed, due to the cognitive and behavioral symptoms that constitute the core and associated features of autism, treatment for autism and PDDs will almost invariably involve educational and clinical professionals at some point. The involvement of a variety of professionals across a range of service-delivery contexts, such as home, school, and clinic, further complicates evaluating the empirical support for many comprehensive treatment approaches. Without careful documentation and measurement of ancillary treatments and therapies, one might erroneously conclude that the treatment of interest accounts for progress when this may not be the case.

INTRODUCTORY COMMENTS ABOUT TREATMENTS FOR AUTISM AND ORGANIZATION OF THE REVIEW

Perhaps no other group of childhood disorders has elicited the vast number and variety of interventions and therapies than autism and PDDs. A brief review of scientific and lay literature will yield a range of highly controversial educational and treatment options for children with autism and PDD, such as hyperbaric oxygen therapy, hippotherapy, secretin, and facilitated communication. In Simpson and colleagues' (2005) impressive review of educational interventions and therapies for PDDs, 37 intervention strategies were identified. Of the 37 treatments, 4 treatment approaches were scientifically based and 13 were identified as promising. The remaining 20 treatments were found to be unsupported.

Due to the overwhelming amount of literature that exists regarding treatments for autism, in terms of both the number of treatments proposed and the number of empirical investigations published, any review will necessarily be selective. We began our own review by consulting several recent comprehensive reviews of empirically supported treatments for children with autism and PDDs. The reviews consisted of the special series published by the *Journal of Autism and Developmental Disorders* in 2002, the National Research Council's (2001) review of educational interventions for children with autism, and Simpson's (2005) recently published text, among others (e.g., Gresham et al., 1999; Rogers, 1998; Smith, 1999). When evaluated against modified versions of Chambless and Hollon's (1998) criteria for empirically supported treatments, no treatments were identified as "well-established" or "probably efficacious" (e.g., Rogers, 1998). In light of these reviews, we chose to focus our review on comprehensive and focal behaviorally based therapies due to the large number of children with autism and PDDs receiving these services.

BEHAVIORAL THERAPIES: APPLIED BEHAVIORAL ANALYSIS

Various reviews of treatments for children with autism and PDD have acknowledged consistently that the forms of treatment enjoying the most extensive empirical support are interventions based on behavioral theory (e.g., Schreibman, 2000). It is also fairly widely held that behavioral treatments are best implemented intensively and early, hence the preponderance of studies examining the effectiveness of early intensive behavioral intervention (EIBI). Lovaas and Smith (1989) proposed a comprehensive behavioral theory to guide treatment for children with autism and PDDs; it focuses on specific behavioral symptoms as opposed to the diagnostic entity of autism, the etiology of which is most likely neurobiological. As such, symptoms exhibited by children with autism are thought to represent a "mismatch" between an impaired neurobiological system and typical learning environments. Treatment and educational progress, therefore, can take place if environments are systematically altered and manipulated.

Applied behavior analysis (ABA) serves as the conceptual and technical basis for different instructional methodologies aimed at improving cognitive, language, communication, and socialization skills for individuals with autism. A variety of intervention techniques exist under the general rubric of ABA therapy, such as discrete trial training (DTT), incidental teaching (IT), pivotal response training (PRT), and peer-mediated interventions. Although techniques may differ, ABA treatments stress intervention at the level of specific behaviors, whether acquiring skills or reducing problem behaviors. ABA therapies are characterized by (1) objective and ongoing measurement of behaviors that are operationally defined and reliably recorded, (2) implementation of individualized curricula, (3) selection and systematic use of reinforcers, (4) use of functional analysis to identify variables that increase or inhibit behaviors, and (5) emphasis on generalization of learned skills (Anderson & Romanczyk, 1999).

Discrete Trial Training or Teaching

Discrete trial training or teaching (DTT) is based on principles of learning theory, primarily operant conditioning, and has been used to intervene with children with autism. DTT incorporates units of instruction used to teach and assess the acquisition of basic skills. Regardless of the skill being taught, a discrete trial incorporates the same sequential components: (1) a discriminative stimulus (S^D) provided by therapist or teacher; (2) a prompt, if necessary, to elicit a response; (3) the individual's response (correct or incorrect); and (4) consequence of the response (S^R; e.g., verbal praise). Typically, generalization to new settings, therapists, stimuli/prompts, and specific tasks occurs after predetermined mastery criteria are met.

Experiments involving DTT formats have provided a foundation for the development of procedures needed to teach discriminative performances that children with autism had not learned on their own (Goldstein, 2002).

Comprehensive DTT Treatment Programs

Lovaas' (1987) Young Autism Project (YAP) is a comprehensive treatment approach based on the extensive application of DTT to the entire range of symptoms expressed by autism and PDDs. Using a quasi-experimental design, Lovaas (1987) documented remarkable outcomes for children with autism (n = 19) enrolled in the 40-hour-per-week YAP program when compared to two matched control groups: one group of children who received 10 hours per week of YAP therapy (n = 19) and another who received unspecified intervention (n = 21). Children in intensive therapy showed significant improvement in intellectual functioning and school placement when compared to both control groups. McEachin et al. (1993) also documented significant long-term improvements (i.e., IQ, adaptive behavior, school placement, and social-emotional adjustment) for the 19 children who received intensive YAP treatment when compared to controls.

Findings reported from the original YAP study have been the subject of intense debate (e.g., Gresham et al., 1999). Criticisms launched at the initial YAP findings have included the use of quasi-experimentation due to the lack of random assignment to treatment conditions, problems with varied measures used to document outcomes over time, lack of external validity of study findings, and incomplete documentation of treatment outcomes. Subsequent scientific study of the YAP program has employed improved methodological controls, such as the use of yoked-pair random assignment and increased documentation of treatment outcomes. Findings have been replicated in varied settings (e.g., schools), and with varied samples of children.

The UCLA YAP treatment approach has been partially replicated in at least five additional studies at treatment sites within and outside the United States, such as the May Institute in Massachusetts and Norway, with similar outcomes (Smith, 1999). The replicated outcomes are described as "partial" due to reduced treatment intensity and length. While the original UCLA YAP consisted of 40 hours per week of treatment, replications ranged in intensity between 18 and 25 hours per week. Similarly, the replication studies assessed outcomes at shorter intervals (12–63 months) than the original follow-up reports (M = 11.5 years).

Smith et al. (1997) examined the utility of YAP for children with PDD through retrospective review of treatment records. The experimental group consisted of 11 children enrolled in YAP at UCLA, Oslo, or Kansas who received 30 hours per week of DTT intervention; the control group consisted of 10 children who received 10 hours per week of DTT based on Lovaas' model. Groups did not differ on intake IQ, chronological age, or use of speech. Follow-up assessments revealed significant improvement in IQ for the experimental group versus the control group and greater use of speech as rated by blind evaluators.

Three prospective studies have supported the efficacy of the UCLA YAP treatment program. Smith et al. (2000) randomly assigned children diagnosed with either autism or PDD-NOS either to (1) 30 hours per week of YAP treatment delivered in the home by trained therapists (n = 15) or (2) parent training in DTT (n = 13). Children assigned to YAP received 25 hours per week of intervention for an average of 33 months, while the parent training group received 3 to 9 months of parent training. Treatment groups were found to be similar on pretreatment measures of intelligence, language, and academic skills. At follow-up, children receiving intensive therapy performed significantly better than the parent training group on measures of intelligence and academic achievement. No differences were found between groups on measures of adaptive behavior or parent- and teacher-rated social-emotional functioning.

Also examining potential differences in delivery of ABA, Sallows and Graupner (2005) randomly assigned 24 children with autism to receive Lovaas-based ABA services that were either clinic-directed (n = 13) or parent-directed (n = 10). The clinic-directed ABA services were identified as an intensive behavioral treatment group with parent-directed service intended to serve as a less intensive form of ABA, similar to Lovaas' (1987) 10-hour-week control group. The clinic-directed group received approximately 38 hours of treatment per week over a 2-year period, while the parent-directed group received approximately 31 hours of treatment per week. Children were followed over a period of more than four years. Posttest scores revealed significant gains for both treatment groups on measures of cognitive functioning, language, adaptive behavior, and autism symptomatology. Outcomes did not differ across treatment groups; however, posttreatment scores were slightly higher in the parent group when compared to the clinic group. Children were subclassified into "rapid learners" versus "moderate learners," with rapid learners achieving better outcomes on all cognitive and clinical measures.

Eikeseth et al. (2002) also evaluated Lovaas' treatment program using a prospective design with older children (aged 4 to 7) in a public school setting. The authors employed a quasi-experimental design comparing Lovaas' DTT approach (n = 13) to eclectic treatment (n = 12), defined as a combination of interventions, such as sensory-motor therapy, TEACCH-based instruction, ABA, and other special education interventions. Assignment to conditions depended on the availability of personnel as opposed to random assignment. At the onset of treatment, groups did not differ on variables such as age, verbal and nonverbal cognitive functioning, language, and adaptive behavior. At one-year follow-up, children receiving DTT outperformed the eclectic treatment group on measures of overall IQ, total language functioning, and adaptive communication.

Further empirical evidence has also supported intensive behavior analytic therapy as superior to both eclectic special education approaches and general educational programming (Howard et al., 2005). Sixty-one preschool children diagnosed with either autism or PDD-NOS participated in either (1) "intensive behavioral treatment" (IBT; n = 29), (2) "eclectic programming (e.g., a combination of DTT; TEACCH-based instruction;

n = 16), or (3) general special education services (n = 16). The IBT condition involved 25–30 hours per week of one-on-one intervention for children below the age of 3 and 35–40 hours per week of one-on-one intervention for children 3 years or older. After 14 months of intervention for each group, children receiving IBT outperformed the other groups on measures of overall IQ, language, and adaptive functioning. Similar to the Eikeseth et al. (2002) study, Howard and colleagues did not randomly assign children to treatment conditions. Taken together, the studies provide initial evidence that intensive ABA yields more favorable outcomes than "eclectic" blends of educational services for children across the PDD spectrum.

Variables Associated with Outcomes in Intensive ABA Therapy

Proposed predictors of positive outcomes for intensive ABA therapy include (1) younger age of child at time of enrollment, (2) pretreatment IQ, (3) treatment intensity, and (4) treatment duration (e.g., Rogers, 1998). Most children in the studies described above were enrolled in treatment services prior to the age of 5, with the exception of Eikeseth et al. (2002). In describing outcomes from the Princeton Child Development Institute (PCDI), a comprehensive ABA treatment program, Fenske et al. (1985) found that nine children with autism enrolled prior to 60 months enjoyed better outcomes than nine children enrolled after 60 months of age. Harris and Handleman (2000) found a significant relationship between age at time of admission and long-term educational placement for 27 children with autism enrolled in the Douglass Developmental Disabilities Center program. Younger age was predictive of regular education placement. Other tests of the relationship between age of enrollment and outcome have yielded nonsignificant findings. For example, Eikeseth et al. (2002) did not find significant relationships between age and outcomes.

In Lovaas' (1987) study, pretreatment mental age was significantly related to outcomes, as measured by educational placement and IQ. Harris and Handleman (2000) also found that IQ functioning at admission was predictive of regular education placement. Eikeseth et al. (2002) found that pretreatment IQ was associated positively with language improvement for children receiving intensive behavioral treatment. Therefore, there is some evidence to suggest a positive relationship between pretreatment IQ and treatment outcomes; however, the association between pretreatment IQ and later outcomes has not been evaluated routinely.

Although Lovaas (1987) found significant differences favoring high-intensity versus low-intensity treatment, follow-up studies have not replicated these findings. The partial replications of Lovaas' original study have yielded improvements with less intensive service. In a direct test of the relationship between intensity of service and outcome, Sheinkopf and Siegel (1998) found no differences between a high-intensity group (28–43 hours per week) and low-intensity group (12–27 hours per week) on cognitive outcomes. Sheinkopf and Siegel suggested that 40 hours per week may not be necessary to produce positive outcomes and that less intensive therapy may be sufficient for significant improvement.

Review of the treatment outcomes presented indicates that significant improvement can occur in as short as a one-year period of intensive treatment. In the only direct test of the relationship between duration of treatment and outcomes, Luiselli et al. (2000) found that *longer* duration of intervention service predicted more favorable communication, cognitive, and social-emotional outcomes. Similar to the other variables discussed, determining the effects of length of treatment on outcome requires additional study.

FOCAL BEHAVIORAL INTERVENTIONS

Focal behavioral interventions have been implemented across a wide range of targeted areas for individuals with autism, such as social skills, language, daily living skills, academic skills, and problem behaviors. In a descriptive review of the published literature, Matson et al. (1996) identified 251 single-case studies describing behavioral interventions for individuals with autism. Matson et al. (1996) described a range of behavioral techniques used in the treatment of children with autism, such as reinforcement-based procedures (e.g., tangible), punishment (e.g., verbal reprimand), extinction (e.g., ignoring undesirable behavior), and combinations of these methods. The efficacy of focal behavioral interventions has been reviewed extensively in several recently published papers including the use of focal interventions to increase communication (Goldstein, 2002), improve social adaptation (McConnell, 2002), and reduce problem behaviors (Campbell, 2003).

Communication Skills

A variety of focal behavioral interventions have been examined to increase the communicative capacity of children with autism. In a review of 60 published studies, Goldstein (2002) found empirical support for the use of sign language, DTT, and milieu teaching procedures (e.g., incidental teaching) to increase the communication skills for children with autism. Within the communication intervention literature, functional communication training (FCT) has been used to reduce the frequency of problem behaviors for individuals with autism. Conceptually, FCT is based on the notion that problem behaviors, such as self-injury, can serve a communicative function that can be replaced with appropriate methods of communication. For example, self-injury might occur when a child is asked to complete an academic task that results in the removal of an undesirable stimulus. In this case, self-injury may serve an escape function via negative reinforcement. In the FCT paradigm, a functional equivalent might be taught, such as teaching the child to request a break or help if the academic task is too difficult.

Facilitated communication (FC) warrants brief mention here. FC is an intervention based primarily on the notion that communicative intent is present for many individuals with autism; however, sensory-motor problems prevent communication. FC requires the assistance of a "facilitator" to assist the individual with autism communicate using a communication board or similar device. When examined rigorously, FC has been shown to be an ineffective intervention (see Simpson, 2005, pp. 62–75, for review).

Social Interaction

McConnell (2002) reviewed 55 published articles examining the intervention literature designed to improve social interaction for young children with autism. Interventions were coded as ecological, collateral skills interventions, child-specific interventions, and peer-based. Ecological intervention, i.e., manipulating the environment to promote social contact with peers, resulted in "weak to moderate effects" (p. 360). Collateral skills interventions are those that consist of teaching a skill in one area of development, such as play, that yields improvement in social interaction. Child-specific interventions are reinforcement- or instructionally based interventions to increase frequency and quality of social behaviors, such as direct instruction in social problem solving. McConnell found empirical support for skill-based interventions but cautioned that such instruction may be limited in isolation. Peer-mediated interventions, such as training peers to initiate social interactions with children with autism, yielded strong and robust treatment effects. McConnell documented that a variety of peer-mediated techniques have demonstrated utility, such as peer tutoring.

Reduction of Problem Behaviors

Epidemiological studies suggest that 13–30% of children with autism engage in problematic behaviors that warrant intervention (Horner et al., 2002). Campbell (2003) reviewed 117 published single-subject experiments targeting reduction of problem behaviors for children and adults with autism. The review documented that, in general, a variety of behavioral treatments are effective in reducing problematic behaviors, including reinforcement-based and punishment-based approaches. Campbell found that treatments based on experimental functional analysis (EFA) produced greater behavioral suppression than treatments without EFA. The most effective behavioral interventions were also associated with higher degree of inter-rater reliability in observing problem behavior.

Pivotal Response Treatment or Training

Pivotal response treatment (PRT) is an intervention grounded in behavioral theory that has received an impressive amount of empirical support. In part, the development of PRT resulted from findings from the DTT literature, which documented improved outcomes for children with autism but only after extensive and costly treatments (Koegel et al., 2001). Koegel et al. (2001) asserted that if one can improve functioning in the areas most disabling for autism (i.e., "pivotal" areas), then treatment effects should extend to other areas. A core idea of PRT is that children with autism are unmotivated to respond to complex social and environmental stimuli (Koegel et al., 2001); therefore, pivotal areas of intervention include (1) teaching children to respond to multiple environmental cues, (2) increasing motivation (e.g., using child-selected reinforcers), (3) increasing capacity for self-management, and (4) increasing self-initiations.

Sherer and Schreibman (2005) analyzed archival data for 28 children who participated in PRT research and identified social, communicative, and behavioral characteristics associated with positive response to treatment. When compared to nonresponders, treatment responders (1) exhibited greater interest in toys, (2) were more tolerant of social proximity of others, (3) engaged in lower rates of nonverbal self-stimulatory behavior, and (4) showed higher rates of verbal self-stimulatory behaviors. The treatment response profiles were applied to six additional children: three responders and three nonresponders. Children with the responder profile showed better gains in appropriate language use, engagement in play behaviors, and appropriate social behaviors when compared to children with the nonresponder profile. The type of research conducted by Sherer and Schreibman is important, in terms of the possible identification of a general "treatment responder profile" as well as possibly identifying an individual-by-PRT treatment "fit" that predicts successful outcome.

BRIEF INTRODUCTION OF THREE ADDITIONAL COMPREHENSIVE TREATMENT APPROACHES

The TEACCH Program

The TEACCH program is a comprehensive assessment, educational, and treatment program for children with autism that is implemented statewide in North Carolina. TEACCH espouses a treatment philosophy grounded in parent-professional collaboration, improvement of the child's adaptation through teaching and environmental accommodation, the use of structured teaching, and lifelong community-based service, among other guiding principles (see Schopler, 1997). The TEACCH philosophy was developed, in part, to counter the prevailing psychoanalytic theories guiding treatment for children with autism.

Panerai et al. (2002) compared the TEACCH program to an integrated educational model in a sample of 16 children diagnosed with autism (M CA = 9.26 year; M IQ = 16). After one year of treatment, authors found that the experimental group showed significant gains in a variety of developmental domains and adaptive behavior (e.g., cognitive performance), while the control group showed gains in only two domains. It was not clear if children were assigned to conditions or whether the study was prospective versus retrospective. Ozonoff and Cathcart (1998) examined the effectiveness of a 10-week TEACCH-based home intervention program for 11 children with autism (M CA = 53.3 months) compared to a control group of 11 age-matched children. Both groups received day treatment services, while only the experimental group received home-based TEACCH services, which were provided once per week for one hour. At four-month follow-up, the experimental group showed significant improvements in imitation, fine motor, gross motor, and cognitive performance areas when compared to the control group. Children were not randomly assigned to conditions.

Learning Experiences...An Alternative Program (LEAP)

The LEAP program is an educational program for children with autism and typical peers that espouses the educational and treatment value of peer-mediated intervention (Kohler et al., 2005). The LEAP program consists of classroom instruction, parent education, and provision of additional services, such as speech-language, within the classroom setting as needed. Instruction is characterized by balance between quiet and active activities, varied group sizes, and child- versus teacher-directed tasks (Kohler et al., 2005). LEAP instruction is individualized, data-driven, and focused on generalizing learning skills across contexts through saturation of learning opportunities throughout the day (Strain & Hoyson, 2000). Families are involved in the LEAP program through supporting instruction within the classroom and participating in curriculum to teach core behavioral principles to increase desirable behaviors and reduce inappropriate behaviors. At the core of the LEAP curriculum is active involvement of peers as intervention agents.

Hoyson et al. (1984) published initial treatment outcomes for six children with autistic-like behavioral presentations (M CA = 39.67 months; M IQ = 71.11). Follow-up evaluations two years out indicated developmental gains beyond that expected given developmental progress at intake (Hoyson et al., 1984). Strain and Hoyson (2000) reported on the same six participants at the age of 10 and found that (1) autistic symptoms were reduced, (2) developmental and cognitive functioning were significantly improved (e.g., M IQ = 101), (3) social interactions were more positive, and (4) five of six participants were being educated in regular classrooms without special education services.

University of Colorado Health Science Center (UCHSC)

The UCHSC program is a center-based program built upon three developmental theories relevant to understanding the core pathology of autism, chiefly, cognitive functioning, language development, social communication, and interpersonal relationships. Piaget's theory of cognitive development, pragmatics theory of language development, and Mahler's theory of the development of interpersonal relationships all contribute to programming in the UCHSC model (Rogers & DiLalla, 1991). The program emphasizes *play* as a primary instructional format to target development and the importance of *positive affect* to increase attention, motivation, and social connection and assist in memory and learning (Rogers & DiLalla). Center-based activities occur within a predictable structure and routine, and inappropriate behaviors are approached from a positive programming perspective. Four published outcomes have documented gains for children with autism and PDDs in the domains of cognitive, language, motor, adaptive behavior, and social-emotional development (Rogers & DiLalla, 1991; Rogers et al., 1986, 1987; Rogers & Lewis, 1989). The program has been replicated in four rural communities (Rogers et al., 1987), and children with autism and PDDs have shown developmental gains equal to a comparison group of children with other behavioral and developmental disorders (Rogers & DiLalla, 1991).

SUMMARY

Although each comprehensive treatment program reviewed has received some empirical support, none currently reaches criteria to be classified as well-established. Based on our review of the literature, interventions grounded in behavioral theory feature the most empirical support in terms of both focal and comprehensive treatment approaches. Support for the use of ABA techniques is found in hundreds of published single-subject experiments, many of which feature appropriate experimental quality in terms of design, describing treatment methods, and incorporating reliable observations across time. Of the group-based experiments, Lovaas' ABA program is the most rigorously evaluated, including replication across sites using randomized controlled trials. The first two published randomized controlled trials have yielded modest support for Lovaas' model by evaluating the effects of intensity of services on outcomes.

Common Components of Comprehensive Treatments

Dawson and Osterling (1997) and Schreibman (2000) identified a shared set of features for the comprehensive treatment programs reviewed that have garnered empirical support. First, intervention begins early (i.e., by age 4 or 5) and is implemented intensively (15–40 hours per week). As demonstrated in the review, intervention that is implemented early in development can be very effective in improving outcomes for children with autism and PDDs; however, outcomes vary widely, with some children experiencing little gain. Within the group of therapies, intervention is tailored to unique characteristics of children treated. The programs emphasize social development and target social communicative development in the areas of attending, imitation, using language, and play.

Instruction and intervention are provided in structured, predictable, and supportive teaching environments with *generalization* a common goal of intervention. Children with autism and PDDs are typically poor at generalizing learned skills to new situations; therefore, generalization of new skills to new persons and environments requires planning and programming (Schreibman, 2000). With this in mind, effective intervention involves parents as collaborators in the treatment and education of their children, thereby fostering generalization of skills to new settings and persons. Programs also approach problem behaviors from a functional perspective, that is, programs attempt to prevent problem behavior from occurring and alter the environment or instructional strategies to reduce its likelihood. Finally, programs anticipate and provide instruction relevant to transition from the program's preschool classroom environment.

RECOMMENDATIONS

There appears to be movement toward improved research design for evaluating the efficacy of comprehensive treatments for children with autism, with an increasing number of randomized clinical trials being published. We identified two such trials evaluating comprehensive ABA therapy. Due to the chronic and severe symptoms of autism, effective psychosocial treatment will need to be implemented comprehensively with at least moderate intensity and over a lengthy period of time (Smith et al., 2007). From a clinical research perspective, this set of circumstances makes treatment evaluation a complex endeavor in terms of both implementing treatment and adequately evaluating its effects. For example, rigorous evaluation of two "competing" treatment approaches would require (1) identification of an adequate number of participants agreeing to random assignment, (2) a large team of interventionists employed over a long period of time, (3) careful documentation of treatment fidelity, (4) standardized assessment procedures, and (5) long-term follow-up. Participant recruitment and enrollment needs grow as potential moderators and mediators of treatment outcome are evaluated, such as gender, pretreatment IQ, and intensity of service delivery. Such circumstances likely require multisite collaboration.

Lord et al. (2005), Schopler (2005), and Smith et al. (2007) identified methodological "tensions" within the autism treatment literature that exist between the traditions of group-based experimentation, exemplified by the randomized controlled trial, and single-subject experimentation. These two paradigms are perhaps most at odds in the quantification and synthesis of single-subject experiments, where group-based statistical methods are employed with individual outcomes. To date, there is no consensus regarding whether such outcomes can be synthesized and interpreted simultaneously. Due to the overwhelming amount of treatment literature being generated for children with autism and PDDs, methods of quantitative synthesis may prove useful in documenting outcomes when treatments are compared and detecting characteristics of responders to treatment. Within the autism treatment literature, quantitative reviews of group-based designs and single-subject experiments have occurred separately; therefore, future conceptual, methodological, and statistical work in the area of synthesizing findings seems warranted.

At present, attempts to identify children who will respond most favorably to treatment have not yielded a clear profile of who is most likely to benefit. The typical heuristic is that long-term outcome is predicted by cognitive functioning and meaningful language use by the age of 5 to 6 years. The present review revealed mixed relationships among pretreatment IQ, age of enrollment in treatment, or intensity of treatment and response to DTT therapy for over 300 children with autism. Encouraging current research within the PRT literature attempts to identify individuals who are likely to respond to treatment. Single-subject experimentation appears to be a useful method for identifying and testing initial hypotheses regarding individual to treatment matching. Hypotheses generated through single-subject designs might then be subjected to group-based research designs (Lord et al., 2005). Regardless of methodology used to guide treatment decisions, understanding why some children with autism respond to therapies will continue to be an area of worthwhile study.

REFERENCES

Anderson, S. R., & Romanczyk, R. G. (1999). Early intervention for young children with autism: Continuum-based behavioral models. *The Journal of the Association for Persons with Severe Handicaps, 24,* 162–173.

Campbell, J. M. (2003). Efficacy of behavioral interventions for reducing problem behavior in persons with autism: A quantitative synthesis of single-subject research. *Research in Developmental Disabilities, 24,* 120–138.

Chambless, D. L., & Hollon, S. D. (1998). Defining empirically supported therapies. *Journal of Consulting and Clinical Psychology, 66,* 7–18.

Dawson, G., & Osterling, J. (1997). Early intervention in autism. In M. J. Guralnick (Ed.), *The Effectiveness of Early Intervention* (pp. 307–326). Baltimore: Brookes.

Eikeseth, S., Smith, T., Jahr, E., & Eldevik, S. (2002). Intensive behavioral treatment at school for 4- to 7-year-old children with autism: A 1-year comparison controlled study. *Behavior Modification, 26,* 49–86.

Fenske, E. C., Zalenski, S., Krantz, P. J., & McClannahan, L. E. (1985). Age at intervention and treatment outcome for autistic children in a comprehensive intervention program. *Analysis and Intervention in Developmental Disabilities, 5,* 49–58.

Fombonne, E. (2005). Epidemiological studies of pervasive developmental disorders. In F. R. Volkmar, R. Paul, A. Klin, & D. Cohen (Eds.), *Handbook of Autism and Pervasive Developmental Disorders,* 3rd ed. (pp. 42–69). New York: Wiley.

Goldstein, H. (2002). Communication intervention for children with autism: A review of treatment efficacy. *Journal of Autism and Developmental Disorders, 32,* 373–396.

Gresham, F. M., Beebe-Frankenberger, & MacMillan, D. L. (1999). A selective review of treatments for children with autism: Description and methodological considerations. *School Psychology Review, 28,* 559–575.

Harris, S. L., & Handleman, J. S. (2000). Age and IQ at intake as predictors of placement for young children with autism: A four- to six-year follow-up. *Journal of Autism and Developmental Disorders, 30,* 137–142.

Horner, R. H., Carr, E. G., Strain, P. S., Todd, A. W., & Reed, H. K. (2002). Problem behavior interventions for young children with autism: A research synthesis. *Journal of Autism and Developmental Disorders, 32,* 423–446.

Howard, J. S., Sparkman, C. R., Cohen, H. G., Green, G., & Stanislaw, H. (2005). A comparison of intensive behavior analytic and eclectic treatments for young children with autism. *Research in Developmental Disabilities, 26,* 359–383.

Howlin, P. C. (2005). Outcomes in autism spectrum disorders. In F. R. Volkmar, R. Paul, A. Klin, & D. Cohen (Eds.), *Handbook of Autism and Pervasive Developmental Disorders*, 3rd ed. (pp. 201–220). New York: Wiley.

Hoyson, M., Jamieson, B., & Strain, P. S. (1984). Individualized group instruction of normally developing and autistic-like children: The LEAP curriculum model. *Journal of the Division for Early Childhood*, *8*, 157–172.

Kanner, L. (1943). Autistic disturbances of affective contact. *Nervous Child*, *2*, 217–250.

Koegel, L. K., Koegel, R. L., & McNerney, E. K. (2001). Pivotal areas in intervention for autism. *Journal of Clinical Child Psychology*, *30,* 19–32.

Kohler, F. W., Strain, P. S., & Goldstein, H. (2005). Learning Experiences...An Alternative Program for preschoolers and parents: Peer-mediated interventions for young children with autism. In E. D. Hibbs & P. S. Jensen (Eds.), *Psychosocial Treatments for Child and Adolescent Disorders: Empirically Based Strategies for Clinical Practice*, 2nd ed. (pp. 659–687). Washington, DC: American Psychological Association.

Lord, C., Wagner, A., Rogers, S., Szatmari, P., Aman, M., Charman, T., et al. (2005). Challenges in evaluating psychosocial interventions for autistic spectrum disorders. *Journal of Autism and Developmental Disorders*, *35*, 695–708.

Lovaas, O. I. (1987). Behavioral treatment and normal educational and intellectual functioning in young autistic children. *Journal of Consulting & Clinical Psychology*, *55*, 3–9.

Lovaas, O. I., & Smith, T. (1989). A comprehensive behavioral theory of autistic children: Paradigm for research and treatment. *Journal of Behavioral Therapy and Experimental Psychiatry*, *20*, 17–29.

Luiselli, J. K., Cannon, B. O., Ellis, J. T., & Sisson, R. W. (2000). Home-based behavioral intervention for young children with autism/pervasive developmental disorder. *Autism*, *4*, 426–438.

Matson, J. L., Benavidez, D. A., Compton, L. S, Paclawskyj, T., & Baglio, C. (1996). Behavioral treatment of autistic persons: A review of research from 1980 to the present. *Research in Developmental Disabilities*, *17*, 433–465.

McConnell, S. R. (2002). Interventions to facilitate social interaction for young children with autism: Review of available research and recommendations for educational intervention and future research. *Journal of Autism and Developmental Disorders*, *32*, 351–371.

McEachin, J. J., Smith, T., & Lovaas, O. I. (1993). Long-term outcome for children with autism who received early intensive behavioral treatment. *American Journal on Mental Retardation*, *97*, 359–372.

National Research Council (2001). *Educating Children with Autism*, C. Lord & J. P. McGee (Eds.). Washington, DC: National Academy Press.

Ozonoff, S., & Cathcart, K. (1998). Effectiveness of a home program intervention for young children with autism. *Journal of Autism and Developmental Disorders*, *28*, 25–32.

Panerai, S., Ferrante, L., & Zingale, M. (2002). Benefits of the Treatment and Education of Autistic and Communication Handicapped Children (TEACCH) programme as compared with a non-specific approach. *Journal of Intellectual Disability Research*, *46*, 318–327.

Rogers, S. J. (1998). Empirically supported comprehensive treatments for young children with autism. *Journal of Clinical Child Psychology*, *27*, 168–179.

Rogers, S. J., & DiLalla, D. L. (1991). A comparative study of the effects of a developmentally based instructional model on young children with autism and young children with other disorders of behavior and development. *Topics in Early Childhood Special Education*, *11*, 29–47.

Rogers, S. J., Herbison, J. M., Lewis, H. C., Pantone, J., & Reis, K. (1986). An approach for enhancing the symbolic, communicative, and interpersonal functioning of young children with autism or severe emotional handicaps. *Journal of the Division for Early Childhood*, *10*, 135–145.

Rogers, S. J., & Lewis, H. (1989). An effective day treatment model for young children with pervasive developmental disorders. *Journal of the American Academy of Child and Adolescent Psychiatry*, *28*, 207–214.

Rogers, S. J., Lewis, H., & Reis, K. (1987). An effective procedure for training early special education teams to implement a model program. *Journal of the Division for Early Childhood*, *11*, 180–188.

Sallows, G. O., & Graupner, T. D. (2005). Intensive behavioral treatment for children with autism: Four-year outcome and predictors. *American Journal on Mental Retardation, 110,* 417–438.

Schopler, E. (2005). Comments on "Challenges in Evaluating Psychological Intervention for Autistic Spectrum Disorders" by Lord et al. *Journal of Autism and Developmental Disorders,* 709–711.

Schopler, E. (1997). Implementation of TEACCH philosophy. In D. Cohen & F. R. Volkmar (Eds.), *Handbook of Autism and Pervasive Developmental Disorders,* 2nd ed. (pp. 767–795). New York: Wiley.

Schreibman, L. (2000). Intensive behavioral/psychoeducational treatments for autism: Research needs and future directions. *Journal of Autism and Developmental Disorders, 30,* 373–378.

Sheinkopf, S. J., & Siegel, B. (1998). Home-based behavioral treatment of young children with autism. *Journal of Autism and Developmental Disorders, 28,* 15–23.

Sherer, M. R., & Schreibman, L. (2005). Individual behavioral profiles and predictors of treatment effectiveness for children with autism. *Journal of Consulting and Clinical Psychology, 73,* 525–538.

Simpson, R. L. (2005). *Autism Spectrum Disorders: Interventions and Treatments for Children and Youth.* Thousand Oaks, CA: Corwin Press.

Smith, T. (1999). Outcome of early intervention for children with autism. *Clinical Psychology: Science and Practice, 6,* 33–49.

Smith, T., Eikeseth, S., Klevstrand, M., & Lovaas, O. I. (1997). Intensive behavioral treatment for preschoolers with severe mental retardation. *American Journal on Mental Retardation, 102,* 238–249.

Smith, T., Groen, A. D., & Wynn, J. W. (2000). Randomized trial of intensive early intervention for children with pervasive developmental disorder. *American Journal on Mental Retardation, 105,* 269–285.

Smith, T., Scahill, L., Dawson, G., Guthrie, D., Lord, C., Odom, S., et al. (2007). Designing research studies on psychosocial interventions in autism. *Journal of Autism and Developmental Disorders, 37,* 354–366.

Strain, P. S., & Hoyson, M. (2000). The need for longitudinal intensive social skill intervention: LEAP follow-up outcomes for children with autism. *Topics in Early Childhood Special Education, 20,* 116–122.

22

Evidence-Based Treatment for Children with Serious Emotional Disturbance

CAMILLE J. RANDALL and ERIC M. VERNBERG

The term *serious emotional disturbance* (SED) describes children and adolescents who have severe difficulties functioning in home, school, and community settings that are thought to be caused in part by one or more underlying psychopathological conditions. Because the common element in SED is impaired functioning, rather than a core set of symptoms, children and adolescents with this label are heterogeneous in terms of psychiatric diagnoses that may also be appropriately applied. In reality, many who meet criteria for SED carry multiple diagnoses (e.g., bipolar disorder, conduct disorder, attention deficit hyperactivity disorder) and show impairment in multiple domains (e.g., thought problems, mood disturbance, conduct problems). Due to the severity of their impairments and concerns regarding comorbidity, many children and adolescents who meet criteria for SED would likely be excluded from randomized controlled trials (RCTs) evaluating treatment outcomes for discrete diagnostic categories, such as those discussed in Section II of this text. Despite the diverse set of serious problems among children and adolescents with SED, some promise is demonstrated by two randomized controlled trials (RCTs) that used SED as a primary selection criterion, as well as by quasi-experimental studies addressing clinical and functional outcomes in this difficult-to-treat population. In this chapter, we discuss this body of research, compare promising programs thematically, and delineate core principles for delivering evidence-based treatments with this diverse population.

CAMILLE J. RANDALL and ERIC M. VERNBERG • University of Kansas

TYPICAL SERVICES AND OUTCOMES
FOR CHILDREN
WITH SED

Comprehensive programs targeting the SED population strive for service delivery models that exceed the piecemeal and inadequate approaches decried by critics of "treatment as usual." These comprehensive services appear to be offered relatively infrequently, although it is not unusual for children and adolescents with SED to be involved with mental health services, social services, special education, and juvenile justice programs. Prognoses for this population appear poor, especially when viewed in terms of educational, occupational, and social functioning. The National Adolescent and Child Treatment Study (NACTS; Greenbaum et al., 1996) defined children with SED as those receiving intense and sustained services intended to serve children with serious [socioemotional] problems and sought to identify outcomes for these children, aged 9 to 17, across a seven-year span. This study did not attempt to evaluate services, nor did it attempt to define exemplary practices. It simply sought to describe the contemporary status of youth with SED sampled from six geographically diverse states in the United States. Almost half of the sample carried two or more psychiatric diagnoses above a mild to moderate level of severity, with disruptive disorders and anxiety disorders being the most prevalent. Psychiatric symptoms, as measured by a broadband behavior rating scale, declined modestly across the study period, though average composite scores below the clinical range were only observed in the oldest cohort. Adaptive behavior scores, however, declined by one standard point per year, per NACTS data, suggesting that participants entered at the sixth and ended at the third percentile relative to the population. Further, minority children fared worse than their Caucasian peers over time. Contact with law enforcement was common (67%), academic achievement was poor, graduation/GED rates were low (40% over age 18), and recidivism to mental health and correctional facilities was common for participants who had been involved in such placements. Given the clinical and functional outcome status just described, it is important to highlight that youth in the NACTS had received many services over the period of the study: mental health (93%), child welfare (32%), juvenile justice (80%), school-based special education (71%), and vocational rehabilitation (12%). More than one-third utilized four of these five services at any point in the study's span (Greenbaum et al., 1996). We may extrapolate from these results that treatment as usual, at best, prevents children with SED from declining in their functioning over time. However, promising approaches described in the next sections illustrate that empirically informed, focused, and cross-system efforts may foster enduring gains in functioning and promote skills helping youth with SED be less dependent on restrictive supports.

EMPIRICAL SUPPORT FOR TREATMENTS ADDRESSING CHILDREN AND ADOLESCENTS WITH SED

Relevant outcomes for children and adolescents with SED can appear different than clinical outcomes otherwise described in Section II of this text in that indicators of adaptive functioning may be most critical. Certainly, symptom alleviation and the reduction of associated distress are goals of many approaches seeking to treat the SED population. However, some have questioned the role of symptom severity versus other risk and protective factors, such as adequate family environments and positive connections to school and community, in predicting outcomes for youth identified with SED (Vance et al., 2002). School-based interventions commonly target improved educational functioning (e.g., reduction in absences and office referrals, reading achievement gains) as a hallmark of outcome (e.g., Sawka et al., 2002; Popkin & Skinner, 2003). Community interventions measure outcomes related to systemic effects and service utilization, such as days in out-of-home placement and recidivism to psychiatric facilities and juvenile justice settings (Henggeler et al., 1999, 2003; Rowland et al., 2005). Finally, a common outcome variable measures return to a less restrictive setting. This is operationalized variably across sites, though it may be expressed as minutes spent in mainstream education settings (e.g., classroom instruction, specials with peers), or community versus institutional placement. Return to less restrictive settings, further, postulates that families, schools, and other community agents have enhanced capacities to manage children with SED as a result of intervention activities (Osher & Hanley, 2001).

Community-Based Treatment Approaches

There has been some criticism of applying a narrow focus on specific disorders to outcome studies on children with SED, who are often served by multiple systems, have received more than one psychiatric diagnosis, and may have problems extending beyond the scope of their individual pathologies (Ringeisen & Hoagwood, 2002). This earlier writing reviewed the effectiveness of case management and multisystemic therapy (MST) models, which still predominate empirically supported community treatments for SED four years later.

Case management approaches, including wraparound care (see Burns & Goldman, 1999) and intensive case management (ICM), establish a case manager for a child with SED. This person functions as a facilitator and gatekeeper of the multiple services provided to and multiple agencies interacting with the identified child and his or her family. Case management can link appropriate services to children as well as ensure that service agents and families are regularly and effectively communicating with one another. ICM can result in reductions in psychiatric hospitalizations (Evans et al., 1994) and can reduce placement changes and elopement in SED populations living in foster care (Clarke et al., 1998;

abstracted from Ringeisen & Hoagwood, 2002). Despite the ability of case management and wraparound approaches to reduce the usage of more costly alternatives and to maintain children with SED in their communities (Grundle, 2002), additional published studies employing sophisticated research designs are needed (see Burns et al., 2000; Cook & Kilmer, 2004).

Application of a successful home-based approach employed with antisocial youth—multisystemic therapy (MST; Henggeler et al., 1998)—poses some benefit for youth identified with SED. Further, of the approaches reviewed here, MST evaluations have met the RCT standard and include one replication study addressing an SED sample. MST is an integrated approach with home-based services at the core, though it involves simultaneous and coordinated services provided by other community agents and in multiple environments (e.g., school, neighborhood, social interactions with peers). MST intends to be a short-term (albeit intense) intervention, with primary goals to augment the practical, coping, and behavioral skills of targeted parents and youth. Individualized therapy supports for child and adolescent SED clients utilize known evidence-based practices (e.g., behavioral and cognitive-behavioral strategies, pragmatic family therapies; Henggeler, 1999).

Specifically addressing an SED population, a randomized trial sought to compare MST with costly psychiatric hospitalization (Henggeler et al., 1999). Random assignment to experimental condition (MST vs. inpatient disposition with typical postdischarge follow-up care) occurred for 116 children and adolescents approved for acute psychiatric hospitalization. Consistent with other MST populations, services for families assigned to the MST condition lasted an average of four months (SD = one month) for this SED population (average of 97 direct contact hours, SD = 57 hours). Although some youth in the MST group required hospitalization at some point across the study period, inpatient days and other out-of-home placement days were significantly fewer for them compared to youth in the hospitalization condition. Similar rates of psychotropic medication usage were observed in both groups. Compared to youth in the hospitalization condition, youth with SED in the MST condition evidenced greater reductions in externalizing symptoms, enjoyed improved cohesion in their family system, spent fewer days out of school, and reported greater treatment satisfaction. Follow-up investigation one year after initial recruitment revealed that, for many participants in the MST condition, comparative gains in symptom presentation and community placement (e.g., with family member or friend, school attendance) were no longer evident (Henggeler et al., 2003). This result suggests that time-limited treatment has difficulty producing sustained improvement among SED populations, many of whom suffer from persistent and severe mental illness.

Detailed economic analyses suggested that the initial reduction in costly psychiatric inpatient services in the MST condition was not offset by increased use of other expensive placement options (e.g., juvenile justice; Schoenwald et al., 2000). Analyses also revealed that costs in treating the SED population, in this example, were more than 50%

higher than those sustained in treating juvenile offenders within the MST framework. Henggeler and colleagues (1999) acknowledged greater complexity than anticipated in their application of the MST model to this sample of vulnerable children and teens. They cited the need for additional clinical resources, such as consultation from child psychiatrists and some inpatient days addressing crisis stabilization, as driving treatment complexity and cost (Schoenwald et al., 2000). These scholars later asserted, based on their follow-up findings, the need to reconceptualize MST services for youths with SED to be more consistent with evidence-based practices serving adults in the severe and persistent mental illness category (Henggeler et al., 2003).

Further enhancing the literature on effective treatments for children and youth with SED, MST investigators joined with a system of care in Hawaii to replicate a randomized clinical trial with a population at risk for out-of-home placement (Rowland et al., 2005). Although the sample size was smaller than prior investigations (Henggeler et al., 1999, 2003), participants were predominately multiracial, including Asian and Pacific Islander heritages. Historical data revealed these youths to be diagnostically complex and to be, on average, acquainted with psychiatric inpatient facilities and the juvenile justice system. Based on prior experiences working with an SED population, the MST condition, in this implementation, expanded the core treatment team to include child and adolescent psychiatrists, crisis caseworkers, and a family resource specialist, who functioned to incorporate local providers into treatment efforts. Additionally, all core MST staff were trained in crisis intervention in anticipation of some of the skills they may need working with an SED population. At six-month follow-up, compared to a treatment-as-usual comparison group, youths in the MST condition reported less internalizing and externalizing symptoms (though their caregivers noted no substantial change) as well as evidenced less arrests and spent more time in general education settings (findings not statistically significant). Youth in the MST and comparison conditions, importantly, averaged 4 and 12 days in restrictive out-of-home placements, respectively, suggesting this trial was most effective at achieving the goal of maintaining youth receiving MST in the community. Treatment fidelity is a hallmark of MST. These authors noted dissatisfaction with model adherence in this example as well as with the ability of the MST team to link with local service providers. Nevertheless, this study highlights the importance of how community-based services portend enhanced community functioning, as well as retention in the community, for youth with complex pathologies.

A limited review cited three examples of model programs responding to the charge of the President's New Freedom Commission on Mental Health (2003) to develop coordinated, family-centered programs linking mental health services with six other systems commonly serving at-risk youth: education, primary health care, juvenile justice, child welfare, vocational rehabilitation, and substance abuse services (Hansen et al., 2004). In addition to noting outcomes for the earlier MST trial cited above, this review described two extensive, innovative metropolitan initiatives, Pennsylvania's family-based mental health services and Wraparound Milwaukee (Lindblad-Goldberg et al.,1998; Grundle, 2002). Pennsylvania's effort is distinguished by its structural family therapy orientation and clinician training emphasizing appreciation of the individual cultures and ideologies of child-serving systems; Milwaukee's program serves a predominately minority population, includes a mobile crisis team to further prevent removal of children and youth to restrictive placements outside their communities, and operates on a funding structure enabled by reorganizing and synthesizing the budgets of child welfare, juvenile justice, and Medicaid. Hansen and colleagues (2004) describe strong outcomes and successes of these programs, yet, at present, associated outcome research is better described as internal program evaluation versus empirical inquiry intended for peer-reviewed publications (e.g., Milwaukee County Behavioral Health Division, Child and Adolescent Services Branch, 2002). Scholarly journals may anticipate additional outcome research from these sites in the near future (e.g., Grundle, 2002).

School-Based Treatment Approaches

Compelling approaches to treating SED that are primarily linked to, or housed in, schools are increasing in number and are gradually garnering empirical support despite methodological weaknesses (compared to RCTs and strong comparison group designs employed by other efficacy and effectiveness studies in the child and adolescent psychology literature). Educational research, from a clinical scientist's perspective, often champions evidence-based support for a particular method or intervention gleaned with far less empirical rigor, at times extrapolating results from a single study or from outcomes related to a dissimilar population. Although no investigations reviewed below employ randomized designs (some intended to employ comparison group designs, yet were foiled), we offer them as approaches worthy of further implementation, in addition to more rigorous empirical study. These school-based approaches are ordered according to ascending involvement of outside partners and/or the intensity of programming on site.

The effectiveness of classroom contingency management in specifically reducing aggressive and disruptive behaviors in children identified with disruptive behavior disorders (e.g., ADHD, conduct problems) is reviewed by Ringeisen and Hoagwood (2002), though cited studies do not specifically target an SED population. These authors, however, identify specific school-based programs that serve to prevent the expression or severity of several liabilities concomitant with SED: depression (Clarke et al., 1995; Gillham et al., 1995) and aggression/conduct problems (LIFT, Reid et al., 1999; FAST Track, Conduct Problems Prevention Research Group, 1999). Though described as targeted prevention, the LIFT and FAST Track programs include collaborative and parent components in addition to behavioral management and skill-building activities targeting the participating children. Like MST, these programs, as some described later, underscore the importance of including home and community systems in the prevention and treatment of debilitating disruptive behaviors.

Responding to a perceived lack of teachers qualified to work with the SED population, the Strengthening Emotional Support Services Model (SESS) targeted teacher training and consultation as a proxy for improving student outcomes in special education classrooms serving students with SED (Sawka et al., 2002). The four-module SESS curriculum was developed from reviews of empirically supported strategies for educating students with emotional and behavioral disorders (EBDs, a parallel construct to SED in educational parlance). Delivered over a three-month span concurrent with associated on-site consultation, the curriculum was measured to be effective in improving knowledge for educational staff participants in an urban district, yet also contributed to specific observed classroom management practices (particularly after site consultation) assumed to be linked to pre-post improvement in the academic engagement of affected students as well as to noticeable pre-post decline in their disruptive behaviors. Follow-up investigation is needed to determine the endurance of these student gains as well as of effective staff practices.

Implicating systems of care and wraparound approaches, scholars emphasizing family involvement for programs treating children with SED note, "The implementation of evidence-based interventions, interagency collaboration, and programs that accept families as equal partners has not been realized at a level of scale sufficient to significantly improve outcomes for this group of children and youth" (Kutash et al., 2002, p. 100). In an initiative to address this concern, the School, Family, and Community Partnership (the Partnership Program) sought to increase family involvement in the education of middle-school students identified with SED and sought to increase access to relevant community supports (e.g., mental health; Kutash et al.). School, family, and community teams were arranged for students and families participating in the treatment school, meeting regularly. These included educators and school providers, child service agents (e.g., mental health, family agencies), community representatives, and other members of the family's support network. Results indicated school staff training in meeting facilitation enhanced requisite team behaviors up to two years postimplementation. Team meeting frequency, additionally, increased by a substantial magnitude across the study period. These structural changes may be associated with functional changes observed in students, whose discipline rates decreased across the two-year study period and whose emotional functioning improved slightly, per rating scale data. Stronger improvements in emotional functioning, however, may have been prevented by the program's inability to increase student involvement with local mental health agencies, despite the intent to accomplish such (Kutash et al., 2002).

Suggesting a movement toward school-based, community-oriented programming for the educational, emotional, and behavioral needs of children identified with SED, evaluations of relatively comprehensive school-based programs have recently been published in the professional psychology literature, though none has enjoyed the experimental rigor of

RCTs or matched control groups. Robinson and Rapport (2002) evaluated a program where students in elementary through high school grades received mental health services in a public school setting. This school-based program provided multimodal interventions in the least restrictive, most naturalistic (environmentally valid) educational setting possible through a collaborative effort of the school district and a local mental health agency. Participating students had been classified as having a severe emotional disorder and had been unsuccessfully treated in outpatient therapy, resource classrooms, and self-contained behavior disorder classrooms prior to admission. Students received academic instruction as well as mental health treatment provided by a multidisciplinary team. Treatment components included behavioral approaches (e.g., token economies, praise, response cost, overcorrection), social skills training, individual therapy (one hour per week), family therapy (weekly), and collaboration across settings to promote generalization. The educational class sessions were six hours per day, five days per week. Employing a broad outcome questionnaire assessing symptoms as the measure of treatment effectiveness, participants demonstrated significant improvements in clinical functioning over the course of treatment, including reductions in both internalizing and externalizing behavioral symptoms. However, scores for a majority of children remained in the clinical range. Cautilli et al. (2004) also report cautious results from their study of a school-based behavioral health program with an SED population. Teacher data suggested a majority of 17 students evidenced clinically significant change over the study period, although no child demonstrated complete recovery.

The Intensive Mental Health Program (IMHP; Vernberg et al., 2002) is a university-public school partnership providing intensive and comprehensive services for elementary school students who have significant emotional and psychological needs and who are not effectively served in traditional special education programs or in traditional mental health settings. The IMHP model focuses on returning children with severe behavioral and psychological impairment to a normalized, less restrictive educational environment; increasing the accessibility of mental health services; coordinating separate services into a coherent, consistent whole; utilizing empirically supported treatments; and increasing the probability of positive outcomes (for additional program descriptions, see Jacobs et al., 2005; Nyre et al., 2003; Roberts et al., 2003). Similar to the school-based approaches described earlier, on-site programming for the IMHP includes behavioral contingency management, emotion education and social skills groups, individual therapy (using empirically supported treatments, as indicated), and individually tailored academic instruction. However, similar to the systemic interventions of MST thought to assist functional gains in targeted children and their families, other key treatment features of the IMHP include regular home visits and bimonthly core team meetings seeking to collaborate with all home, school, and community agents interacting with the child. Importantly, to facilitate maintenance in the least restrictive educational setting possible, IMHP programming is designed to be half-day, with students attending their neighborhood schools the other portion of their school day. Mental health staff and educational staff from the IMHP consult regularly with neighborhood school providers to build resources, transfer skills, and promote transitions.

Evaluative efforts of the IMHP intended to include local "treatment-as-usual" comparison groups, though practical barriers precluded adequate data. Evaluations of outcomes for the IMHP are based on pre-post designs and analyses of individual differences. Significant, clinically meaningful outcomes are reported for discharged students in terms of functioning (Vernberg et al., 2004), adaptive skills, and behavioral symptoms (Vernberg et al., 2005). For example, during the first five years of the IMHP, over 73% of participating students remained in the local public school system through treatment and discharge (average treatment length was 11.9 months; Vernberg et al., 2005). Based on CAFAS ratings (Hodges, 2000), all children entered the program with Level 4 (extensive services needed) or Level 5 (restrictive placement needed) impairments in adaptive functioning. By discharge, 39% exhibited functional impairment at Level 1 (no services needed) or Level 2 (outpatient services indicated) and 37% exhibited Level 3 impairment (outpatient care with some supportive services in school or community). Additionally, behavioral data identified common trajectories typified by initial improvement within the IMHP setting (about one-month postintake), eventual generalization to the neighborhood school, and performance at 95% of behavioral criteria in school settings by discharge (Vernberg et al., 2005).

Examination of specific IMHP services and children's progress suggested that success of the IMHP can be attributed to its particular features. For example, chart reviews indicated that children who displayed stronger participation in individual and group cognitive-behavioral therapy (e.g., greater attendance, positive statements about therapeutic activities, demonstration of specific skills taught in therapy) and who appeared motivated by the individualized behavior management system evidenced greater improvement on indicators of behavioral and emotional impairment. Other findings suggest that skill transfer to parents and other community providers, caregiver satisfaction with IMHP services (Puddy et al., 2005; Lazicki-Puddy, 2006), and the quality and quantity of service coordination activities predicted outcomes (Puddy et al., 2005).

Other Approaches

It may be unlikely for a child or adolescent identified with SED to be successfully treated with pharmacotherapy or behavioral management alone. Nevertheless, outcome studies employing adequate research designs provide support for these important aspects of the treatment array provided to children and adolescents with SED (see Ringeisen & Hoagwood, 2002). Psychostimulants and other classes of psychotropic medications employed in child and adolescent populations (e.g., neuroleptics, atypical antipsychotics, mood stabilizers, antidepressants, adrenergic agents) evidenced moderate to large weighted effect sizes, overall, according to two meta-analyses addressing medication's role in reducing overt and covert aggression in youth identified with ADHD or SED (respectively, Connor et al., 2002, 2003).

Behavioral contingency management is a hallmark of specialized educational environments and other more restrictive settings, such as day programs and residential facilities. Given its prevalence, it is promising that, when done well and consistently, behavioral management is an empirically supported approach. For example, the Good Behavior Game is one positive, classwide program enjoying support in aggressive behavior reduction across time, even for children identified as highly aggressive in first grade (Kellam et al., 1994). Interdependent group contingency procedures helped a middle-school class of five male students with SED improve their math and spelling performance, according to a modified multiple-baseline study (Popkin & Skinner, 2003). Interdependent group contingencies have also demonstrated support in reducing disruptive behaviors in an SED population (Theodore et al., 2001). A potential benefit of behavioral procedures is that teachers themselves may effectively execute them in their classrooms (Ringeisen & Hoagwood, 2002).

DELINEATING EVIDENCE-BASED TREATMENT COMPONENTS AND PRINCIPLES FOR SED

Treatment Components

Reviewing the literature on empirically supported methods that show promise in enhancing the functioning of children with serious emotional disturbance, no broad treatment package enjoys substantial support via replication across sites and clinical populations. Several aspects of promising programs, however, are assumed to be integral ingredients of interventions contributing to successful outcomes for children with SED. Table 1 describes these components and cites programs and other empirical papers supporting their effectiveness. An associated assumption may be that an accumulation or confluence of integral components may procure more substantial and enduring treatment gains. Although this assumption has not been formally investigated (see Cook & Kilmer, 2004), it is important to note that a few promising approaches are cited in Table 1. Sites wishing to develop and adapt programs for children and adolescents with SED might review and weigh these components in terms of expected benefit, site-specific feasibility, and resource allocation. For instance, if extensive home-based supports are deemed too costly and not feasible for a startup school-based program, developers should explore means to bolster family-school communication and other vital components (e.g., behavioral programming, skills groups).

On a cautionary note, some have argued that substantial improvements across multiple functional domains are not likely when only one component of promising treatment approaches with the SED population is delivered. For instance, the Partnership Program succeeded in involving families as stakeholders in student plan development, yet without the

Table 1. Components of Successful Treatments for Children
and Adolescents with SED

Component	Illustrative References
Consistent behavioral programming focusing on skill development	- Cautilli et al. (2004) - Conduct Problems Prevention Research Group (1999) - Vernberg et al. (2002) - Kellam et al. (1994) - Reid et al. (1999) - Robinson and Rapport (2002)
Individualized treatment employing evidence-based practices	- Henggeler (1999) - Vernberg et al. (2002)
Maintenance in community and familiar environments	- Grundle (2001) - Henggeler (1999) - Robinson and Rapport (2002) - Vernberg et al., (2002)
Family involvement as stakeholders	- Grundle (2001) - Henggeler (1999) - Vernberg et al. (2002) - Kutash et al. (2002)
Multiagency collaboration	- Conduct Problems Prevention Research Group (1999) - Henggeler (1999) - Kutash et al. (2002) - Vernberg et al. (2002) - Robinson and Rapport (2002)
Psychopharmacology	- Connor et al. (2002) - Connor et al. (2003) - Rowland et al. (2005) (MST)

expected involvement of community mental health providers (e.g., skill development support, empirically supported individual therapies), affected students largely did not achieve marked gains in functioning (Kutash et al., 2002). Similarly, for a child evidencing severe disruptive behaviors in multiple domains, professionals would not expect the sole provision of classroom-based contingency management procedures to generalize behavioral gains to home and community environments. The addition of home-school collaboration or other mental health supports in the community, however, may promote this child's cross-setting functioning.

Treatment Principles

Given the heterogeneity of presenting problems, life circumstances, and intervention resources for children and adolescents with SED, it is important to articulate overarching principles that might guide evidence-based treatment for this population across a wide range of service delivery models. Drawing from core constructs from develop-mental psychopathology, social-contextual theory, and the evidence-based practice literature for children and adolescents, Vernberg and colleagues (Vernberg et al., 2002, 2006) proposed a set of nine basic principles for working with SED in the context of the IMHP:

1. Children are deeply embedded in their network of relationships, so treatment must attend to cross-setting linkages and events. This requires the establishment of mechanisms for communicating across settings, such as behavior reporting systems that cover both school and home, and interventions that strengthen positive relationships within the family and with friends, classmates, and teachers.

2. Children do best if adults involved in their lives agree, so it is important to collaborate with everyone involved with the child. This requires the persistent use of strategies for engaging family members and service providers in mutually agreed-upon treatment goals and service plans.

3. Personal skills (e.g., self-regulation, perspective taking) are intimately linked to developmental status, so interventions must match the child's developmental level. This requires a clear understanding of the child's or adolescent's current developmental status and cognitive skills. This understanding may be obtained through careful observation and interviewing, but is often enhanced by the use of psychometrically sound measures of cognition and emotion.

4. Children should function in natural social settings, so treatments should be carried out while the child or adolescent remains at home and in school whenever possible. This may require substantial levels of additional supports at school and at home, such as what can be provided by paraprofessional teachers, youth specialists, and respite care providers.

5. Warmth and positive attention are essential, so it is important to cultivate an authoritative style for all adults involved with the child or adolescent. This style may be difficult to sustain in the face of destructive, hostile, or aggressive behavior; lapsing into punitive methods for gaining or maintaining control generally seems counterproductive, however.

6. Evidence-based treatments should be used, so treatments should utilize a core menu of treatment options for syndromes and disorders. We have a reasonable array of evidence-based protocols to address problems that occur commonly in children and adolescents with SED. (e.g., excessive anger, poor emotion regulation, anxiety). These treatment protocols can often be profitably incorporated into broader service plans.

7. Cognitive and behavioral skill development is a key goal, so interventions should focus on the acquisition and use of specific skills that foster adaptive behavior. Skills targeted for growth may span a wide spectrum, such as personal hygiene and grooming, successful work habits, and recreational capabilities that enhance social relationships or self-esteem.

8. The use of cognitive and behavioral skills depends on the social environment, so it is important to devote energy to focused, sustained efforts in real-world settings and to promote treatment generalization.

This typically requires active involvement by service providers in multiple settings in the child or adolescent's life.

9. Multiple outcomes are possible from similar etiologies, and there are multiple pathways to similar outcomes. Service providers should maintain a flexible, data-driven view of the causes and maintainers of SED symptoms. Biological explanations related to persistent mental illness may be warranted in many instances, yet the role of environmental influences on the ebb and flow of symptom severity and adaptive functioning should not be minimized or ignored.

Promising programs and policies for children with SED, critically evaluated by Osher and Hanley (2001), similarly promote the following: (1) positive learning opportunities and results; (2) school and community capacity; (3) appreciation of diversity and culturally competent approaches; (4) collaboration with families; (5) appropriate assessment; (6) ongoing skill development and support; and (7) comprehensive and collaborative systems. Promising approaches were typified by school- and districtwide and agency intervention programs as well as by county- and statewide capacity-building programs. Although the latter approaches are not direct clinical interventions, they are critical inclusions because they have the potential to reduce implementation barriers almost universally lamented by comprehensive treatment models (e.g., Henggeler et al., 1999; Rowland et al., 2005; Vernberg et al., 2006). Further, Osher and Hanley (2001) highlight the importance of maintaining children with SED in their community and regular education settings, when possible. When self-contained programs are necessary, promising programs have a "desire and capacity to prepare students and environments for reintegration and to reintegrate students as soon as [is] clinically and educationally appropriate" (p. 383). For children and adolescents with SED, acquiring real-world functional, coping, and social skills is best done in real-world environments, with real-world feedback and contingencies. Promising programs are ecologically valid, preparing children to function without the need for supports to function for them.

EVIDENCE-BASED TREATMENT FOR SED IN ACTION: ILLUSTRATIVE VIGNETTE AND COMMENTARY

The following case example is loosely based on an 11-year-old elementary student who participated in the school-based Intensive Mental Health Program (IMHP; Vernberg et al., 2002) for less than one academic year and was successfully transitioned to full-day regular education programming, with weekly outpatient psychotherapy in his community. As practitioners working with children with SED surely know, not all students graduate to regular education settings with minimal community supports. Even in a program these authors believe has worked well for its target population, the term "successful outcome" is relative. Success may equate to reduction in days spent in foster care, juvenile justice, inpatient, or residential facilities (e.g., Rowland et al., 2005), or it may be a gradual increase in the amount of minutes spent in regular education settings, without fully exiting self-contained programming. Nevertheless, as in the case of "Evan," intensive, integrated programming may portend substantial skill acquisition and functional improvement for children identified with SED.

Referral

Evan was referred to the IMHP by his neighborhood school secondary to extreme concerns about his social immaturity, aggressive and disorganized tantrum behaviors, and threatening verbalizations (e.g., Armageddon, suicidality). He had been identified with an emotional exceptionality and a specific learning disability much earlier in elementary school. Though related programming in regular and special education settings had been beneficial up to the time of referral, contemporaneous token systems rewarding his positive behaviors and de-escalation strategies had not been preventing Evan's outbursts, which had become markedly more severe. Diagnostic impressions upon referral sought to rule out a pervasive developmental disorder, an anxiety disorder, and attention deficit hyperactivity disorder (ADHD). Prior psychological testing had disconfirmed ADHD, though some impulsive and inattentive symptoms continued to interfere with Evan's school functioning. Evan regularly saw a child therapist in an outpatient clinic and was prescribed an SSRI by his family physician. Strengths included a supportive family system, strong cognitive and verbal abilities, and a keen sense of humor.

Initial Programming

Evan attended the IMHP classroom half of his academic day and attended his neighborhood school the other half of the day. His specialized classroom was limited to six students and was directly staffed by a certified special education teacher with expertise in emotional and behavioral programming, a paraprofessional skilled in behavioral programming, and two half-time child therapists who alternated days throughout the school week. All staffers participated equally and consistently in three aspects of behavioral programming: (1) a token system frequently rewarding students for appropriate behaviors and approximations (upwards of 20 occasions per 3 hours per student); (2) a response-cost system linking negative behaviors to loss of privileges (e.g., computer time, free time, special off-campus activities); and (3) three phases of de-escalation addressing disruptive behaviors (ending in time out from social rewards, or seclusionary time out). Academic instruction, led by the teacher, alternated with an emotion education group and a social skills group, led by the masters-level clinical child psychology therapists. The teacher and paraprofessional assisted skill generalization by noting and rewarding Evan's displays of what he learned in skill groups during academic times, free time, and recess. Though Evan worked with both of the therapists in group activities, one therapist worked with him individually twice per week and met with his family in the home setting every other week. His primary therapist also facilitated a similar behavior system for him in his neighborhood school and organized regular collaborative meetings with his IMHP teacher, neighborhood school staff, outpatient therapist, and parents. From the onset of his inclusion in IMHP programming, Evan responded well to the behavioral system, often earning most of his points and regularly earning reward activities. His disruptive behaviors escalated to the point of requiring seclusionary time outs only three times in the first months of treatment.

Evan's therapist arranged to meet with his parents within the first week he attended the IMHP. This meeting gathered additional history, collected baseline assessment measures, clarified programming, and helped establish an initial treatment plan. A later meeting with Evan's parents, teachers, and school and community providers further discussed programming, identified three specific target behaviors for Evan, and anticipated criteria for Evan's transition back to his neighborhood school. The latter aspect was crucial, as it sought to solidify all partners' involvement and commitment to fulfilling their roles in Evan's treatment plan. Though his therapist assumed a facilitator role in this and subsequent team meetings, the assumption was that, in treating SED, no single entity or site upholds primacy—not the therapist, the specialized program, or the family system—all agents working with him are crucial in supporting his improved functioning in their respective settings.

Therapeutic Interventions

Rating scales gathered at intake noted clinical levels of aggressiveness, hyperactivity, atypicality (IMHP teacher only), attention problems, anxiety, and depression (IMHP teacher and parent). Interestingly, his new regular education teacher noted no concerns in the clinical or at-risk ranges. Excellent behavioral data from his neighborhood school corroborated her report and suggested that Evan's symptoms were managed well by positive supports for him in this environment. Via parent history, school observational and behavioral data, and individual sessions with Evan, his therapist determined anxiety symptoms to underlie his behavioral presentation at school. School situations and tasks, in particular, were anxiety-provoking for Evan. His strong verbal skills and creativity suggested that the *Coping Cat*, an empirically supported treatment for childhood anxiety problems (Kendall, 2000), would be a useful individual approach, combined with relaxation training and other behavioral coping strategies. Evan's therapist noted that he participated well with the *Coping Cat* curriculum. Regular home visits by Evan's therapist addressed anxiety-provoking situations at home, skill generalization, and specific parenting techniques to targeting his impulsive behaviors and lack of organization. Additionally, Evan's parents employed behavioral data from school to advocate for a medication trial with a psychostimulant in addition to his ongoing SSRI prescription. This proved to be successful in alleviating residual hyperactive and inattentive symptoms that had not improved as Evan mastered steps along the *Coping Cat* sequence.

Outcome

Fortunately for Evan, his neighborhood school team applauded his behavioral gains and was eager to add specials (e.g., art, PE) and, eventually, instructional time with his classmates as he became more skilled at managing his emotions. Evan himself often expressed a desire to return to his neighborhood school full-time and was motivated to participate in and benefit from therapeutic exercises. This is important, as many students who are placed in restrictive settings feel safer in these environments because they are freer from stigma or scrutiny from peers who may have witnessed prior outbursts and bizarre behaviors. By mid-spring, Evan was participating in his neighborhood school all day. A functional outcome measure indicated "no noteworthy impairment" (Hodges, 2000), though his IMHP teacher and parents rated depression and anxiety symptoms to remain in the at-risk range. Hence, restrictive school-based services were discontinued and outpatient therapy continued to monitor and treat Evan's internalizing symptoms.

FUTURE DIRECTIONS AND CHALLENGES

Widespread Use of Promising Programs

Some of the most promising treatment frameworks addressing children with serious emotional disturbance are also the most difficult to sustain. An application of the MST model in a community-based continuum of care, for example, invoked substantial structural difficulties contributing to the premature demise of its clinical and empirical venture (Rowland et al., 2005). Difficulties included scarcity of potential therapeutic staff who were proficient in evidence-based practice, lack of MST model adherence and espousal by other continuum partners, and threats to the financial stability of the project by politicized funding agents. Though the university-public school partnership exemplified by the IMHP model poses some benefit in terms of enhancing availability of qualified masters- and doctoral-level clinical staff, it is similarly constrained by related community systems' and agents' slow pace in developing capacities for implementing evidence-based assessments and interventions as well as by constantly shifting funding policies and priorities.

Although community-based programs are less costly than inpatient or residential settings, not to mention more ecologically valid, they are nevertheless expensive (Grundle, 2001; Henggeler, 2001). Comprehensive programming requires substantial outset costs related to staff training, fidelity checks, material procurement, and the like. For sites that will not directly or immediately recoup long-term cost savings (e.g., schools, some community agencies), the adoption of comprehensive programs is simply not feasible unless there is broader investment from other systems. School budgets, for instance, do not directly benefit from reductions in juvenile justice or psychiatric inpatient expenditures. Also, many agencies have learned difficult lessons about funding important programs with "soft monies," for these programs tend to disappear when grants expire. Empirical papers and, importantly, policy briefs for state and federal governments need to link agencies explicitly (e.g., mental health centers, schools) and tacitly (e.g., juvenile justice) treating SED-identified youth in terms of cost sharing and cost offset. Unless supporting economic arguments are recognized and valued by potential funders of comprehensive and promising practices, agencies wishing to adapt them are paralyzed. The MST franchise has begun to tackle such work, and policy collectives have taken notice of cost-effective interventions for difficult clinical populations (e.g., Washington State Institute for Public Policy, 1998). The present task is to deliver this type of information more broadly to local and national government task forces and funding agents. The Milwaukee Project (Grundle, 2002) appears to have a close collaborative relationship with the governmental funders of interrelated children's services, factors that promote its scope and longevity.

Greater Support for Outcomes Research on SED

Although there is a reasonable scientific literature on how to treat and develop good programming for children and adolescents with SED (see Sawka et al., 2002), there are substantial pragmatic hindrances to rigorous treatment outcome research in this area. Problems for children and adolescents with SED tend to be chronic, and treatments are necessarily lengthy, labor-intensive, and expensive. The SED population is heterogeneous, making it more difficult to describe a single treatment approach that might be used within an RCT format. Few communities have the resources to offer comprehensive, integrated services that meet fidelity criteria for rigorous evaluative research, and even fewer could offer two plausible alternative treatments simultaneously. With the current emphasis on RCTs as the gold standard for treatment outcome studies, proposals for outcome studies involving treatments for SED populations that are comprehensive and sustained almost inevitably fare poorly compared to more compartmentalized, relatively brief intervention protocols in terms of elegance of design and measurement of treatment fidelity. Acceptance of alternate research designs, such as comparisons between communities that offer different service models for SED and within-subjects designs offer hope for progress toward more rigorous evaluations of outcomes. Even these require substantial investments of money for both service delivery and evaluative research.

REFERENCES

Burns, B. J., & Goldman, S. K. (Eds.) (1999). *Promising Practices in Wraparound for Children with Serious Emotional Disturbance and Their Families; Systems of Care: Promising Practices in Children's Mental Health* (1998 series, Vol. 4). Washington, DC: Center for Effective Collaboration and Practice, American Institutes for Research.

Burns, B. J., Schoenwald, S. K., Burchard, J. D., Faw, L., & Santos, A. (2000). Comprehensive community-based interventions for youth with severe emotional disorders: Multisystemic therapy and the wraparound process. *Journal of Child and Family Studies, 9*, 283–313.

Cautilli, J., Harrington, N., Gillam, E. V., Denning, J., Helwig, I., Ettingoff, A., et al. (2004). Do children with multiple patterns of problem behavior improve? The effectiveness of an intensive bio-behaviorally oriented school-based behavioral health program. *Journal of Early and Intensive Behavior Intervention, 1*, 75–94.

Clarke, H. B., Prange, M., Lee, B., Steward, E., McDonald, B., & Boyd, L. (1998). An individualized wraparound process for children in foster care with emotional/behavioral disturbances: Follow-up findings and implications from a controlled study. In M. Epstein, K. Kutash, & A. Duchnowski (Eds.), *Outcomes for Children and Youth with Behavioral and Emotional Disorders and Their Families* (pp. 513–542). Austin, TX: PRO-ED.

Conduct Problems Prevention Research Group (1999). Initial impact of the FAST Track prevention trial for conduct problems: II. Classroom effects. *Journal of Consulting and Clinical Psychology, 67*, 648–657.

Connor, D. F., Boone, R. T., Steingard, R. J., Lopez, I. D., & Melloni, R. H., Jr. (2003). Psychopharmacology and aggression: II. A meta-analysis of nonstimulant medication effects on overt behaviors in youth with SED. *Journal of Emotional and Behavioral Disorders, 11*, 157–168.

Connor, D. F., Glatt, S. J., Lopez, I. D., Jackson, D., & Melloni, R. H., Jr. (2002). Psychopharmacology and aggression: I. A meta-analysis of stimulant effects on overt/covert aggression-related behaviors in ADHD. *Journal of the American Academy of Child and Adolescent Psychiatry, 41*, 253–261.

Cook, J. R., & Kilmer, R. P. (2004). Evaluating systems of care: Missing links in children's mental health research. *Journal of Community Psychology, 32*, 655–674.

Evans, M. E., Banks, S. M., Huz, S., & McNulty, T. L. (1994). Initial hospitalization and community tenure outcomes of intensive case management for children and youth with serious emotional disturbance. *Journal of Child and Family Studies, 3*, 225–234.

Gillham, J., Reivich, K., Jaycox, L., & Seligman, M. (1995). Prevention of depressive symptoms in school children: Two-year follow-up. *Psychological Science, 6*, 343–351.

Greenbaum, P. E., Dedrick, R. F., Freidman, R. M., Kutash, K., Brown, E. C., Lardieri, S., & Pugh, A. M. (1996). National Adolescent and Child Treatment Study (NACTS): Outcomes for children with serious emotional and behavioral disturbance. *Journal of Emotional and Behavioral Disorders, 4*, 130–146.

Grundle, T. J. (2002). Wraparound care. In D. T. Marsh & M. Fristad (Eds.), *Handbook of Serious Emotional Disturbance in Children and Adolescents* (pp. 323–333). New York: John Wiley & Sons.

Hansen, M., Litzelman, A., Marsh, D. T., & Milspaw, A. (2004). Approaches to serious emotional disturbance: Involving multiple systems. *Professional Psychology: Research and Practice, 35*, 457–465.

Henggeler, S. W. (1999). Multisystemic therapy: An overview of clinical procedures, outcomes, and policy implications. *Child Psychology and Psychiatry Review, 4*, 2–10.

Henggeler, S. W. (2001). Multisystemic therapy. In S. I. Pfeiffer & L. A. Reddy (Eds.), *Innovative Mental Health Interventions for Children: Programs That Work* (pp. 75–85). New York: Haworth Press.

Henggeler, S. W., Rone, L., Thomas, C., & Timmons-Mitchell, J. (1998). *Blueprints for Violence Prevention: Multisystemic Therapy*. D. S. Elliott (Series Ed.), University of Colorado, Center for the Study and Prevention of Violence. Boulder, CO: Blueprints Publications

Henggeler, S. W., Rowland, M. D., Halliday-Boykins, C., Sheidow, A. J., Ward, D. M., Randall, J., et al. (2003). One-year follow-up of multisystemic therapy as an alternative to the hospitalization of youths in psychiatric crisis. *Journal of the American Academy of Child and Adolescent Psychiatry, 42*, 543–551.

Henggeler, S. W., Rowland, M. D., Randall, J., Ward, D. M., Pickrel, S. G., Cunningham, P. B., & Miller, S. L., et al. (1999). Home-based multisystemic therapy as an alternative to the hospitalization of youths in psychiatric crisis: Clinical outcomes. *Journal of the American Academy of Child and Adolescent Psychiatry, 38*, 1331–1339.

Hodges, K. (2000). *Child and Adolescent Functional Assessment Scale*, 3rd ed. Ypsilanti, MI: Eastern Michigan University.

Jacobs, A. K., Randall, C. J., Vernberg, E. M., Roberts, M. C., & Nyre, J. E. (2005). Providing services within a school-based intensive mental health program. In R. G. Steele & M. C. Roberts (Eds.), *Handbook of Mental Health Services for Children, Adolescents, and Families* (pp. 47–61). New York: Kluwer/Plenum Press.

Kellam, S., Rebok, G., Ialongo, N., & Mayer, L. (1994). The course and malleability of aggressive behavior from early first grade into middle school: Results of a developmental epidemiology-based preventive trial. *Journal of Child Psychology, Psychiatry, and the Allied Disciplines, 35*, 259–281.

Kendall, P. (2000). *Cognitive Behavioral Therapy for Anxious Children: Therapist Manual*, 2nd ed. Ardmore, PA: Workbook Publishing, Inc.

Kutash, K., Duchnowski, A. J., Sumi, W. C., Rudo, Z., & Harris, K. M. (2002). A school, family, and community collaborative program for children who have emotional disturbances. *Journal of Emotional and Behavioral Disorders, 10*, 99–107.

Lazicki-Puddy, T. (2006). The impact of consumer and provider perceptions and consumer involvement upon children's outcomes in a school-based intensive mental health program. Unpublished dissertation project, University of Kansas.

Lindblad-Goldberg, M., Dore, M. M., & Stern, L. (1998). *Creating Competence from Chaos.* New York: Norton.

Milwaukee County Behavioral Health Division, Child and Adolescent Services Branch (2002). Wraparound Milwaukee (Annual Report). Milwaukee, WI.

Nyre, J. E., Vernberg, E. M., & Roberts, M. C. (2003). Serving the most severe of serious emotionally disturbed students in school settings. In M. D. Weist, S. W. Evans, & N. A. Lever (Eds.), *Handbook of School Mental Health: Advancing Practice and Research* (pp. 203–222). New York: Kluwer.

Osher, D., & Hanley, T. V. (2001). Implementing the SED national agenda: Promising programs and policies for children and youth with emotional and behavioral problems. *Education and Treatment of Children, 24*, 374–403.

Popkin, J., & Skinner, C. H. (2003). Enhancing academic performance in a classroom serving students with serious emotional disturbance: Interdependent group contingencies with randomly selected components. *School Psychology Review, 32*, 282–295.

President's New Freedom Commission on Mental Health (2003). *Achieving the Promise: Transforming Mental Health Care in America. Final Report* (DHHS Publication No. SMA-03-3832). Rockville, MD.

Puddy, R. W., Roberts, M. C., & Vernberg, E. M. (2005). Service coordination as a predictor of functioning in a school-based intensive mental health program. In C. Newman, C. J. Liberton, K. Kutash, & R. M. Friedman (Eds.), *The 17th Annual Research Conference. A System of Care for Children's Mental Health: Expanding the Research Base* (pp. 415–417). Tampa, FL: Louis de la Parte Institute.

Reid, J., Eddy, M., Fetrow, R., & Stoolmiller, M. (1999). Description and immediate impacts of a preventive intervention for conduct problems. *American Journal of Community Psychology, 27*, 483–517.

Ringeisen, H., & Hoagwood, K. (2002). Clinical and research directions for the treatment and delivery of children's mental health services. In D. T. Marsh & M. Fristad (Eds.), *Handbook of Serious Emotional Disturbance in Children and Adolescents* (pp. 33–55). New York: John Wiley & Sons.

Roberts, M. C., Jacobs, A. K., Puddy, R., Nyre, J. E., & Vernberg, E. M. (2003). Treating children with serious emotional disturbance in schools and the community. *Professional Psychology: Research and Practice, 34*, 519–526.

Robinson, K. E., & Rapport, L. J. (2002). Outcomes of a school-based mental health program for youth with serious emotional disorders. *Psychology in the Schools, 39*, 661–675.

Rowland, M. D., Halliday-Boykins, C. A., Henggeler, S. W., Cunningham, P. B., Lee, T. G., Kruesi, M. J. P., et al. (2005). A randomized trial of multisystemic therapy with Hawaii's Felix Class youths. *Journal of Emotional and Behavioral Disorders, 13*, 13–23.

Sawka, K. D., McCurdy, B. L., & Mannella, M. C. (2002). Strengthening emotional support services: An empirically based model for training teachers of students with behavior disorders. *Journal of Emotional and Behavioral Disorders, 10*, 223–232.

Schoenwald, S. K., Ward, D. M., Henggeler, S. W., & Rowland, M. D. (2000). Multisystemic therapy versus hospitalization for crisis stabilization of youth: Placement outcomes 4 months postreferral. *Mental Health Services Research, 2*, 3–12.

Theodore, L. A., Bray, M. A., Kehle, T. J., & Jenson, W. R. (2001). Randomization of group contingencies and reinforcers to reduce classroom disruptive behavior. *Journal of School Psychology, 3*, 279–284.

Vance, J., Bowen, N. K., Fernandez, G., & Thompson, S. (2002). Risk and protective factors as predictors of outcome in adolescents with psychiatric disorder and aggression. *Journal of the American Academy of Child and Adolescent Psychiatry, 41*, 36–43.

Vernberg, E. M., Jacobs, A. K., Nyre, J. E., Puddy, R. W., & Roberts, M. C. (2004). Innovative treatment for children with serious emotional disturbance: Preliminary outcomes for a school-based intensive mental health program. *Journal of Clinical Child and Adolescent Psychology, 33*, 359–365.

Vernberg, E. M., Randall, C. J., Gamm, B. K., & Jacobs, A. K. (2005). Positive changes for children in the Intensive Mental Health Program. In C. Newman, C. J. Liberton, K. Kutash, & R. M. Friedman (Eds.), *The 17th Annual Research Conference: A System of Care for Children's Mental Health: Expanding the Research Base.* Tampa, FL: Louis de la Parte Institute.

Vernberg, E. M., Roberts, M. C., & Nyre, J. E. (2002). School-based intensive mental health treatment. In D. T. Marsh & M. Fristad (Eds.), *Handbook of Serious Emotional Disturbance in Children and Adolescents* (pp. 412–427). New York: John Wiley & Sons.

Vernberg, E. M., Roberts, M. C., Randall, C. J., Biggs, B. K., Nyre, J. E., & Jacobs, A. K. (2006). Intensive mental health services for children with serious emotional disturbances through a school-based, community-oriented program. *Clinical Child Psychology and Psychiatry, 11*, 417–430.

Washington State Institute for Public Policy (1998). *Watching the Bottom Line: Cost-Effective Interventions for Reducing Crime in Washington.* Olympia, WA: The Evergreen State College.

23

Evidence-Based Approaches to Social Skills Training with Children and Adolescents

SHARON L. FOSTER and JULIE R. BUSSMAN

Acquisition of the skills required to form and maintain successful interpersonal relationships has long been considered a crucial aspect of child development. Deficits in these skills characterize most forms of child psychopathology, including autism, attention deficit disorder, conduct problems, and social anxiety. In addition, adaptive peer relationships are particularly important to healthy social development: Having friends is associated with a variety of positive correlates (see Bukowski et al., 1996), whereas general dislike in the peer group and association with deviant peers have both been linked to negative short- and long-term outcomes (Bierman, 2004; Gifford-Smith et al., 2005; Parker & Asher, 1987).

Perhaps as a result of early literature linking problems with peers and later maladjustment, investigators have developed and evaluated a variety of approaches for improving children's social skills and peer relationships. This chapter overviews this literature and identifies evidence-based social skills training interventions. In the pages that follow, we draw from three approaches to identify evidence-based practices and principles applicable to social skills training with children. First, we identify specific programs that have been repeatedly shown to produce positive effects on children's social behavior or peer relationships in randomized controlled investigations. Second, we survey the findings of meta-analyses. Third, we integrate conclusions from contemporary qualitative reviews that examined social skills training, looking in particular for areas of convergence. We conclude the chapter by discussing issues in dissemination and suggesting areas for future research.

SHARON L. FOSTER and JULIE R. BUSSMAN • Alliant International University

SPECIFIC EVIDENCE-BASED SOCIAL SKILLS TRAINING
PROGRAMS

Identifying evidence-based programs requires criteria for determining which interventions are effective. These criteria often concern (1) the populations with which the intervention has been evaluated, (2) the quality of the investigations used to examine the intervention (e.g., design of studies, adequacy of measures and statistical analyses), (3) aspects of the intervention that would be required for effective dissemination and widespread use of the intervention, and (4) the degree, type, longevity, and replicability of improvements attributable to the intervention (Biglan et al., 2003).

Determining the population, the nature of the intervention, and what constitutes "improvement" poses particular challenges in the areas of interventions to improve children's social skills because virtually any interpersonal behavior is rightly called "social," so virtually any skill involved in managing one's interpersonal interactions is, in essence, a "social skill." In a related vein, most child difficulties are characterized by interpersonal problems of some sort. Thus, virtually ANY intervention for ANY child population could be construed as a potential social skills intervention.

Gresham et al. (2001) provide a useful framework for understanding this heterogeneity in populations with social skills problems. They suggest that social skills acquisition problems occur when the child has never acquired a particular skill or does not understand when it is and is not appropriate to use the behavior. With a social performance deficit, the child fails to execute the skill in appropriate situations. With a fluency problem, the child performs the skill but does so awkwardly. Finally, competing behaviors are maladaptive responses (e.g., aggression, social withdrawal) that interfere with effective performance. Children may differ in which of these problems interfere with their peer relationships. Similarly, interventions may differ in the extent to which they address each of these areas.

An additional complication that is somewhat unique to social skills interventions for children lies in different possible ways of defining what constitutes a successful or positive outcome of social skills training. Some investigators identify social behavior as the key outcome of social skills training. Others focus on social cognition such as problem solving or empathy.

Many criticize sole reliance on behavioral or cognitive outcomes as an indicator of success, however (e.g., Gresham et al., 2001), largely based on social validity issues. The term "social validity" generally refers to the need to demonstrate that the outcomes or targets of treatment have real-world or applied significance in children's lives (Foster & Mash, 1999). In the peer relations domain, this is often operationalized by assessing whether behavioral or cognitive change is accompanied by improved acceptance or liking by peers or, less frequently, by improvements in the number or quality of a child's friendships. Because of the long-term importance of peer acceptance and friendship (e.g., Bukowski et al., 1996; Parker & Asher, 1987), improvements in social behavior should be accompanied by improved access to positive sources of peer socialization to be considered meaningful changes.

In this chapter, we limit our review to interventions specifically designed and shown to have beneficial effects on children's behavior and relationships with peers, because behavior with peers is the most common target of interventions that identify themselves as social skills training programs. We identified effective social skills training programs based on the following criteria. First, the intervention addressed the youth's (aged 3–18) interpersonal functioning in the peer group. Second, the intervention contained components specifically intended to improve the youth's interpersonal behavioral or social-cognitive skills. Third, investigators measured improvements in social behavior with peers and/or in some aspect of peer acceptance or friendship. Fourth, the intervention was directed toward children who were identified as rejected or friendless (low peer acceptance), were deficient in adaptive social behavior with peers, or showed excessive negative social behavior with peers. Interventions targeting children with a high likelihood of one or more of these characteristics (e.g., children diagnosed with conduct disorder) were also included. Fifth, we required that the intervention have a treatment manual or be sufficiently specified so that it could be replicated. Sixth, the intervention involved the child in the treatment process. Finally, because the social skills literature is so extensive, we required that the intervention had been shown to produce significant benefits relative to a control condition on one or more peer-related dependent variables in either two or more randomized controlled trials or in a multisite evaluation that examined possible site differences. This permitted identification of effects that were most likely to be replicable.

We excluded interventions that specifically targeted children with severe developmental disabilities or autism because these populations differ markedly from other groups with which social skills training has been applied and likely have unique needs for and responses to intervention. We also did not examine interventions that worked solely with the child's caregivers (e.g., parents and teachers) rather than the child. Although these interventions may produce beneficial changes in children's behavior with peers, examining them is beyond the scope of this chapter. Finally, we excluded studies that focused on skills only applicable in a limited set of situations (e.g., drug-refusal skills).

One final note: In the interventions we identified as effective, investigators examined a wide array of outcome variables; their treatment goals often were much broader than solely affecting children's social skills with peers. Here, however, we focus specifically on the effects of interventions on peer-related assessments, because our specific focus is on interventions that affect children's behavior and acceptance in the peer group.

Dinosaur School

Dinosaur School is a social skills and problem-solving intervention for children aged 4 to 7 years (Webster-Stratton, 1977). In Dinosaur School, children with conduct difficulties attend weekly sessions for 24 weeks in small groups. Weekly sessions involve (1) role-plays designed to engage children in using their new skills to resolve interpersonal conflict, (2) group activities (e.g., artwork, games) that incorporate key concepts, and (3) stories describing children solving social problems (Webster-Stratton & Hammond, 1997). Videotape-assisted modeling using vignettes is used to teach children more effective communication skills, friendship skills, conflict-resolution skills, anger control, and empathy. Finally, participants are sent home each week with homework assignments to remind them of key concepts and to encourage practicing. A distinguishing feature of this program is its emphasis on frequent practice and reinforcement of skills taught in the program by parents and teachers, a technique characteristic of effective social skills training programs (Taylor et al., 1999).

In two randomized control trials, Dinosaur School led to a reduction in conduct problems in comparison to control condition (Webster-Stratton & Hammond, 1997; Reid et al., 2003; Webster-Stratton et al., 2001, 2004). The first randomized trial included 97 clinic-referred children diagnosed with conduct disorder, who had a mean age of 5.74 years. Children and their parents were randomly assigned to child training (CT; Dinosaur School), parent training (PT), child plus parent training (CT + PT), or a waitlist control. In the PT condition, parents attended two-hour weekly group sessions addressing parenting and interpersonal skills for 22 to 24 weeks. Assessment occurred prior to the onset of the study, two months after the study ended, and also one year later.

Results indicated that children in the CT and CT + PT conditions suggested more prosocial solutions to hypothetical social problems compared to control children. Children in the PT-alone condition did not differ from control children. Children in all three treatment conditions also showed fewer negative responses in a potentially conflictual situation with a friend in a laboratory setting than control children. Furthermore, as compared to control and PT-only children, those in the CT condition displayed a significantly higher ratio of positive to negative responses to the conflict (Webster-Stratton & Hammond, 1997). Posttreatment gains in children's social problem solving maintained at one-year follow-up. Observational data on peer interactions were not collected at follow-up.

A later study evaluating the effects of parent, teacher, and child (Dinosaur School) training on children's social skills also supported the use of this curriculum (Webster-Stratton et al., 2004) either as a stand-alone program or in combination with parent training. Specifically, only those participants who received child training (with or without parent and teacher training) scored significantly higher than the control groups on a composite score assessing social competence with peers that was based on teacher report and classroom observations; children who received only parent training did not differ from the controls on this score. Together, Webster-Stratton and colleagues' findings indicate that Dinosaur School can produce significant changes in children's interactions and problem-solving skills when used on its own. They also tentatively suggest that parent training alone produces reductions in externalizing behavior problems in the home, but not improvement in children's peer-related social cognition.

These studies of the Dinosaur School curriculum were based samples that consisted primarily of Caucasian middle-income families. Two randomized control studies adapted the Dinosaur School program for Hispanic participants by translating the videotapes and other materials into Spanish (Barrera et al., 2002; Smolkowski et al., 2005). In both studies, Hispanic and European-American children in kindergarten through third grade who were referred by their teachers for having behavioral or reading difficulties participated in the Schools and Homes in Partnership (SHIP) program, which aims to prevent conduct behaviors through the use of parent training, Dinosaur School, classroom interventions to reduce problem behaviors, and supplemental reading instruction.

In the first randomized control study (Barrera et al., 2002), the SHIP intervention was evaluated with 168 Hispanic and 116 European-American children from the United States assessed four times: baseline (T1), at the end of the academic year (T2), at the end of the second academic year (T3), and one year after the intervention ended (T4). Observational data collected at T1, T2, and T3 assessments indicated that by T3, participants referred for aggressive behavior who received the intervention displayed less negative peer-directed behavior than control children. This finding did not hold for children referred because of their reading difficulties, however. The intervention worked equally well for Hispanic and European-American children.

In a more recent study (Smolkowski et al., 2005), the SHIP intervention (Including Dinosaur School) was conducted over the course of two years with 171 Hispanic children and 158 European-American children and their parents. In contrast with Barrera et al.'s (2002) results, neither teacher ratings nor directly observed peer behavior showed significant intervention effects. Although 30% of intervention participants did not actually participate in the social skills training, the intervention students who participated in more social skills training sessions did not have significantly better outcomes than intervention students who received fewer (or no) sessions.

Smolkowski et al. (2005) admitted that one important limitation of their research was that their group leaders did not have the same level of training and were not as experienced as group leaders in the Webster-Stratton studies. However, no formal analyses of assessments of treatment integrity were presented to address this possibility.

In summary, the Dinosaur School treatment program has shown short-term and long-term efficacy and effectiveness with children aged 4–8 years referred for conduct problems in three randomized control group studies (Barrera et al., 2002; Webster-Stratton & Hammond, 1997; Webster-Stratton et al., 2001, 2004). Although often implemented in conjunction with parent training interventions, studies that have examined Dinosaur School in the absence of parent training also support its efficacy for improving peer interactions. Effects on peer acceptance and friendship have not been examined, unfortunately. In addition, Dinosaur School did not produce changes when it was included as one part of a larger effectiveness intervention (Smolkowski et al., 2005). This recent failure to replicate suggests a continued need for effectiveness research that examines intervention integrity, treatment process, and the nature of group leader training and supervision required to implement the intervention successfully in real-world settings.

Coping Power

Another cognitive-behavioral intervention program that targets aggressive children's social problem-solving skills and peer acceptance is Coping Power (Lochman & Wells, 2002a, b), which also addresses parent factors associated with delinquency. Coping Power drew from Lochman's early work with an anger coping intervention (Lochman, 1992) and a social relations training program (Lochman et al., 1993). Both had shown some promise in randomized controlled trials, in reducing substance use among aggressive boys (Lochman, 1992) and in producing immediate posttreatment effects on peer acceptance among aggressive-rejected boys (Lochman et al., 1993).

Two randomized controlled trials have evaluated the effects of Coping Power program on at-risk children's social problem-solving skills (Lochman & Wells, 2002a, b, 2003, 2004). Both included boys from fourth and fifth grades referred because of their high scores on teacher measures of aggressive and disruptive behavior. Participants were predominantly African American. In both studies, boys were assessed at baseline (T1), when the intervention ended (T2), and one year later (T3).

Boys in the child component of the Coping Power program met for 33 weekly group sessions for 40 to 60 minutes. Group sessions focused on a variety of areas including identification of feelings, associated physiological responses, anger-management techniques, perspective taking, social problem solving, and peer pressure. The parent component consisted of 16 group sessions designed to teach parents the skills they needed to parent their children more effectively. Trained interventionists implemented the program.

In the first trial, Lochman and Wells (2002a, 2004) compared (1) Coping Power child training alone, (2) Coping Power with the parenting intervention, and (3) an untreated control group. At the end of intervention, boys in the Coping Power intervention had significantly improved outcome expectations and more internal locus of control relative to controls, but not significantly improved attributions (Lochman & Wells, 2002a). At T3, boys in the combined Coping Power intervention (but not the Coping Power-alone condition) reported less covert delinquency and their parents reported that they were involved in less drug use (Lochman & Wells, 2004). Changes in aggressive boys' hostile attributions, outcome expectancies, schematic beliefs, and parenting processes as a group contributed to the intervention effect in reducing delinquent behavior (but not substance use) one year later (Lochman & Wells, 2002a), although this appeared to be largely the result of improvements in parental consistency, not social cognition.

In their second trial, Lochman and Wells (2002b, 2003) assessed a much wider array of peer-related variables. They compared Coping Power (including child and parent training components), Coping Power plus a classroom intervention, the classroom intervention alone, and a control condition. The classroom intervention consisted of periodic parent and teacher didactic/discussion meetings focused on promoting positive child behavior, problem solving, and school adjustment. Lochman and Wells (2002b) found that teachers rated boys who received Coping Power (with or without the classroom intervention) as significantly more socially competent than boys who did not. In addition, teachers reported the best problem-solving skills among boys who received all components of intervention. Boys' reports of their own attributions and anger did not change significantly. At one-year follow-up (Lochman & Wells, 2003), boys who received Coping Power reported less delinquency. Older boys and boys who had been identified as at moderate risk at pretest also reported significantly less drug use at follow-up, whereas comparable controls showed marked increases over this time period.

In sum, the full Coping Power intervention has shown promising and replicated effects in reducing delinquency and drug use. It is less clear whether the child training component of Coping Power improves social cognition; many studies report marginally significant findings, suggesting these effects may be weak. Effects on observed behavior with peers and peer acceptance have not been assessed, possibly because Coping Power was designed primarily to affect aggression and delinquency rather than peer relationships. Although samples have included African-American and Caucasian males, girls have not been included. Finally, Coping Power appears to have greatest effects when both components—parent and child training—are included, not as a stand-alone child social skills training program.

Fast Track

Fast Track is a comprehensive prevention program that combines social skills, parenting, and academic interventions designed to reduce precursors of conduct problems and delinquency. Portions of the intervention are implemented for all children in participating classrooms, while other components are delivered to children with high rates of aggressive and disruptive behavior. Two components of the intervention explicitly address social skills: (1) PATHS, a teacher-delivered problem-solving and affective education curriculum delivered to entire classrooms, and (2) the Friendship Group, a social skills training intervention specifically aimed at disruptive and aggressive children. Families of high-risk Fast Track youth are also provided with (1) parenting groups that focus on parenting skills and positive parent-school relationships, (2) visits from the program staff to promote generalization of skills, and (3) reading tutoring (see Bierman et al., 1996; CPPRG, 1999a, b, 2002b; Lavallee et al., 2005, for descriptions).

In the Fast Track version of PATHS, teachers in grades 1–5 deliver the PATHS program two to three times per week during the entire school year using a series of structured 20- to 30-minute lessons. PATHS content focuses on friendship, conflict management, and affective and problem-solving skills. Teachers use instruction, role-play, stories, videos, and discussion to implement the curriculum. They also employ generalization techniques to help children apply what they are learning in everyday school situations.

One interesting aspect of the Fast Track program is that it is built upon intervention components shown to be effective in previous studies. This was certainly true of PATHS. Greenberg and Kusché (1998) and Greenberg et al. (1995) evaluated precursor versions of PATHS used in Fast Track in randomized controlled trials. These investigations speak to the effects of PATHS as a viable intervention on its own. Greenberg and Kusché (1998) implemented the program with deaf children, whereas Greenberg et al. (1995) employed PATHS with children with various special needs (e.g., learning disabilities, mild mental retardation, emotional and behavioral problems). In both studies children who received PATHS showed significantly better social problem-solving and affective skills on a variety of indicators after the intervention, relative to controls. Greenberg et al. (1995) did not evaluate whether PATHS changed social behavior or peer acceptance, but Greenberg and Kusché (1998) did. They found that after PATHS, treated children were superior to controls on teacher ratings of emotional adjustment, but not peer relations, social adjustment, or behavior problems. However, children scored fairly high on social adjustment and low on behavior problems prior to intervention.

Kam et al. (2004) examined data collected one and two years after the intervention and found that treatment and control trajectories in teacher ratings of various indicators of social competence did not differ. Children who received PATHS did, however, continue to demonstrate improvements in generating nonconfrontational solutions to hypothetical problems and in negative feelings vocabulary. They also showed declining trajectories in teacher ratings of externalizing behavior compared with the average increases of control children.

In contrast with PATHS, the Friendship Group (Bierman et al., 1996; Lavallee et al., 2005) was designed specifically for aggressive/disruptive children, a group particularly likely to be rejected by peers. Educational coordinators led the one-hour Friendship Groups after school or on weekends using a detailed treatment manual. In evaluations of Fast Track, children identified as aggressive/disruptive met in groups of 5 to 6 for 22 sessions in grade 1, 14 sessions in grade 2, and 9 sessions in grade 3. The Friendship Group curriculum addressed many of the same competencies taught in the PATHS curriculum and used the same sorts of training procedures (modeling, discussion, practice). In addition, participants were paired with different lower-risk classmates for 30 minutes per week "peer-pairing" sessions to practice skills taught in the group and to promote generalization and positive peer contacts. Adult supervisors oversaw the children's activities.

The Conduct Problem Prevention Research Group randomly assigned schools either to receive Fast Track or to serve as a control school and then implemented Fast Track in 191 classrooms in four U.S. sites. All children in participating classrooms received the PATHS curriculum. Educational coordinators also met weekly with each teacher to consult on classroom management and to provide ongoing training and feedback; teachers were compensated for their involvement (CPPRG, 1999b).

In addition to the PATHS curriculum, children identified as high-risk (top 10% of sample, based on teacher and parent ratings of aggression and related behavior in kindergarten and grade 1) were invited to participate in the Friendship Group and the remaining parts of the program in grade 1. CPPRG (1999a) reported that 98% of children attended at least one group; average attendance ranged from 74–83% across sites. This high rate of participation was likely due to extensive efforts to involve the high-risk parents, the fact that parents participated in a parenting group concurrently, and the decision to compensate parents $15 for each session they attended as well as providing travel and child care. Teachers implemented the full PATHS curriculum in grades 2 and 3, and high-risk children and their families received other services (including Friendship Groups and peer pairing) as needed.

CPPRG has examined the outcomes of Fast Track at the end of the grades 1, 3, and 5. Few differences between sites have emerged, suggesting a high degree of replicability of findings. At the end of year 1 (CPPRG, 1999a, b), observational data based on two hours of observation per child indicated that high-risk children showed greater amounts of time in positive peer interaction than controls. Peers also liked them better. Assessments of emotional knowledge and problem solving also favored the Fast Track high-risk groups. Peer nominations and teacher ratings of aggressive behavior and observed aggression did not differ for the Fast Track versus control high-risk groups. However, analyses based on data from all children (not just the high-risk youth) indicated that children in Fast Track classrooms were significantly less aggressive (based on observations and peer nominations) than children in control classrooms. This suggests that the classroom-level PATHS intervention may have had a larger effect on children with lower rates of aggression to begin with, although the cumulative effects of the intervention as a whole and the spillover effects of the improvements in the high-risk children could also be responsible for these effects.

By the end of grade 3, effects on the high-risk group were more modest: Social problem-solving cognitive gains were only marginally significant, and peer-nominated prosocial behavior and liking no longer differentiated the treatment vs. control comparisons. As in grade 1, peer nominations of aggression were comparable in Fast Track and control conditions, but teacher ratings of aggression for the first time showed a significant difference between the Fast Track and control high-risk groups (CPPRG, 2002a). At the end of grade 5, the groups also differed on a composite score that included social-cognitive and teacher-rated social and academic competence indicators.

Although Fast Track has affected peer processes and behavior in significant ways, it is important to keep in mind that Fast Track involved multiple components, many of which did not directly target children's peer relations. These were expected to have synergistic effects. Thus, as with most of the multicomponent interventions reviewed here, the specific components responsible for positive changes cannot be disentangled. How PATHS and the Friendship Group might affect social behavior and peer acceptance either on their own cannot be determined from the Fast Track studies.

In addition, Fast Track effect sizes have been relatively modest, especially considering the large amount of effort expended to engage and retain families and maintain treatment fidelity. These efforts seem essential: Gains in teacher and observer ratings of children in the classroom at the end of the first year of Fast Track were associated with the quality of teacher implementation of the PATHS curriculum (CPPRG, 1999b). Kam et al. (2003) reported similar findings when implementing PATHS on its own in inner-city schools. Furthermore, effects have been more consistent on measures of social cognition and child behavior than on indicators of peer acceptance. Despite these limitations, the Fast Track trial is unique in examining multisite dissemination of social skills interventions and showing social skills gains with large numbers of high-risk youth in diverse communities.

Each of the three intervention programs reviewed here has shown some effectiveness in improving social skills in at-risk populations. However, most were a part of studies examining multicomponent interventions focused on a broad array of outcomes, making it difficult to tease apart the individual program's effects on social skills from the larger intervention. Only Dinosaur School showed that it could successfully affect peer variables when used as a stand-alone program.

In addition, the programs varied in the extent to which they evaluated measures of both social behavior and functioning in the peer group (e.g., peer acceptance or rejection); only Fast Track evaluated both over short- and long-term time periods. This makes it difficult to assess whether significant changes in social behavior or cognition actually result in improved peer relationships. A related issue lies in the need to appraise the clinical significance of peer outcomes. The concept of clinical significance, like social validity, addresses whether changes in child behavior are meaningful or "clinically significant." Assessments of clinical significance often focus on the degree of change in targeted skills (e.g., by examining the percentage of treated children whose scores on a measure of behavior fall within the normative range after treatment; Jacobson et al., 1999; Kendall et al., 1999). Although research on all of the programs just described has addressed clinical significance in some way (e.g., by looking at parent report measures of externalizing problems), none has looked at the clinical significance of changes specifically on measures of peer interactions and functioning.

Despite these limitations, all three of these programs have common features that may contribute to their effectiveness. All consider the child's peer relationship difficulties in the context of the broader array of contributors to children's aggression. All involve adult socialization agents in parallel interventions. All are intensive, allow the child many opportunities for skill acquisition and practice, and explicitly include procedures designed to enhance generalization.

Finally, all focus on reducing aggression and disruption, competing behaviors that interfere with peer acceptance. All also include acquisition components to teach presumably deficient social-cognitive skills. Social skills training programs also exist that address performance deficits, notably those involved in social anxiety (see Greco & Morris, 2001, for review). These have produced more limited and less well-replicated outcomes than interventions for externalizing problems, however.

META-ANALYSES AND QUALITATIVE REVIEWS

The specific programs just described represent only a few of a wide variety of intervention programs aimed at improving children and adolescents' behavior in peer interactions. Many additional programs have produced positive effects but have not been replicated. These programs differ in their intervention focus (e.g., problematic behaviors, affective education, social-cognitive deficits, difficulties in problem solving, poor parenting, etc.), eligibility requirements of participants, the number of intervention sessions delivered, duration of treatment, whether parents are included in treatment or not, type of intervention, measures used to assess the program's effectiveness, and outcome variables. Several meta-analytic and qualitative (narrative) reviewers have synthesized this literature to try to identify general conclusions about the interventions that do and do not work.

Because meta-analysts and qualitative reviewers often examine only a subset of interventions based on the research questions of interest to them, quantitative and qualitative evaluations of social skills training programs sometimes produce different conclusions (see Foster & Crain, 2002). For instance, one meta-analysis of outcome studies examined different cognitive-behavioral techniques (skills development, affective education, problem solving, and eclectic treatments) for children with anger control and social skills problems (Sukhodolsky et al., 2004). Using 21 published and 19 unpublished studies, these authors found greater effect sizes (in the medium to large range) for skills development training and multimodal treatments in their effect on social skills as compared to affective education (relaxation, positive imagery, and education about emotions) or problem-solving approaches.

In contrast, other meta-analytic investigators have found less promising effect sizes regarding social skills interventions with children and/or adolescents (Beelmann et al., 1994; Forness & Kavale, 1996). Beelmann et al. (1994) conducted a meta-analysis of 49 studies of social competence training (SCT), including cognitive-behavioral interventions designed to modify motor, cognitive, and/or affective components of children's behavior. Effect sizes showed that SCT is moderately effective at improving social competence among 3- to 15-year-olds. However, short-term effect sizes were lower than in previous meta-analyses (Schneider, 1992), and there were no significant long-term effects (Beelmann et al., 1994). Furthermore, SCT was found to be more effective with socially deprived, at-risk children than those with internalizing or externalizing disorders. This discrepancy in the effectiveness of social skills training for clinical populations has been found in a more recent meta-analysis as well (Quinn et al., 1999), and Erwin (1994) identified larger effect sizes for classroom-based social skills interventions designed for withdrawn students than for interventions that did not target this population.

Some meta-analyses have found even lower effect sizes for social skills interventions with children. Forness and Kavale (1996; Kavale & Mosten, 2004) conducted a meta-analysis of social skills interventions for children with a specific learning disability, involving 53 studies. Although the calculated effect sizes varied in range, the average effect size was deemed to be small. There were no significant differences in effect sizes as a function of age, treatment length, research quality (rated as low, medium, or high), or type of rater (self, teachers, or peers). Similarly, Gresham et al. (2001) reviewed both qualitative and meta-analytic reviews of social skills training, with a specific focus on children with serious, high-incidence disabilities. They concluded that data to date raise serious questions about the short- and long-term effectiveness of social skills interventions with students with severe difficulties, arguably the students who need intervention the most.

Despite some differences, a few noteworthy consistencies emerge across meta-analyses of the effectiveness of social skills interventions (Foster & Crain, 2002). First, most reviews conclude that the overall effects of social skills training on rejected children, or children identified as deficient in adaptive social behavior with peers, are moderate at best. Second, the largest effect sizes were found when researchers examined different measures of social interaction, as opposed to peer acceptance or rejection (Erwin, 1994; Schneider, 1992), and for measures of social-cognitive skills as opposed to social adjustment or self-related cognitions/affect (Beelmann et al., 1994). Because of these weak effects, some of the strongest early proponents of social skills training have raised concerns about the efficacy and effectiveness of the approach (e.g., Bullis et al., 2001; Gresham et al., 2001). Third, several meta-analytic reviews report a significant degree of heterogeneity in effect sizes across the studies included in their reviews, suggesting variability in the effects produced by different social skills interventions (Beelmann et al., 1994; Erwin, 1994; Schneider, 1992).

Despite the results of meta-analytic studies, reviewers are reluctant to dismiss social skills training as a potentially viable intervention, possibly for two reasons. First, meta-analysts have noted highly variable effect sizes, with some studies producing very large effects on measures of socially important behaviors. This suggests that some programs, implemented under some circumstances, are likely to substantially benefit some children. Because so few programs have been replicated or developed with an eye toward dissemination, however, it is difficult to know which ones work best consistently.

Second, experienced outcome researchers have repeatedly noted the many issues a social skills training approach must address successfully to produce lasting and important changes in child behavior. Poor choices in any of these areas are likely to produce weakened effects. Reviewers have identified several of these:

1. Choice of target behaviors to train (Bullis et al., 2001): The behaviors selected for training should be socially valid—they should include "socially significant behaviors exhibited in specific situations that predict important social outcomes for children and youth" (Gresham et al., 2001, p. 333). If social cognitions or emotion regulation skills are the focus of intervention, improvements in these mechanisms should be associated with improvements in socially significant behaviors. For example, a broad literature on behavioral and cognitive correlates of peer rejection and acceptance (important social outcomes) exists and can form the basis for social skills curricula aimed at children who are actively disliked by peers (see Bierman, 2004, for review). In addition, the focus of intervention should include a sufficient range of behaviors to produce changes in important social outcomes for children, such as their peer relations and friendships. For example, improvements in prosocial behavior may not be sufficient to improve a child's social standing if the child's aggression does not decrease as well.

2. Matching the child's problems to the intervention: Children with social skills problems are remarkably heterogeneous; the same is true among subgroups of these children, such as aggressive or rejected children (Bierman, 2004). As Gresham et al. (2001) point out, different interventions (or combinations of interventions) may be required depending upon the child's social skills profile. For example, a child with acquisition problems but no competing maladaptive behaviors may benefit from modeling and coaching, whereas a child with performance issues and many competing behaviors may need exposure to strategies to reduce problem behaviors as well as contingencies to support performance of appropriate behaviors in relevant situations. Interventionists must therefore determine for whom an intervention is most likely to work and then select children who have those characteristics.

3. Selection of effective intervention strategies that change the child's behavior in the short term: To be effective, the intervention must include components that lead to immediate improvements in behavior. Even if the correct targets are chosen for the right population of children, intervention that relies on ineffective or outmoded strategies will not produce significant change. In addition, the amount or dosage of intervention must be sufficient to produce behavior change (Bierman, 2004; Bullis et al., 2001; Gresham et al., 2001).

4. Intervention strategies must promote generalization and maintenance (Bierman, 2004): A common concern among meta-analysts and qualitative reviewers of social skills training since its inception lies in the need for interventions to produce generalized and lasting change (see

Bierman, 2004, for a historical overview). Principles for promoting generalization have been known since the 1970s and include training multiple exemplars of target skills, training in a broad array of circumstances, ensuring that appropriate responses will be reinforced in the natural environment, and actively encouraging generalized responding (Stokes & Baer, 1977). More recently, social skills researchers have embedded social skills interventions in the context of broader programs (Bierman, 2004) and have included parents (e.g., Frankel, 2004) as possible ways to improve generalization. Bierman (2004) also recommends careful attention to peer reactions in the natural environment to ensure peer support of changed behavior. Whether these strategies actually contribute to either generalized behavior change or to long-term effects has not been completely established, however.

5. Implementation integrity (Bullis et al., 2001; Gresham et al., 2001): Even the most effective program cannot produce good results if it is not implemented properly. With the exception of the Fast Track program (where treatment integrity in PATHS was associated with improved outcomes; CPPRG, 1999b), treatment integrity issues have received little explicit attention in social skills evaluations.

6. Treatment process issues: Most social skills treatment is conducted in groups of children. Bierman (2004) rightly pointed out that managing youth with social skills difficulties can pose great challenges because their social skills problems are evident in the treatment setting, even in groups that include socially high-functioning children. In line with this, Lavallee et al. (2005) found that first-grade high-risk children in the Fast Track program who teachers rated as most aggressive prior to treatment were also rated by social skills trainers as least positively engaged and most disruptive in social skills training groups. The importance of creating this positive engagement was underscored by the fact that high ratings of children's positive behavior in social skills training groups were associated with improvements in classroom aggression at the end of first grade.

Disruptive behavior during intervention sessions makes it more difficult for the social skills trainer to implement the intervention with integrity. In addition, Dishion et al. (1999) warn of the possible negative effects of conducting group interventions with high-risk youth, particularly adolescents: In several studies, youth in these groups have shown worse behavior after treatment than control youth. Although some question the existence and pervasiveness of this effect (Weiss et al., 2005), Kavale and Mostert (2004) reported 22% of the effect sizes they examined in their meta-analysis indicated that controls did better than treated children after SST with youth with learning disabilities. These data suggest that possible iatrogenic effects of SST should not be dismissed. Peer reinforcement of deviant behavior (and conversations about this behavior) is one mechanism by which this might happen (Dishion et al., 2001; Mager et al., 2005). Mager et al. (2005) found that iatrogenic processes and negative outcomes were more likely to occur in groups composed of some 6th- and 7th-grade children with and some without behavior problems than in groups in which all children had behavior problems.

FROM EFFICACY TO EFFECTIVENESS: IMPLEMENTING EVIDENCE-BASED SOCIAL SKILLS TRAINING IN THE REAL WORLD

Social skills training interventions have varied in how closely their evaluations approximated true effectiveness trials. Although SHIP (including Dinosaur School) and Fast Track implementation come closest to "real-world" conditions, most evaluations of social skills training would be characterized as "efficacy" assessments. Efficacy studies examine the intervention under circumstances that are closer to ideal than those typically found in real-world clinical and school settings.

Our experience conducting and supervising various versions of social skills and problem solving training suggests a number of practical issues that must be considered in real-world applications. One involves using evidence-based methods to select youth for the intervention. Although some teacher and parent screening measures used in research settings are practical to administer, other assessment tools are more difficult to implement. In particular, measures such as peer nomination sociometrics require participation by whole classes to identify children who are generally disliked, and such measures may be difficult or impossible to use in nonresearch contexts due to the time and effort required to obtain parent and teacher permission and to administer and score the instruments. Observational measures, too, typically require more resources than the average clinician, teacher, or school counselor has available.

A second set of issues involves establishing and conducting social skills groups. A sufficient number of children must be identified to compose a sufficiently homogeneous group (e.g., in terms of age, presenting problems, etc.) to proceed, and their parents must consent for their participation. Once the intervention begins, interventionists must develop plans to prevent and deal with missed sessions, engage youth in the curriculum, and manage disruptive behavior and attentional issues (see Bierman, 2004, for extended discussion). In particular, some youth may dominate groups, while more withdrawn children may need encouragement to become involved in activities and discussion. Mechanisms to discourage positive peer attention to deviant behavior and conversation about misbehavior need to be firmly in place in light of the possibility that aggregating at-risk youth can have iatrogenic effects if the leader fails to manage group processes successfully. In addition, the need for generalization programming suggests that teachers, parents, and peers be involved in appropriate ways to support the child's newly developing skills in the natural environment. This in turn requires that they be engaged in the treatment process.

A third set of issues involves assessing whether children's difficulties are unique to their peer relationships or are more generalized. Because peer difficulties are implicated in so many forms of child psychopathology, many children's social skills problems are part of a broader set of behavioral excesses or deficits that may be evident with parents, teacher, siblings, etc. This is particularly likely with youth who are clinically referred. In these cases, social skills training should be accompanied by other evidence-based approaches to address the broader problem set of problems in which peer relationship difficulties play a role.

Implementing evidence-based social skills training programs on a broader scale (e.g., as a standard part of school curricula) raises a host of systemic issues as well. Walker (2004) provides an excellent overview of these considerations in school settings. Among the most important of these are (1) the fit between the program and the educational goals of the school and the professionals who will implement the intervention, (2) community and administrative support for adopting and implementing the intervention, (3) careful identification of what is required for treatment integrity, (4) appropriate and high-quality training, supervision, and ongoing technical support for those who will implement the intervention.

Despite many studies of social skills training with children, much has yet to be learned about the core requirements for creating and implementing social skills training interventions in real-world settings in order to make meaningful improvements in the social lives of children who have peer relationship problems. A few programs have replicated effects, however, and some of these have done so in effectiveness contexts. Most of these have designed to reduce aggression rather than to address peer relationships issues specifically. Few programs specifically designed to address performance deficits or fluency problems have the same track records.

Despite limitations in the research to date, existing approaches can form the basis or become the standard of comparison for the next generation of social skills interventions. This "next-generation" research can draw from best practices in past research in several ways. First, treatment outcome research should draw from literature on developmental psychopathology to select targets for social skills training based on an understanding of the deficits, fluency problems, and competing behaviors that (1) characterize the group toward whom the intervention is addressed, and (2) directly contribute to peer acceptance and friendship. The Fast Track model exemplifies this approach. Second, research should explicitly assess changes in target social cognitive skills and social behavior as well as changes in functioning in the peer group. Third, intervention research should routinely examine both clinical as well as statistical significance. Fourth, investigators should evaluate how treatment process variables contribute to treatment outcome by assessing treatment integrity as well as processes that enhance or detract from social skills training done in groups. Finally, intervention researchers should develop the next generation of evidence-based strategies with dissemination in mind (Walker, 2004).

The variable effects of social skills training with many populations suggest that rethinking the models that underlie social skills training may also be necessary to increase the effectiveness and efficacy of social skills intervention. For example, interventions may benefit from devoting more explicit attention to ways of ensuring opportunities for positive peer interactions once treated children's behavior begins to improve (see Bierman's studies as one example of this). Positive consequences for improved behavior with peers in the natural environment may also need to be built into training approaches. Research that takes closer looks at children who fail to benefit from social skills interventions can form the basis for models of factors that contribute to treatment nonresponse. Results of this work will undoubtedly suggest new components for social skills intervention. In testing the new interventions that emerge, investigators should examine whether treatment mechanisms work as theorized; for example, by testing mediation models in the context of randomized controlled trials. Replications in real-world settings with an eye toward cost-benefit analyses will also be important.

In sum, promising approaches for children with social skills difficulties—particularly aggressive children—have emerged in the last three decades. Even the most promising social skills training programs, however, do not produce clinically significant improvement with all of the children enrolled in the intervention. Moving to the next generation of interventions will be challenging but is particularly important in order to increase the pervasiveness, longevity, social validity, and clinical significance of treatment benefits for a larger number of children.

REFERENCES

Barrera, M., Biglan, A., Taylor, T., Gunn, B., Smolkowski, K., Black, C., et al. (2002). Early elementary school intervention to reduce conduct problems: A randomized trial with Hispanic and non-Hispanic children. *Prevention Science, 3*, 83–94.

Beelmann, A., Pfingsten, U., & Losel, F. (1994). Effects of training social competence in children: A meta-analysis of recent evaluation studies. *Journal of Clinical Child Psychology, 23*, 260–271.

Bierman, K. L. (2004). *Peer Rejection: Developmental Processes and Intervention Strategies.* New York: Guilford Press.

Bierman, K., Greenberg, M. T., & the Conduct Problems Prevention Research Group (1996). Social skills training in the Fast Track Program. In R. D. Peters & R. J. McMahon (Eds.), *Preventing Childhood Disorders, Substance Use, and Delinquency* (pp. 65–89). Thousand Oaks, CA: Sage.

Biglan, A., Brennan, P., Foster, S. L., & Holder, H. (2003). *Helping Adolescents at Risk: Prevention of Multiple Problem Behaviors.* New York: Guilford Press.

Bukowski, W. M., Newcomb, A. F., & Hartup, W. W. (1996). *The Company They Keep.* New York: Cambridge University Press.

Bullis, M., Walker, H. M., & Sprague, J. R. (2001). A promise unfulfilled: Social skills training with at-risk and antisocial children and youth. *Exceptionality, 9*, 67–90.

Conduct Problems Prevention Research Group (1999a). Initial impact of the Fast Track prevention trial for conduct problems: I. The high-risk sample. *Journal of Consulting and Clinical Psychology, 67*, 631–647.

Conduct Problems Prevention Research Group (1999b). Initial impact of the Fast Track prevention trial for conduct problems: II. Classroom effects. *Journal of Consulting and Clinical Psychology, 67*, 648–657.

Conduct Problems Prevention Research Group (2002a). Evaluation of the first 3 years of the Fast Track prevention trial with children at high risk for adolescent conduct problems. *Journal of Abnormal Child Psychology, 30*, 19–36.

Conduct Problems Prevention Research Group (2002b). The implementation of the Fast Track program: An example of large-scale prevention science efficacy trial. *Journal of Abnormal Child Psychology, 30*, 1–18.

Conduct Problems Prevention Research Group (2004). The effects of the Fast Track program on serious problem outcomes at the end of elementary school. *Journal of Clinical Child and Adolescent Psychology, 33,* 650–661.

Dishion, T. J., McCord, J., & Poulin, F. (1999). When interventions harm: Peer groups and problem behavior. *American Psychologist, 54,* 755–764.

Dishion, T. J., Poulin, F., & Burraston, B. (2001). Peer group dynamics associated with iatrogenic effects in group interventions with high-risk adolescents. *New Directions in Child and Adolescent Development, 91,* 79–92.

Erwin, P. (1994). Effectiveness of social skills training with children: A meta-analytic study. *Counseling Psychology Quarterly, 7,* 305–310.

Forness, S., & Kavale, K. (1996). Treating social skill deficits in children with learning disabilities: A meta-analysis of the research. *Learning Disability Quarterly, 19,* 2–3.

Foster, S. L., & Crain, M. M. (2002). Social skills and problem solving training. In T. Patterson (Ed.), *Comprehensive Handbook of Psychotherapy,* Vol. 2. New York: John Wiley & Sons.

Foster, S. L., & Mash, E. J. (1999). Social validity issues in clinical treatment research. *Journal of Consulting and Clinical Psychology, 67,* 308–319.

Frankel, F. D. (2004). Parent-assisted children's friendship training. In E. D. Hibbs & P. S. Jensen (Eds.), *Psychosocial Treatments for Child and Adolescent Disorders: Empirically Based Strategies for Clinical Practice,* 2nd ed. (pp. 693–715). Washington, DC: American Psychological Association.

Gifford-Smith, M., Dodge, K. A., Dishion, T. J., & McCord, J. (2005). Peer influence in children and adolescents: Crossing the bridge from developmental science to intervention science. *Journal of Abnormal Child Psychology, 33,* 255–265.

Greco, L. A., & Morris, T. L. (2001). Treating childhood shyness and related behavior: Empirically evaluated approaches to promote positive social interactions. *Clinical Child and Family Psychology Review, 4,* 299–318.

Greenberg, M. T., & Kusché, C. A. (1998). Preventive intervention for school-aged deaf children: The PATHS curriculum. *Journal of Deaf Studies and Deaf Education, 3,* 49–63.

Greenberg, M. T., Kusché, C. A., Cook, E. T., & Quamma, J. P. (1995). Promoting emotional competence in school-aged children: The effects of the PATHS curriculum. *Development and Psychopathology, 7,* 117–136.

Gresham, F. M., Sugai, G., & Horner, R. H. (2001). Interpreting outcomes of social skills training for students with high-incidence disabilities. *Exceptional Children, 67,* 331–334.

Jacobson, N. S., Roberts, L. J., Burns, S. B., & McGlinchey, J. B. (1999). Methods for defining and determining the clinical significance of treatment effects: Description, application, and alternatives. *Journal of Consulting and Clinical Psychology, 67,* 300–307.

Kam, C.-M., Greenberg, M. T., & Kusché, C. A. (2004). Sustained effects of the PATHS curriculum on the social and psychological adjustment of children in special education. *Journal of Emotional and Behavioral Disorders, 12,* 66–78.

Kam, C.-M., Greenberg, M. T., & Walls, C. T. (2003). Examining the role of implementation quality in school-based prevention using the PATHS curriculum. *Prevention Science, 4,* 55–63.

Kavale, K. A., & Mostert, M. P. (2004). Social skills interventions for individuals with learning disabilities. *Learning Disabilities Quarterly, 27,* 31–43.

Kendall, A. E., Marrs-Garcia, A., Nath, S. R., & Sheldrick, R. C. (1999). Normative comparisons for the evaluation of clinical significance. *Journal of Consulting and Clinical Psychology, 67,* 285–299.

Lavallee, K. L., Bierman, K. L., Nix, R. L., & the Conduct Problems Prevention Research Group (2005). The impact of first-grade "Friendship Group" experiences on child social outcomes in the Fast Track program. *Journal of Abnormal Child Psychology, 33,* 307–324.

Lochman, J. E. (1992). Cognitive behavioral intervention for aggressive boys: Three-year follow-up and preventive effects. *Journal of Consulting and Clinical Psychology, 60,* 426–532.

Lochman, J., Coie, J., Underwood, M., & Terry, R. (1993). Effectiveness of a social relations intervention program for aggressive and nonaggressive, rejected children. *Journal of Consulting and Clinical Psychology, 61,* 1053–1058.

Lochman, J. E., & Wells, K. C. (2002a). Contextual social-cognitive mediators and child outcome: A test of the theoretical model in the Coping Power program. *Development and Psychopathology, 14,* 945–967.

Lochman, J. E., & Wells, K. C. (2002b). The Coping Power program at the middle-school transition: Universal and indicated prevention effects. *Psychology of Addictive Behaviors, 16,* S40–S54.

Lochman, J. E., & Wells, K. C. (2003). Effectiveness of the Coping Power program and of classroom intervention with aggressive children: Outcomes at a 1-year follow-up. *Behavior Therapy, 34,* 493–515.

Lochman, J. E., & Wells, K. C. (2004). The Coping Power program for preadolescent aggressive boys ad their parents: Outcome effects at the 1-year follow-up. *Journal of Consulting and Clinical Psychology, 72,* 571–578.

Mager, W., Milich, R., Harris, M. J., & Howard, A. (2005). Intervention groups for adolescents with conduct problems: Is aggregation harmful or helpful? *Journal of Abnormal Child Psychology, 33,* 349–362.

Parker, J. G., & Asher, S. R. (1987). Peer relations and later personal adjustment: Are low-accepted children "at risk"? *Psychological Bulletin, 102,* 357–389.

Quinn, M., Kavale, K., Mathur, S., Rutherford, R., & Forness, S. (1999). A meta-analysis of social skill interventions for students with emotional or behavioral disorders. *Journal of Emotional and Behavioral Disorders, 7,* 54–64.

Reid, M. J., Webster-Stratton, C., & Hammond, M. (2003). Follow-up of children who received the Incredible Years intervention for Oppositional-Defiant Disorder: Maintenance and Prediction of 2-year outcome. *Behavior Therapy, 34,* 471–491.

Schneider, B. (1992). Didactic methods for enhancing children's peer relations: A quantitative review. *Clinical Psychology Review, 12,* 363–382.

Smolkowski, K., Biglan, A., Barrera, M., Taylor, T., Black, C., & Blair, J. (2005). Schools and homes in partnership (SHIP): Long-term effects of a preventative intervention focused on social behavior and reading skill in early elementary school. *Prevention Science, 6,* 113–125.

Stokes, T. F., & Baer, D. M. (1977). An implicit technology of generalization. *Journal of Applied Behavior Analysis, 10,* 349–367.

Sukhodolsky, D., Kassinove, H., & Gorman, B. (2004). Cognitive-behavioral therapy for anger in children and adolescents: A meta-analysis. *Aggression and Violent Behavior, 9,* 247–269.

Taylor, T. K., Eddy, J. M., & Biglan, A. (1999). Interpersonal skills training to reduce aggressive and delinquent behavior: Limited evidence and the need for an evidence-based system of care. *Clinical Child and Family Psychology Review, 2,* 169–182.

Walker, H. M. (2004). Commentary: Use of evidence-based interventions in schools: Where we've been, where we are, and where we need to go. *School Psychology Review, 33,* 398–407.

Webster-Stratton, C., & Hammond, M. (1997). Treating children with early-onset conduct problems: A comparison of child and parent training interventions. *Journal of Consulting and Clinical Psychology, 65,* 93–109.

Webster-Stratton, C., Reid, M., & Hammond, M. (2001). Preventing conduct problems, promoting social competence: A parent and teacher training partnership in Head Start. *Journal of Clinical Child Psychology, 30,* 283–302.

Webster-Stratton, C., Reid, M., & Hammond, M. (2004). Treating children with early-onset conduct problems: Intervention outcomes for parent, child, and teacher training. *Journal of Clinical Child and Adolescent Psychology, 33,* 105–124.

Weiss, B., Caron, A., Ball, S., Trapp, J., Johnson, M., & Weisz, J. R. (2005). Iatrogenic effects of group treatment for antisocial youth. *Journal of Consulting and Clinical Psychology, 73,* 1036–1044.

24

Evidence-Based Treatments for Adolescent Substance Use Disorders

DEBORAH DEAS, KEVIN GRAY, and HIMANSHU UPADHYAYA

INTRODUCTION

Adolescent substance use is a major concern throughout the United States. Despite a slight decline in substance use among adolescents over the past decade, far too many adolescents continue to use alcohol and/or drugs. The Monitoring the Future survey (Johnston et al., 2004) revealed that in 2004, 12th-graders reported 30-day prevalence rates of 48% for alcohol use, almost 20% for marijuana use, 25% for nicotine use, and 2.3% for cocaine use. Even more striking is the rate of binge drinking (five or more drinks in a row during a single sitting) among high school seniors. According to the Youth Risk Behavior survey, almost 40% of male 12th-graders and 34.5% of female 12th-graders reported binge drinking in the 30 days prior to the survey in 2003. There was little to no decline in 2004, where 29.2% of high school seniors reported binge drinking in the 30 days prior to the Monitoring the Future survey (Johnston et al., 2004).

While the aforementioned survey results are not enough to make a diagnosis of a substance use disorder, a nationwide diagnostic survey questionnaire revealed that 10% of 17-year-olds met criteria for alcohol abuse or dependence and 7% met criteria for marijuana abuse or dependence (Kilpatrick et al., 2000). The impact of developing a substance use disorder during adolescence is far-reaching. The single most predictive factor for adult alcohol and other drug dependence is the presence

DEBORAH DEAS • Professor of Psychiatry, Center for Drug and Alcohol Programs, **KEVIN GRAY** • Assistant Professor of Psychiatry, Youth Division and **HIMANSHU UPADHYAYA** • Associate Professor of Psychiatry, Clinical Neurosciences Division

of alcohol and drug use during adolescence (Swadi, 1999). Further, adolescent substance use is associated with motor vehicle accidents (Mayhew et al., 1986), suicide (Brent et al., 1995), homicide (McLaughlin et al., 2000), as well as short- and long-term health problems (Aarons et al., 1999).

The focus of this chapter is evidence-based treatment of adolescent substance use disorders. Unfortunately, substance abuse treatments for adolescents have lagged behind those of adults. In many cases, attempts have been made to directly transfer treatments used in adults to adolescents with little modification. On the other hand, clinicians and researchers treating adolescents with substance use disorders recognize more clearly that "adolescents are not adults" (Deas et al., 2000) and have developed treatments specifically designed for adolescents. This chapter will review treatment modalities tailored for adolescents with substance use disorders that have been studied in a controlled fashion comparing one or more modalities. Treatment modalities for substance use disorders consist of psychosocial therapies and pharmacotherapy. The psychosocial therapies are applicable to various forms of drug use and thus can be modified to target different substance use disorders. Therapies that have targeted specific drugs will also be highlighted.

PSYCHOSOCIAL TREATMENTS

Psychosocial treatments are the mainstay of interventions for substance use disorders, particularly among adolescents since the bulk of the pharmacotherapy interventions for adolescent substance abusers have been conducted in an open-label fashion. The psychosocial treatments that have been explored in a controlled fashion and have been shown to be efficacious in treating adolescents with substance use disorders include behavioral therapy, cognitive-behavioral therapy, contingency management, 12-step programs, motivational enhancement therapy, and family-based interventions.

Behavioral Therapy

Behavioral therapy targets substance use in the context of the individual's environment. Approaches in behavioral therapy are based on classical and operant conditioning. At the crux of this intervention is the identification of behaviors and triggers that promote substance use. Once these behaviors have been identified, it is important for the client/patient to recognize how these behaviors function to perpetuate the alcohol and/or drug use. Skills are then taught that target the triggers for substance use with the goal of abstinence and prevention of relapse. Essential elements in behavioral therapy are functional analysis, skills training, and relapse prevention. The functional analysis explores the triggers for substance use and the stimuli that promote maintenance of use. Once problematic areas have been identified, individual specific skills are taught to prevent relapse. Other areas of focus include stress management, drug refusal skills, assertiveness training, social skills, and self-regulation.

Azrin and colleagues (1994) randomized 26 treatment-seeking adolescents with substance use disorders to either behavioral therapy or supportive counseling. The behavioral therapy group received written assignments and review of in-session assignments, rehearsals, therapist modeling, and self-recording. On the other hand, the supportive counseling group focused on expressions of feelings, self-generated insight into reasons for substance use, and the discussion of drug-related experiences without directives by the counselor. Adolescents in the behavioral therapy condition reported less frequent substance use and had fewer positive drug screens than those in the supportive counseling group. The behavioral therapy group of adolescents also had improved school attendance and performance as well as better conduct ratings than those in supportive counseling.

A nine-month follow-up study of 74 subjects (aged 13–43) with substance use disorders who received behavioral therapy versus supportive therapy (Azrin et al., 1996) revealed that the behavioral therapy group had significantly greater reduction in drug use at the end of treatment as well as the follow-up period. Further, the behavioral therapy group showed greater days worked, less alcohol use, and greater days in school than the supportive therapy group. Behavioral therapy in the treatment of adolescent substance use has been further expanded in the context of the family. Family behavioral therapy has been shown to be as effective as individual-cognitive problem solving in treating adolescents with conduct disorder and substance dependence (Azrin et al., 2001).

While there are so few trials comparing behavioral therapy to other modalities for treating adolescent substance use disorders, the trials to date are very promising.

Cognitive-Behavioral Therapy

Cognitive-behavioral therapy (CBT) expands behavioral therapy by integrating the impact of cognitive elements in addressing substance use. Cognitive-behavioral therapy is based on social learning theories and emphasizes functional analyses by addressing drug use in the context of its antecedents and consequences. The mainstay of CBT is the recognition of high-risk situations and the acquisition of skills aimed to address those high-risk situations.

Kaminer and colleagues (1998) randomized 32 dually diagnosed adolescents to a 12-week treatment of CBT versus interactional group therapy in an outpatient setting. The primary outcome variables were urine drug screens, scores on the Teen Addiction Severity Index (Teen-ASI) (Kaminer, 1991), and self-report of quantity and frequency of drug use. They hypothesized that adolescents with disruptive disorders such as conduct disorder, oppositional defiant disorder, and attention deficit hyperactivity disorder would do better in CBT, while those with internalizing disorders such as depression and anxiety disorders would receive greater benefit from interactional therapy. Although there was no treatment matching effect, adolescents in the CBT group showed a significant reduction in the severity of substance use based on the Teen-ASI. On the other hand, treatment differences were not seen with urine drug screens.

Kaminer and colleagues (2002) completed a larger randomized controlled trial comparing CBT to psychoeducational therapy (PET) in treating adolescents with substance use disorders. Adolescents ($n = 88$) were predominately dually diagnosed and were randomized to eight weeks of either CBT or PET group therapy. The authors hypothesized that both groups would improve from pretreatment to three- and nine-month follow-up; however, adolescents assigned to the CBT group would have better retention rates in treatment and at follow-up. Older adolescents and males in the CBT group had significantly lower rates of positive urine drug screens than those in the PET group at the three-month follow-up. Both conditions revealed improvements in self-reported substance use measures from baseline to three- and nine-month follow-up periods.

Contingency Management

Contingency management (CM) treatment interventions have been largely studied in adult populations, and reviews of its use have been shown to be feasible, acceptable to patients, and efficacious (Budney & Higgins, 1998; Higgins & Silverman, 1999). One of the goals of CM is to create an environmental paradigm so that drug use and abstinence can be measured by urine testing. Rewards are given for drug abstinence, and rewards are immediately lost when drug use is detected. Thus, the reinforcement is increased to compete with the reinforcing effects of the drugs (Higgins et al., 1994).

There are no controlled trials to date comparing CM to another modality in treating adolescents with substance use disorders; however, Corby and associates (2000) explored the feasibility of treating adolescent cigarette smokers. In this small study, contingencies were not placed on adolescents during the baseline phase; however, during the intervention week, the adolescent's payment was contingent on not smoking. CM was effective in increasing the number of total abstinences as well as the consecutive abstinences. The positive results of this small study underscore the need for larger controlled trials in treating substance-disordered adolescents.

Twelve-Step Approaches

Twelve-step approaches have long been used in treating adults with alcohol dependence and drug dependence, although not typically in a controlled fashion. The philosophy of 12-step approaches such as Alcoholics Anonymous (AA) and Narcotics Anonymous (NA) is rooted in the individual's need to recognize that his or her substance use is problematic and to admit to loss of control due to the substance use. To our knowledge, there are no controlled trials comparing 12-step approaches to other modalities in treating adolescents with substance use disorders. From a clinical standpoint, it is advisable that adolescents who are referred to 12-step groups choose groups that are specifically designed for adolescents. The differences in adolescent development and severity of substance use when compared to some adults may undermine treatment when adolescents are placed in adult 12-step groups. For example, when adolescents hear adults in AA and/or NA groups talk about "hitting bottom" or "falling off the wagon," adolescents have difficulty identifying with the major losses in their lives due to substance use. In part, the adolescents have not lived long enough to gain the things that they want to keep protected from loss.

Motivational Enhancement Therapy (MET)

Motivational enhancement treatments have been developed as brief interventions to enhance motivation to change. Common targets of these treatments have been addiction and other high-risk behaviors (Miller & Rollnick, 2002). The five main tenets of motivational interviewing are an empathic, nonjudgmental stance, listening reflectively, developing discrepancy, rolling with resistance and avoiding arguments, and supporting self-efficacy for change. Considering that adolescents with substance use problems rarely seek treatment on their own, a treatment method that targets motivation to change is theoretically appealing (O'Leary et al., 2004). The brief nature of motivational enhancement therapy also lends itself to potential cost-effectiveness and enhanced patient adherence.

McCambridge and Strang (2004) randomized 200 adolescents to one session of motivational interviewing versus no treatment. The motivational interviewing group showed significant reductions in nicotine, alcohol, and marijuana use, with effect sizes of 0.37, 0.34, and 0.75, respectively. Other investigations have revealed that motivational enhancement provides reductions in alcohol consumption and alcohol-related risky behaviors in adolescents when compared with standard care (Monti et al., 1999, 2001a). Marlatt and colleagues (1998) randomized high-risk graduating high school seniors to a brief motivational enhancement intervention versus no treatment, demonstrating declines in drinking rates and alcohol-related problems in the motivational enhancement group. Promising results have also been reported in motivating adolescents for smoking cessation (Colby et al., 1998), revealing 22% abstinence at follow-up of smokers receiving motivational interviewing versus 10% for those who received brief advice. Clinicians and researchers are currently recognizing the benefit of a couple of sessions of motivational interviewing with adolescents before beginning other therapies such as cognitive-behavioral therapy.

Family-Based Interventions

Family-based interventions for adolescent substance use disorders have received considerable research attention. These approaches stem from the family systems theory, which posits that individual functioning occurs in the context of family functioning. Family functioning, in turn, exists within the context of social and community surroundings. As such, it is theorized that individual change requires contextual change, such as patterns of familial behavior and interaction. This theoretical position has been supported by a growing evidence base in treating substance use disorders in adolescents. Excellent reviews (Ozechowski & Liddle, 2000; Liddle, 2004) provide information on the current knowledge base in this area and potential directions for research.

Waldron and colleagues (2001) randomized 114 substance-abusing adolescents to individual cognitive-behavioral therapy, family therapy, combined cognitive-behavioral therapy and family therapy, or group intervention, yielding mixed results. From pretreatment to four months, family therapy and combined treatment subjects reported significantly fewer days of substance use. Significantly more youths in the family therapy, cognitive-behavioral therapy, and combined conditions achieved minimal substance use levels. However, from pretreatment to seven months, reduction in percent days of use was significant only for the combined and group interventions. Changes in minimal use levels were significant for family, combined, and group treatments.

Latimer and colleagues (2003) compared an integrated family therapy and cognitive-behavioral therapy approach (IFCBT) with a drug harm psychoeducation curriculum in 43 youths with substance use disorders. At six months' posttreatment, the IFCBT group displayed improved problem management skills and significantly fewer days of alcohol (2.03 versus 6.06) and marijuana (5.67 versus 13.83) use per month.

The following two studies reveal a greater effect of family therapy when compared to group therapy. Joanning and colleagues (1992) randomized 82 adolescents to structural-strategic family therapy, adolescent group therapy, or family drug education group. The family therapy condition yielded greater improvement in drug use but had no effect on family functioning. At posttest, there was a reduced incidence of drug use and problem behaviors among adolescents in the family therapy condition. Lewis and colleagues (1990) randomized 84 drug-abusing adolescents to brief family therapy and family drug education and reported significantly lower posttreatment drug use for the family therapy group. The adolescents in the brief family therapy condition had significantly lower Index of Drug Severity (IDS) scores.

A number of specific family-based approaches have been studied in recent decades. The most evidence-supported approaches include brief strategic family therapy (BSFT), functional family therapy, multisystemic therapy (MST), and multidimensional family therapy (MDFT).

Brief Strategic Family Therapy (BSFT)

In a structured, problem-focused approach, BSFT focuses on adjusting repetitive maladaptive patterns of family interactions (Robbins et al., 2002). Specifically, the BSFT therapist examines existing networks of interactions within the family and community. While establishing a working alliance, the therapist supports areas of strength and redirects potential problem interactions. The length of treatment varies based on the complexity of cases but typically lasts 12 to 16 sessions over 3 to 4 months.

In a sample of 126 Hispanic behavior-problem and drug-using youths, BSFT was compared with group treatment control. Youth randomized to BSFT showed greater improvement in self-reports of marijuana use, family functioning, and conduct problems (Santisteban, 2003). Equally important, rates for treatment engagement and retention are superior for BSFT when compared to community-based treatments (Coatsworth et al., 2001).

Functional Family Therapy

This approach focuses on enhancing positive aspects of the family environment and improving clarity and consistency of communication (Barton & Alexander, 1981). Families of adolescents receiving outpatient drug abuse treatment were randomly assigned to functional family therapy ($n = 85$) or a parent group ($n = 50$), which focused on teaching communication and assertiveness skills (Friedman, 1989). Treatment lasted for approximately six months and resulted in equal reductions in substance use and improvements in family functioning in both groups. However, treatment engagement was superior for the functional family therapy group (93% vs. 67%).

Multisystemic Therapy (MST)

MST is an intensive treatment designed for families of adolescents with severe social, emotional, and behavioral problems. This modality seeks to reduce problem behaviors by delivering, in concert with families, substantive adjustments to the ecological context of the behaviors. Therapists, working with a small caseload, are available to clients at all hours and typically provide treatment in the home, school, and other community settings (the adolescent's ecology) rather than in the office. A strong evidence base has been developed to support MST in reducing criminal behavior, incarceration, and out-of-home placement (Henggeler et al., 1998; Littell et al., 2005). Recent studies have explored MST as a treatment for substance use disorders in delinquents (Henggeler et al., 1999, 2002). In a group of 118 juvenile offenders randomized to MST or the usual community services, the MST group showed significantly less alcohol, marijuana, and other drug use at the conclusion of treatment and 50% less out-of-home placement at six months' posttreatment. At four-year follow-up, 80 subjects were assessed, revealing significant long-term MST effects for aggressive criminal activity (0.15 vs. 0.57 convictions per year) and marijuana abstinence (55% vs. 28% of young adults). Ongoing work has explored a combination of MST with community reinforcement and vouchers for successful drug abstinence (Randall & Cunningham, 2003; Randall et al., 2001).

Multidimensional Family Therapy (MDFT)

MDFT is a short-term, manualized treatment targeting adolescent and family functioning across a variety of risk and protective factors. In a study by Liddle and colleagues (2001), 182 clinically referred marijuana- and alcohol-abusing 13- to 18-year-olds were randomized to MDFT, adolescent group therapy, or multifamily educational interaction. All treatments yielded improvements, but MDFT was overall significantly superior. Eighty 11- to 15-year-old urban youths were randomized to MDFT or peer group therapy. MDFT resulted in reduced substance use over the course of treatment, as well as positive changes in risk and protective factors in individual, peer, and school domains (Liddle et al., 2004). Efforts are underway to incorporate MDFT into existing community treatment programs for adolescent substance abusers (Liddle et al., 2001).

PHARMACOTHERAPY

Unlike for adult substance using populations, pharmacotherapy for the treatment of adolescents with substance use disorders has been conducted mainly in the context of other psychiatric disorders. To date, two adolescent studies have targeted both the substance use disorder and the psychiatric disorder, and one has targeted opiate use. In a study conducted by Geller and colleagues (1998), 25 adolescents with bipolar disorder and secondary substance use disorder were randomized to six weeks of treatment with either lithium or placebo. Random urine drug screens revealed that the lithium group had significantly fewer positive urine drug screens than the placebo group. While there were no significant differences in mood outcome between the groups, the lithium group had higher scores on the Children's Global Assessment Scale (C-GAS).

In another study, Deas and associates (1998) randomly assigned 10 depressed adolescent alcoholics receiving group cognitive-behavioral therapy to 12 weeks of sertraline (Zoloft) or placebo. Both groups experienced a significant reduction in depression scores, percent days drinking, and drinks per drinking day. The authors concluded that reduction in depression and alcohol use across both groups was likely due to the effectiveness of CBT, which may have masked the drug effect. In both studies, adolescents tolerated the medication without adverse effects.

Marsch and colleagues (2005) randomized 36 opiate-dependent adolescents to buprenorphene versus clonidine detoxification in a 28-day outpatient treatment setting. Adolescents who received buprenorphine had fewer positive urine screens for opiates and better retention rates than those in the clonidine group.

The aforementioned double-blind placebo-controlled medication trials used to treat adolescents with substance use disorders show promise for future exploration of medication trials in this population.

SUBSTANCE-FOCUSED TREATMENTS

While the aforementioned studies targeted adolescents with various substance use disorders, some studies have focused primarily on a given substance of abuse. This section reviews the extant literature of the paucity of studies that demonstrate evidence of efficacious treatment for specific targeted substances of abuse in adolescents.

Alcohol

Alcohol is the most common substance of abuse among adolescents; however, adolescents who meet the criteria for an alcohol use disorder rarely use alcohol alone. Marijuana is the most common substance used concomitantly with alcohol. Adolescents with problematic use usually meet criteria for both an alcohol use disorder and a marijuana use disorder. Adolescent substance use treatment usually targets alcohol and other drugs without focusing on alcohol exclusively. Deas and colleagues (1998) targeted alcohol dependence in their cohort, which is described above.

Marijuana

Marijuana remains the most commonly used illicit substance among adolescents. As such, treatments for adolescent substance abusers generally target marijuana use among outcome measures. However, only a limited number of studies have focused specifically on marijuana-abusing adolescents.

Dennis and colleagues (2004) synthesized results from two randomized trials with 600 adolescent marijuana users which revealed similarly positive outcomes between groups in regards to days of abstinence and days in recovery. The groups included a 5-session combined motivational enhancement therapy and cognitive-behavioral therapy (MET/CBT), a 12-session combined motivational enhancement therapy and cognitive-behavioral therapy (MET/CBT12), family education and therapy (Family Support Network [FSN]), Adolescent Community Reinforcement Approach (ACRA), and multidimensional family therapy (MDFT). The most cost-effective interventions appeared to be MET/CBT, MET/CBT12, and ACRA. This study provides the largest-scale, most comprehensive adolescent marijuana treatment investigation to date. The positive outcome across treatments is encouraging, and further work determining common beneficial treatment factors must be undertaken.

Kamon and colleagues (2005) developed an intervention for adolescent marijuana abusers with comorbid conduct problems. This treatment was composed of (1) a clinic-administered, abstinence-based incentive program, (2) parent-directed contingency management targeting substance use and conduct problems, (3) a clinic-administered incentive program for parent participation, and (4) individual cognitive-behavioral therapy for adolescents. A pilot investigation (nonrandomized, noncontrolled) in 19 adolescents revealed significant pre- to posttreatment improvements in substance use, externalizing behaviors, and negative parenting behaviors. Cannabis abstinence increased from 37% to 74% over the course of treatment and fell to 53% 30 days' posttreatment.

Cannabis withdrawal symptoms have been observed in adolescent treatment-seekers and may complicate treatment, particularly among the heaviest-using adolescents (Vandrey et al., 2005). Cannabis withdrawal and craving may be potential targets for pharmacotherapy. Investigation in this area has occurred among adult subjects, but no randomized trials have been undertaken in adolescents.

Cocaine

Although cocaine abuse has been included among entrance criteria and outcome measures of existing randomized trials, no study to our knowledge has specifically targeted adolescent cocaine abuse.

Nicotine Dependence

At present, the U.S. Food and Drug Administration (FDA) has approved nicotine replacement therapies (NRT; e.g., transdermal patch) and bupropion sustained release (SR) for smoking cessation in adult smokers. Although not approved by the FDA, other medications that have been shown to be efficacious for smoking cessation in controlled trials include nortriptyline, doxapine, and clonidine (George & O'Malley, 2004). In addition, several medications are currently under study (e.g., rimonabant, verinecline, selegeline, mecamylamine, and topiramate).

There are very few controlled studies of pharmacological treatments for smoking cessation in adolescents. NRT (mainly transdermal nicotine patch) and bupropion SR are mostly studied for adolescent smokers. The efficacy of NRT has been modest among adolescents, with one open-label study reporting a 5–18% short-term abstinence rate (Hurt et al., 2000; Smith et al., 1996). One study reported a short-term abstinence rate of 18% using NRT in adolescent smokers, which did not show a statistically significant difference from the placebo group (Hanson et al., 2003). The main limitation in the study was that the cognitive-behavioral therapy and contingency management provided to both groups may have overwhelmed the medication effects. In a controlled study using the transdermal nicotine patch (TNP), the abstinence rate was highest among the TNP group at three months (17.6% vs. 6.5% for the gum and 2.5% for placebo), and only the TNP group had a statistically significant higher abstinence rate, better retention, and greater medication adherence than the placebo group (Moolchan, 2004). In addition, adolescents on inpatient units may have nicotine withdrawal symptoms; therefore, NRT (preferably TNP) may need to be provided to these nontreatment-seeking adolescent smokers to alternate their withdrawal symptoms while hospitalized (Upadhyaya et al., 2005).

A recent study of combined bupropion SR + TNP vs. placebo + TNP for adolescent smokers did not show an added benefit of bupropion SR over placebo (Killen et al., 2004). The limitations of this study included the use of only 150-mg dosage of bupropion SR as well as poor medication adherence.

Opioid Use Disorder

FDA-approved medications for substitution therapy in opioid dependence include methadone, L-α-acetylmethadol (LAAM), and buprenorphine. The use of these agents in adolescents has not been systematically studied. In addition, substitution therapy in adolescents is limited by parent/legal guardian consent issues and federal requirements of at least two documented treatment failures with detoxification or psychosocial treatments in the past year (Schottenfeld, 2004).

A report of 37 adolescents and young adults with opiate dependence revealed an abstinence rate of 35% postdetoxification with methadone (DeAngelis & Lehman, 1973). Buprenorphine has received significant attention as a treatment among adults due to its partial agonism of the opioid receptor, making it harder to overdose. Furthermore, the combination of buprenorphine with naloxone (an opiate antagonist) makes it difficult to abuse intravenously. Naloxone is absorbed poorly by sublingual oral route (buprenorphine is taken sublingually), and if someone tries to inject the medication, naloxone blocks the opiate receptors and hence the reinforcing property of buprenorphine (Collins & Kleber, 2004). A recent double-blind, double-dummy trial of buprenorphine versus clonidine detoxification in a 28-day outpatient setting involving 36 adolescents with opiate dependence reported that those on buprenorphine had better retention and fewer positive urine tests for opiates as compared to clonidine (Marsch et al., 2005). In addition, 61% chose longer-term naltrexone as opposed to 5% of those on clonidine. Currently, a National Institute of Drug Abuse–sponsored controlled trial of buprenorphine substitution therapy in adolescents is underway.

Other Substances (Stimulants, Sedative/Hypnotics, Club Drugs)

Currently, there is practically little to no evidence for pharmacotherapy of stimulant, sedative/hypnotic, and club drug use disorders in adolescents. Hence, psychosocial treatment is the first line of treatment for these disorders.

TREATMENT RESOURCES

Several treatment manuals or reviews specifically targeting adolescents with substance use disorders are available online. The National Institute on Drug Abuse (NIDA) has a Web site for the use of brief strategic family therapy for adolescent drug abuse. The manual can be found at http://www.nida.nih.gov/TXManuals/bsft/bsftindex.html.

The Substance Abuse and Mental Health Services Administration (SAMHSA) has a Web site focusing on the treatment of cannabis abuse/dependence. The manuals have been used in treatment trials and are accessible for public use. Two Web sites that focus on the treatment of cannabis users are http://www.kap.samhsa.gov/products/manuals/cyt/pdfs/cyt5.pdf and http://www.kap.samhsa.gov/products/manuals/cyt/pdfs/cyt1.pdf.

Although there is only one controlled trial exploring the use of buprenorphine treatment of adolescents with opiate dependence, the SAMHSA/CSAT Web site provides a link to a chapter that specifically addresses the treatment of adolescents with opiate dependence. This information can be found at http://www.ncbi.nlm.nih.gov/books/bv.fcgi?rid=hstat5.chapter.72248.

Monti and colleagues (2001b) described brief interventions for treating adolescents with substance use disorders. Empirical illustrations and clinical applications of brief interventions are presented. Step-by-step instructions are outlined emphasizing strategies in the treatment as well as case studies. This body of work may serve as a practitioner guide for using brief interventions to treat adolescents with substance use disorders.

SUMMARY

Despite the decline in prevalence rates of substance use among adolescents, problematic use remains a concern. Adolescents with problematic substance use should be treated with interventions that are empirically based. Unfortunately, treatment advances for adolescents with substance use disorders have lagged behind advances in adult populations. Efforts have been made to develop treatments specifically designed for adolescent substance abusers. There is a growing literature of evidence-based treatments for adolescent substance use disorders (Deas & Thomas, 2001; Kaminer & Slesnick, 2005; Elliott et al., 2005), and much progress has been made since Catalano's (1990) review more than a decade ago. The evidence-based treatments described in this chapter have been shown to be feasible, acceptable, and efficacious in treating adolescents with substance use disorders. Clinicians and researchers are encouraged to utilize these available treatments, especially the Web-based manuals and guides available for public use.

ACKNOWLEGEMENT. The authors wish to thank Natalie Johnson and Courtney Merritt for their assistance with preparation of this manuscript.

REFERENCES

Aarons, G. A., Brown, S. A., Coe, M. T., Myers, M. G., Garland, A. F., Ezzert-Lofstraum, R., et al. (1999). Adolescent alcohol and drug abuse and health. *Journal of Adolescent Health*, *24*, 412–421.

Azrin, N., Acierno, E., Kogan, B., Donohue, B., Besalel, V. A., & McMahon, P. T. (1996). Follow-up results of supportive versus behavioral therapy for illicit drug use. *Behaviour Research and Therapy, 34*(1), 41–46.

Azrin, N., Donohue, B., Besalel, V., et al. (1994). Youth drug abuse treatment: A controlled outcome study. *Journal of Child and Adolescent Substance Abuse, 32*, 857–866.

Azrin, D., Donohue, B., Teichner, G., Crum, T., Howell, J., & DeCato, L. A. (2001). A controlled evaluation and description of individual-cognitive problem solving and family-behavior therapies in dually-diagnosed conduct-disordered and substance-dependent youth. *Journal of Child and Adolescent Substance Abuse, 11*(1), 1–43.

Barton, C., & Alexander, J. (1981). Functional family therapy. In A. Gurman & D. Kniskern (Eds.), *Handbook of Family Therapy* (pp. 403–443). New York: Brunner/Mazel.

Brent, D. A. (1995). Risk factors for adolescent suicide and suicidal behavior: Mental and substance abuse disorders, family environmental factors, and life stress. *Suicide & Life-Threatening Behavior, 25*, 52–63.

Budney, A. G., & Higgins, S. T. (1998). *Therapy Manuals for Drug Addiction: A Community Reinforcement Plus Voucher Approach for Treating Cocaine Addiction.* Rockville, MD: National Institute on Drug Abuse.

Catalano, R. F., Hawkins, J. D., Wells, E. A., Miller, J., & Brewer, D. (1990). Evaluation of the effectiveness of adolescent drug abuse treatment, assessment of risks for relapse, and promising approaches for relapse prevention. *The International Journal of the Addictions, 25*, 1085–1140.

Center for Substance Abuse Treatment (2004). Clinical guidelines for the use of buprenorphine in the treatment of opioid addiction. *Treatment Improvement Protocol (TIP) Series 40.* [DHHS Publication No. (SMA) 04-3939]. Rockville, MD: Substance Abuse and Mental Health Services Administration. Retrieved December 9, 2006, from http://www.ncbi.nlm.nih.gov/books/bv.fcgi?rid=hstat5.chapter.72248.

Coatsworth, J. D., Santisteban, D. A., McBride, C. K., & Szapocznik, J. (2001). Brief strategic family therapy versus community control: Engagement, retention, and an exploration of the role of adolescent symptom severity. *Family Process, 40*(3), 313–332.

Colby, S. M., Monti, P. M., Barnett, N. P., Rohsenow, D. J., Weissman, K., Spirito, A., et al. (1998). Brief motivational interviewing in a hospital setting for adolescent smoking: A preliminary study. *Journal of Consulting and Clinical Psychology, 66*, 574–578.

Collins, E. D., & Kleber, H. D. (2004). Opioids. In M. Galanter & H. D. Kleber (Eds.) *Textbook of Substance Abuse Treatment* (pp. 265–289). Washington, DC: American Psychiatric Publishing.

Corby, E. A., Roll, J. M., Ledgerwood, D. M., & Schuster, C. R. (2000). Contingency management interventions of treating the substance abuse of adolescents: A feasibility study. *Experimental and Clinical Psychopharmacology, 8*(3), 371–376.

DeAngelis, G., & Lehmann, W. (1973). Adolescents and short-term, low-dose methadone maintenance. *The International Journal of Addictions, 8*(5), 853–863.

Deas, D., Riggs, P., Langenbucher, M., & Brown, S. (2000). Adolescents are not adults: Developmental considerations in alcohol users. *Alcoholism: Clinical and Experimental Research, 24*(2), 232–237.

Deas, D., & Thomas, S. (2001). An overview of controlled studies of adolescent substance abuse treatment. *The American Journal on Addictions, 10*, 178–189.

Deas-Nesmith, D., Randall, C., Roberts, J., et al. (1998). Sertraline treatment of depressed adolescent alcoholics: A pilot study. *Alcoholism: Clinical and Experimental Research, 22*, 74A.

Dennis, M., Godley, S. H., Diamond, G., Tims, F. M., Babor, T., Donaldson, J., et al. (2004). The cannabis youth treatment (CYT) study: Main findings from two randomized trials. *Journal of Substance Abuse Treatment, 27*, 197–213.

Elliott, L., Orr, L., Watson, L., & Jackson, A. (2005). Secondary prevention interventions for young drug users: A systematic review of the evidence. *Adolescence, 40*(157), 1–22.

Friedman, A. (1989). Family therapy vs. parent groups: Effects on adolescent drug abusers. *The American Journal of Family Therapy, 17*, 335–347.

Geller, B., Cooper, T., Sun, K., Zimerman, B., Frazier, J., Williams, M., et al. (1998). A double-blind and placebo-controlled study of lithium for adolescent bipolar disorders with secondary substance dependence. *Journal of the American Academy of Child and Adolescent Psychiatry, 37,* 171–178.

George, T. P., & O'Malley, S. S. (2004). Current pharmacological treatments for nicotine dependence. *Trends in Pharmacological Sciences, 25*(1), 42–48.

Hanson, K., Allen, S., Jensen, S., & Hatsukami, D. (2003). Treatment of adolescent smokers with the nicotine patch. *Nicotine and Tobacco Research, 5,* 515–526.

Henggeler, S. W., Clingempeel, W. G., Brondino, M. J., & Pickrel, S. G. (2002). Four-year follow-up of multisystemic therapy with substance-abusing and substance-dependent juvenile offenders. *Journal of the American Academy of Child and Adolescent Psychiatry, 41*(7), 868–874.

Henggeler, S. W., Pickrel, S. G., & Brondino, M. J. (1999). Multisystemic therapy of substance-abusing and dependent delinquents: Outcomes, treatment, fidelity, and transportability. *Mental Health Services Research, 1*(3), 171–184.

Henggeler, S. W., Schoenwald, S. K., Borduin, C. M., Rowland, M. D., & Cunningham, P. B. (1998). *Multisystemic Treatment of Antisocial Behavior in Children and Adolescents.* New York: Guilford.

Higgins, S. T., Budney, A. J., & Bickel, W. K. (1994). Applying behavioral concepts and principles to the treatment of cocaine dependence. *Drug and Alcohol Dependence, 34,* 87–97.

Higgins, S. T., & Silverman, K. (Eds.) (1999). *Motivating Behavior Change Among Illicit-Drug Abusers.* Washington, DC: American Psychological Association.

Hurt, R. D., Croghan, G. A., Beede, S. D., Wolter, T. D., Croghan, I. T., & Patten, C. A. (2000). Nicotine patch therapy in 101 adolescent smokers: Efficacy, withdrawal symptoms relief, and carbon monoxide and plasma cotinine levels. *Archives of Pediatric and Adolescent Medicine, 154,* 31–37.

Joanning, H., Quinn, Q., Thomas, F., & Mullen, R. (1992). Treating adolescent drug abuse: A comparison of family systems therapy, group therapy, and family drug education. *Journal of Marital and Family Therapy, 18,* 345–356.

Johnston, L. D., O'Malley, P. M., Bachman, J. G., & Schulenberg, J. E., (2004). *Monitoring the Future National Results on Adolescent Drug Use: Overview of Key Findings, 2003* (NIH Publication No. 04-5506). Bethesda, MD: National Institute on Drug Abuse.

Kaminer, Y., Buckstein, O. G., & Tarter, R. E. (1991). The teen addiction severity index: Rationale and reliability. *International Journal of Addiction, 26,* 219–226.

Kaminer, Y., Burleson, J., Blitz, C., Sussman, J., & Rounsaville, B. J. (1998). Psychotherapies for adolescent substance abusers: A pilot study. *The Journal of Nervous and Mental Disease, 186,* 684–690.

Kaminer, Y., Burleson, J., & Goldberger, R. (2002). Psychotherapies for adolescent substance abusers: Short- and long-term outcomes. *Journal of Nervous and Mental Disease, 190,* 737–745.

Kaminer, Y., & Slesnick, N. (2005). Evidence-based cognitive-behavioral and family therapies for adolescent alcohol and other substance use disorders. *Recent Developments in Alcoholism, 17,* 383–405.

Kamon, J., Budney, A., & Stanger, C. (2005). A contingency management intervention for adolescent marijuana abuse and conduct problems. *Journal of the American Academy of Child and Adolescent Psychiatry, 44*(6), 513–521.

Killen, J. D., Robinson, T. N., Ammerman, S., Hayward, C., Rogers, J., & Stone, C. (2004). Randomized clinical trial of the efficacy of bupropion combined with the nicotine patch in the treatment of adolescent smokers. *Journal of Consulting and Clinical Psychology, 72,* 729–735.

Kikpatrick, D. G., Acierno, R., Saunders, B., Resnick, H. S., Best, C. L., & Schnurr, P. P. (2000). Risk factors for adolescent substance abuse and dependence: Data from a national sample. *Journal of Consulting and Clinical Psychology, 68*(1), 19–30.

Latimer, W. W., Winters, K. C., D'Zurilla, T., & Nichols, M. (2003). Integrated family and cognitive-behavioral therapy for adolescent substance abusers: A stage I efficacy study. *Drug and Alcohol Dependence, 71,* 303–317.

Lewis, R. A., Piercy, F. P., Sprenkle, D. H., & Trepper T. S. (1990). Family-based interventions for helping drug-abusing adolescents. *Journal of Adolescent Research, 5,* 82–95.

Liddle, H. A. (2002). *Multidimensional Family Therapy for Adolescent Cannabis Users, Cannabis Youth Treatment Series, Vol. 5* (DHHS Publication no. 02-3660). Rockville, MD: Center for Substance Abuse Treatment, Substance Abuse and Mental Health Services Administration. Retrieved December 9, 2006, from http://www.kap.samhsa.gov/products/manuals/cyt/pdfs/cyt5.pdf.

Liddle, H. A. (2004). Family-based therapies for adolescent alcohol and drug use: Research contributions and future research needs. *Addiction, 99*(S2), 76–92.

Liddle, H. A., Dakof, G. A., Parker, K., Diamond, G. S., Barrett, K., & Tejeda, M. (2001). Mulitdimensional family therapy for adolescent drug use: Results of a randomized clinical trial. *American Journal of Drug and Alcohol Abuse, 27*(4), 651–688.

Liddle, H. A., Rowe, C. L., Dakof, G. A., Ungaro, R. A., & Henderson, C. E. (2004). Early intervention for adolescent substance abuse: Pretreatment to posttreatment outcomes of a randomized clinical trial comparing multidimensional family therapy to peer group treatment. *Journal of Psychoactive Drugs, 36*(1), 49–63.

Littell, J. H., Popa, M., & Forsythe, B. (2005). Multisystemic therapy for social, emotional, and behavioral problems in youth aged 10–17. *Cochrane Database Systems Review, 20*(3).

Marlatt, G. A., Baer, J. S., Kivlahan, D. R., Dimeff, L. A., Larimer, M. E., Quigley, L. A., et al. (1998). Screening and brief intervention for high-risk college student drinkers: Results from a 2-year follow-up assessment. *Journal of Consulting and Clinical Psychology, 66*, 604–615.

Marsch, L. A., Bickel, W. K., Badger, G. J., Stcothart, M. E., Quesnal, K. J., Stanger, C., et al. (2005). Comparison of pharmacological treatments for opioid-dependent adolescents. *Archives of General Psychiatry, 62*, 1157–1164.

Mayhew, D. R., Donelson, A. C., Beirness, D. J., & Simpson, H. M. (1989). Youth alcohol and relative risk of crash involvement. *Accident; Analysis and Prevention, 18*(4), 273–287.

McCambridge, J., & Strang, J. (2004). The efficacy of single-session motivational interviewing in reducing drug consumption and perceptions of drug-related risk and harm among young people: Results from a multi-site cluster randomized trial. *Addiction , 99*(S2), 63–75.

McLaughlin, C. R., Daniel, J., & Joost, T. F. (2000). The relationship between substance use, drug selling, and lethal violence in 25 juvenile murderers. *Journal of Forensic Sciences, 45*, 349–353.

Miller, W. R., & Rollnick, S. (2002). *Motivational Interviewing: Preparing People for Change*, 2nd ed. New York: Guilford Press.

Monti, P. M., Barnett, N. P., O'Leary, T. A., & Colby, S. M. (2001a). Motivational enhancement for alcohol-involved adolescents. In P. M. Monti, S. M. Colby, & T. A. O'Leary (Eds.), *Adolescents, Alcohol, and Substance Abuse: Reaching Teens Through Brief Interventions* (pp. 145–182). New York: Guilford Press.

Monti, P. M., Colby, S. M., Barnett, N. P., Spirito, A., Rohsenow, D. J., Myers, M., et al. (1999). Brief intervention for harm reduction with alcohol-positive older adolescents in a hospital emergency department. *Journal of Consulting and Clinical Psychology, 67*, 989–994.

Monti, P. M., Colby, S. M., & O'Leary, T. A. (2001b). *Adolescents, Alcohol, and Substance Abuse: Reaching Teens Through Brief Interventions.* New York: Guilford Press.

Moolchan, E. T., Robinson, M. L., Ernst, M., Cadet, J. L., Pickworth, W. B., Heishman, S. J., et al. (2004). Safety and efficacy of the nicotine patch and gum for the treatment of adolescent tobacco addiction. *Pediatrics, 115*, 407–414.

O'Leary, T. T., & Monti, P. M. (2004). Motivational enhancement and other brief interventions for adolescent substance abuse: Foundations, applications, and evaluations. *Addiction, 99*(S2), 63–75.

Ozechowski, T. J., & Liddle, H. A. (2000). Family-based therapy for adolescent drug abuse: Knowns and unknowns. *Clinical Child and Family Psychology Review, 3* (4), 269–298.

Randall, J., & Cunningham, P. B. (2003). Multisystemic therapy: A treatment for violentsubstance-abusing and substance-dependent juvenile offenders. *Addictive Behaviors, 28* (9), 1731–1739.

Randall, J., Henggeler, S. W., Cunningham, P. B., Rowland, M. D., & Swenson, C. C. (2001). Adapting multisystemic therapy to treat adolescents substance abuse more effectively. *Cognitive and Behavioral Practice, 8* (4), 359–366.

Robbins, M. S., Bachrach, K., & Szapocznik, J. (2002). Bridging the research-practice gap in adolescent substance abuse treatment: The case of brief strategic family therapy. *Journal of Substance Abuse Treatment, 23* (2), 123–132.

Sampl, S., & Kadden, R. (2001). *Motivational Enhancement Therapy and Cognitive Behavioral Therapy for Adolescent Cannabis Users: 5 Sessions, Cannabis Youth Treatment Series, Vol. 1* (DHHS Publication No. 01-3486). Rockville, MD: Center for Substance Abuse Treatment, Substance Abuse and Mental Health Services Administration. Retrieved December 9, 2006, from http://www.kap.samhsa.gov/products/manuals/cyt/pdfs/cyt1.pdf.

Santisteban, D. A., Coatsworth, J. D., Perez-Vidal, A., Kurtines, W. M., Schwartz, S. J., LaPerrier, A., et al. (2003). Efficacy of brief strategic family therapy in modifying hispanic adolescent behavior problems and substance use. *Journal of Family Psychology, 17*(1), 121–133.

Schottenfeld, R. S. (2004). Opioids: Maintenance treatment. In M. Galanter & H. D. Kleber (Eds.), *Textbook of Substance Abuse Treatment* (pp. 291–304). Washington, DC: American Psychiatric Publishing.

Smith, T. A., House, R. F., Croghan, I. T., Gauvin, T. R., Colligan, R. C., Offord, K. P., et al. (1996). Nicotine patch therapy in adolescent smokers. *Pediatrics, 98*, 659–667.

Swadi, H. (1999). Individual risk factors for adolescent substance use. *Drug and Alcohol Dependence, 55*, 209–224.

Szapocznik, J., Hervis, O., & Schwartz, S. (2003). *Brief Strategic Family Therapy for Adolescent Drug Abuse. Therapy Manuals for Drug Addiction* (NIH Publication No. 03-4751). Retrieved December 9, 2006, from http://www.nida.nih.gov/TXManuals/bsft/bsftindex.html.

Upadhyaya, H. P., Deas, D., & Brady, K. T. (2005). A practical clinical approach to the treatment of nicotine dependence in adolescents. *Journal of American Academy of Child and Adolescent Psychiatry, 44*, 942–946.

Vandrey, R., Budney, A. J., Kamon, J. L., & Stanger, C. (2005). Cannabis withdrawal in adolescent treatment seekers. *Drug and Alcohol Dependence, 78*, 205–210.

Waldron, H. B., Slesnick, N., Brody, J. L., Turner, C. W., & Peterson, T. R. (2001). Treatment outcomes for adolescent substance abuse at 4- and 7-month assessments. *Journal of Consulting and Clinical Psychology, 69*(5), 802–813.

III

Implementation Issues

25

Dissemination of Evidence-Based Manualized Treatments for Children and Families in Practice Settings[1]

MICHAEL A. SOUTHAM-GEROW, ALYSSA M. MARDER, and A. AUKAHI AUSTIN

With prevalence estimates of mental health problems in childhood ranging as high as 20% (Hoagwood & Olin, 2002), identifying effective ways to treat mental health and substance use problems is a federal public health policy priority (USPHS, 2000). Evidence supporting the efficacy of psychological treatments for youth exists; several promising interventions have emerged, including cognitive-behavioral therapy (CBT) and interpersonal therapy (Kazdin & Weisz, 2003). Despite this growing knowledge, efficacious interventions are not being systematically used within community service settings (e.g., Weiss et al., 2000), and only recently have efforts been made to disseminate evidence-based treatments (EBTs) in such settings (e.g., Chorpita et al., 2002).

This gap between science and practice represents a critical public health issue (e.g., Hoagwood & Olin, 2002); many have posited explanations for the discrepancy between what is known to be useful in research

[1] This project was supported in part through the Research Network on Youth Mental Health, sponsored by the John D. and Catherine T. MacArthur Foundation. In addition, preparation of this article was supported by National Institute of Mental Health Grant K23 MH69421.

MICHAEL A. SOUTHAM-GEROW and ALYSSA M. MARDER • Virginia Commonwealth University and **A. AUKAHI AUSTIN** • University of Hawai'i at Mānoa

settings and what is done in real-world settings. Although a review of the explanations is beyond the scope of this chapter, they include contentions that (1) evidence-based treatments (EBTs) have been tested with cases that do not represent real-world cases, (2) EBTs have been tested with providers (graduate students) who are different from real-world providers, (3) EBTs have been tested in settings (university-based research clinics funded through grant monies) that differ from real-world service agencies, and (4) there is reluctance among providers to adopt EBTs (e.g., Southam-Gerow et al., 2003; Weisz et al., 2004). As an initial step toward reducing the discrepancy between science and practice, policy makers and funding sources have encouraged the rapid development of mental health dissemination research (e.g., Schoenwald & Hoagwood, 2001).

The challenges posed by dissemination of mental health treatments are formidable. One obstacle is that few discussions are aimed at both researchers and providers that cover the relevant conceptual and practical issues involved in conducting dissemination research. This chapter addresses this problem by delineating our field of inquiry (including description of a developmental model of clinical research), briefly reviewing several major conceptual models guiding dissemination research, and discussing the practical implications of dissemination research, for researchers, for mental health providers (hereafter providers[2]), and for mental health services administrators.

THE SCOPE OF THIS CHAPTER AND KEY DEFINITIONS

We begin by discussing what we view as the spectrum of clinical studies, presented in Table 1. The first three columns in the table are defined using traditional terms and progression (cf. Friedman et al., 1998), whereas the latter two columns are more reflective of work by Schoenwald et al. (e.g., Schoenwald & Hoagwood, 2001; Weisz et al., 2003). We briefly describe each stage, with a focus on the research questions and research designs common to each.

Clinical testing of a new treatment begins with *early clinical research* using single-case and open-trial studies that establish the safety and preliminary (positive) effects of the new treatment. If the treatment is successful at this level, *efficacy studies* are the next step. Applying randomized controlled trial (RCT) methodology, the primary goal of efficacy studies is to determine if the treatment produces good outcomes in controlled settings when compared to a control group. Typically, the passage of time (i.e., waitlist) or a placebo represents an initial control group. If the treatment passes this test, active treatments are used as comparators. Once supportive data are amassed, the stage of *effectiveness studies* begins.

---

[2] Throughout this chapter, we use the term "provider" as a synonym for "therapist" or "practitioner" (i.e., any professional providing mental health services to children and families).

Table 1. A Continuum of Treatment Development Stages

Stage Name	Early Clinical Studies (cf. Phase I & II Trials)	Efficacy Studies (cf. Phase III Trials)	Effectiveness Studies	Transportability Studies	Dissemination Studies
Focus of inquiry	Safety, feasibility of the treatment in tightly controlled setting, estimate of the effect size	Comparative effects of the treatment in a tightly controlled setting	Comparative effects of treatment in a new, less controlled setting; cost-effectiveness	Identifying factors related to successful implementation of the treatment in a variety of settings	Testing different strategies to get the end user to use your intervention, including the implementation strategy
Primary research questions	-Does the treatment work?-Can the treatment be delivered reliably? -What is the expectable effect size? -Is the treatment safe?	-Is the treatment superior to a control treatment?	-Does the treatment work in a practice setting? -Is the treatment cost-effective?	-What processes are needed to make the treatment work in practice settings?	-What dissemination strategies are most effective? -How does the implementation model fare when disseminated on a large scale (e.g., service system-wide)?
Outcomes	-Preliminary, safe, feasible treatment model	-Treatment model with an evidence base	-Treatment model with cost-effectiveness evidence -Treatment model with evidence of effectiveness in an alternate setting	-Implementation model	-Dissemination model

The *efficacy/effectiveness* distinction has generated controversy (cf. Barlow, 1996; Donenberg et al., 1999; Nathan et al., 2000). The primary research question for both efficacy and effectiveness studies remains on the effects of the treatment for the client/patient. However, effectiveness studies[3] go beyond the efficacy studies by testing the mettle of the treatment under real-world conditions, including the use of providers who work in the setting (vs. graduate students in research labs), inclusion of clients referred through typical channels (vs. research recruitment procedures), and therapy provided in clinical setting (vs. research setting). Furthermore, effectiveness studies often include an analysis of cost-effectiveness (see also Chapter 3).

Once an innovation is shown to produce beneficial and cost-effective effects outside the lab, a next step for many products (e.g., cell phones, medications) is wide-scale dissemination. However, for psychosocial treatments, some have argued that an intermediate step between effectiveness and dissemination studies is needed: *transportability studies.* Moving hastily from a few effectiveness studies to widespread dissemination ignores potentially critical contextual factors and may yield a host of problems that decrease the chances that a treatment will be successfully integrated into new systems (Schoenwald & Hoagwood, 2001). Transportability studies avoid this mistake by identifying processes involved in moving the treatment into community settings. For example, which provider, organizational, or service system variables impact the execution and outcomes of an innovation in community settings? A key issue is the identification of the strategies needed to encourage the *adoption* and *effective execution* of innovations. Such strategies include (1) identifying the appropriateness of dissemination settings, (2) securing and maintaining needed funding and referral streams, (3) making needed changes at the agency and system levels, (4) establishing training and supervision procedures, and (5) creating administrative supports needed for outcome monitoring. Transportability research results in an *implementation intervention:* the methods and procedures needed to make the treatment work in new settings. The implementation intervention involves a shift in focus from client-level outcomes in earlier research stages to provider, agency, and system variables (e.g., Southam-Gerow et al., 2006)

Finally, research shifts to the *dissemination* stage, with a focus on how to disseminate both the treatment *and* the implementation strategies to achieve widespread adoption. Thus, another intervention is being developed and tested: a *dissemination intervention.* This intervention is a set of procedures and methods that encourage adoption of *both* the

---

[3] Rounsaville and colleagues (e.g., Carroll & Rounsaville, 2003; Rounsaville et al., 2001) have argued that efficacy research involves initial safety and feasibility testing, whereas effectiveness research must "address issues of transportability of treatments whose efficacy has been demonstrated" (Carroll & Rounsaville, 2003, p. 334). As we describe in this chapter, however, there are advantages to moving beyond a dichotomous division of clinical research. Thus, although we agree with the general thrust of Rounsaville and colleagues' arguments, we have created a model that expands on the efficacy-effectiveness paradigm.

treatment and the implementation procedures that appear needed. During the dissemination phase, the treatment program (already tested across four phases) and the implementation intervention are tested, though the focus is on the dissemination intervention.

In summary, Table 1 presents the treatment development model that guides this chapter, a model starting with small-scale safety studies to test the effects of a new treatment and ending with large-scale dissemination studies where the effectiveness of the means of dissemination is a key outcome. In this chapter, our emphasis is on transportability and dissemination research.

One last note about Table 1 is warranted. The linear layout suggests systematic progression through the stages. Though possible in theory, progress is more likely to occur "in fits and starts." As an example, one may proceed to the effectiveness stage only to find that the evidence for the treatment program is weak. At that stage, one may have also identified some moderators of treatment that suggest adaptations of the program. It may be desirable to go back and test the adapted program at the efficacy (and in some cases safety) "level" before returning to the effectiveness level. Similar events will occur throughout all stages, making the overall process more iterative and recursive than linear.

Before discussing conceptual models that guide research that bridges the science-practice gap, we offer definitions of several terms used throughout the chapter.[4] *Diffusion*, *dissemination*, and *implementation* are three terms that are at times used synonymously to refer to the spread of an innovation (e.g., treatment program). For our purposes, we see the words as having distinct meanings and have followed and extended conceptual work by Schoenwald and Hoagwood (2001) and Chambers et al. (2005) in defining them. First, consistent with their having been used as synonyms in the past, we consider all three on a spectrum representing the *level of organization* involved in the effort to spread the innovation. At one end of the spectrum is *diffusion*, the unplanned or spontaneous spread of an innovation. Diffusion refers to the *natural* distribution of a new idea. On the other end of the spectrum we place the terms *implementation* and *dissemination* as referring to the directed and planned spread of an innovation. However, we view the two words as distinct. Extending work by Chambers et al. (2005), we view implementation as the "specific effort to fit a program [or] treatment ... within a specific care context" (Chambers et al., 2005, p. 324). As described earlier, implementation is the study of how to make the treatment program work across settings. Dissemination is the "targeted distribution of a well-designed set of information" (p. 323). Again, as we outlined earlier, dissemination represents how a treatment is marketed *after* the means for implementing it successfully have been identified.

Our definition of *implementation* is comparable to the one provided by Fixsen et al. (2005, p. 5): "a specified set of activities designed to put into

---

[4] Our definitions, though based on a careful reading of the literature, may generate controversy. Because dissemination research is an emerging field, specific meanings of key terms remain in flux. Our hope is to offer clear definitions that will guide and clarify future work.

practice an activity or program of known dimensions." Fixsen et al. (2005) also distinguished among different degrees of implementation, ranging from paper (i.e., enacting policies consistent with the innovation) to process (i.e., creating procedures that enable training and supervision in the use of a new innovation) to performance implementation (i.e., creating procedures that identify ways to ensure that the innovation is being used properly *and* that its use is having the expected consequence—that is, benefit for the consumer).

Not all past work concurs with our definition of *implementation*. In her recent exposition on the diffusion of mental health and substance abuse treatments, Gotham (2004) referred to implementation as the third of three steps in what she calls the "diffusion process" (see our discussion later). In her model, the first step is treatment development, and the second is dissemination (by which Gotham uses Orlandi's definition of "deliberate efforts to spread an innovation" [p. 123]). According to Gotham, implementation is "how technologies are used in practice and how that [use] influences the effect of the technology" (2004, p. 167). Thus, Gotham does not necessarily view implementation as involving a planned strategy, whereas we (and others) have construed it that way.

A few other terms often used in relation to dissemination research warrant brief mention. *Technology transfer* is a term that has long been applied to the process of taking scientific findings and turning them into products that are consumed in the commercial sector. Along these lines, then, dissemination research is viewed as a specific example of technology transfer. Another term used in the literature is *deployment;* this term is typically used as a synonym of "dissemination" as we are defining it here, though its use is less widespread.

FRAMEWORKS GUIDING DISSEMINATION RESEARCH

Because dissemination of psychological treatments is a relatively new enterprise, frameworks and models are needed to guide the work. Although several models have been described in the literature, we focus on three: (1) Diffusion of Innovations theory; (2) Mental Health System Ecological theory; and (3) the Implementation Research Framework. The interested reader can find a more comprehensive review elsewhere (e.g., Southam-Gerow et al., in press).

Diffusion of Innovations Theory

Rogers developed *Diffusion of Innovations* theory (2003) based upon research on social change from many different disciplines including anthropology, sociology, marketing, and public health. On a fundamental level, Rogers' theory describes the process associated with social change. From his perspective, the degree to which social change successfully occurs in any setting can be predicted by four main factors: (1) characteristics of the innovation; (2) the nature of communication channels in the system; (3) the passage of time; and (4) the social system itself.

Innovation Characteristics

Several characteristics of the innovation affect its acceptability to individuals in a system, including the perceived newness of the idea, its relative advantage over existing ideas or ways of doing things, its compatibility with existing values, past experiences and needs of individuals, its complexity, its trialability, and the observability of its results. These aspects are largely within the control of the innovation developer.

Communication Channels

The communication channels within any system determine the type and speed of transmission of information within a system. When one intends to bring a new idea into a system, different communication channels are necessary to reach the various potential adopters of an innovation into the system (Rogers, 2003). Mass media channels are particularly effective at increasing knowledge and awareness within a system. They are relatively easy to access and involve a unidirectional communication stream. Interpersonal channels, on the other hand, are more effective in persuading an individual to accept a new idea because of their bidirectional nature where group members can exchange ideas about an intervention rather than simply accepting what is being presented. Interpersonal channels are most effective when they involve individuals with similar socioeconomic status, education, and belief systems. At the same time, in the diffusion and dissemination process, individuals are necessarily dissimilar in their knowledge or attitude toward an innovation if one of the individuals is promoting or has adopted an innovation and the other has not. This creates a challenge for individuals seeking to introduce an innovation into a social system in that the individual promoting change has to be viewed as similar by group members and yet be able to promote the innovation and provide a unique perspective on the benefits of its adoption. This can be achieved by recruiting and training community partners to work with the dissemination team, by hiring staff that are similar in some ways to the targeted social system, or by partnering with existing community agencies.

Time

One of the most important elements of Rogers' model is his discussion of the role of time in the diffusion of innovations. Time, in the way that Rogers (2003) uses it, describes the decision-making course taken by all group members and the tendency for individuals with different traits to complete this process earlier or later than other members of their group. The innovation-decision process involves five steps that typically occur in sequence: knowledge, persuasion, decision, implementation, and confirmation. Because individuals differ in their openness to new ideas, several individual differences are posited explanations for differential speed moving through the innovation-decision process. Individuals most likely to move rapidly through to adoption include those who are more educated, are able to cope with greater uncertainty, and have greater exposure to mass media (Rogers, 2003). Typically, the number of individuals adopting an innovation follows an S-shaped curve over time, with only a few individuals quickly adopting an innovation, followed by increasing adoption rates as early adopters communicate their experiences to more and more members of the system. The majority of individuals in a system will not adopt the innovation until they are able to observe how the change has affected individuals in the system they can relate to and hear face-to-face descriptions about the costs and benefits associated with adopting the new idea. Once the majority of individuals in a system have adopted an innovation, the rate of adoption slows until only the last few individuals in the system who are least likely to change make their decision to adopt or reject the innovation completely.

Social System

The speed at which an innovation spreads throughout a social system depends both on the speed of communication channels and on the structure and norms of a social system. Social norms can impact the success of a dissemination effort both if they relate directly to a group's attitude toward change or if they relate to a belief or practice that is congruent with the innovation being presented. These social norms are often represented by opinion leaders in the community who are at the center of communication channels within the system. Opinion leaders can be extremely influential in the success or failure of a dissemination effort through their approval or rejection of an innovation. When innovations are presented by change agents outside the system or developed by unpopular or highly different members of the system, opinion leaders can be the critical link between group members and change agents who may be viewed as too different to be trusted by the majority of the group.

This view of the opinion leader as central to a social system has implications for the dissemination of psychological treatments to new settings. It suggests that the primary recruitment targets for applying new treatments should be individuals (e.g., service providers, clients) who are community opinion leaders. This idea also presents some challenges, as opinion leaders are not always the most innovative members of a social system and may be less likely to be early adopters of a new intervention. Given Rogers' point that the majority of group members decide to adopt an innovation only after they have seen it work for someone they know, identifying the few most innovative members of a group who would be willing to try a new intervention may be another starting point.

Another element of the social system that impacts the rate of dissemination is the decision-making structure of the system. If decisions are made by a single powerful member of a group who can mandate compliance (e.g., clinical director at a mental health center), then adoption of an innovation can happen very quickly. However, the risk of individuals circumventing these efforts is potentially high. If, instead, individual group members are allowed to decide whether to adopt an innovation, adoption happens more slowly and relies more heavily on interpersonal communication channels and opinion leaders to move the group to choose adoption. Finally, if adoption of an innovation relies on collective decision making, where all members of a group must arrive at a consensus about whether or not to adopt an innovation, adoption tends to happen more slowly than with individuals each deciding for themselves.

Taken together, several recommendations for dissemination researchers arise from diffusion theory (Rogers, 2003). Successful dissemination of psychological treatments may involve presenting treatments as compatible with the social system's norms, in line with a community need, and an improvement on existing services or interventions. Such efforts could use both mass media and interpersonal communication channels. Further, gaining support from opinion leaders and innovative group members may be helpful to support systemwide adoption. Because reinvention is a key step in the adoption of innovations process (Rogers, 1993), mental health treatments designed to support reinvention may fare better. Last, diffusion theory emphasizes thinking of the dissemination of psychological treatments as an effort toward changing a whole system rather than thinking of individual group members as the target, an emphasis that has influenced the other models we discuss.

Mental Health System Ecological Model

Schoenwald and Hoagwood's mental health system ecological model (2001) depicts multiple levels of variables that should be considered when planning to disseminate a mental health treatment: (1) client, (2) provider, (3) agency, and (4) service system. Although the point here is that treatments may need to be sensitive to context, it is not common for treatments to be contextualized in this way. Development work in the early research phases considers the relevance of client variables, often narrowly focused on symptoms and/or diagnoses. The Schoenwald and Hoagwood model implies that dissemination necessitates a much broader focus at each level (e.g., Southam-Gerow, 2004). The Schoenwald and Hoagwood model emphasizes the importance of considering the *whole* ecology involved in the mental health services system before embarking on large-scale dissemination projects. They also highlight the important step of transportability research and its focus on the development of an implementation model. Unlike Rogers' model, the Schoenwald and Hoagwood model was developed specifically to address mental health. As such, the model offers guidance to the mental health treatment dissemination researcher. There is no question that the model has had considerable impact on transportability and dissemination researchers already.

Implementation Research Framework

Although Rogers' model of innovation diffusion is arguably the best known, Fixsen et al.'s (2005) recent treatise on implementation research may be the most comprehensive examination of diffusion of evidence-based practices (EBPs) in mental health services. Their basic conceptual framework is straightforward, including five essential components: (1) a source (i.e., a program to be implemented); (2) a destination (i.e., the context in which the context will be implemented); (3) a communication link [i.e., a "purveyor" of the program—the primary implementer(s)]; (4) a feedback mechanism (i.e., a specified manner in which information is shared and used among the first three components); and (5) a sphere of influence favorable to the program (i.e., social, political, etc., forces). Further, Fixsen et al. (2005) elaborated a Stages of Implementation model similar to Rogers' but with less focus on the adoption phase and more on the postadoption phase. The stages move from exploration and adoption through program installation, initial implementation, and full operation to innovation and sustainability. As they noted, most of the research literature has focused on the early stages of dissemination, with very little attention to what happens after an initial implementation effort is made.

In addition to these two conceptual models, Fixsen et al. (2005) identified two other constructs relevant to this chapter: (1) core intervention components and (2) core implementation components. Core intervention components represent the crucial elements in the treatment program to be implemented; in other words, those techniques or principles that both are replicable and make a difference (Fixsen et al., 2005). Because most treatment programs have so many elements, one of the first jobs of the "purveyor" (i.e., the implementer) is to focus the implementation on those that will get the job done.[5]

More relevant to the focus of this chapter, Fixsen et al. (2005) also outlined core implementation components. They define these as the "drivers" of good implementation, that is, techniques or procedures that lead to "high-fidelity practitioner behavior" (p. 28). The components range from careful selection of staff as the "destination" to training and ongoing consultation of staff to methods for evaluating the effects of the program and provider fidelity to it (see Fixsen et al., 2005). Furthermore, they identified administrative and systems-level supports that impact implementation, akin to the Schoenwald and Hoagwood (2001) model discussed earlier.

Research on these various components was reviewed by Fixsen et al. (2005). For example, descriptive studies and case examples have

---

[5] Of course, when considering the mental health treatment literature, it would be an understatement to say that there is a lack of consensus as to what these core components might be. Across the adult and child/adolescent literatures, there are only a few evidence-based treatment programs for which any evidence of the "key ingredients" exists. A particularly good example of this is multisystemic therapy (MST; Henggeler et al., 1998, 2002). The treatment program includes nine principles, adherence to which has been directly linked to positive outcomes (Huey et al., 2000; Schoenwald et al., 2003).

been published describing how some implementation projects have conducted staff selection (e.g., Fisher & Chamberlain, 2000), though little experimental research exists. Research on training suggests that passive approaches (e.g., providing education alone) are ineffective alone as an implementation strategy (Grimshaw et al., 2001); ongoing consultation/coaching of providers and a quality assurance system are critical. Unfortunately, the paucity of experimental studies precludes firm conclusions. Finally, evidence on the importance of administrative and systems supports exists, including research on organizational culture and climate (e.g., Glisson, 2000) as well as work documenting the importance of remaining aware of funding sources available to the implementation site.

Similar to the Schoenwald and Hoagwood model, Fixsen et al.'s approach was developed to address mental health treatments specifically. And not surprisingly, the similarities between the two are many, especially the broad ecological focus. The model also has parallels to the Diffusion of Innovations model and its focus on the processes involved in adopting, adapting, and becoming adept (or not) at using innovations. An intriguing aspect of the Fixsen et al. focus concerns the importance of identifying *drivers* at the intervention and implementation level. The model lends itself nicely to the posing of research questions at multiple stages of the dissemination process.

PRACTICAL ISSUES IN DISSEMINATION OF EBTS

In this section, we discuss a variety of practical issues that may be unique to treatment dissemination, beginning with those relevant to researchers conducting dissemination research. Next, we focus on issues relevant to (1) providers who want to use evidence-based practices or (2) administrators who want to implement evidence-based practices in their agency.

Research-Related Issues

There are many issues facing dissemination researchers; an exhaustive discussion of them is beyond the scope of this chapter. We focus our present discussion on two important considerations: (1) the roles of the researcher and community partners in transportability and dissemination research and (2) the need for a variety of research designs in transportability and dissemination research.

Roles in Transportability and Dissemination Research

Moving out of the lab and into community settings increases the complexity of the roles of researchers and participants, posing many challenges to researchers used to the "safety" of the lab (Southam-Gerow, 2005). That is not to say that the roles played by researcher and participant in the first two to three phases of clinical research in Table 1 are not complex. However, beginning with effectiveness research, new stakeholder groups emerge, including agencies and their staff, third-party payors, other systems (e.g., juvenile justice, child welfare), advocacy groups, and policy makers. Thus, how to integrate these stakeholders into the research process becomes a central question. However, involving stakeholders in research is challenging because most clinical research is conducted with a primary decision maker, the principal investigator (PI) or, more recently, a group of co-investigators, all of whom have scientific backgrounds. As research moves out of the lab and into the community, such an approach may not be feasible (e.g., Southam-Gerow, 2005), as most service agencies would not permit a researcher (or group of researchers) to come in and "take over."

So what are the alternatives? Clearly, involving other stakeholders in the research endeavor is critical. The questions become *how* and *how much* to involve them. Methodology from participatory action research (PAR; Jason et al., 2004) provides a useful context for this question. PAR represents a diverse set of strategies with the goal of *empowering and giving voice* to a group or groups of citizens to *create social action* (Taylor et al., 2004). Varying levels of stakeholder involvement occur across multiple dimensions: (1) degree of partner control over research process (ranging from no control to equal partnership in the process); (2) amount of collaboration (from minimal to highly active); and (3) degree of partner commitment (none to full ownership of the process by the partner; see Suarez-Balcazar et al., 2004). At low levels of involvement, a small number of stakeholders may serve as occasional advisors, whereas at high levels of involvement, stakeholders would be active in the planning, implementation, and ongoing operation of the research project. The level of partnership will be determined by the goals of the project as well as practical aspects (e.g., funding limitations, time restrictions). At greater levels of stakeholder involvement, sustainability of the project may be more likely, but control over its direction is less certain. As stakeholder commitment and involvement decrease, researcher control increases, but sustained change becomes less likely.

Although increasing stakeholder involvement may yield significant benefits especially concerning the sustainability of a dissemination effort, doing so is not a common (or comfortable) experience for many researchers whose training has emphasized the importance of control over the research project. Despite this challenge, several recent exemplars of partnership research have emerged. For example, Southam-Gerow (2005) described a project applying a partnership model to adapt and test evidence-based treatments for childhood mental health problems, including components such as an advisory board and the use of qualitative research elements to assess and include the voices of multiple stakeholders. As another example, McKay and colleagues (2004) have been engaged in an impressive project that involved a partnership among community parents, school staff, community-based agency representatives, and university-based researchers organized to reduce HIV exposure of fourth- and fifth-grade children. McKay et al. indicated that their project involved the highest level of stakeholder involvement. To accomplish this, they created an advisory board (the CHAMP Collaborative Board) through which the direction, leadership, and evaluation of the prevention research project were accomplished. These examples demonstrate the emergence of partnership studies in the literature. As researchers move out of the laboratory and into the community, involving stakeholders will become an integral ingredient to these efforts. We anticipate that such partnerships will be fruitful fields for innovation in the coming years.

Using a Variety of Research Designs

In transportability and dissemination research, there is a need for a variety of research designs because of the variety of research questions asked (see Table 1). This is unlike most efficacy research, which typically involves randomized controlled trial (RCT) design. Although RCT design has been used often in transportability and dissemination research, other strategies abound as well. Thus, the researcher involved in dissemination research must have design flexibility. In this section, we describe RCT design, benchmarking strategies, and several other designs used in transportability and dissemination research.

RCT Strategies: Definitions and Uses

The essential ingredients of an RCT are (1) an "experimental" treatment group, (2) at least one control group, and (3) random assignment of participating clients/patients to one of the treatment groups. RCT design affords many methodological advantages including control of variety of confounding factors that plague uncontrolled research. A typical design might compare an evidence-based treatment to a "standard" treatment, most commonly what has been called "usual care" (e.g., Weisz et al., 2003).

RCTs have applicability throughout the whole range of clinical studies in Table 1. In an effectiveness study, Addis and colleagues (2004) compared an EBT for adult panic disorder to a usual-care control group in a community mental health center. The focus of the study was on patient/client outcomes; hence, random assignment was made of clients to treatment group. Results suggested better outcomes for the EBT. Transportability and dissemination studies also employ RCT methodology. For example, Gerrity et al. (1999) randomly assigned physicians to an education intervention (designed to increase physician sensitivity to major depressive disorder) or to a no-education control group. Outcomes included level of physician knowledge about depression as well as physician behavior (e.g., asking about depression symptoms) during a "standardized" office visit. Transportability and dissemination studies often focus on outcomes such as provider behaviors in addition to more traditional patient-level outcomes. Despite the advantages and applications of the RCT design, downsides of their use merit consideration. Discussion of these is beyond the scope of this chapter; the interested reader is referred to recent reviews (e.g., Borkovec & Castonguay, 1998; Westen et al., 2004).

Benchmarking Strategies

Benchmarking studies represent a low-cost and relatively simple method for the dissemination researcher. The basic notion in benchmarking is to use outcome data achieved at a research site as a benchmark for outcomes achieved in a practice setting. To the extent that the outcomes in the practice setting approach the benchmark, the treatment is considered to have support. Several examples of this approach have appeared in the literature in the last 10 years (e.g., Franklin et al., 2000; Persons et al., 1999; Wade et al., 1998; Warren & Thomas, 2001). In one of the earliest such studies, Wade et al. (1998) found that adults with panic disorder in a community mental health center who received an EBT for panic (Barlow & Craske, 1994) fared about as well as those who were treated in two separate RCTs.

Using the literature as a benchmark provides a tremendous advantage when conducting research in the field. It does not require several design elements that make research in community settings difficult, including random assignment, training and supervising providers in at least two separate treatment protocols, and assessment of treatment differentiation. However, benchmarking has several disadvantages. Most prominently, the absence of a control group does not provide adequate information about the value added by the new treatment over "usual care." As we have discussed, "usual care" is typically viewed as ineffective, though well-designed examinations of this assertion are few (e.g., Weiss et al., 2000) and some contrary evidence has been reported (e.g., Clarke et al., 2002). Without some estimate of the effect of "usual care" in a particular community, a benchmarking strategy will not inform stakeholders about the relative advantages of implementing a particular EBT for that setting. Another problem with the benchmarking strategy is that it does not easily permit statistical tests. Thus, comparisons between the achieved outcome and the benchmark are subjective.[6] The problem is more pronounced if apparent differences in outcomes are detected, but differences in sample sociodemographic characteristics and/or symptomatology are also present.

A benchmarking approach has several potential uses throughout the treatment development model we outlined earlier. During the effectiveness research phase, for example, a benchmarking strategy represents a useful and inexpensive method to identify EBTs with promise for use in service settings. Later in the sequence (see Table 1), particularly once the effectiveness of usual care is known, benchmarking could also be valuable. As an example, presume that usual care in a CMHC resulted in an effect size (ES) of 0.30 for youth with depression. If an EBT for youth depression resulted in an ES of 0.65, stakeholders would have good data on which to base adoption and/or continuation decisions.

---

[6] Weersing and Weisz (2002) have used 95% confidence intervals to gauge if effects in a practice setting were in the range of those achieved in a benchmark study. This strategy offers more power for a researcher to describe the effects of a treatment tested in a practice setting, as it provides some basis for comparison, though it comes short of a statistical test.

Other Research Designs

As described earlier, although RCTs (and to a lesser extent bench-marking strategies) represent a primary design in transportability and dissemination research, other designs also play important roles. These designs include clinical methods such as single-case and pre-post design. In addition, the correlational (observational) research paradigm is used. As there are chapters in this volume devoted to describing these method-ological approaches, we will not discuss them here. However, we will provide a few examples of how these designs can and have been used in transportability and dissemination research.

A study by Schoenwald et al. (2003) provides an excellent example of how pre-post design can be used in transportability research. In the study, Schoenwald and colleagues were interested in identifying factors associated with adequate implementation of multisystemic therapy (MST) outcomes. The design included pre-post measurement of outcomes of youth treated with MST at 39 clinic sites as well as pretreatment measurement of potential implementation factors including organizational climate and organizational structure. Further, the researchers measured treatment adherence as a key mechanism of ensuring positive outcomes, as identified in previous studies. The primary focus of the study concerned the relation-ships among the organizational variables, the adherence measure, and the child outcomes.

Hemmelgarn et al. (2001) recently conducted a study also focused on organization-level constructs that involved a correlational research design. The project involved a mixture of qualitative and quantitative methods used to understand how organizational culture (i.e., behavioral norms and expectations that exist within an organization) and organizational climate (i.e., shared perception of the psychological impact of the work environment on his or her own well-being) were related to the implemen-tation of one component (emotional support) of a broader initiative referred to as "Family-Centered Care" in hospital emergency rooms. Evidence from quantitative interviews and structured questionnaires were used to examine these relationships.

In addition, surveys and qualitative research methods (e.g., focus groups, interviews) with relevant stakeholders may lend data that forecast how easy (or challenging) a dissemination effort will be in a particular setting. The Southam-Gerow (2005) study described earlier is an example of a mixed-methods (quantitative/qualitative) project that applies a partnership model and uses qualitative data to guide a transportability study. In short, transportability and dissemination research involves the use of multiple research designs including, but not limited to, the RCT. We now turn to issues in transportability and dissemination research that concern providers and mental health administrators.

Practice-Related Issues

The dissemination process poses formidable challenges to researchers, providers, and mental health administrators alike. As discussed earlier, researchers must use creativity and flexibility when working outside traditional "lab" settings. Likewise, engaging in partnerships for the purposes of dissemination may require providers to operate outside their normal routine and clinical mindset. Further, administrators must consider the operational consequences of choosing to implement evidence-based treatments in the context of almost no data to guide them in *how* to accomplish such a goal. Although many issues are relevant here, we focus on two: (1) provider training and (2) treatment acceptability.

Provider Training

The perspectives and attitudes held by providers related to theoretical orientation are rooted in their graduate training and subsequent clinical experiences. Statistics representing the distribution of theoretical orientations held by mental health providers are scarce, a task made more difficult because the mental health workforce is composed of a variety of training backgrounds (e.g., social work, rehabilitation counseling, MA/MS in clinical or counseling psychology, Psy.D. and Ph.D. in clinical or counseling psychology, MFT, MA in art therapy, etc.). Training experiences across and within these groups vary widely, leading to different core beliefs about the etiology and maintenance of mental health problems as well as the best ways to treat clients. Thus, although the vast majority of evidence-based treatments are cognitive-behavioral (or, to a lesser extent, interpersonal; Kazdin & Weisz, 2003), a large proportion of providers have not had much experience with such orientations or techniques. Indeed, national surveys indicate that most practicing psychologists and social workers identify as having an approach other than behavioral, such as eclectic, multitheory, or psychoanalytic (e.g., Jayaratne, 1982; Norcross & Prochaska, 1988). Therefore, one of the initial challenges for providers during dissemination may be learning about techniques that are prescribed by an unfamiliar orientation and are vastly different from or perceived to be incompatible with the "usual care" they provide. For a provider, the implementation of such techniques may challenge long-standing beliefs about what is necessary to create change, and in so doing may be perceived as a threat to their well-established identity and style.

Whereas the training background of providers may not have included the techniques or guiding orientations of current EBTs, this does not necessarily mean that providers are altogether opposed to acquiring competencies in new areas. For those providers interested in learning EBTs, access to training may be an obstacle. Identifying efficient, comprehensive, and affordable training may be a difficult task, particularly for those practicing in rural communities. One opportunity may come through participation in clinical research using EBTs in their community setting, wherein they may receive didactic instruction, test cases, and supervision within this new area. However, the current number of such trials is not sufficient to train the large numbers of existing providers. Further, clinical trials are not likely to be held in all settings where providers are found.

A second opportunity may come through attendance of a continuing education (CE) course or workshop on the topic of an EBT. Psychologists in most states are mandated to attend between 10–20 CE credits per year (Sharkin & Plageman, 2003), and other licensed mental health providers have similar requirements. However, the effectiveness of this training method alone has been called into question (e.g., Davis et al., 1999), and some researchers have suggested that CE should increase its focus on specific applied skills to increase its acceptability and usefulness for providers.

Granted that CE courses are not the answer, other options are needed. Comprehensive training is costly (Strosahl, 1998), and individual agencies may not have adequate funds to do the job right. Instructional Design Technologies (e.g., computer training programs, supervision via computer) provide some potential alternatives to the traditional CE route of "teaching" new skills, though this method has its own limitations, including the time necessary to complete online courses, the need for strong intrinsic motivation to complete them, and potential threats to unchecked treatment integrity (Lane & Addis, 2004). Further, several state governments have begun developing initiatives to provide more funding for training in EBTs.

Clearly, training availability is the first hurdle. Another and perhaps more pressing question is how much training is needed—and in what form(s). Research on this is sparse but suggests that education (e.g., provided in a CE course) in combination with ongoing consultation and/or a quality assurance system leads to more lasting changes (e.g., Grimshaw et al., 2001). Thus, an interested provider will need to consider how best to learn a new technique to proficiency. And interested administrators will need to weigh the costs and benefits of less costly education-only training approaches versus more intensive (and expensive) training approaches.

Finally, considering that there is diversity in theoretical orientation and training background of providers and a large number of identified EBTs, one must ask, "How many EBTs can one provider be expected to master?" Arriving at a comfortable and competent level of practice within one specialty area is considered a lengthy and effortful process. Establishing competency within multiple treatment programs for multiple problems poses a daunting task. This issue has ramifications for providers and administrators alike. A provider may ask, "Which treatment programs are most relevant to the population(s) I serve?" and "How long will it take to master a new treatment program?" Although Addis et al. (1999) suggest that providers might strive for proficiency in one EBT for each broad problem area (e.g., mood, anxiety, externalizing problems) and further training would depend on specialized needs of the individual provider in her practice, it is not clear how valid this supposition is. From an administrator's point of view, maximization of competency coverage in the areas most relevant to the agency and its consumers may become a guiding principle for the organization of programs and the hiring of staff. Further, such guidelines could inform training (and retraining) plans. Still, many administrators may not have an adequate "pipeline" of applicants for jobs at the agency to fill all relevant areas with evidence-based expertise. Thus, training is a critical (and understudied) phase for dissemination.

Treatment Acceptability

Access to and the format of training opportunities represent an important challenge for providers and administrators in the process of dissemination of evidence-based treatments. As discussed above, attitudes and beliefs about evidence-based treatment may influence willingness to seek and/or receive training in this area. The term "treatment acceptability" represents the degree to which a treatment is perceived to be appropriate, fair, reasonable, and unintrusive (Kazdin, 1980). Traditionally, treatment acceptability has been rated by client consumers of treatment (Reimers et al., 1992; Sterling-Turner & Watson, 2002). However, within the dissemination process, the assessment of treatment acceptability during training and implementation on the part of provider consumers are also relevant. For example, a recent study aimed at implementing a school-based treatment for attention deficit hyperactivity disorder (Evans et al., 2005) included the assessment of treatment acceptability and feasibility among school staff, and their feedback was used to modify the mode of delivery to fit the needs of the system.

Some research has examined provider attitudes regarding the general use of manualized treatments, though not within the context of any current training experience. Addis et al. (1999) summarized some of the most common concerns held by providers, grouping them into six categories: (1) The therapeutic relationship will be compromised or ineffective; (2) client (individual, multiple, or emotional) needs may not be met; (3) concerns about competence and job satisfaction, (4) credibility of the treatments; (5) the restriction of clinical innovation; and (6) feasibility of training, implementation, and client acceptability. A recent survey of providers (Addis & Krasnow, 2000) indicated that while many of them have heard of treatment manuals, only around half reported having a clear idea of what they are. Further, these surveys show that provider opinions on manualized treatments were largely based on consultation with colleagues or on reading literature, rather than on actual hands-on experience with the manuals (Addis & Krasnow, 2000).

Whereas many providers recognize the value of evidence-based practice, they have legitimate concerns about their professional autonomy, identity, and ability to maintain competent, ethical service delivery in a system increasingly challenged by managed care restraints (Addis & Krasnow, 2000). Providers perceive significant loss of control to managed care companies in the area of clinical care decisions, particularly within the area of caps on total treatment sessions (Murphy et al., 1998). Fears that managed care companies will use evidence-based recommendations to enforce more restrictions on clinical care decisions may contribute to provider attitudes.

Further investigation of provider attitudes toward EBTs is warranted, particularly during the process wherein providers within a common setting are trained in specific treatments (e.g., Evans, Green & Serpell, 2005; Schmidt & Taylor, 2002). Qualitative research (e.g., interviews and focus groups) related to treatment acceptability and provider concerns about EBTs have the potential to provide insights into the dissemination process beyond what can be detected under the constraints of quantitative measures (Addis et al., 1999). Such qualitative information would be helpful in guiding efforts to increase treatment acceptability by addressing provider concerns within EBT trainings.

It is less clear to what extent the attitudes of administrators are relevant in the uptake of EBTs, but it does seem likely that there is an important effect. As discussed earlier, Glisson and his colleagues have demonstrated the importance of organizational variables (such as leadership) in the adoption of innovations like treatment programs (e.g.,Gilsson & Green, 2006; Glisson & Hemmelgarn, 1998; Glisson, 2002). Furthermore, Rogers' (2003) diffusion model suggests the importance of opinion leaders in dissemination. Assuming that administrators are opinion leaders in their agencies, the importance of their attitudes toward a new treatment is clearly critical. Moreover, administrators generally have the power to directly affect the chance of the uptake of a new treatment through staff selection and training offerings. Thus, the treatment acceptability of administrators merits future research attention.

Dissemination of mental health treatments presents challenges to researchers, providers, and administrators. Given the profusion of state and national efforts to promote the uptake of evidence-based treatments and practices, we will all need to face and overcome the challenges. As we have discussed in the chapter, we think that the mental health fields are at an exciting and potentially fruitful juncture wherein collaborations among the many stakeholders in the child mental health system will yield great gains for the children and families in need of mental health services.

CONCLUSIONS

This chapter has provided an overview of the new and growing area of dissemination and transportability clinical research in child mental health. Because researchers and policy makers have begun to focus efforts beyond efficacy trials, the importance of clarifying the methodological and conceptual issues has become a particular challenge. Unlike some technologies, mental health treatments have proven to be difficult to transport in a simple manner from one context to another (e.g., Southam-Gerow, 2004). Thus, we anticipate tremendous growth in the amount of dissemination and transportability research over the years as researchers grapple with the complex variables associated with successful implementation of treatments with an evidence base. Furthermore, we anticipate that this new fieldwork will yield many innovations, including changes to current treatments as well as the development of novel interventions.

However, it is more likely that innovations will come at the implemen-tation and dissemination intervention level, as the field begins to study the processes involved in integrating new treatments into a variety of practice settings. In the end, we hope that these emerging fields of transportability and dissemination research will be the bridge that closes the science-practice gap and makes effective treatment available to all who need them.

ACKNOWLEGEMENT. We thank Sonja K. Schoenwald for her thoughtful and instructive feedback on an earlier version of this manuscript.

REFERENCES

Addis, M. E., Hatgis, C., Krasnow, A. D., Jacob, K., Bourne, L., & Mansfield, A. (2004). Effec-tiveness of cognitive-behavioral treatment for panic disorder versus treatment as usual in a managed care setting. *Journal of Consulting & Clinical Psychology, 72* , 625–635.

Addis, M. E., & Krasnow, A. D. (2000). A national survey of practicing psychologists' attitudes toward psychotherapy treatment manuals. *Journal of Consulting & Clinical Psychology, 68*, 331–339.

Addis, M. E., Wade, W. A., & Hatgis, C. (1999). Barriers to dissemination of evidence-based practices: Addressing practitioners' concerns about manual-based psychother-apies. *Clinical Psychology: Science & Practice, 6*, 430–441.

Barlow, D. H. (1996). The effectiveness of psychotherapy: Science and policy. *Clinical Psychology: Science & Practice, 3*, 236–240.

Barlow D. H., & Craske, M. (1994). *Mastery of Your Anxiety and Panic.* San Antonio, TX: Psychological Corporation.

Borkovec, T. G., & Castonguay, L. G. (1998). What is the scientific meaning of "Empirically Supported Therapy?" *Journal of Consulting and Clinical Psychology, 66*, 136–142.

Carroll, K. M., & Rounsaville, B. J. (2003). Bridging the gap: A hybrid model to link efficacy and effectiveness research in substance abuse treatment. *Psychiatric Services, 54*, 333–339.

Chambers, D. A., Ringeisen, H., & Hickman, E. E. (2005). Federal, state, and foundation initiatives around evidence-based practices child and adolescent mental health. *Child and Adolescent Psychiatric Clinics of North America, 14*, 307–327.

Chorpita, B. F., & Nakamura, B. J. (2004). Four considerations for dissemination of inter-vention innovations. *Clinical Psychology: Science & Practice, 11*, 364–367.

Chorpita, B. F., Yim, L. M., Donkervoet, J. C., Arensdorf, A., Amundsen, M. J., McGee, C., et al. (2002). Toward large-scale implementation of empirically supported treatments for children: A review and observations by the Hawai'i Empirical Basis to Services Task Force. *Clinical Psychology: Science & Practice, 9*, 165–190.

Clarke, G. N., Hornbrook, M., Lynch, F., Polen, M., Gale, J., O'Connor, E., et al. (2002). Group cognitive-behavioral treatment for depressed adolescent offspring of depressed parents in a health maintenance organization. *Journal of the American Academy of Child & Adolescent Psychiatry, 41*, 305–313.

Davis, D., Thomson, M. A., Freemantle, N., Wolfe, F. M., Mazmanian, P., & Taylor-Vaisey, A. (1999). Impact of formal medical continuing education: Do conference workshops, rounds, and other traditional continuing education activities change physician behavior or health outcomes? *Journal of the American Medical Association, 282*, 867–874.

Donenberg, G. R., Lyons, J. S., & Howard, K. I. (1999). Clinical trials versus mental health services research: Contributions and connections. *Journal of Clinical Psychology, 55* , 1135–1146.

Evans, S. W., Green, A. L., & Serpell, Z. N. (2005). Community participation in the treatment development process using community development teams. *Journal of Clinical Child & Adolescent Psychology, 34* , 765–771.

Fisher, P. A., & Chamberlain, P. (2000). Multidimensional treatment foster care: A program for intensive parenting, family support, and skill building. *Journal of Emotional & Behavioral Disorders, 8* , 155–164.

Fixsen, D. L., Naoom, S. F., Blasé, K. A., Friedman, R. M., & Wallace, F. (2005). *Implementation Research: A Synthesis of the Literature*. Tampa, FL: University of South Florida, Louis De la Parte Florida Mental Health Institute, The National Implementation Research Network.

Franklin, M. E., Abramowitz, J. S., Kozak, M. J., Levitt, J. T., & Foa, E. B. (2000). Effectiveness of exposure and ritual prevention for obsessive-compulsive disorder: Randomized compared with nonrandomized samples. *Journal of Consulting & Clinical Psychology, 68*, 594–602.

Friedman, L., Furberg, C., & DeMets, D. L. (1998). *Fundamentals of Clinical Trials*, 3rd ed. New York: Springer-Verlag.

Gerrity, M. S., Cole, S. A., Dietrich, A. J., & Barrett, J. E. (1999). Improving the recognition and management of depression: Is there a role for physician education? *Journal of Family Practice, 48*, 949–957.

Glisson, C. & Green, P. (2006). The effects of organizational culture and climate on the access to mental health care in child welfare and juvenile justice systems. Administration and Policy in Mental Health and Mental Health Service Research, *33*, 433–458.

Glisson, C. (2000). Organizational culture and climate. In R. Patti (Ed.), *The Handbook of Social Welfare Management* (pp. 195–218). Thousand Oaks, CA: Sage Publications.

Glisson, C., & Hemmelgarn, A. (1998). The effects of organizational climate and interorganizational coordination on the quality and outcomes of children's service systems. *Child Abuse & Neglect, 22*, 401–421.

Grimshaw, J. M., Shirran, L., Thomas, R., Mowatt, G., Fraswer, C., Bero, L., et al. (2001). Changing provider behavior: An overview of systematic reviews of interventions. *Medical Care, 39*, II-2–II-45.

Gotham, H. J. (2004). Diffusion of mental health and substance abuse treatments: Development dissemination, and implementation. *Clinical Psychology: Science and Practice, 11*, 161–176.

Hemmelgarn, A. L., Glisson, C., & Dukes, D. (2001). Emergency room culture and the emotional support component of family-centered care. *Children's Health Care, 30* , 93–110.

Henggeler, S. W., Schoenwald, S. K., Borduin, C. M., Rowland, M. D., & Cunningham, P. B. (1998). *Multisystemic Treatment of Antisocial Behavior in Children and Adolescents*. New York: Guilford Press.

Henggeler, S. W., Schoenwald, S. K., Rowland, M. D., & Cunningham, P. B. (2002). *Serious Emotional Disturbance in Children and Adolescents: Multisystemic Therapy*. New York: Guilford Press.

Hoagwood, K., & Olin, S. (2002). The NIMH blueprint for change report: Research priorities in child and adolescent mental health. *Journal of the American Academy of Child & Adolescent Psychiatry, 41*, 760–767.

Huber, T. P., Godfrey, M. M., Nelson, E. C., Mohr, J. J., Campbell, C., & Batalden, P. B. (2003). Microsystems in health care: Part 8. Developing people and improving work life: What front-line staff told us. *Joint Commission Journal on Quality and Safety, 29*, 512–522.

Huey, S. J., Henggeler, S. W., Brondino, M. J., & Pickrel, S. G. (2000). Mechanisms of change in multisystemic therapy: Reducing delinquent behavior through therapist adherence and improved family and peer functioning. *Journal of Consulting and Clinical Psychology, 68*, 451–467.

Jason, L. A., Keys, C. B., Suarez-Balcazar, Y., Taylor, R. R., & Davis, M. I. (Eds.) (2004). *Participatory Community Research: Theories and Methods in Action*. Washington, DC: American Psychological Association.

Jayaratne, S. (1982). Characteristics and theoretical orientations of clinical social workers: A national survey. *Journal of Social Service Research, 4*, 17–30.

Kazdin, A. E. (1980). Acceptability of alternative treatments for deviant child behavior. *Journal of Applied Behavior Analysis, 13*, 259–273.

Kazdin, A. E., & Weisz, J. R. (2003). *Evidence-Based Psychotherapies for Children and Adolescents*. New York: Guilford Press.

Lane, J. M., & Addis, M. E. (2004). Pros and cons of educational technologies as methods for disseminating evidence-based treatments. *Clinical Psychology: Science & Practice, 11*, 336–338.

McKay, M. M., Chasse, K. T., Paikoff, R., McKinney, L., Baptiste, D., Coleman, D., et al. (2004). Family-level impact of the CHAMP Family Program: A community collaborative effort to support urban families and reduce youth HIV risk exposure. *Family Process, 43,* 79–93.

Murphy, M. J., DeBernardo, C. N., & Shoemaker, W. E. (1998). Impact of managed care on independent practice and professional ethics: A survey of independent practitioners. *Professional Psychology: Research & Practice, 29,* 43–51.

Nathan, P. E., Stuart, S. P., & Dolan, S. L. (2000). Research on psychotherapy efficacy and effectiveness: Between Scylla and Charybdis? *Psychological Bulletin, 126 ,* 964–981.

Norcross, J. C., & Prochaska, J. O. (1988). A study of eclectic (and integrated) views revisited. *Professional Psychology: Research & Practice, 19,* 170–174.

Persons, J. B., Bostrom, A., & Bertagbolli, A. (1999). Results of randomized controlled trials of cognitive therapy for depression generalize to private practice. *Cognitive Therapy & Research, 23 ,* 535–548.

Reimers, T. M., Wacker, D. P., Cooper, L. J., & DeRaad, A. O. (1992). Acceptability of behavioral treatments for children: Analog and naturalistic evaluations by parents. *School Psychology Review, 21,* 628–643.

Rogers, E. M. (1993). Diffusion and the re-invention of Project D.A.R.E. In T. E. Backer & E. M. Rogers (Eds.), *Organizational Aspects of Health Communication Campaigns: What Works?* Thousands Oaks, CA: Sage Publications.

Rogers, E. M. (2003). *Diffusion of Innovations,* 5th ed. New York: The Free Press.

Rounsaville, B. J., Carroll, K. M., & Onken, L. S. (2001) A stage model of behavioral therapies research: Getting started and moving on from stage I. *Clinical Psychology: Science and Practice, 8,* 133–142.

Schmidt, F., & Taylor, T. K. (2002). Putting empirically-supported treatments into practice: Lessons learned in a children's mental health center. *Professional Psychology: Research & Practice, 33,* 483–489.

Schoenwald, S. K., & Hoagwood, K. (2001). Effectiveness and dissemination research: Their mutual roles in improving mental health services for children and adolescents. *Emotional & Behavioral Disorders in Youth, 2 ,* 3–4, 18–20.

Schoenwald, S. K., Sheidow, A. J., Letourneau, E. J., & Liao, J. G. (2003). Transportability of multisystemic therapy: Evidence for multilevel influences. *Mental Health Services Research, 5 ,* 223–239.

Sharkin, B. S., & Plageman, P. M. (2003). What do psychologists think about mandatory continuing education? A survey of Pennsylvania practitioners. *Professional Psychology: Research & Practice, 34,* 318–323.

Southam-Gerow, M. A. (2004). Some reasons that mental health treatments are not technologies: Toward treatment development and adaptation outside labs. *Clinical Psychology: Science & Practice, 11,* 186–189.

Southam-Gerow, M. A. (2005). Using partnerships to adapt evidence-based mental health treatments for use outside labs. *Report on Emotional & Behavioral Disorders in Youth, 5,* 58–60, 77–79.

Southam-Gerow, M. A., Austin, A. A., & Marder, A. M. (in press). Transportability and dissemination of psychological methods. In D. McKay (Ed.), *Handbook of Research Clinical Psychology.* Newbury Park, CA: Sage Publications.

Southam-Gerow, M. A., Ringeisen, H. L., & Sherrill, J. T. (2006). Introduction to Special Issue: Integrating interventions and services research: Progress and prospects. *Clinical Psychology: Science and Practice, 13,* 1–8.

Southam-Gerow, M. A., Weisz, J. R., & Kendall, P. C. (2003). Childhood anxiety disorders in research and service clinics: Preliminary examination of differences and similarities. *Journal of Clinical Child and Adolescent Psychology, 32,* 375–385.

Sterling-Turner, H. E., & Watson, T. S. (2002). An analog investigation of the relationship between treatment acceptability and treatment integrity. *Journal of Behavioral Education, 11,* 39–50.

Strosahl, K. D. (1998). The dissemination of manual-based psychotherapies in managed care: Promises, problems, and prospects. *Clinical Psychology: Science & Practice, 5,* 382–386.

Suarez-Balcazar, Y., Davis, M. I., Ferrari, J., Nyden, P., Olson, B., Alvarez, J., et al. (2004). University-community partnerships: A framework and an exemplar. In L. A. Jason, C. B. Keys, Y. Suarez-Balcazar, R. R. Taylor, & M. I. Davis (Eds.), *Participatory Community*

Research: Theories and Methods in Action (pp. 105–120). Washington, DC: American Psychological Association.

Taylor, R. R., Jason, L. A., Keys, C. B., Suarez-Balcazar, Y., Davis, M. I., Durlak, J. A., et al. (2004). Introduction: Capturing theory and methodology in participatory research. In L. A. Jason, C. B. Keys, Y. Suarez-Balcazar, R. R. Taylor, & M. I. Davis (Eds.), *Participatory Community Research: Theories and Methods in Action* (pp. 3–14). Washington, DC: American Psychological Association.

U.S. Public Health Service (2000). *Report of the Surgeon General's Conference on Children's Mental Health: A National Action Agenda.* Washington, DC: Department of Health and Human Services.

Wade, W. A., Treat, T. A., & Stuart, G. L. (1998). Transporting an empirically supported treatment for panic disorder to a service clinic setting: A benchmarking strategy. *Journal of Consulting & Clinical Psychology, 66* , 231–239.

Warren, R., & Thomas, J. C. (2001). Cognitive-behavior therapy of obsessive-compulsive disorder in private practice: An effectiveness study. *Journal of Anxiety Disorders, 15* , 277–285.

Weersing, V. R., & Weisz, J. R. (2002). Community clinic treatment of depressed youth: Benchmarking usual care against CBT clinical trials. *Journal of Consulting and Clinical Psychology, 70,* 299–310.

Weiss, B., Catron, T., & Harris, V. (2000). A 2-year follow-up of the effectiveness of traditional child psychotherapy. *Journal of Counseling and Clinical Psychology, 68,* 1094–1101.

Weisz, J. R., Chu, B. C., & Polo, A. (2004). Treatment dissemination and evidence based practice: Strengthening intervention through clinician-researcher collaboration. *Clinical Psychology: Science and Practice, 11,* 300–307.

Weisz, J. R., Southam-Gerow, M. A., Gordis, E. B., & Connor-Smith, J. (2003). Primary and secondary control enhancement training for youth depression: Applying the deployment focused model of treatment development and testing. In A. E. Kazdin & J. R. Weisz (Eds.), *Evidence-Based Psychotherapies for Children and Adolescents* (pp. 165–183). New York: Guilford Press.

Westen, D., Novotny, C. M., & Thompson-Brenner, H. (2004). The empirical status of empirically supported psychotherapies: Assumptions, findings, and reporting in controlled clinical trials. *Psychological Bulletin, 130* , 631–663.

26

Client, Therapist, and Treatment Characteristics in EBTs for Children and Adolescents

STEPHEN SHIRK and DANA MCMAKIN

A substantial body of evidence has emerged over the last 20 years supporting the efficacy of multiple, psychosocial treatments for child and adolescent disorders (Weisz, 2004). However, closer inspection of the literature reveals variations in treatment outcomes, even within treatments deemed efficacious. In some cases, nearly one in three youngsters treated with an evidence-based treatment (EBT) fails to attain an adequate response (Fonagy et al., 2002). Research on predictors of treatment response is at an early stage of development. Similarly, little is known about therapist variables that might affect treatment outcome. Although variation in therapist effects is assumed to be reduced by manual-guided therapy, therapists are likely to vary in flexibility, interpersonal style, and overall competence, thereby potentially resulting in variation in outcomes. Finally, despite evidence for positive treatment *outcomes*, research on treatment *processes* remains quite limited (Shirk & Karver, 2006). In fact, the specific active ingredients of most treatments have not been identified.

By no means do these gaps in the literature undermine the significance of progress that has been made in child and adolescent treatment research. Instead, questions about client, therapist, and treatment characteristics that predict outcome are the logical next step in treatment research. In this chapter, we review the existing literature on client, therapist, and treatment variables in EBTs for youth. We recognize from the outset that research in this area is just beginning to emerge and that part of our task will be to identify important questions for the next wave of studies. The chapter is

STEPHEN SHIRK and DANA MCMAKIN • University of Denver

organized into three sections; within each we focus on three of the most common referral problems—anxiety, depression, and disruptive behavior—as they relate to client, therapist, and treatment variables.

CLIENT CHARACTERISTICS

Because of within-treatment variation in outcomes, investigators have begun to search for predictors of treatment response (or nonresponse) in an effort to improve treatment specificity and efficacy. In this section, we review pretreatment characteristics that have been examined as predictors of outcome in the treatment of anxiety, depression, and disruptive behavior problems. Suggestions for treatment adaptation and modification are presented, and potential but unexamined predictors are considered.

Comorbidity

Among client characteristics, there has been considerable interest in the impact of comorbidity on treatment outcome. The prevailing assumption in the field is that comorbidity complicates treatment of primary disorders and is likely to result in poorer treatment response. However, emerging evidence suggests that both the type of comorbidity and the type of primary disorder must be part of any consideration of the impact of comorbidity.

Consistent with the view that comorbidity compromises treatment response, results indicate that anxious youngsters with co-occurring depression or mixed depression and anxiety show poorer treatment response than youth without these co-occurring conditions (Berman et al., 2000; Southam-Gerow et al., 2001), though at least one study did not show this pattern of results (Kendall et al., 1997, 2001). Similarly, one treatment study of depression revealed poorer responses among adolescents with comorbid anxiety disorder (Brent et al., 1998), but the opposite effect was found in a second CBT trial (Rohde et al., 2001). Among youngsters with conduct disorder, comorbid attention deficit hyperactivity disorder appears to attenuate treatment response (e.g. Hinshaw & Melnick, 1995; e.g., Lynam et al., 2000), and this response appears to be more pronounced among older than younger children (Hartman et al., 2003). It is possible that the severe and pervasive symptoms associated with early-onset conduct disorder and attention deficit hyperactivity disorder could, over time, lead to highly entrenched problems with behavior across multiple settings (school, home, and community; Lynam et al., 2000). In fact, adolescents with attention and conduct symptoms frequently have a history of early-onset behavior problems, academic underachievement (see Hinshaw, 1992), and poor peer relations (Hinshaw & Melnick, 1995). Clearly, intervening as early as possible is indicated in this population.

Because of their prevalence among clinic referrals (Southam-Gerow et al., 2001), the impact of co-occurring disruptive behavior problems on successful treatment of other primary disorders deserves special attention. Comordid disruptive disorders, especially oppositional-defiant disorder and conduct disorder, could complicate the treatment of other primary disorders because of the high rates of noncompliance. Evidence on the impact of comorbid disruptive problems is relatively limited because such youth are often underrepresented or excluded from efficacy trials of other primary disorders (Southam-Gerow et al., 2003) For example, Rohde et al. (2001) did *not* find a lifetime history of disruptive behavior disorders to predict response to CBT for depression, but youth with *current* conduct disorders are typically excluded from depression trials. One exception is a study by Rohde et al. (2004), who found CBT to be more effective than an active control condition but also less effective than CBT for depression in trials without youth with co-occurring conduct problems. With regard to anxiety, Kendall et al. (2001) found that anxious youth with and without co-occurring externalizing symptoms responded equally well to CBT for anxiety. However, this study grouped externalizing symptoms together for the majority of the analyses. Furthermore, the sample included only two participants with conduct disorder, and only 42 disruptive behavior diagnoses out of 310 total comorbid diagnoses. Additional research with larger sample sizes is necessary to investigate the potential moderation of treatment outcome.

Contrary to the view that comorbidity attenuates treatment effects, some evidence suggests that comorbidity actually *improves* treatment response. Youngsters with comorbid anxiety and depression respond better to treatment for conduct disorder than children or preadolescents without these comorbidities (Beauchaine, 2000; Beauchaine et al., 2005). Interestingly, boys with high collateral anxiety/depression were responsive to all active forms of treatment (parent training, child-focused cognitive training, teacher training), whereas boys with low anxiety/depression were most amenable to parent training (Beauchaine et al., 2005). Thus, the assessment of comorbid internalizing symptoms may inform treatment selection.

As these results suggest, the impact of comorbidity varies as a function of type of comorbidity and type of primary disorder. What, then, are the implications for treatment? As is so often the case, it depends. For example, hopelessness has been shown to attenuate treatment response among depressed adolescents (Brent et al., 1998) and could contribute to poorer response among anxious youth with collateral depression. In order to address hopelessness among anxious youth, additional attention might be given to building positive expectations or to challenging pessimistic cognitions about treatment. Anhedonia, also found among depressed youth, may interfere with engagement or with completing homework assignments such as planned exposures in the treatment of anxiety. The inclusion of specific cognitive-behavioral interventions to increase activity level might be necessary for anxious youth with comorbid depressive symptoms, particularly those that involve fatigue and lethargy. On the other hand, youth with depression and co-occurring anxiety might be disengaged for different reasons, including increased arousal in sessions or social avoidance outside sessions. For such youth, relaxation training could improve treatment outcome by reducing anxious arousal. Finally, the most important treatment strategy for youth with conduct disorder and co-occurring attention symptoms is to provide intervention as early as possible and to add a Teacher Training component (Beauchaine et al., 2005). In summary, treatment modification for youth with comorbid problems must consider the type of comorbidity and whether it exerts a facilitating or limiting effect.

Developmental Characteristics

The most common developmental predictor of treatment outcome is age. However, age and other important variables such as symptom severity or cognitive sophistication often overlap, resulting in inconsistencies in the literature. For example, some research suggests that older children respond less favorably to CBT for anxiety (Southam-Gerow et al., 2001), but counterevidence also exists in the literature (Berman et al., 2000; Kendall et al., 1997). An early meta-analysis indicated that age was positively related to CBT outcomes (Durlak et al., 1991). The authors concluded that age was a proxy for developmental processes, specifically cognitive level, that enabled youth to benefit from cognitive techniques.

Age has also been shown to be related to outcome in the treatment of disruptive disorders. Age effects for parent training suggest that younger children respond better to parent management training than older children (Ruma et al., 1996). However, age is confounded with duration and severity of symptoms (Dishion & Patterson, 1992; Ruma et al., 1996) such that older children often present with more deeply entrenched, maladaptive patterns of behavior than their younger counterparts. This is consistent with research showing that youth with more severe symptoms of conduct disorder make fewer gains in treatment and are less likely to generalize positive behavioral changes across settings (Ruma et al., 1996; Webster-Stratton, 1996).

Disentangling age and its confounding variables is an important research agenda. For now, mental health professionals can surmise that younger children are not as well suited for cognitive methods as older children and that modeling and other behavioral techniques might be better suited to younger clients. But age is not always yoked to cognitive sophistication, and these two factors should be considered independently. Children with early-onset conduct disorder, for example, may evidence greater cognitive deficits (see Nigg & Huang-Pollock, 2003) than other children with conduct disorder. Perhaps cognitive therapy is not well suited for these individuals despite their chronological age. The relationship between age and increased severity of disruptive behavior symptoms suggests that the earlier mental health professionals can intervene with children with disruptive behavior symptoms, the better the prognosis.

Family Characteristics

Given the significant role of family factors in the development of psychopathology, it is not surprising that they are influential in treatment response as well. Nevertheless, the role of family factors in predicting treatment response is not simple and appears to vary with disorder. For example, in the treatment of anxiety, a range of maternal symptoms has predicted poor treatment outcome (Berman et al., 2000; Southam-Gerow et al., 2001). The strongest effects are revealed at long-term follow-up (Southam-Gerow et al., 2001), suggesting that a maladaptive pattern of interaction is degrading treatment effects over time. Of course, it is possible that children of highly anxious mothers could have greater genetic liability for anxiety and more susceptibility to treatment deterioration than other anxious youth.

Family factors have been shown to play an integral role in the development of conduct problems (Patterson et al., 1992) and in the prediction of treatment response. Higher parenting stress and depression scores among mothers, lower marital satisfaction, adverse child-rearing practices, dysfunctional family environment, single-parent family status, and lower SES are all associated with poorer response to parent management training (Dumas, 1984; Ruma et al., 1996; Webster-Stratton, 1985, 1990) and youth-focused cognitive-behavioral therapy (Kazdin & Crowley, 1997). Improved parenting over the course of treatment successfully mediates treatment response among young children (Beauchaine et al., 2005; Webster-Stratton et al., 2004) and indicates that treatment can successfully address critical aspects of family functioning.

Research on family processes and youth depression has revealed important longitudinal connections between parent-adolescent conflict, family adversity, and depressive outcomes (Sheeber et al., 2001). However, little research has been directed to family predictors of treatment response. Parent-adolescent conflict is a prominent treatment target in IPT for adolescent depression, but evidence regarding the potential impact of family conflict and parent psychopathology on outcomes in IPT has yet to be presented. There is some evidence that higher levels of psychosocial adversity predict poorer treatment response (Wood et al., 1996), and the fact that referred youth have been shown to respond less favorably than recruited youth could reflect differences in psychosocial adversity. Adversity represents a potentially critical variable for investigation in light of findings showing extremely high levels of stress among mothers of depressed youth, and in depressed youth themselves, who are treated in community outpatient clinics (Hammen et al., 1999). In a recent benchmark study of CBT for adolescent depression, Shirk, Crisp, Gudmundsen (under review) found that adolescent stress, but not parent-adolescent conflict, predicted treatment outcome. Parent-adolescent conflict should be assessed as a potential moderator of treatment response in future trials and as a potential treatment target in clinical practice.

What, then, are the implications for clinical practice? It is tempting to assume that the addition of a family component will uniformly enhance treatment outcomes. However, the literature is mixed relative to this assumption. For example, research supports the efficacy of a family component in the treatment of childhood anxiety (Barrett et al., 1996;

Cobham et al., 1998; Diamond & Josephson, 2005). However, the addition of a family component does not consistently improve outcomes and may only be relevant for families with highly anxious mothers (Barmish & Kendall, 2005) or with younger children (Barmish & Kendall, 2005; Barrett et al., 1996). The added benefit of a family component can be substantial. Cobham et al. (1998) reported that an individual child treatment with no family component worked *poorly* for families with anxious mothers such that only 37% of child clients improved, as opposed to 77% in treatment with a family component.

In the treatment of disruptive behavior problems, the inclusion of a family or parent component is strongly indicated. Several studies indicate that parent management training (PMT) in combination with individual CBT leads to more marked improvements than either approach alone (Dishion & Andrews, 1995; Webster-Stratton & Reid, 2003). Based on research demonstrating the robustness of PMT (as compared to child training and teacher training) across seven moderating variables of treatment outcome, Beauchaine (2005) suggests that PMT should be the base treatment for all children with conduct problems and that additional components should be added as needed. Parent treatment attendance and adherence may also require intervention for some families (Nock & Kazdin, 2005) if we are to recommend PMT for all youth with conduct problems.

Evidence is mixed for the inclusion of a family component in the treatment of adolescent depression. In a comparison of group CBT versus group CBT plus parent group, Clarke, Rohde, Lewinsohn, Hops, & Seeley (1999) did not find enhanced benefits in the parent augmented condition. In contrast, Brent et al. (1997) found that a family-focused intervention produced comparable outcomes as individually focused CBT for adolescent depression. Admittedly, the family components in these studies are quite different and suggest that involving parents per se may not enhance outcomes. At this point, research is needed to identify family character-istics that predict treatment response in IPT and CBT. With the identifi-cation of factors such as high criticism or conflict, specific family-focused interventions could be developed for recalcitrant cases.

Summary

As this review indicates, the identification of predictors of treatment response is in an early stage of development. Comorbidity, developmental factors, and family characteristics represent promising variables for further consideration. It is evident that these characteristics do not have a uniform effect across disorders, and existing research provides few clear guide-lines for the modification of evidence-based protocols. Although it may seem intuitive to customize and modify evidence-based protocols to fit specific characteristics of clients, there is virtually no evidence to support the superiority of customized over standardized treatments for youth. As evidence for predictors of treatment response emerges, guidelines for treatment modification and flexibility can be developed.

THERAPIST CHARACTERISTICS

The study of therapist effects has roots in the child and adolescent treatment literature. Over 30 years ago, Ricks (1974) contrasted the characteristics of an exceptional therapist, dubbed "supershrink," who worked with seriously troubled adolescents at a child guidance clinic with those of a less successful therapist. However, the provocative results of this early study failed to stimulate research on the characteristics of effective *therapists* in the child and adolescent literature. Instead, researchers have focused their attention on the search for effective *therapies* (APA, 1995).

The effort to identify EBTs is based on the assumption that technical procedures designed to remedy specific pathogenic processes in specific disorders are the core elements of the change process. In the logic of clinical trials, the therapist is assumed to be secondary to the procedures, rather than viewed as the central figure in the change process (Okiishi et al., 2003). Efforts are made to minimize variability due to differences in therapists through specific training, manualization, close supervision, and adherence checks. In fact, a review of therapist effects in the adult literature suggests that such effects are relatively limited when treatments are structured and monitored (Crits-Christoph & Mintz, 1991).

Not surprising then, research on therapist variables in child and adolescent therapy, especially in treatments based on evidence from clinical trials, is essentially missing. Yet therapist effects should not be neglected for two reasons: one methodological and one practical. When therapist effects are ignored in our statistical analyses, we essentially assume that the sampling of therapists has nothing to do with the observed differences in treatments. But if some therapists produce better outcomes than others, the sampling of therapists clearly makes a difference. In this case, differences between treatments could be a function of the sampling of therapists, and generalization to other therapists might not be warranted (Crits-Christoph & Mintz, 1991). Further, failure to consider therapist effects can lead to overestimation of treatment effects if therapists are not equally effective across conditions (Kenny & Judd, 1986). Thus, results from clinical trials should be evaluated for therapist effects, and the impact of therapists should be reported.

From a practical perspective, therapist effects are likely to swell as practitioners with different levels of training, experience, and supervision attempt to implement EBTs in clinical settings. In practice, the exact features of clinical trials that minimize therapist effects are typically limited or completely absent. Evidence indicates substantial therapist effects in routine clinical practice (Lambert & Okiishi, 1997; Okiishi et al., 2003), in less structured treatments (Crits-Christoph & Mintz, 1999), and among less experienced therapists (Perry & Howard, 1989). In some studies, therapist effects accounted for up to 50% of the outcome variance!

One of the only therapist characteristics to be examined in the child and adolescent literature has been level of therapist training. At first glance, the results appear to be counterintuitive. In their meta-analysis of 150 outcome studies, Weisz et al. (1995) found that paraprofessionals produced *larger* treatment effects than either students or full professionals. That is, treatment response appears to be inversely related to level of therapist training! Moreover, students and professionals did not differ in their efficacy. Although this pattern of results might be seen as an indictment of clinical training, Weisz et al. (1995) point out that most treatments delivered by paraprofessionals, such as parent management training, followed training and supervision provided by professionals. Similarly, student delivery of treatment typically is supervised by professionals. In addition, it is possible that professionals might be assigned more difficult cases than therapists with less experience or training. There were, in fact, two areas where therapist training appeared to enhance outcomes. Professionals generated larger effects than other therapists when treating internalizing problems, but not externalizing, and when treating adolescents. Although it is tempting to conclude that professional training is uniquely critical for adolescent internalizing problems, it is likely that the efficacy of parent and teacher management training for children with externalizing problems contributes to this pattern of results.

Given the paucity of research on therapist effects, and the potential importance of such variables in child clinical practice, what characteristics might be useful to consider in future studies? Two immediately come to mind: therapist competence and relational capacity. It seems obvious that competence should be related to outcomes, and substantial therapist differences in both the magnitude and rapidity of change point in this direction (Okiishi et al., 2003). Nevertheless, research on EBTs has focused almost exclusively on therapist *adherence* to treatment procedures or principles, despite evidence indicating that therapist competence predicts outcomes (Trepka et al., 2004).

Within the child treatment literature, Kendall and Chu (2000) have shown that therapists vary in how flexibly they deliver a manualized treatment. Similarly, it is quite likely that therapists vary in how competently they deliver prescribed treatment components, especially when components are relatively complex or demand nuanced application. For example, cognitive restructuring, an important component in the treatment of adolescent depression, can be done in a relatively mechanical way by encouraging teens to generate alternative views of situations or can involve the integration of metaphors and language that actively reframe particular events. In brief, therapist coverage of components is not equivalent to therapist competence in their delivery and requires a different measure for assessment.

A second therapist variable to consider is relational capacity. Substantial evidence indicates that relationship processes such as the therapeutic alliance are related to outcomes with both adult (Martin et al., 2000) and child clients (Shirk & Karver, 2003). In fact, in the child and adolescent literature, relationship variables predict outcomes in both manualized and nonmanualized therapies (Shirk & Karver, 2003). Although research has shown that client characteristics are related to alliance development (Eltz et al., 1995), it is likely that therapists differ in their ability to engage clients and maintain working relationships in therapy. An important question, then, is whether there are therapist effects in alliance formation. Given the association between alliance and outcome, such effects could account for variation in treatment response.

Summary

Research on the contribution of therapist characteristics to outcomes has paled in comparison to the focus on specific treatment protocols. It is likely, however, that therapist variables will contribute to outcomes under clinically representative conditions that involve limited supervision and monitoring. Consequently, the search for effective therapies should be complemented with investigations of effective therapists under clinically representative conditions. Examination of therapist competence and relational capacity represents a good starting point for these analyses.

TREATMENT CHARACTERISTICS

At the heart of research on treatment processes is the question, "What are the active ingredients of effective therapy?" That is, what are the components, processes, or interactions that contribute to beneficial effects? Given the multicomponent nature of most evidence-based treatments as well as the focus on evaluations of whole treatments, the field remains some distance from understanding what makes our evidence-based treatments work (Shirk & Karver, 2006). In fact, very few studies have formally evaluated mediators of change in child and adolescent therapy, and those that have have focused on changes in *pathogenic* processes rather than specific *treatment* processes (Shirk & Karver, 2006). Consequently, evidence for the active ingredients *within* effective therapies is very thin, indeed.

There are, however, a few studies that point in a promising direction. The first concerns the role of treatment adherence. Huey et al. (2000) examined the association between therapist adherence to treatment principles and changes in hypothesized pathogenic mechanisms—in this case, parental monitoring and delinquent peer affiliation—among youth treated with multisystemic therapy (MST). This study is unique in its linking of treatment processes to pathogenic mechanisms, and then mechanisms to treatment outcomes. In brief, therapist adherence to the MST protocol, measured from multiple participant perspectives, was predictive of changes in family functioning (family cohesion, parent monitoring) at the end of treatment. In turn, changes in family functioning were both directly and indirectly related to changes in delinquent behavior. Although therapist adherence had both a direct and an indirect association with outcome, adherence principally operated on delinquency through the more proximal mechanism of improved family functioning.

The study does have a number of limitations. First, the process variable was assessed during the fourth and sixth weeks of treatment; consequently, early change in treatment or initial family characteristics could be driving therapist adherence. Second, measures of change in pathogenic mechanisms did not precede measures of change in outcomes, thereby making it difficult to disentangle direction of effect. Nevertheless, the study is unique in the EBT literature in that it actually demonstrated associations among therapist adherence, pathogenic process, and treatment outcomes.

Complementing research on therapist behavior, several studies have addressed children's participation in therapy. Chu and Kendall (2004) evaluated the association between variations in child involvement and treatment outcome in CBT—Coping Cat—for anxious children. The level of child involvement in therapy was based on ratings of two 10-minute segments of therapy sessions. Raters coded child "enthusiasm for the task," "self-disclosure," "verbal initiation," and "verbal elaboration" as indicators of positive involvement. Negative involvement codes included "child withdrawal or passivity" and "child inhibition or avoidance." Good to excellent reliability was demonstrated for the *Child Involvement Rating Scale.* The level of child involvement measured at mid-treatment was predictive of positive treatment outcomes as indexed by the absence of an anxiety disorder diagnosis and by reductions in impairment. The *maintenance* of a working relationship that includes the child's active involvement may be as critical as, or more so than, the initial building of the relationship. As Chu and Kendall (2004) observe, "growing signs of withdrawal, avoidance, and diminished participation may signal to the therapist that strategies to re-engage the child may be required."

Consistent with the foregoing results, Shirk et al. (2003) reported associations between youth involvement, measured as collaboration with problem-solving training, and change in depressive symptoms in a small controlled trial with suicidal adolescents. A unique feature of this study involved the measurement of involvement in terms of adolescents' responses to a specific therapy task, namely, generating alternative solutions for social problems. This approach to assessing involvement has the advantage of gauging participation across different components of therapy.

These two studies suggest that a youngster's active involvement in therapy may be critical for beneficial outcomes, and they are consistent with results from the adult process research literature (Martin et al., 2000). The results also indicate that treatment involves more than passive exposure to a protocol, even one that is delivered with fidelity. Further, they point to an additional aspect of therapy dose, namely the degree to which the child or adolescent actively participates in treatment procedures presented by the therapist. In this respect, a more complex model of therapy dose involves both the degree to which a component is faithfully delivered *and* the degree to which the client is actively involved. To borrow from pharmacology, a dose is not simply a function of milligrams of active ingredient in a pill, but also involves patient compliance with taking the medication. Consequently, blood levels are a better indicator of therapeutic dose than the dispensed prescription.

To the degree that active involvement is essential for beneficial effects across EBTs, research on processes that promote or impede treatment involvement appears to be critical. Relatively little attention has been directed to this issue. Creed and Kendall (2005) examined a set of therapist behaviors hypothesized to promote or interfere with alliance formation during the first three sessions of CBT for anxious children. Child and therapist reports were used to assess the alliance at sessions 3 and 7. Child-reported alliance at session 3 was positively associated with therapist collaboration strategies including presenting therapy as a team effort, building a sense of togetherness by using words like "we," "us," and "let's," and helping the child set goals for treatment. "Pushing the child to talk" about anxiety and "emphasizing common ground," that is, where the therapist makes comments like "me too!" predicted weaker child-reported alliance. Efforts to push the child to talk about anxiety predicted a poor alliance at session 7 as well. For therapist-reported alliance, none of the therapist behaviors predicted alliance scores at session 3, but collaborative strategies predicted better alliances at session 7, and being "overly formal," that is, talking to the child in a way that is overly didactic, stuffy, or patronizing, predicted a weaker alliance. Other therapist behaviors were not predictive of child or therapist reports of alliance, including being playful, providing hope and encouragement, and general conversations.

Shirk et al. (2003) presented initial results linking therapist behaviors and early alliance in CBT for depressed adolescents who made a suicide attempt. To evaluate the therapist contribution to alliance formation, Shirk et al. (2003) proposed a heuristic model that organized therapist behaviors into four broad clusters: experience-focused, motivation-focused, negotiation-focused, and efficacy-focused interventions. Experience-focused interventions emphasize the provision of empathy, validation, and support and tend to focus on eliciting event descriptions and internal state responses. Motivation-focused interventions involve strategies for mobilizing the adolescent's intent to change and tend to involve eliciting self-motivating statements. Negotiation-focused interventions revolve around the establishment of treatment goals and linking these goals to treatment participation. Finally, efficacy-focused interventions involve establishing positive expectations for change, including the provision of a recovery model and statements about the utility of the treatment for adolescents.

Initial results based on coding the first two sessions of therapy for 22 depressed adolescents showed that the specific behavioral codes could be reliably rated but that some behaviors were quite rare, e.g., eliciting self-motivating statements. Of equal importance, close analysis of the tapes revealed a set of *therapist lapses* that occurred despite careful training of these doctoral-level therapists. Three lapses were identified: therapist criticizes; therapist fails to understand; and therapist fails to respond to expressed emotion. Although criticism was quite rare, the other two lapses were the best predictors of adolescent alliance at session 3. In brief, none of the positive alliance building behaviors reliably predicted strength of alliance, but both therapists' misunderstanding of adolescents' comments and therapists' failure to respond when teens expressed emotion were associated with poorer alliances.

Clearly, the results of both of these studies need to be replicated. However, they do suggest that successful engagement strategies may differ by age and disorder. Furthermore, both studies relied on a "frequency" approach to process in which the frequency or extensiveness of therapist behaviors are tallied and related to other variables. Alternatives to this approach should be considered. For example, Patterson and Forgatch (1985) evaluated the conditional probabilities of client resistance and therapist behaviors in parent management training, and Stoolmiller et al. (1993) showed that *patterns* of resistance over the course of treatment were better predictors of outcome than a static measure of early resistance. Examination of the context and pattern of therapist behaviors rather than frequency alone is likely to yield important insights into the engagement process.

Summary

Although the foregoing studies of therapy process illustrate promising directions, research on treatment variables is so slim that it is premature to speculate which treatment characteristics are critical for outcomes in EBTs. In fact, Jensen et al. (2005) have exposed the "soft" evidence base for many of our evidence-based treatments. Although these treatments uniformly beat waitlist controls in efficacy trials, evidence demonstrating clear benefits over equally intense control conditions is less compelling. In their review of studies that included comparable attention control groups that presumably did not contain active components of the evidence-based treatment, roughly half showed superior outcomes for evidence-based treatments. This "split decision" raises serious concerns about the potency of evidence-based treatments relative to generic therapies that include support, alliance, and attention. The absence of compelling evidence for *specific* treatment factors is startling and represents the most pressing question to be addressed by process researchers. Do EBTs loaded with *specific* treatment procedures actually outperform credible, but nontechnical, therapies with high levels of nonspecific factors such as alliance and rapport?

CONCLUSION

There has been substantial progress in the development and evaluation of efficacious treatments for child and adolescent disorders. Although much more work needs to be done to demonstrate the utility of EBTs under clinically representative conditions, progress has positioned the field for a new wave of studies on client, therapist, and treatment characteristics. Our review indicates that work in this area is at an early stage of development, with somewhat more research on client factors than therapist or treatment variables. Overall, the literature is somewhat piecemeal, not entirely consistent, and stocked with suggestive findings begging for replication. At this point, it is clearly premature to attempt to identify client, therapist, or treatment variables that consistently relate to outcome across different disorders. Although it is possible that a core set of variables will ultimately predict or moderate outcomes across disorders—for example, high levels of parental psychopathology might undermine treatment across disorders or factors that make for a "good" therapist hold across types of clients—at present it appears that these factors may be disorder-specific.

Systematic research on client, therapist, and treatment characteristics will be a sound investment for improving psychosocial treatments for youth. Identification of client characteristics that moderate treatment response provides the foundation for treatment adaptation. Similarly, identification of therapist characteristics carries important implications for the selection, training, and supervision of effective therapists. And finally, the identification of active treatment components provides the basis for "streamlining" therapies and maximizing impact. Advances in these areas are likely to be of great relevance to practitioners who need to tailor treatments to diverse clients, know when they are competent to treat a specific problem, and maximize the impact under time and resource constraints.

REFERENCES

American Psychological Association (1995). Training in and dissemination of empirically validated psychological treatments: Report and recommendations. *Clinical Psychologist, 48,* 3–27.

Barmish, A. J., & Kendall, P. C. (2005). Should parents be co-clients in cognitive-behavioral therapy for anxious youth? *Journal of Consulting & Clinical Psychology, 34*(3), 569–581.

Barrett, P., Rapee, R., Dadds, M., & Ryan, S. (1996). Family enhancement of cognitive styles in anxious and aggressive children. *Journal of Abnormal Child Psychology, 24,* 187–203.

Beauchaine, T. P. (2000). Comorbid depression and cardiac function as predictors of inpatient treatment response by conduct-disordered, ADHD boys. Poster session presented at the meeting of the Society for Research in Child Development.

Beauchaine, T. P., Webster-Stratton, C., & Reid, J. M. (2005). Mediators, moderators, and predictors of 1-year outcome among children treated for early-onset conduct problems: A latent growth curve analysis. *Journal of Consulting & Clinical Psychology, 73*(3), 371–388.

Berman, S. L., Weems, C. F., Silverman, W. K., & Kurtines, W. M. (2000). Predictors of outcome in exposure-based cognitive and behavioral treatments for phobic and anxiety disorders in children. *Behavior Therapy, 31,* 713–731.

Brent, D. A., Kolko, D. J., Birmaher, B., Baugher, M., Bridge, J., Roth, C., & Holder, D. (1998). Predictors of treatment efficacy in a clinical trial of three psychosocial treatments for adolescent depression. *Journal of the American Academy of Child & Adolescent Psychiatry, 37*(9), 906–914.

Chu, B., & Kendall, P. C. (2004). Positive association of child involvement and treatment outcome within a manual-based cognitive-behavioral treatment for children with anxiety. *Journal of Consulting & Clinical Psychology, 72*(5), 821–829.

Clarke, G., Rohde, P., Lewinsohn, P., Hops, H., & Seeley, J. (1999). Cognitive–behavioral group treatment of adolescent depression: Efficacy of acute treatment and booster sessions. *Journal of the American Academy of Child and Adolescent Psychiatry, 38,* 272–279.

Cobham, V., Dadds, M., & Spence, S. (1998). The role of parental anxiety in the treatment of childhood anxiety. *Journal of Consulting & Clinical Psychology, 66,* 893–905.

Creed, T., & Kendall, P. C. (2005). Therapist alliance building behavior within a cognitive-behavioral treatment for anxiety in youth. *Journal of Consulting & Clinical Psychology*, *73*, 498–505.

Crits-Christoph, P., & Mintz, J. (1991). Implications of therapist effects for the design and analysis of comparative studies of psychotherapies. *Journal of Consulting & Clinical Psychology*, *50*(1), 20–26.

Diamond, G., & Josephson, A. (2005). Family-based treatment research: A 10-year update. *Journal of the American Academy of Child & Adolescent Psychiatry*, *44*(9), 872–888.

Dishion, T. J., & Andrews, D. W. (1995). Preventing escalation in problem behaviors with high-risk young adolescents: Immediate and 1-year outcomes. *Journal of Consulting & Clinical Psychology*, *63*, 538–548.

Dishion, T. J., & Patterson, G. R. (1992). Age effects in parent training outcome. *Behavior Therapy*, *23*, 719–729.

Dumas, J. E. (1984). Interactional correlates of treatment outcome in behavioral parent training. *Journal of Consulting & Clinical Psychology*, *52*(6), 946–954.

Durlak, J., Fuhrman, T., & Lampman, C. (1991). Effectiveness of cognitive-behavioral therapy for maladapting children: A meta-analysis. *Psychological Bulletin*, *110*, 204–214.

Eltz, M., Shirk, S., & Sarlin, N. (1995). Alliance formation and treatment outcomes among maltreated adolescents. *Child Abuse and Neglect*, *19*, 419–431.

Fonagy, P., Target, M., Cottrell, D., Phillips, J., & Kurtz, Z. (2002). *What Works for Whom? A Critical Review of Treatments for Children and Adolescents*. New York: Guilford Press.

Hammen, C., Rudolph, K., Weisz, J., Rao, U., & Burge, D. (1999). The context of depression in clinic-referred youth: Neglected areas in treatment. *Journal of the American Academy of Child & Adolescent Psychiatry*, *38*(1), 64–71.

Hartman, R. R., Stage, S. A., & Webster-Stratton, C. (2003). A growth curve analysis of parent training outcomes: Examining the influence of child risk factors (inattention, impulsivity, and hyperactivity problems), parental and family risk factors. *Journal of Child Psychology and Psychiatry*, *44*(3), 388–398.

Hinshaw, S. P. (1992). Externalizing behavior problems and academic underachievement in childhood and adolescence: Causal relationships and underlying mechanisms. *Psychological Bulletin*, *111*, 127–155.

Hinshaw, S. P., & Melnick, S. M. (1995). Peer relationships in boys with attention-deficit hyperactivity disorder with and without comorbid aggression. *Development & Psychopathology*, *7*, 627–647.

Huey, S., Henggeler, S., & Brondino, M. (2000). Mechanisms of change in multisystemic therapy: Reducing delinquent behavior through therapist adherence and improved family and peer functioning. *Journal of Consulting & Clinical Psychology*, *68*, 451–467.

Jensen, P. S., Weersing, R. V., Hoagwood, K. E., & Goldman, E. (2005). What is the evidence for evidence-based treatments? A hard look at our soft underbelly. *Mental Health Services Research*, *7*(1), 53–74.

Kendall, P. C., Brady, E. U., & Verduin, T. L. (2001). Comorbidity in childhood anxiety disorders and treatment outcome. *Journal of the American Academy of Child & Adolescent Psychiatry*, *40*(7), 787–794.

Kendall, P. C., & Chu, B. (2000). Retrospective self-reports of therapist flexibility in a manual-based treatment for youths with anxiety disorders. *Journal of Clinical Child Psychology*, *29*(2), 209–220.

Kendall, P. C., Flannery-Schroeder, E. C., Panichelli-Mindel, S. M., Southam-Gerow, M. A., Henin, A., & Warman, M. (1997). Therapy for youths with anxiety disorders: A second randomized clinical trial. *Journal of Consulting & Clinical Psychology*, *65*(3), 366–380.

Kenny, D. A., & Judd, C. M. (1986). Consequences for violating the independence assumption in analysis of variance. *Psychological Bulletin*, *99*(3), 422–431.

Lambert, M., & Okiishi, J. (1997). The effects of the individual psychotherapist and implications for future research. *Clinical Psychology: Science and Practice*, *4*(1), 66–75.

Lynam, D. R., Caspi, M., T. E., Wikstrom, P. H., Loeber, R., & Novak, S. (2000). The interaction between impulsivity and neighborhood context on offending: The effects of impulsivity are stronger in poorer neighborhoods. *Journal of Abnormal Child Psychology*, *109*, 563–574.

Nigg, J. T., & Huang-Pollock, C. L. (2003). An early-onset model of the role of executive functions and intelligence in conduct disorder/delinquency. In B. B. Lahey, T. E. Moffitt,

& A. Caspi (Eds.), *Causes of Conduct Disorder and Juvenile Delinquency* (pp. 227–253). New York: Guilford Press.

Nock, M. K., & Kazdin, A. E. (2005). Randomized controlled trial of a brief intervention for increasing participation in parent management training. *Journal of Consulting & Clinical Psychology, 73*(5), 872–879.

Okiishi, J., Lambert, M., Nielsen, S. L., & Ogles, B. M. (2003). Waiting for supershrink: An empirical analysis of therapist effects. *Clinical Psychology and Psychotherapy, 10*(6), 361–373.

Patterson, G., & Forgatch, M. (1985). Therapist behavior as a determinant of client noncompliance: A paradox for the behavior modifier. *Journal of Consulting & Clinical Psychology, 53*, 846–851.

Perry, K., & Howard, K. (1989). Therapist effects: The search for the therapist contribution to psychotherapy outcome. Paper presented at meeting of the Society for Psychotherapy Research, Toronto, Canada, June.

Ricks, D. (1974). Supershrink: Methods of a therapist judged to be successful on the basis of adult outcomes of adolescent patients. In D. Ricks, M. Rott, & A. Thomas (Eds.), *Life History Research in Psychopathology* (pp. 275–297). Minneapolis: University of Minnesota Press.

Rohde, P., Clarke, G., & Lewinsohn, P. M. (2001). Impact of comorbidity on a cognitive-behavioral group treatment for adolescent depression. *Journal of the American Academy of Child & Adolescent Psychiatry, 40*(7), 795–802.

Rohde, P., Clarke, G. N., Mace, D. E., Jorgensen, J. S., & Seeley, J. R. (2004). An efficacy/effectiveness study of cognitive-behavioral treatment for adolescents with comorbid major depression and conduct disorder. *Journal of the American Academy of Child & Adolescent Psychiatry, 43*(6), 660–668.

Ruma, P. R., Burke, R. V., & Thompson, R. W. (1996). Group parent training: Is it effective for children of all ages? *Behavior Therapy, 27*(2), 159–169.

Sheeber, L., Hops, H., & Davis, B. (2001). Family processes in adolescent depression. *Clinical Child and Family Psychology Review, 4*, 19–35.

Shirk, S. R., & Karver, M. (2003). Prediction of treatment outcome from relationship variables in child and adolescent therapy. *Journal of Consulting & Clinical Psychology, 71*, 462–471.

Shirk, S. R., & Karver, M. (2006). Process issues in cognitive-behavioral therapy for youth. In P. Kendall (Ed.), *Child and Adolescent Therapy: Cognitive-Behavioral Procedures* (pp. 465–491). New York: Guilford Press.

Shirk, S., Karver, M., & Spirito, A. (2003). Relationship processes in youth CBT: Measuring alliance and collaboration. Paper presented at meeting of the Association for the Advancement of Behavior Therapy, Boston, August.

Shirk, S., Crisp, H., & Gudmundsen, G. (Under review). Benchmarking School-based CBT for adolescent depression.

Southam-Gerow, M. A., Kendall, P. C., & Weersing, R. V. (2001). Examining outcome variability: Correlates of treatment response in a child and adolescent anxiety clinic. *Journal of Consulting and Clinical Psychology, 30*(3), 422–436.

Southam-Gerow, M. A., Weisz, J. R., & Kendall, P. C. (2003). Youth with anxiety disorders in research and service clinics: Examining client differences and similarities. *Journal of Clinical Child and Adolescent Psychology, 32*(3), 375–385.

Stoolmiller, M., Duncan, T., Bank, L., & Patterson, G. (1993). Some problems and solutions to the study of change: Significant patterns of client resistance. *Journal of Consulting & Clinical Psychology, 61*, 920–928.

Trepka, C., Rees, A., Shapiro, D. A., Hardy, G. E., & Barkham, M. (2004). Therapist competence and outcome of cognitive therapy for depression. *Cognitive Therapy and Research, 28*(2), 143–157.

Webster-Stratton, C. (1985). Predictors of treatment outcome in parent training for conduct disordered children. *Behavior Therapy, 16*(2), 223–243.

Webster-Stratton, C. (1990). Long-term follow-up of families with young conduct problem children: From preschool to grade school. *Journal of Clinical Child Psychology, 19*, 144–149.

Webster-Stratton, C. (1996). Early-onset conduct problems: Does gender make a difference? *Journal of Consulting & Clinical Psychology, 64*(3), 540–551.

Webster-Stratton, C., & Reid, J. M. (2003). *The Incredible Years Parents, Teachers and Children Training Series*. New York: Guilford Press.

Webster-Stratton, C., Reid, J. M., & Hammond, M. (2004). Treating children with early-onset conduct problems: Intervention outcomes for parent, child and teacher training. *Journal of Clinical Child and Adolescent Psychology, 33*(1), 105–124.

Weisz, J. R. (2004). *Psychotherapy for Children and Adolescents*. Cambridge: Cambridge University Press.

Weisz, J., Weiss, B., Han, S. S., & Granger, D. A. (1995). Effects of psychotherapy with children and adolescents revisited: A meta-analysis of treatment outcome studies. *Psychological Bulletin, 117*(3), 450–468.

Wood, A., Harrington, R., & Moore, A. (1996). Controlled trial of a brief cognitive-behavioral intervention in adolescent patients with depressive disorders. *Journal of Child Psychology and Psychiatry, 37*(6), 737–746.

27

Implementing Evidence-Based Treatments with Ethnically Diverse Clients

BETH A. KOTCHICK and RACHEL L. GROVER

The utility and validity of evidence-based treatments (EBTs) for families and clients of ethnic minority status have been the topics of spirited dialogue since the publication of practice guidelines based on the findings of the Division of Clinical Psychology (Division 12) of the American Psychological Association Task Force on Promotion and Dissemination of Psychological Procedures (1995; Chambless et al., 1996). The central issue in this debate is whether those therapies deemed efficacious by virtue of meeting the criteria set forth by this task force[1] are indeed universally valid for all clients with a specific presenting problem, regardless of ethnic, cultural, or socioeconomic background. As noted by Bernal and Scharron-del-Rio (2001), the studies used to develop the list of treatments originally proposed as having the most empirical support for their efficacy paid little, if any, attention to cultural diversity, with participants being almost exclusively European-American, middle-class, and English-speaking. As a result, the

---

[1] The Division 12 Task Force on Psychological Interventions criteria for a "well-established" treatment include at least two between-group design experiments conducted by different research teams that demonstrate that treatment is more beneficial than a rival treatment or placebo control. Treatments may also qualify as well established if at least nine well-designed single-case experiments find that the treatment is superior to an alternative treatment. Other criteria include the use of a treatment manual and clearly defined client samples. Treatments may be qualified as "probably efficacious" with at least two studies demonstrating superiority to an untreated control group or at least three single-case design experiments (Chambless & Hollon, 1998).

BETH A. KOTCHICK and RACHEL L. GROVER • Loyola College in Maryland

generalizability of findings regarding treatment efficacy to clients of ethnic minority status has been called into question (Hall, 2001).

The purpose of this chapter is to provide a context in which to digest and interpret the ongoing conversation regarding diversity and empiricism in evidence-based practice. We first summarize some of the key arguments against the unqualified use of treatments deemed efficacious solely according to the established empirical criteria with clients of diverse ethnic and social class backgrounds. Second, we discuss the "next steps" needed to more adequately address questions of cultural validity for evidence-based practices in child clinical psychology. Third, we review how two commonly utilized evidence-based treatments—parent training for noncompliant behavior and cognitive-behavioral therapy for anxiety—may be influenced by cultural factors, and we discuss how issues of diversity have been addressed within those interventions in clinical research and practice. Finally, we offer guidelines for clinicians who wish to use EBTs with children and families from diverse ethnic and sociocultural backgrounds.

A CRITIQUE OF TREATMENT OUTCOME RESEARCH WITH ETHNIC MINORITIES

Critics of the movement to identify empirically supported treatment guidelines highlight several issues that may limit the utility and validity of EBTs for cultural minorities. As previously noted, the lack of diversity within the samples on which efficacy trials were conducted for most of the empirically supported treatments identified by the Division 12 Task Force severely limits the external validity of their findings. Bernal and Scharron-del-Rio (2001) contend "that having a list of treatments for a specific disorder considered to be established in efficacy … that were actually based on predominantly White, middle-class, English-speaking women is of questionable use for ethnic minorities" and go on to note that there is little, if any, evidence to suggest that such therapies are "appropriate, even efficacious, for communities of color" (p. 329).

Advocates of EBTs, while acknowledging these limitations, would argue that the principles and methods upon which manualized treatment programs are based are universally valid, and thus, treatments that have demonstrated efficacy with European-American clients or families should be equally as effective with ethnic minority groups (Hall, 2001). The fact remains, however, that few studies have investigated that contention. In practice, clinical scientists and therapists are often caught between assuming *either* that treatments found to be efficacious for European-American, middle-class populations will also be efficacious for ethnically diverse populations and within varied socioeconomic contexts because the essential ingredients of those therapies are universally effective agents of change *or* that without cultural validation and/or modification, those ingredients are not likely to effect therapeutic change for clients who differ in cultural background from those on whom the treatment was initially developed and tested.

Proponents of the latter assumption argue that there are many reasons why culture, ethnicity, and socioeconomic status should have an important impact on the treatment of emotional and behavioral problems among children, adolescents, and families. First, culture has a profound impact on the conceptualization of psychopathology and the definition of abnormal or problematic behavior. Simply put, what is considered acceptable behavior in one cultural context may be considered pathological in another context (Hall, 2001). Second, culture and ethnicity play an important role in how interventions are received and implemented, which ultimately affects their efficacy. For example, minority clients are less likely to access mental health services (National Institute of Mental Health, 1999; Surgeon General, 2000) as well as more likely to end treatment prematurely (Sue & Sue, 1990). Further, there is some evidence to suggest that, overall, ethnic minorities experience worse outcomes in psychotherapy than do European-American clients (Lam & Sue, 2001). One explanation for these findings is that conceptualizations of problems and their prescribed interventions are likely not sensitive to cultural and ethnic factors and thus fail to engage ethnic minority families successfully (Wong et al., 2003).

Third, ethnicity is often confounded with socioeconomic status. As a disproportionate number of ethnic minorities also live in poverty, many of the findings regarding ethnic group differences in service utilization and treatment outcome are more accurately conceptualized as being related to financial means, not ethnicity per se. Poverty is a key obstacle to effective psychological intervention for children (e.g., Dumas & Wahler, 1983), and considerable attention has been devoted to making treatment more accessible to lower-income families, including offering flexible times and locations for services, as well as transportation and child care (e.g., Reid et al., 2001).

Simple comparisons of treatment utilization and response across ethnic groups, however, still obscure the psychological constructs or processes that serve as the mechanisms through which these group differences across ethnicities emerge and which may offer a better explanation for any ethnic differences found in studies of treatment efficacy (Wong et al., 2003). For example, Hall (2001) highlighted *interdependence*, *spirituality*, and *discrimination* as three important constructs that may differentiate ethnic minority from majority persons in the United States and highlighted how they might influence the therapeutic process. According to Bernal and Scharron-del-Rio (2001), most of the traditional, mainstream treatment approaches (which would include those deemed empirically supported and efficacious) are based on individualistic values, rather than interdependence, and thus may not resonate with persons of ethnic minority cultures. Likewise, issues relating to spirituality or the experience of discrimination, both of which may play crucial roles in therapy with ethnic minority clients, often are not addressed in manualized treatments developed on and for a nonminority client population.

The great variability that exists within cultures also must not be overlooked. Individuals and families within a particular ethnic group vary along several dimensions, which would affect how they respond to therapeutic interventions, including allegiance to cultural values and history, acculturation and assimilation within the mainstream culture, experiences of discrimination, emphasis on religion and spirituality, financial resources, and access to support and services. It is likely, then, that therapies found to be efficacious for middle-class European-Americans will be the most effective for ethnic minority clients who are most similar to that reference group: those who are more acculturated and less strongly identified with their ethnic group, more educated, English-speaking, and not impoverished (Hall, 2001).

Although proponents of evidence-based practice do not disagree with the importance of cultural factors, the fact remains that very little research that focuses on ethnic or socioeconomic diversity has met the rigorous criteria set by the Division 12 Task Force, and thus few treatments developed for minority clients are formally designated as being empirically supported (Hall, 2001). In the absence of such evidence, the Task Force has made the recommendation that the treatments found to be efficacious with majority clients be used with ethnic minorities. As noted by Bernal and Scharron-del-Rio (2001), despite being well-intentioned, this recommendation is inherently contradictory: "One the one hand, the agenda is to disseminate the available ESTs on the basis of their empirical support. On the other hand, in the absence of data of their generalization, the call is to make a leap of faith and use these treatments in the belief that they will work as well with everyone else including ethnic minorities" (p. 331).

MAKING EVIDENCE-BASED PRACTICE MORE CULTURALLY RELEVANT

Clearly, there is a need to incorporate culture, ethnicity, and socioeconomic diversity into scientific and clinical discussions of treatment outcome research. Several points of consideration for practitioners who wish to implement empirically supported treatments with culturally diverse clients are provided at the end of this chapter. We turn now to a brief discussion of what clinical researchers can do to advance the scientific study of therapy and extend the validity of findings to more diverse client populations.

Most importantly, research is desperately needed to determine which therapies are most effective in treating childhood disorders among ethnic minority populations. Simply including more ethnic minorities in clinical trials would represent a step toward improving external validity and would be in keeping with public policy attempts to address ethnic disparities in mental health and access to treatment (Hohmann & Parron, 1996, as cited in Hall, 2001). However, including more ethnic minorities in clinical trials does not adequately address the complex questions of cultural validity and would not likely generate the sample sizes needed to evaluate ethnicity as a potential moderator of treatment outcome. To do so, comparison of treatment efficacy across ethnic groups must be an explicit goal of research and thus requires targeted recruitment of participants of various ethnicities and cultural identities.

Several criteria have been developed to guide the study of treatment efficacy across diverse ethnic groups (see Sue, 1998). Such criteria require that (1) pre- and posttreatment data be collected from clients from two or more ethnic groups, (2) clients from all ethnic groups be randomly assigned to treatment conditions, (3) multiple and culturally cross-validated measures of outcome be used, and (4) treatment type be crossed with ethnicity when comparisons of outcomes by treatment and ethnicity are made (Sue, 1998, as cited in Hall, 2001). Thus, one possible method for addressing the utility of currently available therapies with ethnic minorities would be to conduct trials that directly compare treatment outcome across diverse ethnic groups. An alternative method would be to test therapies, as they were developed and manualized with nonminority populations, with culturally diverse clients and determine whether outcomes achieved are similar to those obtained with European-American clients.

As noted previously, however, examining ethnicity as a potential moderator of treatment outcome does not speak to *how* a given treatment approach works, or fails to work, within a specific ethnic minority population (Hall, 2001). For example, a clinical trial that finds a given treatment to be more successful for one ethnic group than for another offers little explanation of why those differences emerged and obscures the great variability within cultural groups. More informative would be research that identifies relevant predictors of outcome or change within each ethnic group, such as ethnic identity, acculturation, discrimination experiences, socioeconomic status, symptom severity, comorbidity, and other factors related to the process of psychotherapy.

A different approach involves the development of new treatments designed specifically for clients of a given ethnic group based on cultural theory and research. An excellent example of this approach is *Cuento therapy*, an intervention for Puerto Rican children exhibiting maladaptive behavior in school (Costantino et al., 1986). The therapy uses *cuentos*, or cultural folktales, to model adaptive behavior and promote healthy coping strategies. Developed exclusively for Puerto Rican children and delivered by bilingual therapists from the local community, Cuento therapy represents one of the few culturally specific treatments that have been empirically evaluated and qualifies as a "probably efficacious therapy" (Lam & Sue, 2001).

A compromise between using empirically supported therapies designed for a nonminority population and developing culturally specific therapies designed for a specific ethnic minority population is to tailor or modify existing therapies to meet the needs of culturally diverse clients (Hall, 2001). Such an approach would include the key components of an empirically supported treatment but would make modifications to the materials or methods used to deliver the intervention so that it is packaged in a more culturally relevant manner (e.g., Barrett et al., 1996; Martinez & Eddy,

2005). For example, Barrett et al. (1996) modified a child anxiety treatment manual used in the United States (i.e., Coping Cat; Kendall, 2002) for use in Australia by adapting the examples and pictures in the workbooks to represent Australian culture while still preserving the core cognitive-behavioral therapy components. Very likely, this is the approach taken by many clinicians in their practice of psychotherapy with diverse clients; however, relatively little empirical investigation of cultural modification of evidence-based practice has been conducted.

Finally, in order to further advance the field, clinical scientists need to reevaluate their reliance on randomized controlled trials (RCT) in treatment outcome research. As described by Steele, Mize Nelson, and Nelson (Chapter 3), the very features of RCT that result in high internal validity by controlling or eliminating potential confounds that could account for differences between groups on outcome measures severely limit external and ecological validity, or the degree to which the results of the study could be expected to generalize to clients, settings, and situations beyond the confines of the research lab (Levant, 2004). Certainly, this is one of the key arguments against the universal application of treatments developed and evaluated with one ethnic group (most often European Americans) to clients of other ethnic backgrounds. But this criticism extends far beyond culture; essentially, treatment outcome research typically says little about how various treatments would work for real clients, in the real world, as utilized by real practitioners (Levant, 2004; Deegear & Lawson, 2003).

In contrast, effectiveness trials present clinical researchers with an opportunity to evaluate whether an intervention is likely to be beneficial for "typical" clients under "ordinary practice conditions" (Weisz & Jensen, 2001, p. 1/12). Relative to the number of studies that have examined the efficacy of various child and adolescent therapies using an RCT approach, very few effectiveness trials have been conducted and the results have not been promising (Weisz & Jensen, 2001). Generally speaking, effectiveness studies reveal that most of the treatments found to be efficacious in the laboratory have a negligible effect when implemented under typical community circumstances (Weisz & Jensen, 2001). Such disappointing findings highlight the important contribution that "real life"—which, for minority clients, would include ethnic identity and acculturation, racism, and socioeconomic stressors—makes to the success or failure of therapy. Further research on the factors that affect effectiveness in the field would greatly enhance the scope of empirical evidence by which therapies are judged to be "evidence-based" or "empirically supported."

CULTURAL DIVERSITY AND EVIDENCE-BASED PRACTICE WITH CHILDREN: TWO EXAMPLES

In order to examine further the complexity of applying EBTs to diverse clients, we present two examples of how issues related to ethnicity or culture may influence the delivery and efficacy of commonly used empirically supported therapies. Parent training and cognitive-behavioral therapy for childhood anxiety are frequently used manualized EBTs; thus, the efficacy of their use with ethnically diverse clients is of paramount clinical importance.

Parent Training

As noted by McMahon and Kotler (Chapter 13), "behavioral parent training" has been established as an efficacious therapy for children with externalizing behavior problems. Despite being the primary intervention for families raising "strong-willed" children (Forehand & Long, 2002), parent training has been criticized for its lack of attention to culture (Forehand & Kotchick, 1996). Parent training, and the conceptual models of parenting on which it is based, were developed with mostly middle-class families of European-American descent. Relatively little is known about the effectiveness of parent training with particular ethnic groups or about which factors best predict success in parent training with ethnically diverse populations (Kotchick et al., 2003). Even less empirical attention has been devoted to the development of culturally informed parenting programs (Martinez & Eddy, 2005).

Culture and ethnicity are part of the broader social, economic, and historical context in which children are raised and, as such, have a large impact on childrearing values and practices. Cross-cultural research documents the ways in which cultural values, heritage, and traditions shape the competencies that are valued in children within a particular cultural niche and the parenting strategies designed to promote them (Harkness & Super, 1995; Ogbu, 1981). Within Western industrialized societies, a long history of research has documented how authoritative parenting practices characterized by positive reinforcement, open displays of warmth or affection, active monitoring of children's activities, and consistent but not overly harsh disciplinary strategies relate to various measures of adaptive child psychosocial adjustment, including academic competence, high self-esteem, positive peer relations, and fewer child behavior problems (e.g., Baumrind, 1978; Patterson et al., 1992).

It is upon these empirical foundations that parent training was developed. As such, the skills taught in parent training are those that foster authoritative parenting styles. Subsequent parenting research, however, has revealed that one size does not necessarily fit all when it comes to effective parenting. For example, several studies have noted that authoritarian parenting, characterized by high levels of parental control and discipline, has been found to have positive effects for some African-American (e.g., Lamborn et al., 1996) and Asian-American youth (Chao, 1996). It is likely, then, that the key parenting skills emphasized in traditional parent training programs may actually be inconsistent with the parenting norms or expectations among some ethnic minorities.

The experience of discrimination faced by ethnic minorities in a multicultural society such as the United States is another factor likely to have a profound influence on parenting, yet these experiences are rarely addressed in the context of parent training (Coard et al., 2004).

Ward (2000, as cited by Coard et al., 2004) proposes that part of the parenting role within African-American families is to help children understand and deal with the hostility, prejudice, and discrimination they face as an ethnic minority within American society. African-American parents use various "racial socialization" strategies to help protect and teach children how to succeed (Coard et al., 2004). However, these parenting strategies may be at odds with some of the methods and principles espoused by parent training. For example, African-American parents report more frequent use of spanking than parents of other ethnic backgrounds (e.g., Bradley et al., 2001). Several authors suggest that African-American parents, particularly those from a lower socioeconomic background, use physical discipline to foster obedience and respect for authority, values that may protect children from dangers in their environment and promote their chances for survival and success in a cultural context marked by great disparity in the power held by minority and majority persons (Kelly et al., 1992). Parent training, on the other hand, generally discourages the use of physical punishment and instead promotes the use of alternative methods of discipline, including positive reinforcement of desirable behavior, ignoring minor undesirable behavior, and using time out as a form of punishment (McMahon & Forehand, 2003). Implementing these techniques with minority families who traditionally rely on more physical means of discipline without discussion of their beliefs regarding the role of discipline in their cultural history and personal experiences is virtually doomed to fail and represents a concrete example of how evidence-based practices may not generalize to minority populations without some cultural adaptation.

Because culture has such an important influence on parenting, it seems logical, if not essential, that cultural factors be considered when designing and implementing parenting interventions (Forehand & Kotchick, 1996). Yet, little empirical attention has been devoted to exactly how parent training may be modified to be more culturally specific. In one of the earlier examples found in the literature, parent training was modified to be "more culturally and contextually appopropriate" for African-American parents in a program called Effective Black Parenting (Myers et al., 1992, p. 133). The program, created by Alvy (1987), situates behavioral parent training techniques within a group intervention that highlights the unique historical and cultural context of African-American parenting and family life. For example, a module entitled "The Meaning of Disciplining Children: Traditional Black Discipline Versus Modern Black Self-Discipline" considers the historical context of physical discipline within African-American culture and offers a rationale for why alternative discipline strategies may better prepare children within current society. As Alvy (1987) wrote, "By moving black parents toward a modern perspective they will be more inclined to utilize the parenting skills from the standard [parenting] programs" (p. 136). In addition, Effective Black Parenting openly discusses the current and historical experiences of discrimination and oppression experienced by African Americans. The program explicitly focuses on instilling "pride in Blackness" as an important parenting goal and offers parents guidance on how to communicate with their children about issues such as ethnic identity and how to cope with racism (Myers et al., 1992). Several techniques employed in the program are also clearly culturally referenced, such as the use of a group discussion technique similar to the call-and-response interchange that characterizes many African-American church services (Alvy, 1987).

To evaluate the short- and long-term effectiveness of the Effective Black Parenting program, Myers and colleagues (1992) compared scores on measures of family functioning, parenting practices, and child behavior at pre-, post-, and one-year follow-up for two cohorts of families who were nonrandomly assigned to either the treatment or control condition. Results indicated that participation in the program was associated with improvements in parent-child relationships, increases in the use of praise and decreases in the use of spanking, and some reductions in externalizing behavior problems for both boys and girls. However, the results were inconsistent across cohorts, and most short-term gains were not sustained one year later. It should also be noted that the program was developed and tested as a prevention program, not as an intervention for youth already experiencing clinically significant levels of behavior problems, which may contribute to the subtlety and instability of the results. Still, the findings suggest that parent training programs can be modified to be more culturally relevant without compromising fidelity to the basic tenets and techniques of the original intervention.

More recently, *Nuestras Familias: Anadand Entre Culturas* (Our Families: Moving Between Cultures) was developed as a parent training program designed for Spanish-speaking immigrant parents (Martinez & Eddy, 2005). The Nuestras Familias intervention is grounded in both social learning theory, upon which traditional parent training approaches are based, and ecodevelopmental theory (Szapocznik & Coatsworth, 1999), which emphasizes the interaction between various systems and contexts (e.g., culture, community, family, peers) in the development of youth problem behavior. Acculturation is also emphasized as a process that plays an important role in the development of youth problem behavior as well as in the effectiveness of parent training techniques (Martinez & Eddy, 2005). In a randomized controlled trial with 73 Latino families having a child in middle school, Martinez and Eddy (2005) found that their culturally adapted parent training program produced significant improvements in parents' use of "effective" parenting practices, which included positive parental involvement, monitoring, engagement in the child's homework and schooling, and appropriate discipline, as compared to a no-treatment control group. Youth externalizing and substance abuse outcomes were likewise improved for those children whose parents participated in the parenting program. Children's nativity status (i.e., whether or not they were born in the United States) moderated several outcomes, with most findings highlighting the added risk associated with being born in the United States. The authors speculated that parenting children born in the United States poses several challenges for immigrant parents who may differ from their children in terms of ethnic identity and acculturation (Martinez &

Eddy, 2005). Such findings underscore the complex role culture plays in parenting and, in turn, in working with parents of troubled youth.

Perhaps more enlightening than the outcome results, however, is the delineation of the process by which Martinez and Eddy (2005) modified traditional parent training to be more culturally relevant for Latino immigrant parents. These authors described a two-year collaboration among parent training researchers, Latino family intervention researchers, a state social service agency serving Latino clients, and other community partners in which empirically supported intervention components from the parent training literature were adapted to more specifically address the needs and experiences of Latino parents, and new components or content areas were added to enhance the relevance of the program for Latino immigrant families. Cultural adaptation was described as a two-part process—first, the collaborative team considered whether a process or skill was theoretically relevant (e.g., whether contingent positive reinforcement was an appropriate strategy to encourage prosocial behavior). Next, they considered whether the technique or method used to teach that skill was culturally relevant (e.g., didactic instruction, modeling, role-play). The adapted intervention was then presented to focus groups of Latino parents and further modified based on their feedback concerning the program's relevance, salience, and cultural validity (Martinez & Eddy, 2005).

The development, evaluation, and dissemination of culturally specific parenting programs certainly represent an important next step in the cultural validation of parent training. However, there still remains a lack of research that suggests that all evidence-based treatments, such as parent training, *must* be culturally adapted in order to be effective with ethnic minority clients. As noted by Martinez and Eddy (2005) in their discussion of their findings, positive results for culturally specific treatments alone (relative to a nontreated control group) do not indicate whether similarly positive outcomes would have been achieved if families had participated in an intervention that had not been culturally adapted. Research that directly compares culturally adapted treatment to nonadapted treatment for a particular ethnic minority population is needed to address the question of whether cultural adaptation is required for efficacious intervention. Indeed, there is evidence to suggest that parent training, presented as a culturally universal program (as opposed to culturally specific), may be effective with ethnic minority families, at least in the prevention of conduct problems among high-risk children. Reid and colleagues (2001) evaluated the effectiveness of the Incredible Years Parenting Program among a sample of low-income, multi-ethnic families with a child enrolled in Head Start. All materials (e.g., video vignettes of parent-child interactions, written documents) were designed to represent multiple cultural backgrounds, and all parents attending the program were exposed to the same content, regardless of ethnicity. Cultural relevance and sensitivity were fostered by open collaboration between parents and group facilitators during goal setting and program solving, so that issues related to ethnicity were addressed uniquely for each parent in the group. Reid et al. (2003, p. 210) noted, "In this way, generic content can be individualized to fit with the specific experiences and backgrounds of group members, without the need for different curricula for participants of different backgrounds." Ethnic differences in treatment response were limited and did not exceed the number expected by chance; thus, the authors concluded that the Incredible Years program was universally valid for families of diverse backgrounds.

Cognitive-Behavioral Treatment for Childhood Anxiety

Anxiety disorders[2] remain one of the most common psychological disorders in childhood and are associated with significant concurrent and long-term impairment in academic, social, and psychological domains of functioning (see Silverman & Ginsburg, 1998, for review). In response, the last decade has seen an increase in the development, empirical evaluation, and widespread availability of evidence-based manualized cognitive-behavioral therapies (CBT) focused on ameliorating anxiety symptoms and behaviors in children (Silverman & Piña, Chapter 5). Empirical support for the efficacy of CBT for anxiety disorders in children is quite substantial, with a recent systematic review of 10 randomized controlled trials yielding evidence that CBT was over three times more effective than no treatment (Cartwright-Hatton et al., 2004). One weakness in this otherwise strong body of literature, however, is the relative lack of studies that include minority participants. Thus, the efficacy of CBT for childhood anxiety in minority populations is currently unclear. The small body of literature that examines the efficacy of CBT for anxious youth across ethnic and cultural groups is promising; however, additional research is needed to qualify the treatment as "efficacious" for minority groups.

Treatment research comparing CBT for anxious youth across diverse samples was spurred by early findings of differences in symptom expression. As treatments are targeted toward specific symptoms, if the expression or experience of anxiety varies across groups, then perhaps treatment efficacy varies as well. The first few studies comparing African-American and European-American children revealed significant differences in the amount and types of fears experienced; however, due to disparate samples, these early findings were likely confounded with socioeconomic factors (Neal & Turner, 1991). Recent research that utilizes clinical rather than community samples and controls for socioeconomic status documents more similarities than differences between the two groups. In a comparison of African-American and European-American youth referred for treatment, Last and Perrin (1993) documented similar rates of the majority of diagnoses. Also using a clinical sample, Treadwell et al. (1995) found no significant differences between African-American and European-American youth on child, parent, teacher, or clinician reports of anxiety

---

[2] In this section, "anxiety disorders" refer to social phobia, generalized anxiety disorder, and separation anxiety disorder. Both obsessive-compulsive disorder and posttraumatic stress disorder require a slightly different treatment approach.

or general functioning. Moreover, 8 out of 10 of the most frequently cited fears were the same between the two groups.

Research comparing Latino and European-American youth has seen a more mixed pattern of results. Some studies obtain evidence for increased somatic symptoms among minority youth, whereas other studies find comparable symptom and diagnostic presentation across ethnic groups. Utilizing many of the same outcome measures as Last and Perrin (1993) and Treadwell et al. (1995) above, Ginsburg and Silverman (1996) found few differences between Latino and European-American anxious youth. Both groups presented with the same top four anxiety diagnoses and obtained similar mean scores on parent and child measures of anxiety and depression. Two recent studies of anxiety-disordered Latino and European-American youth yielded similar results in terms of anxiety diagnoses; however, both studies reported significantly higher levels of somatic symptoms in the minority youth (Piña & Silverman, 2004; Varela et al., 2004).

In sum, the above research represents a useful foundation on which to build treatment research. Research on prevalence confirms that anxiety disorders are just as common among minority as nonminority youth and, therefore, represent a serious health issue. The literature on symptom presentation suggests that although all youth (both minority and nonminority) appear to exhibit similar symptoms, some differences may need to be addressed in treatment (e.g., African-American youth may experience different types of fears depending on their environment; Latino youth may report more somatic symptoms).

The majority of research on the application of CBT to treat anxious youth of diverse ethnic and/or cultural backgrounds compares the standard treatment package across two ethnic/cultural groups. Treadwell et al. (1995) conducted one of the first studies to compare the efficacy of the Coping Cat program across diverse groups and found that all children (regardless of ethnicity) improved on self-, parent-, and teacher-reported measures of anxiety and general functioning at posttreatment. In a similar design, Ferrell et al. (2004) compared the efficacy of Social Effectiveness Therapy for Children (SET-C) for African-American and European-American socially phobic children. From pre- to posttreatment, the researchers compared self-reported measures of social phobia, internalizing and externalizing symptoms, observer ratings of social skill, as well as diagnostic status between the two ethnic groups. Both groups exhibited comparable decreases in symptomatology and increases in observed social skill. In addition, the groups did not significantly differ on the percentage of children who achieved responder status (58% of European-American and 30% of African-American children). Both groups exhibited continued improvement at a six-month follow-up assessment, but a direct comparison between ethnic groups was not presented at the follow-up, perhaps due to reduced sample size.

In the Treadwell et al. (1995) and Ferrell et al. (2004) studies, no systematic alterations were made to the treatment manuals specifically for use with African-American youth; however, the Coping Cat manual itself is highly adaptable. Designed to be a flexible manual, Coping Cat has planned ideographic modifications at each step (Kendall & Chu, 2000). For instance, generating anxious thoughts and creating a hierarchy of feared situations are inherently individual. Alteration of the workbooks (the package comes with ancillary materials for both children and adolescents) has been evaluated in Australia (i.e., Coping Koala) with positive results (Barrett et al., 1996). To create the Coping Koala program, Barrett et al. (1996) preserved the core CBT components in the original and adapted the workbooks to reflect Australian culture. In the United States, the Coping Cat has also been translated into Spanish.[3] As of this time, however, we know of no clinical trial that has expressly evaluated the Spanish version of the Coping Cat.

In contrast, Ginsburg and Drake (2002) culturally adapted an established group CBT manual to conduct a pilot study for treating anxious African-American youth in schools. African-American adolescents were randomly assigned to the CBT intervention or to an attention-support control condition. The CBT condition addressed the core components of CBT for anxiety but utilized examples that were culturally modified to address situations that the sample youth were likely to encounter (e.g., violence, drug use, financial hardship). Even with a small sample size, students in the CBT group exhibited significantly greater improvement on a measure of clinician-reported severity of anxiety and one out of two self-reported measures of symptoms of anxiety relative to the control group. No comparison to a traditional CBT intervention was made, however, so it is not clear that the improvements shown by the culturally modified CBT group exceeded those that would have been obtained with the traditional CBT.

Fewer studies have evaluated differences in efficacy of CBT for anxiety between Latino and European-American youth. In post-hoc analyses of two previous clinical trials of individual and group CBT treatment for anxiety, Piña et al. (2003) examined treatment effects and maintenance across the two groups. No systematic modifications were made to the intervention for the Latino youth; however, therapists were sensitized to cultural factors that could play a role in treatment (e.g., different models of coping, possible feared objects). Results revealed that the two groups were statistically equivalent at posttreatment in terms of no longer meeting diagnostic criteria (84.2% Hispanic/Latino and 83.9% European American). Moreover, mean effects sizes for treatment gains on parent- and child-reported measures of anxiety were remarkably similar. Importantly, both groups maintained treatment gains and continued to obtain lower scores on parent and child reports of anxiety over 3-, 6-, and 12-month follow-up.

Although only a handful of studies have evaluated the efficacy of CBT for anxiety among samples of ethnic minority youth, the existing results suggest that minority youth make comparable gains in response

---

[3] The Spanish version of the Coping Cat manual can be obtained by contacting Workbook Publishing at (610) 896-9797 or www.workbookpublishing.com.

to the intervention with minimal cultural adaptation. It is important to note, however, that this may be due to the inherent flexibility of most anxiety treatment manuals and does not absolve researchers of the responsibility to develop and investigate more culturally specific interventions. Although response results are similar across ethnic groups when clinicians employ the standard treatment, the question of whether minority groups would exhibit greater improvement with culturally specific interventions remains unanswered. Moreover, the current research leaves several additional questions unaddressed. For example, although most of the studies controlled for the effects of socioeconomic status, the relative impact of ethnicity and social class on successful treatment is currently unclear. Furthermore, the level of acculturation as well as the origin of ethnic group (e.g., Cuban American vs. Mexican American) likely affects treatment success.

A CLINICIAN'S GUIDE TO USING EBTS WITH DIVERSE FAMILIES

Driven by the goal of delineating efficacious therapies, research has focused on developing and disseminating EBTs for the broad variety of emotional and behavioral problems of youth. Over the last decade, as the list of efficacious treatments grew, it became apparent that the research concerning a majority of empirically supported treatments was based primarily on European-American middle-class youth. Although research suggests that EBTs are effective for treating many clients, clinicians are left with a dilemma when presented with children and families of ethnic minority backgrounds. The following are specific recommendations for the selection and implementation of EBTs in the treatment of culturally diverse families.

1. *Use EBTs wisely.* Despite their limitations with respect to cultural diversity, existing EBTs remain clinicians' best resource for treatment guidelines. Whenever possible, use manuals that have empirical support for use with diverse populations. When such research is not available, consider how treatment manuals may be modified to fit the needs of individual clients. Many therapists misperceive manuals as rigid prescriptions for treatment. In contrast, treatment manuals provide an overall structure of treatment and session goals along with helpful tips for therapists (Kendall et al., 1998). Within that structure, there is often room for adaptation to the specific needs of the case, including cultural issues. In an investigation of the effects of the flexible application of a treatment manual, Kendall and Chu (2000) found no significant relationship between retrospective therapist reports of flexibility and treatment outcome, thus indicating that minor adaptations from the manual do not compromise the efficacy of the treatment.

2. *Be flexible, but remain faithful to the "active ingredients."* Based on their work with depressed and anxious youth, Connor-Smith and Weisz (2003) recommend adapting the structure of the intervention

and/or the session content to meet the needs of the client. In adapting the structure, the clinician may need to add extra rapport-building sessions, additional meetings with support persons, or other treatment components based on the needs of the child. Regarding session content, therapists should use their knowledge of culture to add relevant examples and activities or remove those examples or activities that seem inappropriate.

3. *Address diversity.* This is a two-pronged call to clinicians to address diversity in their own continued training as well as to address the issue in the session with the client. First, as diversity initiatives in training are relatively new (Magyar-Moe et al., 2005), clinicians are encouraged to seek additional training in diversity issues through continuing education programs, books and articles, and/or peer supervision. Second, when treating diverse youth and families, clinicians are encouraged to discuss cultural topics with clients. For example, in treating a socially anxious Latina adolescent who desires to increase peer interaction, the therapist could discuss this goal with the parents to establish culturally acceptable peer activities as therapy goals.

4. *Be your own scientist.* Finally, as with any experimentation, clinicians are encouraged to collect data. Weekly symptom checks, daily symptom diaries, or simply verbal feedback from the client as to their satisfaction with treatment can facilitate the selection and implementation of the most effective and culturally sensitive intervention.

CONCLUSIONS

The recent movement in the field of clinical psychology to identify evidence-based treatments has sparked research and clinical interest in the application of those treatments to youth of diverse backgrounds. Both theoretical and empirical writings call for more substantial research concerning whether EBTs are effective with diverse populations. However, many empirically supported treatment manuals may be used flexibly to accommodate the cultural history and experience of ethnically diverse clients and their families. The stage is now set for more efficacy and effectiveness research concerning treatments for ethnically diverse children and adolescents; until that process comes to fruition, clinicians must continue to combine information from the available treatment outcome research, research and theory about how culture and other issues of diversity may be addressed in the context of psychotherapy, and careful clinical judgment when using EBTs with clients of diverse ethnic backgrounds.

REFERENCES

Alvy, K. T. (1987). *Black Parenting: Strategies for Training.* New York: Irvington Publishers.
Barrett, P. (2000). Treatment of childhood anxiety: Developmental aspects. *Clinical Psychology Review, 20,* 479–494.

Barrett, P., Dadds, M., & Rapee, R. (1996). Family treatment of childhood anxiety: A controlled trial. *Journal of Consulting and Clinical Psychology, 64,* 333–342.

Barrett, P. M., Lowry-Webster, H., & Turner, C. (2000). *FRIENDS Program for Children: Group Leaders' Manual.* Brisbane: Australia Academic Press.

Baumrind, D. (1978). Parental disciplinary patterns and social competence in children. *Youth and Society, 9,* 239–276.

Bernal, G., & Scharron-del-Rio, M. R. (2001). Are empirically supported treatments valid for ethnic minorities? Toward an alternative approach for treatment research. *Cultural Diversity and Ethnic Minority Psychology, 7,* 328–342.

Bradley, R. H., Corwyn, R. F., McAdoo, H. P., & Garcia-Coll, C. (2001). The home environments of children in the United States. Part I: Variations by age, ethnicity, and poverty status. *Child Development, 72,* 1844–1867.

Cartwright-Hatton, S., Roberts, C., Chistabesan, P., Fothergill, C., & Harrington, R. (2004). Systematic review of the efficacy of cognitive behaviour therapies for childhood and adolescent anxiety disorders. *British Journal of Clinical Psychology, 43,* 421–436.

Chambless, D. L., & Hollon, S. D. (1998). Defining empirically supported therapies. *Journal of Consulting and Clinical Psychology, 66,* 7–18.

Chambless, D. L., Sanderson, W. C., Shoham, V., Johnson, S. B., Pope, K. S., Crits-Christoph, P., et al. (1996). An update on empirically validated therapies. *Clinical Psychologist, 49,* 5–18.

Chao, R. K. (1996). Chinese and European American mothers' beliefs about the role of parenting in children's school success. *Journal of Cross-Cultural Psychology, 27,* 403–423.

Coard, S. I., Wallace, S. A., Stevenson, H. C., & Brotman, L. M. (2004). Towards culturally relevant preventive interventions: The consideration of racial socialization in parent training with African American families. *Journal of Child and Family Studies, 13,* 277–293.

Connor-Smith, J. K., & Weisz, J. R. (2003). Applying treatment outcome research in clinical practice: Techniques for adapting interventions to the real world. *Child and Adolescent Mental Health, 8,* 3–10.

Costantino, G., Malgady, R. G., & Rogler, L. H. (1986). Cuento therapy: A culturally sensitive modality for Puerto Rican children. *Journal of Counseling and Clinical Psychology, 54,* 639–645.

Deegear, J., & Lawson, D. M. (2003). The utility of empirically supported treatments. *Professional Psychology: Research and Practice, 34,* 271–277.

Dumas, J. E., & Wahler, R. G. (1983). Predictors of treatment outcome in parent training: Mother insularity and socioeconomic disadvantage. *Behavioral Assessment, 5,* 301–313.

Ferrell, C. B., Beidel, D. C., & Turner, S. M. (2004). Assessment and treatment of socially phobic children: A cross cultural comparison. *Journal of Clinical Child and Adolescent Psychology, 33,* 260–268.

Forehand, R., & Kotchick, B. A. (1996). Cultural diversity: A wake-up call for parent training. *Behavior Therapy, 27,* 187–206.

Forehand, R., & Long, N. (2002). *Parenting the Strong-Willed Child,* 2nd ed. Chicago: Contemporary Books.

Ginsburg, G. S., & Drake, K. L. (2002). School-based treatment for anxious African-American adolescents: A controlled pilot study. *Journal of the American Academy of Child and Adolescent Psychiatry, 41,* 768–775.

Ginsburg, G. S., & Silverman, W. K. (1996). Phobic and anxiety disorders in Hispanic and Caucasian youth. *Journal of Anxiety Disorders, 10,* 517–528.

Hall, G. C. N. (2001). Psychotherapy research with ethnic minorities: Empirical, ethical, and conceptual issues. *Journal of Consulting and Clinical Psychology, 69,* 502–510.

Harkness, S., & Super, C. M. (1995). Culture and parenting. In M. H. Bornstein (Ed.), *Handbook of Parenting: Biology and the Ecology of Parenting,* Vol. 2 (pp. 211–234). Mahwah, NJ: Lawrence Erlbaum.

Kashdan, T. B., & Herbert J. D. (2001). Social anxiety disorder in childhood and adolescence: Current status and future directions. *Clinical Child and Family Psychology Review, 4,* 37–61.

Kelley, M. L, Power, T. G., & Wimbush, D. D. (1992). Determinants of disciplinary practices in low-income Black mothers. *Child Development, 63,* 573–582.

Kendall, P. C. (2000). *Coping Cat Workbook.* Ardmore, PA: Workbook Publishing.

Kendall, P. C., & Chu, B. C. (2000). Retrospective self-reports of therapist flexibility in a manual-based treatment for youths with anxiety disorders. *Journal of Clinical Child Psychology*, 29, 209–220.

Kendall, P. C., Chu, B., Gifford, A., Hayes, C., & Nauta, M. (1998). Breathing life into a manual: Flexibility and creativity with manual-based treatments. *Cognitive & Behavioral Practice*, 5, 177–198.

Kendall, P. C., Flannery-Schroeder, E., Panichelli-Mindel, S. M., Southam-Gerow, M., Henin, A., & Warman, M. (1997). Therapy for youths with anxiety disorders: A second randomized clinical trial. *Journal of Consulting and Clinical Psychology*, 65, 366–380.

Kotchick, B. A., Shaffer, A., Dorsey, S., & Forehand, R. (2003). Parenting antisocial children and adolescents. In M. Hoghughi & N. Long (Eds.), *Handbook of Parenting: Theory and Research for Practice* (pp. 256–275). London: Sage Publications.

Labellarte, M. J., Ginsburg, G. S., & Riddle, M. A. (1999). The treatment of anxiety disorders in children and adolescents. *Biological Psychiatry*, 46, 1567–1578.

Lam, A. G., & Sue, S. (2001). Client diversity. *Psychotherapy*, 38, 479–486.

Lamborn, S. D., Dornbusch, S. M., & Steinberg, L. (1996). Ethnicity and community context as moderators of the relations between family decision making and adolescent adjustment. *Child Development*, 67, 283–301.

Last, C. G., & Perrin, S. (1993). Anxiety disorders in African-American and White children. *Journal of Abnormal Child Psychology*, 21, 153–165.

Levant, R. (2004). The empirically validated treatments movement: A practitioner/educator perspective. *Clinical Psychology: Science and Practice*, 11, 219–224.

Magyar-Moe, J. L., Pedrotti, J. T., Edwards, L. M., Ford, A. I., Petersen, S. E., Rasmussen, H. N., et al. (2005). Perceptions of multicultural training in predoctoral internship programs: A survey of interns and training directors. *Professional Psychology: Research and Practice*, 36, 446–450.

Martinez, C. R., & Eddy, J. M. (2005). Effects of culturally adapted parent management training on Latino youth behavioral health outcomes. *Journal of Consulting and Clinical Psychology*, 73, 841–851.

McMahon, R. J., & Forehand, R. (2003). *Helping the Noncompliant Child: A Clinician's Guide to Effective Parent Training*, 2nd ed. New York: Guilford Press.

Myers, H. F., Alvy, K. T., Arrington, A., Richardson, M. A., Marigna, M., Huff, R., et al. (1992). The impact of a parent training program on inner-city African American families. *Journal of Community Psychology*, 20, 132–147.

National Institute of Mental Health (1999). *Strategic Plan on Reducing Health Disparities*. Rockville, MD.

Neal, A. M. & Turner, S. M. (1991). Anxiety disorder research with African Americans: Current status. *Psychological Bulletin*, 109, 400–410.

Ogbu, J. (1981). Origins of human competence: A cultural-ecological perspective. *Child Development*, 52, 413–429.

Patterson, G. R. (1975). *Professional Guide for "Families" and "Living with Children."* Champaign, IL: Research Press.

Patterson, G. R., Reid, J. B., & Dishion, T. J. (1992). *Antisocial Boys*. Eugene, OR: Castalia.

Piña, A. A., & Silverman, W. K. (2004). Clinical phenomenology, somatic symptoms, and distress in Hispanic/Latino and Euro-American youths with anxiety disorders. *Journal of Clinical Child and Adolescent Psychology*, 33, 227–236.

Piña, A. A., Silverman, W. K., Fuentes, R. M., Kurtines, W. M., & Weems, C. F. (2003). Exposure-based cognitive-behavioral treatment for phobic and anxiety disorders: Treatment effects and maintenance for Hispanic/Latino relative to European-American youths. *Journal of the American Academy of Child and Adolescent Psychiatry*, 42, 1179–1187.

Reid, M. J., Webster-Stratton, C., & Beauchaine, T. P. (2001). Parent training in Head Start: A comparison of program response among African American, Asian American, Caucasian, and Hispanic mothers. *Prevention Science*, 2, 209–227.

Sue, D. W., & Sue, D. (1999). *Counseling the Culturally Different: Theory and Practice*, 3rd ed. New York: Wiley.

Sue, S. (1998). In search of cultural competence in psychotherapy and counseling. *American Psychologist*, 53, 440–448.

Surgeon General (2000). *Supplement to "Mental Health: A Report of the Surgeon General." Disparities in Mental Health Care for Racial and Ethnic Minorities.* Washington, DC: U.S. Public Health Service.

Task Force on Promotion and Dissemination of Psychological Procedures (1995). Training in and dissemination of empirically-validated psychological treatments. *Clinical Psychologist, 48,* 3–23.

Varela, E. R., Vernberg, E. M., Sanchez-Sosa, J. J., Riveros, A., Mitchell, M., & Mashunkashey, J. (2004). Anxiety reporting and culturally associated interpretation biases and cognitive schemas: A comparison of Mexican, Mexican American, and European families. *Journal of Clinical Child and Adolescent Psychology, 33,* 237–247.

Weisz, J. R., & Jensen, A. L. (2001). Child and adolescent psychotherapy in research and practice contexts: Review of the evidence and suggestions for improving the field. *European Child and Adolescent Psychiatry, 10*(1), 12–18.

Westen, D., Novotny, C. M., & Thompson-Brenner, H. (2004). The empirical status of empirically supported psychotherapies: Assumptions, findings, and reporting in controlled clinical trials. *Psychological Bulletin, 130,* 631–663.

Wong, E. C., Kim, B. S. K., Zane, N. W. S., Kim, I., & Huang, J. S. (2003). Examining culturally based variables associated with ethnicity: Influences on credibility perceptions of empirically supported interventions. *Cultural Diversity and Ethnic Minority Psychology, 9,* 88–96.

28

Evidence-Based Therapy and Ethical Practice

WILLIAM A. RAE and CONSTANCE J. FOURNIER

Because of the special vulnerabilities inherent in the treatment of children and the complexities involved in treating multiple family members, the importance of ethical practice in the psychological treatment of children, adolescents, and families has been described as the greatest responsibility of any therapist (Rae & Fournier, 1999). Ethical practice is the cornerstone of trust in a psychotherapeutic relationship. Without ethical practice, the vulnerabilities of children, adolescents, and families could be exploited. If this were to occur, the therapeutic relationship would be rendered impotent.

Evidence-based therapy (EBT) is an approach to treatment that assumes that the clinician is using interventions that evidence has indicated is effective. When one thinks about EBT with children and families, it seems intuitively obvious that EBTs would be the only possible type of therapy that would be ethical. In fact, EBTs have become such a powerful notion that in the last decade scores of books and articles have been published on EBTs and other related terms. The Ethical Principles of Psychologists and Code of Conduct of the American Psychological Association (Ethics Code; APA, 2002) clearly state that the only therapies to be practiced by psychologists must be effective while at the same time not being harmful. Unfortunately, appropriate ethical practice is never nearly so clear-cut because one must deal with the inherent complexity in the human interaction that is psychotherapy.

This situation is exacerbated by the fact that the "standard of practice" in psychology is never static; it is constantly changing. Professionals commonly learn a "solid fact" in graduate school only to learn later that the "fact" was patently untrue. The half-life of knowledge in psychology has been estimated to be about seven years, which means that about half of the knowledge base in psychology will change during that timeframe

WILLIAM A. RAE and CONSTANCE J. FOURNIER • Texas A&M University

(Koocher, 2005). Additionally, the practitioner must integrate disparate research findings on child mental health effectiveness and efficacy. Treatment with children, adolescents, and families is fraught with complexities. Making an informed judgment about what intervention to apply to an idiosyncratic case is often complicated. Ethical decision making under these circumstances can be especially fraught with difficulty, and the appropriate "standard of practice" is not always clearly defined.

The purpose of this chapter is to discuss the ethical dilemmas inherent in practicing evidence-based therapies with children, adolescents, and families. An attempt will be made to discuss ethical issues in a practitioner-oriented manner, which may be helpful both to trainees and to seasoned professionals. The multifaceted nature of EBTs will be discussed as well as how the EBTs interface with the psychotherapy practice. Specific areas of ethical sensitivity addressed in the APA Ethics Code will also be discussed. Finally, specific guidelines for ethical practice using EBTs will also be provided.

THE NATURE OF PSYCHOTHERAPY AND EVIDENCE-BASED THERAPY

Evidence-based therapies (EBTs) are considered the optimal standard of practice for interventions with children and adolescents. The use of EBTs is not only the standard in professional psychology but is also the standard in medicine and in other mental health disciplines (e.g., social work, nursing). Professional psychology has always been concerned with the effectiveness of interventions, but the focus on empirically supported treatments became paramount in the 1990s after the profession became very concerned with economic viability. With the advent of managed care, payors wanted assurance that they were paying for treatments that were effective in treating mental disorders. This led to several defined criteria for "empirically supported" treatments (Task Force on Promotion and Dissemination of Psychological Procedures, 1995; Chambless & Hollon, 1998), which state that there must be demonstrated research in which the benefits of treatment observed are due to the effects of the treatment and not due to confounding factors such as nonequivalent treatment groups, passage of time, and artifacts of psychological assessment.

Evidence for efficacious treatment can be provided by many forms of research, which may include clinical observation, qualitative research, and single-case designs or case studies. Although there are provisions for determining efficacy using single-case design experiments, the "gold standard" for psychological intervention research is the randomized controlled trial (RCT) of the psychological treatment in which the treatment is compared to psychological placebo, pill, or another psychological treatment. For a treatment to be considered empirically validated according to the Task Force (1995) criteria, a product of APA's Division 12 (Clinical Psychology), it must have been shown to be superior to one of these conditions in an RCT. In addition, to be considered a true treatment effect, the results should be replicated by a different research team and optimally should be conducted via a manual (Chambless & Hollon, 1998; Lonigan et al., 1998). Although the use of the internally valid, randomized control trails for determining if an intervention is efficacious became widely accepted, this medical model-derived form of research has been criticized because it limits the demonstration of effectiveness for other forms of psychotherapy not easily tested by the RCT approach (Bryceland & Stam, 2005). In the same way, Bohart (2005) argued that many other therapeutic approaches can be construed as evidence-based that are safe and helpful but do not fit into the randomized controlled clinical trial criteria. In contrast to the "empirically supported" criteria for treatment efficacy, the EBT definition evolved over the next few years to take into account other factors that are also important for treatment effectiveness.

In its resolution on evidence-based practice, the APA (2005) acknowledged that interventions must be tempered by clinical expertise and the inclusion of patient values before deciding on a specific treatment. In fact, the APA (2006) clarified that evidence-based practice must integrate research evidence with clinical data as well as take into account patient characteristics, culture, and preferences that should improve overall outcome. Although sometimes the literature uses terms such as "empirically validated," "empirically supported," and "evidence-based practice" interchangeably, this chapter will use the term "evidence-based treatment" (EBT), which includes elements of each of the definitions.

How then is the clinician to evaluate, first, the research underlying an EBT in general and, then, whether or not the research "fits" the client in question? The first four chapters in this book address in detail the costs and benefits of EBT, optimal criteria for EBT, and methodological issues in the evaluation of therapies. Suffice it to say that empirical studies are important to consider when the clinician chooses a psychological intervention for a particular client/patient. The clinician must, however, also take into account contextual issues surrounding the transportability, the dissemination, and the systemic evaluation of the intervention (Chorpita, 2003). The focus of this chapter will be on considering the EBT, how it is operationalized and applied ethically in clinical situations.

CLINICIAN JUDGMENT AND EBTS

A key issue in determining treatment efficacy requires clinician judgment. First, the rigor of the methodology and the appropriateness of research techniques used in the published studies are examined. After evaluating the appropriateness and rigor of the study on which a particular intervention is based, the clinician must make a decision about whether or not to use a particular intervention with a client. The clinician must also consider the utility of the intervention. The APA Task Force on Psychological Intervention Guidelines (1995) addressed the clinical utility of an intervention that includes issues of feasibility, generalizability, and costs and benefits.

Feasibility

In regards to feasibility, the client/patient needs to accept the possible untoward effects of the treatment (e.g., duration, cost, pain, etc.), accept the treatment in comparison to other choices, and be willing to comply with the treatment regime. More recently, the APA Task Force on Evidence-Based Practice (2006) not only acknowledged the importance of clinical expertise in identifying and integrating research evidence with information about the client, but also highlighted the importance of knowing what intervention will be effective to specific clients based on the client's characteristics, culture, and preferences. Once these factors are considered, the clinician must explain the intervention to the parent/guardian and the client.

After the client and parent weigh the untoward effects, accept the treatment, and consent or assent to the treatment, they must be motivated. The best way to motivate a client (or parent) depends on how the clinician understands the client's unique clinical circumstances, culture, and wishes. In these circumstances, it is not only incumbent on the clinician to "sell" the treatment regime, but also to "sell" the concept of the client working toward a behavioral change. Many clients have a vague notion of wanting to change their behavior but often are ambivalent about engaging in the hard work of making any meaningful change to their behavior. Although the analytically-laden term "resistance" has been used to describe this process, we believe that the term "motivation" more accurately describes this factor. The motivated client or the parent will more likely follow the therapeutic directives of the clinician and may also find novel opportunities for appropriate behavior change. For example, oppositional defiant disorder for preadolescents is often effectively treated using EBTs with techniques such as engaging in positive parent-child inter-action time (e.g., Barkley, 1997). Unless the parent is willing to spend all the time necessary to engage in the structured activities, change is unlikely to occur. In the same way, a motivated, astute parent will be able to find many teachable moments to improve his or her child's behavior well beyond the scope of the structured program that will add to the positive behavior pattern, such as extending positive interactions that occur spontaneously.

Generalizability

In regards to generalizability, the client or parent needs to have characteristics compatible to the intervention population (e.g., gender, cultural background, presenting symptoms). The therapist needs to have compatible therapist characteristics to those described in the intervention (e.g., gender, cultural background, theoretical orientation), the contextual factors of the setting need to be similar with the intervention (e.g., type of clinical setting, geographic location, urban vs. rural setting), and the timeframes of treatment must also be taken into account (APA Task Force on Psychological Intervention Guidelines, 1995). Clinicians must always take into account how well the intervention will generalize to the unique characteristics of their client as well as the family.

Although a number of treatments are available with empirical support, not all potential situations have been investigated. Consequently, there may not be an appropriate intervention for every clinical situation. In particular, the underlying conditions of diagnosis and methodology used in randomized controlled trials may not always apply to children, adolescents, and families in a clinical practice. Westen et al. (2004) argued that when reporting meta-analytic studies of treatment efficacy, the authors should report a range of outcome data with indications of generalizability, which would help other researchers to develop a more nuanced view of treatment efficacy. Obviously, there can be a schism between the researcher's evidence of efficacy and the clinician's experience of clinical effectiveness. In some ways, the schism that occurs between highly controlled research with good internal validity often leads to low external validity in the clinical setting (Chorpita et al., 1998). For example, an intervention that requires 20 visits may not be feasible in a practice setting that emphasizes short-term intervention.

Weisz (2004) argued for the importance of doing research where generalizability would be better for the kinds of problems that are presented in a naturalistic clinical setting. In particular, Weisz (2000) recommended that clinics test interventions to be sure that they work in a real-life setting. In fact, it is often the case that when trainees encounter their first clinical cases, they are often disheartened that the purported empirically supported intervention does not generalize to their setting or to their client. Many intervention studies have been performed in controlled research environments (e.g., university psychology clinics) with clients chosen for only the problem being researched (i.e., without accompanying comorbid conditions). The novice clinician may find that the client has different symptoms and perhaps even comorbid conditions. While this might seem a daunting challenge, use of empirically supported treatments can be justified. Jensen Doss and Weisz (2006) noted that even when comorbid conditions exist, the intervention applied to the most salient condition can be effective overall.

Costs and Benefits

Costs and benefits are another important consideration. The clinician must be aware of the costs of delivering the intervention to the client and family. These costs include, but are not limited to, time, money, and, most importantly, the client's own sense of well-being. In the same way, the clinician must be aware of the costs of withholding effective intervention to his or her client/patient (APA Task Force on Psychological Intervention Guidelines, 1995). The costs of doing the intervention must be weighed with the potential and real benefits of the intervention. This can be problematic if the benefits are short-term, or if the benefits are not immediately seen. The clinician must have a good understanding of how the intervention will relate to the client and potential outcome.

Other risks may be inherent in the traditional method of diagnosis. Wampold (2001) argued that traditional psychotherapy research has inappropriately relied on a medical model paradigm to diagnosis and treatment. This paradigm requires that the first step categorize the child/patient via a diagnosis, usually by the DSM-IV. Most child and adolescent clinicians would acknowledge that not all children of the same age with the same diagnosis should be treated the same. For example, two 13-year-old boys diagnosed with a major depressive disorder (MDD) may require very different interventions when taking into account idiosyncratic personal factors (e.g., motivation) and contextual factors (e.g., family). From a developmental psychopathology standpoint, one child's depression could have evolved from ongoing family conflict (i.e., contextual influences) and the other child's depression could have evolved from endogenous, genetically influenced biological factors (i.e., personal influences). The astute clinician would know that each adolescent could require very different treatment approaches in order to provide appropriate and effective treatment. In fact, the use of a rigidly applied treatment based solely on the diagnosis without regard to context might be considered unethical and antithetical to EBT approaches.

The APA guidelines on practice regard clinical expertise as an important factor in determining an appropriate intervention (APA, 2005). Clinical expertise is difficult to describe and quantify because it involves many factors, including "clinical and scientific training, theoretical understanding, experience, self-reflection, knowledge of current research, and continuing education and training" (APA, 2005, p. 2). The therapist must use his or her clinical judgment to determine what aspects of clinical expertise are important in making a final treatment determination. Spirito and Kazak (2006) described the overzealous adherence to a particular theoretical model and the lack of appreciation of individual differences as major constraints on clinical judgment. As a clinician, deciding what to do and when to do it is not a simple, linear, decision-tree-type process. Thus, the *how* of applying an efficacious treatment is important, but not nearly as important as knowing *when* to apply a particular treatment. Kendall and Beidas (2007) have described using flexibility within fidelity as a method by which empirically supported treatments can be appropriately disseminated from research clinics to service clinics.

Psychological treatment is not only performing a therapeutic procedure but also dealing with the interpersonal and intrapersonal complexities of a person, which are taken into account in EBTs. Powerful therapist factors have been argued to be as important as adherence to a treatment protocol. That is, the particular therapist delivering the treatment is crucial to positive outcome, which argues against the medical model and for the contextual model of psychotherapy (Wampold, 2001). For example, the therapist's ability to join with the client, sometimes called the working alliance, may enhance the client's motivation. Other therapist characteristics such as experience, expertise, and reputation may also influence the intervention. These elements have been shown to provide powerful effects in a psychotherapy relationship (Frank & Frank, 1991). Wampold (2001) and Bohart (2005) have argued that these other factors or "nonspecific" components of therapy may be more powerful than specific procedures for specific DSM-IV diagnoses. Thus, the treatment cannot and must not be evaluated without careful consideration of these nonspecific components concurrent with the EBT.

SPECIFIC ETHICAL ISSUES IN EVIDENCE-BASED THERAPY

The Ethical Principles of Psychologists and Code of Conduct (Ethics Code; APA, 2002) do not directly address EBT, but they clearly suggest ethical concerns that must be addressed in the provision of psychological treatment. Although the sections of the Preamble and General Principles are not in themselves enforceable rules, they give some general directions for the psychologist using EBTs. Obviously, the interpretation of this section of the Ethics Code requires considerable professional judgment by the psychologist, who must be guided by the intent of the Ethics Code.

In the Preamble of the Ethics Code (APA, 2002), psychologists are reminded that they should be "committed to increasing scientific and professional knowledge of behavior and people's understanding of themselves and others and to the use of such knowledge to improve the condition of individuals, organizations, and society" (p. 1062). This sentiment is also reflected in Standard 2.04, which addresses bases for scientific and professional judgment. Although most clinicians have a working understanding of the term "professional judgment," there continues to be debate about what is meant by "scientific." In some ways, scientific evidence may at first glance seem easier to prove, because of operational definitions and a problem-solving process that is tied to being "scientific." This sense of security, however, must be challenged in that conclusion validity (e.g., under what circumstances the treatment is efficacious) is always conjecture until proven. Proof in every instance is impossible. This is when professional judgment comes to the forefront. Both professional and scientific judgment have a role in the adaptation of the EBT to a unique clinical situation.

The Ethics Code (APA, 2002) includes the General Principles section, where Principle A (Beneficence and Nonmaleficence) indicates that psychologists should "strive to benefit those with whom they work and take care to do no harm" (p. 1062). This sentiment is also reflected in Standard 3.04, which discusses avoiding harm. While the obvious concept of harm can be thought of as intentional, harm can also be construed as unintentional. Harm may occur when an intervention is applied inappropriately; alternately, harm may occur when an appropriate intervention is not applied, including EBTs. Obviously, any treatment that is not effective would have the potential of being harmful because it would prevent clients/patients from getting needed effective interventions for their mental disorders. In practice, all interventions have the potential of harming the individual, because by their nature the psychologist is attempting to change current patterns in the life functioning of another person. For example, vigorous cognitive-behavioral, client-centered, or psychodynamic therapy can create emotional distress in some individuals since they are being confronted with their inappropriate behaviors and thoughts.

This issue becomes very complex when treating a child because of the context of the family situation in which the child resides. For example, while treating the behavior problems of a child, the therapist may need to help the parents confront their own lack of consistency or the therapist might reveal a marital issue that gets in the way of them working together. The "do no harm" standard makes it clear that the psychologist should minimize any harm when it can be recognized as such and can be avoided. Unfortunately, the possibilities of unforeseen negative effects of any intervention are always possible.

Several of the standards in the Ethical Code pertain to the issue of practitioners using EBT. For example, psychologists must be careful not to take on a professional role in treatment that might impair effectiveness, competence, or objectivity (Standard 3.06, Conflict of Interest). Also contained in Standard 3.06 is the prohibition from exploiting or harming the client/patient. Psychologists who adhere to a strongly held theoretical orientation or philosophy of treatment may be blinded by their theoretical orientation or philosophy of treatment and not be open to other evidence-based approaches that do not share their philosophy. Thus, the psychologist may not be delivering the most effective treatment for a particular patient/client. Although not meaning to harm a client/patient, the psychologist could inadvertently treat the client/patient with an ineffective treatment because of the psychologist's strongly held belief that a particular treatment modality based on his or her chosen theory or training background is the most effective one.

Another conflict of interest can occur when the psychologist must decide when treatment should be terminated. Standard 10.10 (Terminating Therapy) states that therapy should be terminated when it is recognized that the client/patient is not likely to benefit, is being harmed, or no longer needs the service. Unfortunately, the decision to terminate treatment is not always easily determined since multiple factors go into that decision. Professional standards would require that if an ineffective treatment is continued and the client/patient is not likely to benefit from treatment, the psychologist should terminate treatment immediately. For example, a therapist using EBT that is thought to be appropriate could adhere to the treatment regimen without recognizing changing therapeutic conditions that could result in continuing with a course of treatment when the outcome would be unfavorable to the client. Premature termination may occur in the same way if the therapist is unfamiliar with how the intervention progresses in the typical case. For example, a therapist might be tempted to stop treatment during an extinction burst of inappropriate behavior. Conversely, a therapist may assume a set of behaviors is within the limits of the intervention when it may, in fact, be an artifact of another event that should take precedence in the treatment regimen (e.g., acting-out behaviors may mask abuse or a learning disability). An unaware psychologist might terminate the client when a treatment has been completed without considering the need for further treatment. In the same way in a fee-for-service environment, psychologists might be tempted to continue with less-than-optimal treatment because they are being financially rewarded for continuing treatment. Termination is an important part of treatment and must always be part of the EBT process.

The importance of professional competence is well articulated in the Ethical Code. Psychological services should only be provided within the boundaries of professional competence of the psychologist based on his or her training, education, professional experience, consultation, study, and supervised experience (Standard 2.01, Boundaries of Competence). Unfortunately, therapeutic approaches are often characterized by being complicated and multifaceted. Many require the understanding of complex sequences in treatment manuals and require learning many steps for appropriate implementation. For the practicing clinician, it is not always clear when he or she might be "competent" in a new treatment approach. At every level of experience, the therapist faces challenges in mastering complex treatments. For novice practitioners, not every new treatment will be mastered (or addressed) at the beginning of practice, although it is likely that the newer practitioner may have more extensive training in particular treatment approaches. More senior psychologists must obtain continuing education and consultation in order to be truly competent in providing newer treatments. However, workshops, in-service training, and reading can only go so far in providing the expertise needed in mastering a new treatment. New treatments may not be routinely disseminated in the child area, because of organizational, personnel, and systemic constraints within the profession. Treatment manuals may not always be readily available, continuing education is not always accessible, and graduate programs have not always provided training in the most up-to-date treatments (Herschell et al., 2004) even though maintaining competence is an important principle in the Ethics Code (Standard 2.03, Maintaining Competence). The most recent APA criteria for accreditation in professional psychology (i.e., clinical, counseling, and school psychology) clearly specify a requirement for training in empirically supported procedures (APA, Committee on Accreditation, 2005).

CONSIDERATIONS OF EBT AND CONSENT

Psychologists must inform the client/patient about aspects of therapy (Standard 10.01, Consent to Therapy). Besides limits of confidentiality, fees, and the involvement of third parties, the psychologist must inform the client/patient about the nature of the therapeutic intervention and the anticipated course of the therapy. When the treatment does not have established efficacy, the psychologist must inform the child and family about the developing nature of the treatment, what potential risks might be involved, and what kinds of alternative treatment could be offered. Unfortunately, when working with children and families, there are added complications. Because of their age-related diminished capabilities and their lack of experience, children have significant limitations in their ability to understand what is meant by the anticipated course of psychological treatment. Of course, the psychologist must also explain the details of the treatment to parents/guardians. These issues of evaluating the risks of, benefits of, and alternatives to a particular intervention are often hard for the practitioner to fully comprehend. Trying to communicate these issues to an unapprised parent can be very complex. In addition, there may be some significant impediments to explaining a complex treatment intervention to both the child (client/patient) and his or her parents/guardians. Many children and family experience considerable psychological distress, which may interfere with their ability to understand the treatment. Competently obtaining informed consent from children and families requires the highest standard of practice (Rae & Fournier, 1999), yet providing clear and understandable information about EBTs can be daunting.

The APA Ethical Code specifies that the psychologist must accurately report the nature of the service provided to payors or insurance companies. This information should include the clinical findings and the diagnosis. Accurately diagnosing child and adolescent disorders is sometimes difficult because of the developmental nature of childhood problems and the fact that many child, adolescent, or family problems do not always lend themselves to a simple DSM-IV diagnostic category. Use of an EBT can help the psychologist meet this standard because these treatments are clearly defined and tied to specific diagnoses. At the same time, complications arise related both to the appropriateness of assigning diagnoses to particular clients and to the availability of EBTs for children with multiple diagnoses or with obscure diagnoses. Given the pressure to diagnose tied to EBTs, accurately diagnosing children and adolescents can also get distorted in the environment of managed care because of the covert pressure endemic to the reimbursement policies of some insurance companies (Davidson & Spring, 2006). Insurance companies demand that clinicians use only evidence-based treatments, many of which are tied to specific DSM-IV diagnoses. Because the astute clinician knows that certain treatments will be disallowed under certain diagnoses (Roberts & Hurley, 1997), the clinician might be tempted to alter a diagnosis in order to improve the likelihood of being paid for services. In the same way, a clinician might alter a diagnosis in order to fit a favored treatment that matches the psychologist's knowledge or theoretical orientation.

PRESCRIPTIVE ETHICAL GUIDELINES FOR THE CLINICIAN USING EVIDENCE-BASED THERAPY

Because of the allowance of flexibility tempered by clinical expertise, client characteristics, client culture, and client preferences, the APA Presidential Task Force on Evidence-Based Practice (2006) articulated an approach to EBTs for children, adolescents, and families that is inherently ethical. Many clinicians may continue to be drawn to a more narrow interpretation of treatment that only allows for treatments based on the highest scientific standard for research (i.e., "gold standard" of the randomized controlled clinical trial). There may be times when the "gold standard" treatment will not be the appropriate treatment for every client/patient, because individual and contextual circumstances vary widely. The implementation of EBTs with all due regard to ethical practice is essential. The following are 10 guidelines for the ethical treatment of children and adolescents using evidence-based treatments.

Step 1: Conceptualize Case Using a Developmental and Contextual Framework

Although the choice of treatment for child and adolescent cases is usually influenced by the DSM-IV diagnosis, cases should be understood not only by their nosology, but also by the multiple underlying causes of their problems. The DSM-IV diagnostic categories do not indicate a specific etiology, but rather just report on a constellation of grouped symptoms that make up the disorder. This DSM-IV categorization often sets the direction of the evidence-based treatment approach. We believe the most ethical approach to determining the treatment approach is to understand the case using a developmental and contextual framework. Using this framework, the clinician can understand how problems have emerged, how they have changed over time, and how they have been influenced by environmental and developmental processes. This conceptualization often leads to unique treatment approaches that are specific to the child, adolescent, and/or family and that do not rely exclusively on DSM-IV categorizations. For example, in using a developmental framework, the therapist may determine that an EBT established for 4- to 10-year-old children would fit the needs of an 11-year-old who functions more like a younger child. On the other hand, in considering the context of behavior, an EBT designed to assist parents with a defiant child may be inappropriate if the behavior is related to frustration at school because of ineffective teaching. Many treatments are developed for clinic settings, which may leave out a key context for children, specifically schools. Clinical judgment is essential in order to generalize EBTs to other settings that are an integral part of children's lives.

Step 2: Be Adequately Trained in EBTs

Clinicians should be broadly trained in EBTs. Unfortunately, many clinicians are out of date in their skills regarding EBTs shortly after their formal graduate training. Therapeutic techniques including evidence-based treatment approaches (and accompanying treatment manuals) are often difficult to learn and require large amounts of time (often with supervised practice) to learn adequately. It is incumbent upon the ethical clinician to learn as many EBTs offered as part of his or her ongoing continuing education; however, there can be issues with the fidelity of the intervention. The typical avenues of instruction that include workshops, in-service training, and reading the professional literature may not be enough. In some cases, the senior practitioner may be the student of the newer and more comprehensively trained practitioner. Addis (2002) has described numerous obstacles to dissemination of EBT, which include the practical constraints on practitioners' ability to use research and the lack of research on training in the integration of science and practice.

Step 3: Consider the EBT from "Gold Standard" Scientific Research

Clinicians should always consider the "gold standard" of research using a randomized controlled clinical trial of the psychological treatment when choosing an EBT. Obviously, generalizing controlled research to the clinical setting can be problematic, but the most scientifically valid research should always be considered first.

Step 4: Use Clinical Expertise in Judging the Appropriateness of Efficacious Treatments

The most important single ethical guideline for child and adolescent clinicians is to provide the most effective treatment while at the same time doing no harm. The APA (2005, 2006) has clearly recognized that clinical expertise is an important factor in determining appropriate evidence-based practice. Clinical expertise involves much more than knowledge of research findings; it also involves experience and training. Many factors can contribute to the failure of a well-established, research-based, empirically validated, efficacious treatment (e.g., motivation, context, comorbidity, client characteristics). The ethical clinician should use his or her carefully developed clinical expertise in judging the appropriateness of a well-researched efficacious treatment to the individual situation along with a clearly articulated case conceptualization.

Step 5: Modify the Treatments to Unique Circumstances of the Clinical Situation

Clinicians should begin by following an empirically supported treatment approach; however, judgment must be exercised to fit the treatment to the unique clinical case. Manualized treatment programs often have multiple components that work together to change behavior, but the astute clinician should be able to use pieces of the manualized treatment that seem to fit the unique clinical circumstance. Again, if the clinician conceptualizes the case via a developmental and contextual framework, it can give some valuable clues to therapeutic direction by using other evidence that forms the basis of selecting, using, and perhaps modifying the EBT.

Step 6: Use the Other "Rogerian" Approach

The astute and ethical clinician may need to consider changing the treatment approach if that approach is not working effectively and be continually assessing therapeutic effectiveness. We describe this responsive therapeutic flexibility as the other "Rogerian" approach since it is based on the philosophy described in the Kenny Rogers song "The Gambler." Specifically, the clinician must know when to continue to use a technique that is working ("know when to hold 'em") and when to discontinue using a technique that is not working ("know when to fold 'em"). The timing of the intervention is crucial. In fact, effective clinicians often do not know every empirically supported treatment technique, but they may know *when* to apply a specific treatment at the right time. Clinicians must not be afraid to discard a theoretical approach or an empirically supported technique if it is not showing a positive outcome.

Step 7: Use the Nonspecific Effects in Psychotherapy

Evidence exists pointing to the powerful positive effects that nonspecific factors have in psychotherapy (Wampold, 2001). All psychotherapy involves these "nonspecific factors" such as therapeutic relationship and expectancy, which most likely contribute to positive outcome. The ethical clinician should use these powerful factors, which are inherent (if not always specified) in empirically supported treatments and EBTs to enhance treatment outcome.

Step 8: Inform Patient About the Pros and Cons of Treatment

The child or adolescent patient and the patient's family should be fully informed about the nature of the treatment, including the risks and benefits. In addition, the clinician should inform the client and his or her family of the developing nature of a treatment if the treatment has not been "scientifically" established. It is recognized that psychology does not have proven efficacy for all treatments. The clinician must be truthful with the client but, at the same time, be sensitive to the potentially detrimental effects that might occur by providing a range of outcome expectations. The clinician must be truthful and realistic about what might happen in therapy, yet the notion of hopefulness about change should also be included regardless of treatment approach.

Step 9: Motivate Client and Family in EBT

Motivating a client/patient and the family is crucial to positive outcome in psychotherapy. Many accepted effective treatments may not work if there is a lack of patient adherence and follow-through. Untoward family dynamics can also contribute to the sabotaging of therapy. Most behavioral interventions with children and adolescents are effective, but not if the child or adolescent does not follow the therapeutic regimen. Salesmanship is not a concept that is part of most graduate training programs, but selling the concept of changing behavior has broad implications for therapeutic effectiveness. After deciding on an EBT, the ethical clinician should motivate the client to adhere to the treatment and follow through with the established plan.

Step 10: Evaluate Effectiveness

While EBT has some degree of effectiveness implied by the very nature of design, reliability, and validity report, and by peer-reviewed publication, the final verdict is in the hands of the clinician. Assuming fidelity and appropriate application of the EBT to the client, the effectiveness must be judged. If the clinician is making a good-faith effort to competently apply the EBT, and results are not as expected, then the efficacy of the EBT itself must be considered. Just because the EBT worked "in the lab," it may or may not translate into the realm of clinical practice. Of course, the EBT that has been modified to meet the needs of a particular client may not be effective, and this must also be taken into consideration as the modification may inadvertently negate the effects of the EBT. Using a standardized approach to evaluation can be aided by EBT research; the practitioner can use the measures developed by the researchers on the specific target behaviors of interest. Alternatively, if these measures are not readily available (e.g., unpublished instrument) or are not practical to implement (e.g., home-based behavioral observation), other means of evaluation should be considered (e.g., symptom checklist). In all cases, the clinician should make an effort to use standardized and objective methods of evaluation to assist in judging clinical effectiveness.

CONCLUSION

Psychotherapy is often considered both a science and an art (Shapiro et al., 2006). Evidence-based treatments contribute much to the scientific aspect of psychology; however, even the most carefully designed and delivered treatment may not fit the situations the clinician faces. When clinical judgment, contextual issues, and patient values are taken into account, EBTs should be helpful to many children, adolescents, and families. The challenge then becomes how to ethically and effectively use EBTs to best assist clients presenting to psychologists and other mental health practitioners. Considering that children can be the most vulnerable of the populations that psychologists work with, the standard of practice must be at the highest level. Knowing the what, the how, and the when of EBT is essential to the ethical practice by the child-oriented clinician.

REFERENCES

Addis, M. E. (2002). Methods for disseminating research products and increasing evidence-based practice: Promises, obstacles, and future directions. *Clinical Psychology: Research and Practice, 9*, 367–378.

American Psychological Association (2002). Ethical principles of psychologists and code of conduct. *American Psychologist, 57*, 1060–1073.

American Psychological Association (2005). *Policy Statement on Evidence-Based Practice in Psychology.* Washington, DC.

American Psychological Association, Committee on Accreditation (2005). *Guidelines and Principles for Accreditation for Programs in Professional Psychology.* Washington, DC.

American Psychological Association Presidential Task Force on Evidence-Based Practice (2006). Evidence-based practice in psychology. *American Psychologist, 61*, 271–285.

American Psychological Association Task Force on Psychological Intervention Guidelines (1995). *Template for Developing Guidelines: Interventions for Mental Disorders and Psychosocial Aspects of Physical Disorders.* Washington, DC: American Psychological Association.

Barkley, R. A. (1997). *Defiant Children: A Clinician's Manual for Assessment and Parent Training,* 2nd ed. New York: Guilford Press.

Bohart, A. C. (2005). Evidence-based psychotherapy means evidence-informed, not evidence-driven. *Journal of Contemporary Psychotherapy, 35*, 39–53.

Bryceland, C., & Stam, H. J. (2005). Empirical validation and professional codes of ethics: Description or prescription? *Journal of Constructivist Psychology, 18*, 131–155.

Chambless, D. L., & Hollon, S. D. (1998). Defining empirically supported therapies. *Journal of Consulting and Clinical Psychology, 66*, 7–18.

Chorpita, B. F. (2003). The frontier of evidence-based practice. In A. E. Kazdin & J. R. Weisz (Eds.), *Evidence-Based Psychotherapies for Children and Adolescents* (pp. 42–59). New York: Guilford Press.

Chorpita, B. F., Barlow, D. H., Albano, A. M., & Daleiden, E. L. (1998). Methodological strategies in child clinical trails: Advancing the efficacy and effectiveness of psychosocial treatments. *Journal of Abnormal Psychology, 26*, 7–16.

Davidson, K. W., & Spring, B. (2006). Developing an evidence base in clinical psychology. *Journal of Clinical Psychology, 62*, 259–271.

Frank, J. D., & Frank, J. B. (1991). *Persuasion and Healing: A Comparative Study of Psychotherapy,* 3rd ed. Baltimore, MD: The Johns Hopkins University Press.

Herschell, A. D., McNeil, C. B., & McNeil, D. W. (2004). Clinical child psychology's progress in disseminating empirically supported treatments. *Clinical Psychology: Science and Practice, 11*, 267–288.

Jensen Doss, A., & Weisz, J. R. (2006). Syndrome co-occurrence and treatment outcomes in youth mental health clinics. *Journal of Consulting and Clinical Psychology, 74*, 416–425.

Kendall, P. C., & Beidas, R. S. (2007). Smoothing the trail for dissemination of evidence-based practices for youth: Flexibility within fidelity. *Professional Psychology: Research and Practice, 38*, 13–20.

Koocher, G. P. (2005). *Ethical implications of evidence-based treatments for practice.* Symposium conducted at the meeting of the American Psychological Association, Washington, DC, August.

Lonigan, C. J., Elbert, J. C., & Johnson, S. B. (1998). Empirically supported psychosocial interventions for children: An overview. *Journal of Clinical Child Psychology, 27*, 138–145.

Rae, W. A., & Fournier, C. J. (1999). Ethical and legal issues in the treatment of children and families. In T. Ollendick & S. Russ (Eds.), *Handbook of Psychotherapies with Children and Families* (pp. 67–84). New York: Plenum Press.

Roberts, M. C., & Hurley, L. K. (1997). *Managing Managed Care.* New York: Plenum Press.

Shapiro, J. P., Friedberg, R. D., & Bardenstein, K. K. (2006). *Child and Adolescent Therapy: Science and Art.* Hoboken, NJ: Wiley.

Spirito, A., & Kazak, A. E. (2006). *Effective and Emerging Treatments in Pediatric Psychology.* New York: Oxford University Press.

Task Force on Promotion and Dissemination of Psychological Procedures (1995). Training in and dissemination of empirically-validated psychological treatments. *The Clinical Psychologist, 48*(1), 3–23.

Wampold, B. E. (2001). *The Great Psychotherapy Debate: Models, Methods, and Findings.* Mahwah, NJ: Erlbaum.

Weisz, J. R. (2000). Lab-clinic differences and what can we do about them. I. The clinic-based treatment development model. *Clinical Child Psychology Newsletter, 15*(1), 1–3.

Weisz, J. R. (2004). *Psychotherapy for Children and Adolescents: Evidence-Based Treatments and Case Examples.* New York: Cambridge University Press.

Westen, D., Novotny, C. M., & Thompson-Brenner, H. (2004). The empirical status of empirically supported psychotherapies: Assumptions, findings, and reporting in controlled clinical trials. *Psychological Bulletin, 130*, 631–663.

29

Adoption of Evidence-Based Treatments in Community Settings: Obstacles and Opportunities

JULIANNE M. SMITH-BOYDSTON and TIMOTHY D. NELSON

Although the field has witnessed an increase in evidence-based treatments targeting mental illness in youth (Chorpita, 2003; Weisz et al., 1995), a considerable gap between this knowledge and the dissemination of such information into community-based settings remains apparent. This so-called science-practice gap has been widely acknowledged and often lamented in psychology (e.g., Beutler et al., 1995; Chorpita, 2003; Ollendick & Davis, 2004). In the area of child treatment, a wide range of efficacious approaches is now available (Chambless & Ollendick, 2001; Kazdin & Weisz, 2003); however, these treatments are rarely used in clinical practice (Kazdin, 2000, Kazdin et al., 1990). For example, Weisz and Kazdin (2003) reported that most evidence-based programs are behavioral or cognitive-behavioral, while nonbehavioral models are most widely used in clinical practice. This disconnect between science and service has stimulated considerable debate within the field regarding the value of most clinical research (e.g., Persons & Silberschatz, 1998) and the role of research in treatment selection (Beutler, 2004; Levant, 2004). Although a wide range of attitudes exists in the field, the debate has often pitted researchers calling for increased use of evidence-based approaches (e.g., Ollendick & Davis, 2004) against practitioners criticizing these approaches and highlighting clinical judgment as a more appropriate foundation of practice (e.g., Levant, 2004).

JULIANNE M. SMITH-BOYDSTON • Bert Nash Community Mental Health Center and **TIMOTHY D. NELSON** • University of Kansas, Clinical Child Psychology Program

Despite the sometimes contentious exchanges between outspoken researchers and practitioners, professional psychology recently took a step toward consensus on the issue of evidence-based treatments. The American Psychological Association (APA) has formally approved a policy statement defining and supporting evidence-based practice in psychology (EBPP; APA, 2005, 2006). The APA statement closely reflects the Institute of Medicine's (2001) definition of evidence-based practice, highlighting the importance of best research evidence, clinical expertise, and patient values. Although this statement is seen as an important step toward the use of EBTs for psychologists in applied settings, it is perhaps best understood as the most recent evidence of the general movement toward evidence-based practice in mental health care services.

While recent developments give reasons for optimism, considerable work in transporting EBTs to community settings is still needed. This chapter will outline some of the challenges associated with moving EBTs into a community-based treatment context as well as some of the unique opportunities of using EBTs in these settings. We will review some efforts to facilitate the adoption of EBTs in community settings and offer recommendations for future work to increase the likelihood of successfully transporting EBTs into community settings.

UNIQUE CHARACTERISTICS OF COMMUNITY SETTINGS

Mental health care in community settings can involve a range of settings including private clinics, medical centers, traditional private practice offices, and community mental health centers (CMHCs). In this chapter, we will concentrate on CMHCs because they show a wider range of client problem presentation, operate under federal and state mandates to serve children with severely emotional disturbances (SED), and maintain a team-based approach with a range of professionals guiding treatment. In considering the movement of EBTs from research settings to CMHCs, some important differences must be considered. These differences include the structure of treatment, the presentation of clients, and the training of therapists (Smith-Boydston, 2005). In terms of structure, many EBTs are designed for use by a qualified individual therapist in a one-on-one setting. In contrast, community settings more often employ team-based approaches, with team members having different defined roles in working with the child and family. As we will discuss later, such differences in the structure of services are important factors to be considered when transporting an EBT to a community-based context.

Another important potential difference between typical research and community settings can be found in the presentation of clients. Children present to CMHCs with a wide range of referral problems and symptom severity. On the one hand, some youth present with relatively mild symptoms and can be treated with short-term outpatient therapy. On the other hand, youth may present with severe symptoms, comorbid disorders, and major family disruptions. These children may be identified as severely emotionally disturbed (SED), which indicates that (1) the youth has a diagnosable disorder as defined by the *Diagnostic and Statistical Manual-IV-TR* [DSM-IV-TR, American Psychiatric Association (APA), 2000] and (2) this condition affects the child's functioning in at least one area such as within the family, at school, or in the community. Children designated as SED tend to have more severe symptoms and greater comorbidity than children seen in treatment research studies. However, many researchers have taken note of this potential discrepancy, and research using children with presentations more similar to those served in CMHCs has begun to emerge (see Steele et al., Chapter 3, for review).

Because CMHCs serve a wide and diverse array of problems, a variety of services are required. Outpatient services may include individual, family, group treatment, and, potentially, medication services. In light of the trend toward the decreased use of inpatient hospitalization, increasing demands have been placed on community-based services in treating the most problematic youth (Saxe et al., 1988). Community-based services incorporate a wide range of mental health professionals in varying capacities. Although differences exist between centers, treatment teams often consist of masters- and Ph.D.-level psychologists, bachelor- and masters- level social workers, counselors, psychiatrists, and/or nurses (Smith-Boydston, 2005). This team-based approach allows for intensive community-based services but also requires considerable communication and collaboration among team members.

CHALLENGES OF ADOPTING EBTs IN COMMUNITY SETTINGS

Several professionals have discussed the challenges involved in disseminating validated treatment protocols to community settings (Weisz et al., 1995, 2000). First, professionals in community settings may not "buy in" to the importance of implementing evidence-based treatments (Weisz et al., 1995, 2000). Several reasons have been posited for this suspected indifference, including differential educational training of staff that does not include a background of evidence-based treatment, belief systems of staff that clinical practice is more of an art than science, and thoughts that outcome research cannot capture the most applicable pieces of clinical change. In addition, there are concerns regarding the applicability of evidence-based practice that has been researched primarily on homogeneous samples with a primary disorder to comorbid disorders that are often seen in community settings. In addition, most of these protocols are developed for therapists and do not include roles for other treatment team members to implement, such as case managers, who usually have the most interaction with children and families.

Even for those professionals interested in EBTs, they may not have the sources to access information on what evidence-based programs are available (Ollendick & Davis, 2004). Oftentimes, community agencies use sources for treatment protocols that are not written by academic institutions, including local treatment newsletters or Web sites. Except for completing continuing education licensing requirements (CEUs) and the intrinsic benefits of gaining new knowledge, few real incentives for learning new approaches are currently in place (Weisz et al., 2000). In addition, community settings may have difficulty finding training protocols that meet their current client population and current training needs (Chorpita & Donkervoet, 2005).

Second, administrative factors are critical when examining drawbacks to implementation of evidence-based programs (Henggeler, 2003; Henggeler et al., 1995). Henggeler et al. (1995) outlined specific factors that must be initially addressed in community settings that differ from academic settings, including therapist caseloads, diverse referral issues on caseloads, and supervisory support. More focus in community settings on productivity standards and heterogeneous caseloads can make it difficult to focus more intensively on specific cases. As a result, time is a major factor in managing the ability to learn new skills and implementing these new skills with clients. In addition, funding considerations can make a difference regarding the amount of staff time spent in training for new procedures and ongoing protocol support. Support from community partners, including social service, juvenile justice, and families, can also become key as shifts are being made in treatment programs. Without this support, new programs may become stymied before they are able to show their effectiveness with problem youth. Also, some evidence-based practices may be underfunded or not reimbursable by different payor sources (Henggeler, 2003). Staff turnover and funding training of new staff in evidence-based protocols can also be a formidable challenge in community settings (Hoagwood et al., 1995).

Third, community settings often have limited resources to address the sustainability of a treatment program, especially if funds were originally garnered through time-limited state or federal grants (Henggeler, 2003). In addition, although treatment adherence and client outcomes are often assessed in research settings when analyzing EBTs, this process is usually discontinued in community settings, which has made it more difficult to advance effectiveness research (Henggeler et al., 1995; Weisz et al., 2000).

Emerging research supports the importance of some of these challenges. Preliminary findings from focus groups with community mental health practitioners (Nelson et al., 2006) suggest several challenges to implementing EBTs in community settings. Specifically, practitioners identified characteristics of many EBTs (e.g., highly structured formats and detailed manuals), characteristics of many practitioners (e.g., training), and characteristics of community settings (e.g., heavy client loads) that make implementing EBTs into regular practice difficult. Many practitioners also expressed concern that treatments tested in highly controlled studies with strict exclusion criteria may not be appropriate for severe clients seen in community settings. While the legitimacy of such concerns is somewhat unclear currently, the consistent expression of such concerns on the part of CMHC practitioners is worth noting. Efforts to implement EBTs in community settings will need to consider such practitioner concerns and work to facilitate adequate buy-in from both front-line clinicians and supervisors.

BENEFITS OF ADOPTING EBTs IN COMMUNITY SETTINGS

Although several challenges have been highlighted, community settings are an important venue for implementing and evaluating evidence-based treatments. Recognizing this opportunity, many in the field have suggested focusing on how to transport efficacious treatments from research contexts to applied settings. While highly controlled "efficacy" studies have dominated treatment research to date, an increased emphasis on "effectiveness" research that tests treatments in clinical settings has become apparent (Hoagwood & Olin, 2002). Notably, NIMH funding priorities have undergone a shift toward effectiveness research (NIMH, 2001), and such evaluations are now becoming increasingly available in the literature (e.g., Flannery-Schroeder et al., 2004). A more detailed discussion on trends in EBT research can be found in Steele et al. (Chapter 3); however, we mention the growing importance of effectiveness research here because it is central to our discussion of transporting EBTs to community settings.

Unfortunately, little research on adapting EBTs to community settings is currently available. Of particular interest is how efficacious one-on-one treatment protocols can be implemented within a community-based team approach. While treatment in a community setting presents numerous challenges not usually present in highly controlled research settings (Weersing & Weisz, 2002), we contend that this reality need not diminish the benefits of treatment. Instead, the unique advantages of community-based treatment might provide an opportunity for *increasing* the potency of a given EBT. Community-based teams are able to work with children and adolescents in their natural environment and can provide support for interventions made in individual or family treatment. For example, a CMHC's use of an anxiety protocol such as the *Coping Cat* (Kendall, 1990) might incorporate community-based professional involvement during exposure tasks to support the skills learned during individual therapy.

In the same way, many clients present to CMHCs with comorbid issues that need to be addressed. This population challenges the use of EBTs across a diverse range of problems that are seen in clinics (Doss & Weisz, 2006; Weisz et al., 1995). Also, the use of EBTs in cases with comorbid conditions can add to the effectiveness literature, examining the potential for combining elements of different treatments to meet the needs of clients (Weisz & Kazdin, 2003).

Administrative issues, specifically financial issues, are often primary for CMHCs when approaching the issue of staff training. Incorporating EBTs can be an efficient and cost-effective way to change youth problem behavior and worth CMHCs' investing staff training time. Therefore, CMHCs may need to look more and more to local resources as state and federal money becomes less available for these purposes. For example, at our CMHC, money was donated by a local resident in memory of his wife to develop the Nancy Shontz Educational Fund for ongoing staff training in evidence-based techniques. Local foundations may also be an option for centers to locate resources for training.

OVERVIEW OF TRAINING MODELS

The current gap between science and practice in community settings suggests that traditional models of training and dissemination are in need of revision. Traditional approaches such as sending individual therapists to one-time workshops do not appear to generalize to change in day-to-day clinical practice (Weisz et al., 2000). This is unfortunate, because state licensure requirements are often based on certain hours of workshop attendance or training, and many workshops have been set up to introduce evidence-based assessment and treatment across a variety of disorders (see www.catietraining.org for one example from a training institute).

Different models for generalizing and sustaining training have been proposed in the literature. Dissemination manuals are being developed for community settings, such as "Turning knowledge into practice: A manual for behavioral health administrators and practitioners about understanding and implementing evidence-based practices" developed by the Technical Assistance Collaborative, Inc., the John D. and Catherine T. MacArthur Foundation Network on Mental Health Policy Research, and the American College of Mental Health Administration (2003; www.tacinc.org or www.acmha.org). This manual provides information on how to select and implement EBTs; how to work with practitioners, organizations, and programs around EBTs; and how to sustain adopted programs. Manuals have also been developed to summarize treatment protocols (e.g., Kendall, 1990). However, some studies have found that exclusively using therapist manuals for training purposes does not lead to practice behavior change (Miller et al., 2005; Sholomskas et al., 2005). In contrast, some support has been found for Web-based training of core treatment strategies (Sholomskas et al., 2005).

Often agencies may use a top-down approach in identifying and incorporating training needs, which involves developing administrative support first and then offering benefits to staff implementing new approaches. However, one study found it helpful also to use key opinion leaders from line staff to facilitate buy-in and implementation of a model as well as using indigenous resources to address sustainability (Atkins et al., 2003). In addition, administering a needs assessment to guide workshop development has been shown to be useful in addition to developing a treatment manual to guide therapists to generalize skills following the training workshop (Roberts et al., 1990). Providing training and ongoing consultation from the treatment developers has also shown some support (Chorpita & Donkervoet, 2005). In fact, the strongest results have been found for participants attending a workshop and having some sort of follow-up coaching or individual feedback related to the treatment protocol to maintain clinical proficiency (Miller et al., 2004).

The comprehensive training model employed by the Multi-systemic Treatment of Juvenile Offenders (MST) program is an example of a treatment program that has actively considered training and implementation issues. MST is a short-term, intensive, community-focused family preservation treatment that was designed to reduce the recidivism of juvenile offenders (Henggeler et al., 1998). It is listed as an evidence-based program for conduct disorder (Kazdin & Weisz, 1998) and as a model program for juvenile offenders by several government agencies (e.g., U.S. Department of Health and Human Services, 2001; OJJDP, www.ojjdp.ncjrs.org; SAMSHA, www.samhsa.gov). Some evidence suggests that the MST model can be successfully extended to psychiatric crises, as an alternative to inpatient hospitalization (Sondheimer et al., 1994), and to youth with severe emotional disturbance (SED; Henggeler et al., 2002).

In order to disseminate MST while maintaining adherence to the original model, the developers of the MST program created a training institute entitled "MST Services" that trains and monitors new and ongoing community MST programs both nationally and internationally. A major feature of the dissemination of MST has been quality assurance measures, including therapist and supervisor adherence to the MST model (Schoenwald et al., 2000). Training in MST involves several levels of influence, beginning with community and institutional needs assessment and sustainability assessment. After this, there is an initial one-week intensive training series regarding the main principles and treatment aspects of MST, followed by weekly consultations from MST Services, quarterly treatment workshops for MST staff, and regular review of treatment adherence and clinical outcomes.

Clearly, MST has developed a comprehensive plan that addresses administrative, therapist, and training issues regarding disseminating an EBT into community settings. However, there are some drawbacks to such an approach. This comprehensive plan is based only on one EBT model to address the treatment of juvenile offenders. Although the model has been used with other populations, there is much staff time, training, and follow-up based on a potentially small client population in a community setting. This is most likely why many of the MST programs are based in juvenile justice settings, where there is maximum use of the model. Also, high start-up and maintenance costs associated with ongoing licensure and consultation services by MST are often prohibitive for community settings. Without substantial and ongoing outside funding, basic training budgets for CMHCs would have considerable difficulty incorporating this model in its entirety while also addressing other training needs.

A TRAINING MODEL FOR ADOPTING EBTs IN COMMUNITY SETTINGS

Building on past research and training models, we offer a model that aims to incorporate some of the most efficient and effective aspects of previous models while also considering financial limitations of many community settings (see Figure 1). Within this model, we incorporate not only the buy-in and needs of the setting but also the effective training of staff in order to generalize the skills, sustain the program, and allow for changes in evidence-based treatment standards. To many community settings, the task of constructing a comprehensive staff training program may seem

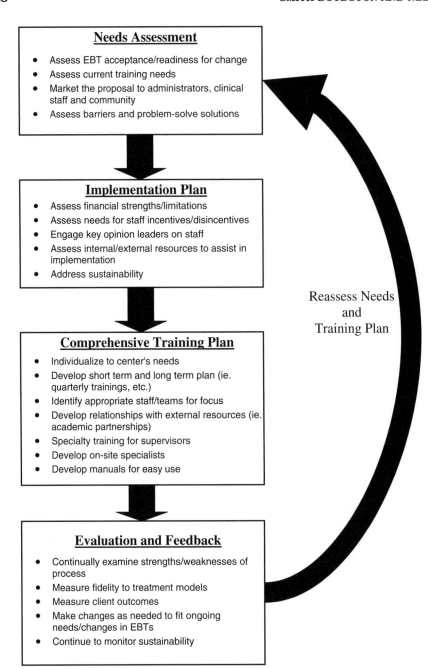

Figure 1. Model for the adoption of EBTs in community settings.

overwhelming. However, we also suggest that CMHCs assess their current training plans and use this model to discuss potential next steps. As others have suggested, planning for and implementing change can take time, especially when sustained system change is the goal (Chorpita &

Donkervoet, 2005). Therefore, we recommend that centers take the time to consider their unique challenges and opportunities process before implementation of major changes.

NEEDS ASSESSMENT

A dissemination plan focusing on assessing agency clinical needs, assessing acceptance of EBTs and change, and "marketing" the plan to administrative and line staff is critical in developing new programs. As a first step, it is key to have administration buy-in, particularly if incentives or disincentives can be used to support the use of the new treatments and plan implementation. Within this process, the needs of the community and agency should be assessed in order to match these needs to evidence-based interventions. Assessing the readiness for EBTs at all levels will help in developing a plan for change. Including key clinical personnel involved, or opinion leaders, to support the plan and treatment implementation will facilitate staff involvement in the project. This can be done by gathering current gaps in meeting client needs and interest training in new procedures to address particular client populations. An intervention can also have more powerful backing if individuals involved with the agency, including community leaders, agency partners, and clients, are a part of the planning and implementation of the program. Addressing barriers as they arise will help to make the next step of implementation more straightforward.

A useful example of this is the statewide implementation of an evidence-based training model used recently in Hawaii (Chorpita & Donkervoet, 2005; Chorpita et al., 2002). Although the initial impetus for the change in program resulted from a federal class-action suit, the developers of the statewide implementation made it a priority to engage critical stakeholders, including administrators, local case managers, and client families, at the beginning of the process to assess needs and how treatment approaches fit with their own client population.

IMPLEMENTATION PLAN

At the next level, we propose that CMHCs carefully develop an implementation plan to support the training program and facilitate an effective transition to the new model. Financial strengths and limitations are often primary in assessment of the range of training that is manageable for the setting. Evaluating these resources can set the boundaries of possibilities regarding modalities such as sending staff to workshops, the ability to bring national professionals to the center, considering local specialists, or potentially Web-based or internal resources. Administration should assess the ability to offer staff incentives and/or disincentives to present practice that may reinforce the adoption of new practices. In particular, having a positive and collaborative approach with staff from the onset regarding barriers to change and pulling in opinion leaders to assist in implementation will make the change smoother. Making early assessments of current practice and finding ways to incorporate changes into an already-functioning structure are also important. For example, CMHCs often have levels of meetings, including individual supervision, team meetings, and area meetings, that can be used in ways to support training goals.

We propose two unique aspects of internal and external resources of training to support implementation and strengthen the sustainability of a training program. First, we suggest a more formal union of community settings and academic settings to form a more synergistic partnership regarding the identification, instigation, and maintenance of programs. This suggestion is consistent with others who have discussed finding ways to bridge the apparent discrepancies between clinical work in academic versus community settings (Weisz et al., 1995). In contrast to the present disjointedness felt between these two settings, we think community-academic partnerships may yield great benefits for both entities and advance knowledge of treatments for children and families. Second, we think it is key to the success of new training programs to have on-site experts to facilitate understanding, guide implementation, and problem-solve potential roadblocks. Having experts who are accessible and part of the existing culture in the CMHC will likely prove helpful as clinicians attempt to learn and implement new treatment strategies.

An ideal community-academic partnership would involve several aspects. Academic departments could assist community settings in identifying evidence-based treatments that could meet the identified client needs. Then community settings could give feedback regarding the strengths and challenges in implementing the given protocol and ways that the protocol may need to be adapted to meet certain demographic or therapist requirements (i.e., certain minority populations without much evidence-based research; meeting productivity standard requirements). A training program could then be adapted to the community setting that takes into account the need for expert workshops as well as consultation by local academic departments. It would be most helpful to develop a plan that hosts different evidence-based techniques at specific intervals (i.e., quarterly) to learn new techniques but then have a chance to practice them, give feedback on the pros and cons of implementation in order to problem-solve difficulties, and then be able to work on new skills. Ongoing consultation and feedback will help to increase the buy-in from staff, which would be different from forcing manualized approaches on teams without feedback, which may encounter more opposition.

Academic settings can also be very useful to community settings regarding developing easy-to-use manuals for therapists to implement skills and assist in collecting fidelity and outcome data (we will explain later) to be used to assess if interventions are effective with client populations. Many academic professors and graduate students in clinical psychology and social work are very interested at this time in forming relationships with community partners to extend treatment research into the field. Also, the American Psychological Association (APA) and National Institute of

Mental Health (NIMH) have expressed interest in increasing academic-community partnerships to extend the effectiveness of treatment interventions (NIMH, 2001). In turn, community settings can be helpful to academic partners by providing them with data to evaluate training programs, ease of program use, fidelity, and the relationship of these factors to client outcomes. Working together in this way will facilitate more positive and productive relationships between academic institutions and community providers, leading to improvement in both clinical services and research.

In addition to academic/clinical linkages, it is important to develop on-site specialists to support ongoing implementation of evidence-based treatment. For some sites, this may be supervisors who become specialists in particular areas. However, if CMHCs have the resources, this person can be an additional staff position available to collect resources, continually assess and monitor training progress, and be a liaison to outside resource. This "go-to person" could interact with academics and clinical staff to assess training needs and assist in developing and coordinating on-site trainings with the goal of learning techniques important across the treatment team and training the supervisors who will assist in sustaining the program after implementation. This person could be key in assisting treatment teams and supervisors in generalizing information they have used and in being an on-site consultant dealing with a variety of implementation issues.

At this point, a detailed plan for the program's sustainability is also needed. This is often the most difficult part of incorporating new programs into standard practice, particularly if money is given for the start-up of a particular program but not promised for ongoing support. This is why having on-site consultants and/or indigenous trainers can be so important to agencies. Also, ongoing connections with academic professionals can be helpful not only in choosing potential evidence-based programs and collecting data, but also in keeping abreast of the latest research and programs to treat clinical problems and to lead to agency training next steps.

COMPREHENSIVE TRAINING PLAN

As stated previously, most professional trainings to develop new skills have focused on one-time workshops for individual therapists or groups of therapists to be trained off-site. For CMHCs, the difficulties with this model are that it tends to focus only on the licensed professional and skills taught do not appear to generalize to day-to-day practice. In contrast, it is important to maximize the training time to include all staff who work with children and families, from licensed professionals to case managers and other youth team members. In order to do this, trainings should be individualized to a center's needs, which represent the clientele served. Therefore, we suggest incorporating the strongest aspects that have been shown to work for dissemination of skills, including focused trainings for teams that will work together, developing manuals for ease of use of the evidence-based technique, and specialty training and support for supervisors who will need to maintain skills over time.

EVALUATION AND FEEDBACK

With the busyness of day-to-day work in CMHCs, this last step in the model is often overlooked. However, this step is very important to have ways to assess if a center's training plan is working for staff as well as the client population being served.

Therapist fidelity to the treatment model can sometimes be difficult to assess with new treatment models. However, without some mechanism to assess this, it is very difficult to determine potential changes in client outcomes. Many evidence-based treatment protocols have methods to assess therapist fidelity to the model. For example, the MST program has developed a Therapist Adherence Measure (TAM) that families in the program complete monthly regarding actions of their therapist, as well as a Supervisor Adherence Measure (SAM) that therapists complete regarding supervisor practices. Both of these measures assess fidelity by asking questions related to the program's core principles. In addition, research outcome studies have shown that these fidelity models are tied to positive client outcomes (Schoenwald et al., 2004). Other programs include review and/or coding of therapist treatment sessions (Miller et al., 2004). Some programs have more limited assessment of fidelity that relies on therapist report of gains or difficulties. Finding ways to incorporate measures across different treatment modalities may be the most efficient way for centers to incorporate this step (Chorpita & Donkervoet, 2005).

Measuring client outcomes can be used as the ultimate indicator of successful implementation of evidence-based practices, especially when connected to therapist fidelity to certain treatment models. Community settings have become more familiar with collecting outcome data partially due to increased pressures from state and insurance organizations, such that most community settings have some form of client outcomes they are collecting. For example, each family that enters our mental health center is asked to complete a Child Behavior Checklist (CBCL; Achenbach, 1991) related to the identified youth. For those children who receive intensive community-based services, the CBCL is collected every six months and submitted to the state for outcome. In addition, the Child and Adolescent Functional Assessment Scale (CAFAS; Hodges et al., 1998) is also completed on a subset of clients. Since most agencies have some form of outcome collected for their identified youth, it would not be too difficult to examine outcomes by treatment modality. Again, the assistance of an academic partnership could facilitate these types of analyses.

As stated before, receiving continual feedback from staff and clients can assist in assessing strengths and barriers to the new treatment plan and also lead to changes that will make it more workable for the CMHC. In addition, sustainability issues should also be addressed to be sure the training protocol can continue to be supported and does not become a victim to funding cuts or other administrative issues.

As can be seen from this model, it is important that agencies take time to consider several aspects of implementation as they are contemplating changing their present form of treatment practice. We have developed a model that will hopefully be useful to community settings that are interested in implementing EBTs into their training plan. Our plan involves a comprehensive strategy that begins with assessing the CMHC's current needs in order to effectively plan implementation. Ideally, the CMHC needs to consider how the training plan will be implemented and how to get buy-in from both administrators and clinical staff. The next step involves the actual comprehensive training plan with our suggestions of ways to make the best use of internal and external resources not only to have the most effective training plan but also to look to the sustainability of the program after the initial training. Finally, we emphasize the need to assess training outcomes and reassess needs for future training programs. Because different CMHCs may have different needs, training programs may look different, but these common elements should be helpful in creating a workable plan.

Implementing EBTs in community settings will require an intensive and ongoing effort by administrators, CMHC staff, and community partners. Although this is a formidable task, we believe that it is also an important one. With the recent movement toward EBTs in mental health services, community centers will come under increasing pressure to incorporate evidence-based approaches in a systematic and effective way. This situation provides both a challenge and an opportunity for CMHCs. We encourage community providers to meet this challenge with a thoughtful implementation of the suggestions we have outlined in this chapter.

REFERENCES

Achenbach, T. M. (1991). *Integrative Guide to the 1991 CBCL, YSR, and TRF Profiles.* Burlington, VT: University of Vermont, Department of Psychiatry.

American Psychiatric Association (2000). *Diagnostic and Statistical Manual of Mental Disorders,* 4th ed. (text revision). Washington, DC.

American Psychological Association (2005). Policy statement on evidence-based practice in psychology. Retrieved September 9, 2005, from http://www.apa.org/practice/ebpstatement.pdf.

American Psychological Association (2006). Evidence-based practice in psychology. *American Psychologist, 61,* 271–285.

Atkins, M. S., Graczyk, P. A., Frazier. S. L., & Abdul-Adil, J. (2003). Toward a new model for promoting urban children's mental health: Accessible, effective, and sustainable school-based mental health services. *School Psychology Review, 32,* 503–514.

Beutler, L. E. (2004). The empirically supported treatments movement: A scientist-practitioner's response. *Clinical Psychology: Science and Practice, 11,* 225–229.

Beutler, L. E., Williams, R. E., Wakefield, P. J., & Entwistle, S. R. (1995). Bridging scientist and practitioner perspectives in clinical psychology. *American Psychologist, 50,* 984–994.

Chambless, D. L., & Ollendick, T. H. (2001). Empirically supported psychological interventions: Controversies and evidence. *Annual Review of Psychology, 52,* 685–716.

Chorpita, B. F. (2003). The frontier of evidence-based practice. In A. E. Kazdin & J. R. Weisz (Eds.), *Evidence-Based Psychotherapies for Children and Adolescents* (pp. 42–59). New York: Guilford Press.

Chorpita, B. F., & Donkervoet, C. (2005). Implementation of the Felix Consent Decree in Hawaii. In R. G. Steele & M. C. Roberts (Eds.), *Handbook of Mental Health Services for Children, Adolescents, and Families* (pp. 317–332). New York: Kluwer Academic/Plenum Publishers.

Chorpita, B. F., Yim, L. M., Donkervoet, J. C., Arensdorf, A., Amundsen, M. J., McGee, C., et al. (2002). Toward large-scale implementation of empirically supported treatments for children: A review and observations by the Hawaii Empirical Basis to Services Task Force. *Clinical Psychology: Science and Practice, 9,* 1–36.

Doss, A. J., & Weisz, J. R. (2006). Syndrome co-occurrence and treatment outcomes in youth mental health clinics. *Journal of Consulting and Clinical Psychology, 74,* 416–425

Flannery-Schroeder, E., Suveg, C., Safford, S., Kendall, P. C., & Webb, A. (2004). Comorbid externalising disorders and child anxiety treatment outcomes. *Behaviour Change, 21,* 14–25.

Henggeler, S. W. (2003). Advantages and disadvantages of multisystemic therapy and other evidence-based practices for treating juvenile offenders. *Journal of Forensic Psychology Practice, 3,* 53–59.

Henggeler, S. W., Schoenwald, S. K., Borduin, C. M., Rowland, M. D., & Cunningham, P. B. (1998). *Multisystemic Treatment of Antisocial Behavior in Youth.* New York: Guilford Press.

Henggeler, S. W., Schoenwald, S. K., & Pickrel, S. G. (1995). Multisystemic therapy: Bridging the gap between university- and community-based treatment. *Journal of Consulting and Clinical Psychology, 63,* 709–717.

Henggeler, S. W., Schoenwald, S. K., Rowland, M. D., & Cunningham, P. B. (2002). *Serious Emotional Disturbance in Children and Adolescents.* New York: Guilford Press.

Hoagwood, K., & Olin, S. (2002). The NIMH blueprint for change report: Research priorities in child and adolescent mental health. *Journal of the American Academy of Child and Adolescent Psychiatry, 41,* 760–767.

Hodges, K., Wong, M. M., & Latessa, M. (1998). Use of the Child and Adolescent Functional Assessment Scale (CAFAS) as an outcome measure in clinical settings. *Journal of Behavioral Health Services and Research, 25,* 325–336.

Institute of Medicine (2001). *Crossing the Quality Chasm: A New Health System for the 21st Century.* Washington, DC: National Academy Press.

Kazdin, A. E. (2000). *Psychotherapy for Children and Adolescents: Directions for Research and Practice.* New York: Oxford University Press.

Kazdin, A. E., Siegel. T. C., & Bass, D. (1990). Drawing upon clinical practice to inform research on child and adolescent psychotherapy: A survey of practitioners. *Professional Psychology: Research and Practice, 21,* 189–198.

Kazdin, A. E., & Weisz, J. R. (1998). Identifying and developing empirically supported child and adolescent treatments. *Journal of Consulting and Clinical Psychology, 66,* 19–36.

Kazdin, A. E., & Weisz, J. R. (2003). Introduction: Context and background of evidence-based psychotherapies for children and adolescents. In A. E. Kazdin & J. R. Weisz (Eds.), *Evidence-Based Psychotherapies for Children and Adolescents* (pp. 3–20). New York: Guilford Press.

Kendall, P. C. (1990). *Coping Cat Workbook.* Ardmore, PA: Workbook Publishing.

Levant, R. F. (2004). The empirically validated treatments movement: A practitioner's perspective. *Clinical Psychology: Science and Practice, 11,* 219–224.

Miller, W. R., Yahne, C. E., Moyers, T. B., Martinez, J., & Pirritano, M. (2004). A randomized trial of methods to help clinicians learn motivational interviewing. *Journal of Counseling and Clinical Psychology, 72,* 1050–1062.

National Institute of Mental Health (2004). *Bridging Science and Service: A Report by the National Advisory Mental Health Council's Clinical Treatment and Services Research Workgroup.* Bethesda, MD: National Institutes of Health.

Nelson, T. D., Steele, R. G., & Mize, J. A. (2006). Practitioner attitudes toward evidence-based practice: Themes and challenges. *Administrative Policy in Mental Health and Mental Health Services Research, 33,* 398–409.

Ollendick, T. H., & Davis, T. E. (2004). Empirically supported treatments for children and adolescents: Where to from here? *Clinical Psychology: Science and Practice, 11*, 289–294.

Persons, J. B., & Silberschatz, G. (1998). Are results of randomized controlled trials useful to psychotherapists? *Journal of Consulting and Clinical Psychology, 66*, 126–135.

Roberts, M. C., Blount, R. L., Lyman, R. D., & Landolf-Fritsche, B. (1990). Collaboration of a university and state mental health agency: Curriculum for improving services for children. *Professional Psychology: Research and Practice, 21*, 69–71.

Saxe, L., Cross, T., & Silverman, N. (1988). Children's mental health: The gap between what we know and what we do. *American Psychologist, 43*, 800–807.

Schoenwald, S. K., Brown, T. L., & Henggeler, S. W. (2000). Inside multisystemic therapy: Therapists, supervisory, and program practices. *Journal of Emotional and Behavioral Disorders, 8*, 113–127.

Sholomskas, D. E., Syrause-Siewert, G., Rounsaville, B. J., Ball, S. A., Nuro, K. F., & Carroll, K. M. (2005). We don't train in vain: A dissemination trial of three strategies of training clinicians in cognitive-behavioral therapy. *Journal of Consulting and Clinical Psychology, 73*, 106–115.

Smith-Boydston, J. M. (2005). Providing a range of services to fit the needs of youth in community mental health centers. In R. G. Steele & M. C. Roberts (Eds.), *Handbook of Mental Health Services for Children, Adolescents, and Families* (pp. 103–116). New York: Kluwer.

U.S. Department of Health and Human Services (2001). *Youth Violence: A Report of the Surgeon General*. Rockville, MD: U.S. Department of Health and Human Services, Centers for Disease Control and Prevention, National Center for Injury Prevention and Control, Substance Abuse and Mental Health Services Administration, Center for Mental Health Services, and National Institutes of Health, National Institute of Mental Health.

Weersing, V. R., & Weisz, J. R. (2002). Community clinic treatment of depressed youth: Benchmarking usual care against CBT trials. *Journal of Consulting and Clinical Psychology, 70*, 299–310.

Weisz, J. R., Donenberg, G. R., Han, S. S., & Weiss, B. (1995). Bridging the gap between laboratory and clinic in child and adolescent psychotherapy. *Journal of Consulting and Clinical Psychology, 63*, 688–701.

Weisz, J. R., Hawley K. M., Pilkonis, P. A., Woody, S. R., & Follette, W. C. (2000). Stressing the (other) three Rs in the search for empirically supported treatments: Review procedures, research quality, relevance to practice and public interest. *Clinical Psychology: Science and Practice, 7*, 243–258.

Weisz, J. R., & Kazdin, A. E. (2003). Present and future of evidence-based psychotherapies for children and adolescents. In A. E. Kazdin & J. R. Weisz (Eds.), *Evidence-Based Psychotherapies for Children and Adolescents* (pp. 439–451). New York: Guilford Press.

30

Evidence-Based Assessment for Children and Adolescents

VICKY PHARES and JESSICA CURLEY

Throughout this book, evidence-based therapies (EBTs) for children and adolescents have been delineated for different disorders and clinical problems. Before clinicians can decide on an evidence-based therapy, however, they must identify the problems to target in treatment. Thus, the use of an evidence-based therapy is contingent upon a reliable and valid evidence-based assessment (EBA) of the problems that are to be addressed in treatment (Kazdin, 2005; Weisz & Addis, 2006). If an evidence-based therapy is chosen based on inaccurate diagnostic information or if treatment progress is assessed with inaccurate assessment procedures, then even the best evidence-based therapy may not work well because it was applied to the wrong target problem. Thus, evidence-based assessment is essential for the appropriate use of evidence-based therapy. As Achenbach (2005) summarized, "Without accurate identification and measurement of the problems to be treated and of outcomes following treatment, the potential benefits of EBT cannot be achieved" (p. 541).

This chapter will first address the background and rationale for the use of evidence-based assessment and will then discuss a number of issues related to identifying what constitutes an evidence-based assessment. Because diagnostic tools and evaluation methods specific to individual disorders are discussed throughout this book in the context of each evidence-based therapy, this chapter will approach the issue from a broader perspective that is not disorder-driven. For measures specific to a disorder, each chapter can be reviewed to identify measures that were used to establish symptom reduction for that disorder. In addition, a special section of the *Journal of Clinical Child and Adolescent Psychology* provides an excellent resource for evidence-based assessments, including articles focused on anxiety (Silverman & Ollendick, 2005), depression (Klein et al., 2005), pediatric bipolar disorder (Youngstrom et al., 2005), attention deficit

VICKY PHARES and JESSICA CURLEY • University of South Florida

hyperactivity disorder (Pelham et al., 2005), conduct problems (McMahon & Frick, 2005), learning disorders (Fletcher et al., 2005), and autism spectrum disorders (Ozonoff et al., 2005).

BACKGROUND AND HISTORICAL ISSUES

With all of the focus on evidence-based therapies in both the adult and child literatures, it is quite surprising that professionals have only recently turned their attention to evidence-based assessment within the context of evidence-based therapies. Empirically based and evidence-based treatments have been the focus of widespread attention for over a decade (Task Force on Promotion and Dissemination of Psychological Procedures, 1995), and yet there has not been a concomitant focus on evidence-based assessments until recently (Mash & Hunsley, 2005). Of course, the concept of using empirically derived evaluation methods is not new (Achenbach, 1985; Achenbach & McConaughy, 1987), but the field-wide attention to evidence-based assessment and the linking of evidence-based assessment to evidence-based interventions appear to be recent trends.

Like the history of therapies and interventions, the history of assessment has been riddled with widely used techniques that have not had an empirical basis. Likely the biggest controversy in the history of assessment regards the use of the Rorschach inkblot test (Garb et al., 2005). Whether with adults or children, the use of the Rorschach inkblot test has been routinely questioned on empirical grounds (Lilienfeld et al., 2000; Wood et al., 2003). In a chapter entitled "Controversial and Questionable Assessment Techniques," Hunsley et al. (2003) listed the Rorschach inkblot test as the first of five questionable assessment procedures that are used widely by clinical psychologists. The other questionable assessment techniques were the Thematic Apperception Test (TAT), projective drawings, anatomically detailed dolls (ADDs), and the Myers–Briggs Type Indicator (MBTI). Regarding the Rorschach inkblot test, Hunsley and colleagues (2003) reviewed the empirical data for standardization, norms, reliability, and validity and concluded that "there is insufficient scientific evidence to justify the continued use of the test in clinical settings" (p. 50). This conclusion applies to both child and adult populations. There is a need to increase the emphasis on evidence-based assessment in the context of the evaluation of evidence-based treatments. Unfortunately, the national and international dialogues about evidence-based treatments for children and adolescents have largely ignored any commentary on the necessity to identify and utilize assessment techniques that are based on empirical evidence.

RATIONALE FOR EVIDENCE-BASED ASSESSMENTS

The underlying rationale for using evidence-based assessments is ultimately the same as the underlying rationale for using evidence-based therapies: Professional psychologists need to know that their clinical techniques are accurate, and evidence needs to serve as the cornerstone of these techniques. Our definition of evidence relies on knowledge that is gained through empirical research studies that are well controlled and carefully carried out. In the interventions literature, the "gold standard" of empirical evidence focuses on randomized clinical trials that show that one treatment is more effective than a placebo or another treatment (Task Force on Promotion and Dissemination of Psychological Procedures, 1995). Thus, by definition, evidence-based treatments are more effective than placebo procedures or other treatments including treatment as usual (Ollendick & King, 2006).

In the assessment literature, it is more difficult to establish a firm basis for which assessment tools are or are not evidence-based. At a minimum, assessment techniques should be reliable and valid, but Mash and Hunsley (2005) pointed out that measures may have stronger evidence for some uses in certain populations and weaker or no evidence for other uses in different populations. For example, one measure may have strong norms for the general population, less strong but adequate norms for outpatient clinical populations, and weak norms for inpatient clinical populations. The internal consistency, test-retest reliability, content validity, concurrent validity, predictive validity, discriminant validity, incremental validity, diagnostic utility, and treatment utility may also vary for the same measure across these different populations (Mash & Hunsley, 2005). Thus, categorizations of certain measures or assessment techniques must be cognizant of the specific use of the measure and the intended population to be evaluated.

Unlike the criteria put forth by Chambless and Hollon (1998) that codified the definitions of empirically supported therapies, there is currently no formal framework by which to judge whether a measure meets criteria as an evidence-based assessment technique. There are, however, guidelines and standards for the development and use of psychological assessment techniques that are well known. The publication *Standards for Educational and Psychological Testing* (1999) is widely used as the national standard for the development and use of psychological tests; the publication focuses on the establishment of empirical data in test development and use. Mash and Hunsley (2005) argued that additional guidelines should be developed that are specific to evidence-based assessment. They noted that guidelines need to take into account evidence-based methods (e.g., the types of assessment techniques used) as well as the assessment process (e.g., how assessment data are used and how divergent information is combined and ultimately utilized in the treatment process).

In addition to needing more standardized criteria for defining evidence-based measures and for developing more standardization in the assessment process, a number of issues must be considered when trying to formalize a more evidence-based assessment process that is linked to the evaluation of evidence-based treatments. These issues include the need for assessments of both broad and specific problems, considerations of both categorical as well as dimensional aspects of behavior, the use of multiple informants that represent children's behavior in multiple contexts, the use of multiple methodologies, the need to assess strengths as well as problems, the use of assessment techniques that are sensitive to diversity, the use of assessments that are sensitive to child and adolescent functioning over time, and assessments that explore the context and environment as they relate to children's and adolescents' functioning.

ISSUES IN CONDUCTING EVIDENCE-BASED ASSESSMENTS

Assessments of Both Broad and Specific Problems

A thorough evidence-based assessment process should include the evaluations of both the referral problem and other potential problems that were not identified initially by the child, his or her parents, his or her teachers, and other professionals. Comorbidity is the rule rather than the exception in child and adolescent clinical populations (Angold et al., 1999). Thus, an evidence-based assessment process must go beyond the exploration of the referral problem in order to identify other possible problems that are related to the child's functioning. Certainly, a referral for depressive symptoms in a child would call for the use of a measure like the Children's Depression Inventory (Kovacs, 1992), but other symptoms would need to be assessed with broader measures such as the Child Behavior Checklist (Achenbach & Rescorla, 2001) to ascertain whether there were any comorbid problems such as anxiety or conduct problems (Klein et al., 2005).

Parallel examples could be given for structured clinical interviews that result in psychiatric diagnoses. One of the advantages of using a diagnostic interview like the Diagnostic Interview Schedule for Children (DISC; Shaffer et al., 2000) is that the clinician is able to assess a wide array of potential diagnoses. However, the advantages of the global nature of the DISC are not always maximized by clinical researchers and clinicians, perhaps because of the extensive amount of time that it takes to administer a thorough diagnostic interview (Weisz & Addis, 2006).

In a system of evidence-based assessment, it would be ideal to include measures that assess both broadly and specifically. These same issues are relevant to the assessment of children's and adolescents' functioning through categorical versus dimensional approaches.

Assessments of Both Categorical and Dimensional Aspects of Behavior

There have long been debates on the nature of children's behavior and whether it is best conceptualized in a categorical taxonomy [e.g., using the *Diagnostic and Statistical Manual of Mental Disorders, 4th edition, Text Revision (DSM-IV-TR)*; American Psychiatric Association, 2000] or dimensional taxonomy [e.g., using the Achenbach System of Empirically Based Assessment (ASEBA; Achenbach & Rescorla, 2001)]. With an eye toward revisions for the fifth edition of *DSM*, a special section of the *Journal of Abnormal Psychology* was devoted to dimensionally based taxonomies of psychopathology (Krueger et al., 2005). In addition, a number of researchers have explored the empirical evidence in the structure of developmental psychopathology and have concluded that many childhood problems are best conceptualized in a continuous rather than a dichotomous fashion (Achenbach et al., 2003; Hankin et al., 2005).

With all of this debate, it should be noted that dimensional and categorical conceptualizations of children's functioning need not be considered incongruent. Achenbach (2005) argued that categorical and quantitative or dimensional approaches can inform each other and can add to the richness of data gathered about children's and adolescents' functioning. In fact, most randomized clinical trials include assessments from both categorical and dimensional conceptualizations of child functioning [e.g., Treatment for Adolescents with Depression Study (TADS) Team, 2004]. Thus, it would be ideal if evidence-based assessments included evaluations of behavior from both a categorical and dimensional perspective.

Assessments of Multiple Informants in Different Settings

It would also be ideal if children's and adolescents' behavior were assessed by different informants who can report on behavior in different settings, such as in the home and at school. One of the unique features in working with youth as opposed to adults is that child clinicians can easily gather information about children in the form of self-reports as well as from collateral informants. Using multiple informants of children and adolescents has been a well-established practice for decades (DeLosReyes & Kazdin, 2004).

The challenge, however, is that informants often do not agree on their conceptualizations of the child's or adolescent's behavior. These differences are common in both the identification of problems to be targeted for therapeutic intervention and in more global ratings of behavior (Hawley & Weisz, 2003; Yeh & Weisz, 2001). Overall, there is a fair amount of disagreement among youth, parents, and therapists about the target problems of therapy.

This same issue is relevant when using standardized assessment measures. In their classic meta-analysis, Achenbach et al. (1987) found that informants' ratings of children and adolescents differed largely based on the comparability of the role of the informant in relation to the child (e.g., parent with parent vs. parent with teacher). They found that informants in the same role and in the same situations, such as parents with parents in the home, had an average correlation of 0.60. Informants in different situations, such as parents and teachers, correlated 0.28 on average. Across informants, there appeared to be stronger inter-rater associations for externalizing rather than internalizing behaviors and for children in contrast to adolescents. More recent studies have found comparable results whereby different informants, such as mothers and fathers, often show significant correspondence in reporting on their children's behavior, but the correlations are modest and account for relatively small amounts of variance (DeLosReyes & Kazdin, 2004; Duhig et al., 2000).

There are many possible explanations for these differences in perceptions of children's and adolescents' behavior, including situational specificity (Achenbach et al., 1987), differing experiences of what is distressing
(Phares & Compas, 1990), or differing tolerance levels for defining
behavior as problematic (Weisz et al., 1988). Parents' own psychological
functioning has also been found to be related to their reports of children's
emotional/behavioral problems (Kurdek, 2003).

Thus, a number of factors can influence informants' reports of
children's and adolescents' emotional/behavioral problems. No set of informants, including even trained observers, is considered a "gold standard"
for use in assessing children's and adolescents' emotional/behavioral
problems (DeLosReyes & Kazdin, 2004). Thus, evidence-based assessment
protocols should consider using multiple informants in order to gather a
comprehensive overview of the child's or adolescent's functioning.

Assessments with Multiple Methodologies

In addition to the use of multiple informants in evidence-based assessment,
there is also empirical evidence to support the use of multiple methodologies in the assessment of children and adolescents. Methodologies such
as interviews, behavior checklists, and direct observations have all been
investigated in relation to the different types of information that can be
collected about the referred child or adolescent.

The use of interviews with children and parents is usually evaluated
separately depending on whether the interviews are unstructured or
structured. There is little empirical support for the use of unstructured
interviews for the purpose of psychiatric diagnosis. Unstructured clinical
interviews are used widely in clinical practice, with the overwhelming
majority of clinicians using an unstructured interview to begin the
assessment process with a parent or child or both (Jensen & Weisz, 2002).
Unfortunately, unstructured interviews are not terribly reliable or valid
(Jensen & Weisz, 2002).

Although unstructured clinical interviews do not have strong empirical
support for diagnostic purposes, they can be beneficial in developing
rapport with child and adolescent clients (Sattler & Hoge, 2006). Given
that rapport is essential for completion of a full evaluation and that
rapport is linked to therapeutic alliance, which, in turn, is linked to therapeutic outcome (Karver et al., 2006; Shirk & Karver, 2003), it seems that
unstructured clinical interviews may have a place within an evidence-based
assessment if only to help develop rapport and to gather background information (Sattler & Hoge, 2006). There continues to be support for the use
of structured clinical interviews to ascertain psychiatric diagnoses (Shaffer
et al., 2000).

Behavior checklists have been used extensively in the assessment
of children and adolescents, and many behavior checklists have strong
psychometric properties. Behavior checklists can be used for rating broad
spectrums of behavior, such as with the Child Behavior Checklist (CBCL;
Achenbach & Rescorla, 2001) and the Behavior Assessment System for

Children–2 (BASC-2; Reynolds & Kamphaus, 2004), or they can be used for the assessment of specific symptoms, such as the Children's Depression Inventory (CDI; Kovacs, 1992) or the Multidimensional Anxiety Scale for Children (MASC; March, 1998). Because of their ease of use and their strong psychometric properties, behavior rating checklists will likely remain a cornerstone of evidence-based assessment.

Structured observations are also a potentially useful tool in evidence-based assessment if the target behavior is observable (e.g., overactivity vs. suicidal ideation). The majority of structured observational systems are geared toward use in the classroom. The Direct Observation Form (DOF; Achenbach, 1986) and the Student Observation System (SOS; Reynolds & Kamphaus, 2004) are both well-standardized observational systems that can be used for assessing children's behavior in the classroom. Functional behavior assessment is often used within the context of applied behavior analysis, with the idea of identifying the causes of the maladaptive behavior before designing an intervention to change the behavior (Weber et al., 2005). Depending on the target problem and the resources available for the assessment procedures, structured observations can be a useful part of evidence-based assessment.

Thus, in order to secure a thorough evaluation of children and adolescents, evidence-based assessments should use multiple methodologies in the assessment of children and adolescents. These methodologies can be used to assess problematic features of youth as well as strengths and competencies.

Assessments of Strengths as Well as Problems

In addition to assessing emotional/behavioral problems in children and adolescents, it makes sense also to assess competencies and strengths. Hopefully, clinicians who use evidence-based treatments are seeking not only to decrease emotional/behavioral problems but also to enhance competencies and strengths within youth (Cavell et al., 2003).

There are a number of evidence-based measures of competencies and strengths, including the competence scores from multiple informants with the ASEBA system (Achenbach & Rescorla, 2001) and the BASC-2 system (Reynolds & Kamphaus, 2004). In addition, other measures such as the Strengths and Difficulties Questionnaire (Goodman, 1997) and the series of measures by Harter (1985, 1988) that measure perceived competence can be a good way to assess the positive aspects of children's and adolescents' functioning. Ideally, a thorough evidence-based assessment would help to document both the problems and the strengths of children and adolescents in treatment.

Assessments That Are Sensitive to Diversity

One of the cornerstones of using measures that are consistent with evidence-based assessment is choosing measures that are sensitive to diversity. At a minimum, measures should be sensitive to developmental considerations and gender differences in behavior, but there is also evidence to support the use of measures that have been investigated regarding racial/ethnic considerations and socioeconomic status issues.

Depending on the target behavior being assessed, age and gender may play a large role in the understanding of behavior. Because age and gender are so meaningful in understanding the normative basis of behavior, most standardized measures take gender and age into account during the standardization process (e.g., Achenbach & Rescorla, 2001; Kovacs, 1992; Reynolds & Kamphaus, 2004).

There is equivocal evidence as to the relevance of racial/ethnic differences and socioeconomic status issues in the use of standardized assessments. For example, out of 663 analyses of specific items and total scores on the CBCL and YSR, only two items showed over 1% of the variance accounted for by race/ethnicity or SES (Achenbach & Rescorla, 2001). These analyses suggest that race/ethnicity and SES have very little influence in the assessment process. There is, however, evidence that some standardized measures have different factor structures for different racial/ethnic populations (Politano et al., 1986; Steele et al., 2005). Thus, it makes sense to use only measures that have been investigated in diverse groups and that have been validated for a variety of racial/ethnic and socioeconomic groups. These points are part of providing high-quality assessments, but they are also consistent with providing evidence-based assessments.

Assessments That Are Sensitive to Changes over Time

Another aspect of evidence-based assessment that is inherent in any high-quality assessment process is to assess children and adolescents over a period of time. Measures that are sensitive to changes over time are especially relevant when clinicians are evaluating the progress of a child or adolescent in evidence-based treatment. At a minimum, there should be a thorough assessment of the child before and after treatment, but there is good reason to assess the child even more frequently than that in order to make sure that the expected treatment effects are occurring (VanAcker et al., 2004). Mash and Hunsley (2005) highlighted the need to select assessment measures that are sensitive to change over time in order to make sure that changes in children's behavior are not due to measurement error but are in fact due to improvements in the child's behavior.

One measure that has gained great popularity across the United States in evaluation outcome studies is the Youth Outcome Questionnaire (YOQ; Dunn et al., 2005). With both parent-reported and self-reported versions, the YOQ has been used extensively in outcome studies in a variety of different settings (Russell, 2003). Overall, clinicians who are interested in using evidence-based assessment techniques should also be cognizant of assessing children and adolescents at more than one time point.

Assessments Beyond the Child or Adolescent

In addition to assessing emotional/behavioral problems and strengths/ competencies, a number of other aspects are relevant to children's and adolescents' functioning. For example, maternal and paternal behavior (Greco & Morris, 2002), parental psychopathology (Connell & Goodman, 2002; Kane & Garber, 2004; Marmorstein & Iacono, 2004), interparental conflict (Fincham, 1998), parent-child conflict (Marmorstein & Iacono, 2004), and family stressors (McMahon et al., 2003) have all been linked to developmental psychopathology, so there is good reason for clinicians to consider assessing these aspects in relation to a child's well-being. Different environments, such as the family and the school, can influence children's behavior and can be assessed as part of a comprehensive evaluation of children's functioning (Carlson, 2003; Liaupsin et al., 2004).

Within the therapeutic environment, there is growing evidence of the importance of therapeutic alliance in the effectiveness of treatment. Based on a meta-analysis of 23 studies, Shirk and Karver (2003) concluded that the connection between the therapeutic relationship and treatment outcome was significant across all developmental levels studied. Specific characteristics such as the clinician's interpersonal skills and the clinician's use of direct influence skills are strongly associated with positive therapeutic outcomes for children and adolescents (Karver et al., 2006). Thus, these characteristics may be relevant to assess when conducting a thorough evaluation of treatment outcome.

A number of promising measures are being used within the study of mental health service utilization, including the Services Assessment for Children and Adolescents (SACA; Horwitz et al., 2001) and the Therapy Procedures Checklist (Weersing et al., 2002). Overall, further exploration of therapeutic alliance and the use of mental health services by children and adolescents should strengthen the ties between evidence-based assessment and evidence-based therapies.

FUTURE DIRECTIONS IN EVIDENCE-BASED ASSESSMENT

In reflecting on the somewhat brief history of evidence-based assessment, it is important to realize that there are still many unanswered questions as to how to make evidence-based assessment techniques the predominant, and perhaps only, mode of assessment. There is certainly a need to develop more practice-friendly measures for evidence-based assessments, such as computerized log-in systems that provide a quick screen of clients' functioning when clients and their parents show up to the clinician's office (Mash & Hunsley, 2005). There has also been a call for more time-efficient problem scales that are quicker and more user-friendly for the assessment of children's and adolescents' emotional/behavioral problems (Lucas et al., 2001). For example, Item Response Theory procedures can be used to shrink lengthy questionnaires into shorter, circumscribed measures that are still psychometrically sound and that have strong clinical utility (Lambert et al., 2003).

Finally, probably the biggest challenge in the future use of evidence-based assessment is a problem common to the use of evidence-based therapies. Specifically, clinical scientists develop well-standardized procedures for evidence-based assessments and therapies that are investigated extensively and they present to each other at conferences and cite each others' published work, but clinicians in the community are often still not using these techniques (Weisz, 2004). This problem has been discussed throughout this book and is relevant to evidence-based assessment as well as evidence-based interventions.

SUMMARY

Overall, the issues discussed throughout this chapter (assessments of broad vs. specific problems, categorical vs. dimensional conceptualizations, multiple informants, multiple methodologies, assessment of strengths and competencies, sensitivity to diversity, sensitivity to functioning over time, and environmental context for children's and adolescents' behavior) are not specific to the study of evidence-based assessments, but they provide the foundation for providing assessments that are grounded in empirical research. These features are important to consider in conducting an evidence-based assessment that can help to identify the problems to be addressed and the progress of evidence-based therapies.

REFERENCES

Achenbach, T. M. (1985). *Assessment and Taxonomy of Child and Adolescent Psychopathology.* Thousand Oaks, CA: Sage Publications.

Achenbach, T. M. (1986). *The Direct Observation Form of the Child Behavior Checklist (Rev. Ed.).* Burlington, VT: University of Vermont, Department of Psychiatry.

Achenbach, T. M. (2005). Advancing assessment of children and adolescents: Commentary on evidence-based assessment of child and adolescent disorders. *Journal of Clinical Child and Adolescent Psychology, 34,* 541–547.

Achenbach, T. M., Dumenci, L., & Rescorla, L. A. (2003). DSM-oriented and empirically based approaches to constructing scales from the same item pools. *Journal of Clinical Child and Adolescent Psychology, 32,* 328–340.

Achenbach, T. M., & McConaughy, S. H. (1987). *Empirically Based Assessment of Child and Adolescent Psychopathology: Practical Applications.* Thousand Oaks, CA: Sage Publications.

Achenbach, T. M., McConaughy, S. H., & Howell, C. T. (1987). Child/adolescent behavioral and emotional problems: Implications of cross-informant correlations for situational specificity. *Psychological Bulletin, 101,* 213–232.

Achenbach, T. M., & Rescorla, L. A. (2001). *Manual for ASEBA School-Age Forms and Profiles.* Burlington, VT: University of Vermont, Research Center for Children, Youth, and Families.

American Psychiatric Association (2000). *Diagnostic and Statistical Manual of Mental Disorders,* 4th ed. (text revision). Washington, DC.

Angold, A., Costello, E. J., & Erkanli, A. (1999). Comorbidity. *Journal of Child Psychology and Psychiatry, 40,* 57–87.

Carlson, C. I. (2003). Assessing the family context. In C. R. Reynolds & R. W. Kamphaus (Eds.), *Handbook of Psychological and Educational Assessment of Children: Personality, Behavior, and Context,* 2nd ed. (pp. 473–492). New York: Guilford Press.

Cavell, T. A., Meehan, B. T., & Fiala, S. E. (2003). Assessing social competence in children and adolescents. In C. R. Reynolds & R. W. Kamphaus (Eds.), *Handbook of Psychological and Educational Assessment of Children: Personality, Behavior, and Context,* 2nd ed. (pp. 433–454). New York: Guilford Press.

Chambless, D. L., & Hollon, S. D. (1998). Defining empirically supported therapies. *Journal of Consulting and Clinical Psychology, 66,* 7–18.

Connell, A. M., & Goodman, S. H. (2002). The association between psychopathology in fathers versus mothers and children's internalizing and externalizing behavior problems: A meta-analysis. *Psychological Bulletin, 128,* 746–773.

DeLosReyes, A., & Kazdin, A. E. (2004). Measuring informant discrepancies in clinical child research. *Psychological Assessment, 16,* 330–334.

Duhig, A. M., Renk, K., Epstein, M. K., & Phares, V. (2000). Interparental agreement on internalizing, externalizing, and total behavior problems: A meta-analysis. *Clinical Psychology: Science and Practice, 7,* 435–453.

Dunn, T. W., Burlingame, G. M., Walbridge, M., Smith, J., & Crum, M. J. (2005). Outcome assessment for children and adolescents: Psychometric validation of the Youth Outcome Questionnaire 30.1 (Y-OQ-30.1). *Clinical Psychology and Psychotherapy, 12,* 388–401.

Fincham, F. D. (1998). Child development and marital relations. *Child Development, 69,* 543–574.

Fletcher, J. M., Francis, D. J., Morris, R. D., & Lyon, G. R. (2005). Evidence-based assessment of learning disabilities in children and adolescents. *Journal of Clinical Child and Adolescent Psychology, 34,* 506–522.

Garb, H. N., Wood, J. M., Lilienfeld, S. O., & Nezworski, M. T. (2005). Roots of the Rorschach controversy. *Clinical Psychology Review, 25,* 97–118.

Goodman, R. (1997). The Strengths and Difficulties Questionnaire: A research note. *Journal of Child Psychology and Psychiatry, 38,* 581–586.

Greco, L. A., & Morris, T. L. (2002). Paternal child-rearing style and child social anxiety: Investigation of child perceptions and actual father behavior. *Journal of Psychopathology and Behavioral Assessment, 24,* 259–267.

Hankin, B. L., Fraley, R. C., Lahey, B. B., & Waldman, I. D. (2005). Is depression best viewed as a continuum or discrete category? A taxometric analysis of childhood and adolescent depression in a population-based sample. *Journal of Abnormal Psychology, 114,* 96–110.

Harter, S. (1985). *Manual for the Self-Perception Profile for Children.* Denver: University of Denver.

Harter, S. (1988). *Manual for the Self-Perception Profile for Adolescents.* Denver: University of Denver.

Hawley, K. M., & Weisz, J. R. (2003). Child, parent, and therapist (dis)agreement on target problems in outpatient therapy: The therapist's dilemma and its implications. *Journal of Consulting and Clinical Psychology, 71,* 62–70.

Horwitz, S. M., Hoagwood, K., Stiffman, A. R., Summerfeld, T., Weisz, J. R., Costello, E. J., et al. (2001). Reliability of the services assessment for children and adolescents. *Psychiatric Services, 52,* 1088–1094.

Hunsley, J., Lee, C. M., & Wood, J. M. (2003). Controversial and questionable assessment techniques. In S. O. Lilienfeld, S. J. Lynn, & J. M. Lohr (Eds.), *Science and Pseudoscience in Clinical Psychology* (pp. 39–76). New York: Guilford Press.

Jensen, A. L., & Weisz, J. R. (2002). Assessing match and mismatch between practitioner-generated and standardized interview-generated diagnoses for clinic-referred children and adolescents. *Journal of Consulting and Clinical Psychology, 70,* 158–168.

Kane, P., & Garber, J. (2004). The relations among depression in fathers, children's psychopathology, and father-child conflict: A meta-analysis. *Clinical Psychology Review, 24,* 339–360.

Karver, M. S., Handelsman, J. B., Fields, S., & Bickman, L. (2006). Meta-analysis of therapeutic relationship variables in youth and family therapy: The evidence for different relationship variables in the child and adolescent treatment outcome literature. *Clinical Psychology Review, 26,* 50–65.

Kazdin, A. E. (2005). Evidence-based assessment for children and adolescents: Issues in measurement development and clinical application. *Journal of Clinical Child and Adolescent Psychology, 34,* 548–558.

Klein, D. N., Dougherty, L. R., & Olino, T. M. (2005). Toward guidelines for evidence-based assessment of depression in children and adolescents. *Journal of Clinical Child and Adolescent Psychology, 34,* 412–432.

Kovacs, M. (1992). *Children's Depression Inventory Manual.* North Tonawanda, NY: Multi-Health Systems, Inc.

Krueger, R. F., Watson, D., & Barlow, D. H. (2005). Introduction to the special section: Toward a dimensionally based taxonomy of psychopathology. *Journal of Abnormal Psychology, 114,* 491–493.

Kurdek, L. A. (2003). Correlates of parents' perceptions of behavioral problems in their young children. *Applied Developmental Psychology, 24,* 457–473.

Lambert, M. C., Schmitt, N., Samms-Vaughan, M. E., An, J. S., Fairclough, M., & Nutter, C. A. (2003). Is it prudent to administer all items for each Child Behavior Checklist cross-informant syndrome? Evaluating the psychometric properties of the Youth Self-Report dimensions with confirmatory factor analysis and item response theory. *Psychological Assessment, 15,* 550–568.

Liaupsin, C. J., Jolivette, K., & Scott, T. M. (2004). Schoolwide systems of behavior support: Maximizing student success in schools. In R. B. Rutherford, M. M. Quinn, & S. R. Mathur (Eds.), *Handbook of Research in Emotional and Behavioral Disorders* (pp. 487–501). New York: Guilford Press.

Lilienfeld, S. O., Wood, J. M., & Garb, H. N. (2000). The scientific status of projective techniques. *Psychological Science in the Public Interest, 1,* 27–66.

Lucas, C. P., Zhang, H., Fisher, P. W., Shaffer, D., Regier, D. A., Narrow, W. E., et al. (2001). The DISC predictive scales (DPS): Efficiently screening for diagnoses. *Journal of the American Academy of Child and Adolescent Psychiatry, 40,* 443–449.

March, J. (1998). *Manual for the Multidimensional Anxiety Scale for Children (MASC).* Toronto: Multi-Health Systems, Inc.

Marmorstein, N. R., & Iacono, W. G. (2004). Major depression and conduct disorder in youth: Associations with parental psychopathology and parent-child conflict. *Journal of Child Psychology and Psychiatry, 45,* 377–386.

Mash, E. J., & Hunsley, J. (2005). Evidence-based assessment of child and adolescent disorders: Issues and challenges. *Journal of Clinical Child and Adolescent Psychology, 34,* 362–379.

McMahon, R. J., & Frick, P. J. (2005). Evidence-based assessment of conduct problems in children and adolescents. *Journal of Clinical Child and Adolescent Psychology, 34,* 477–505.

McMahon, S. D., Grant, K. E., Compas, B. E., Thurm, A. E., & Ey, S. (2003). Stress and psychopathology in children and adolescents: Is there evidence of specificity? *Journal of Child Psychology and Psychiatry, 44,* 107–133.

Ollendick, T. H., & King, N. J. (2006). Empirically supported treatments typically produce outcomes superior to non-empirically supported treatment therapies. In J. C. Norcross, L. E. Beutler, & R. F. Levant (Eds.), *Evidence-Based Practices in Mental Health: Debate and Dialogue on the Fundamental Questions* (pp. 308–317). Washington, DC: American Psychological Association.

Ozonoff, S., Goodlin-Jones, B. L., & Solomon, M. (2005). Evidence-based assessment of autism spectrum disorders in children and adolescents. *Journal of Clinical Child and Adolescent Psychology, 34,* 523–540.

Pelham, W. E., Fabiano, G. A., & Massetti, G. M. (2005). Evidence-based assessment of attention deficit hyperactivity disorder in children and adolescents. *Journal of Clinical Child and Adolescent Psychology, 34,* 449–476.

Phares, V., & Compas, B. E. (1990). Adolescents' subjective distress over their emotional/behavioral problems. *Journal of Consulting and Clinical Psychology, 58,* 596–603.

Politano, P. M., Nelson, W. M., Evans, H. E., & Sorenson, S. B. (1986). Factor analytic evaluation of differences between Black and Caucasian emotionally disturbed children on the Children's Depression Inventory. *Journal of Psychopathology and Behavioral Assessment, 8,* 1–7.

Reynolds, C. R., & Kamphaus, R. W. (2004). *Behavior Assessment System for Children, 2nd ed. Manual.* Circle Pines, MN: AGS Publishing.

Russell, K. (2003). An assessment of outcomes in outdoor behavioral healthcare treatment. *Child and Youth Care Forum, 32,* 355–381.

Sattler, J. M., & Hoge, R. D. (2006). *Assessment of Children: Behavioral, Social, and Clinical Foundations,* 5th ed. La Mesa, CA: Jerome M. Sattler, Publisher.

Shaffer, D., Fisher, P., Lucas, C. P., Dulcan, M. K., & Schwab-Stone, M. E. (2000). NIMH Diagnostic Interview Schedule for Children Version IV (NIMH DISC-IV): Description, differences from previous versions, and reliability of some common diagnoses. *Journal of the American Academy of Child and Adolescent Psychiatry, 39,* 28–38.

Shirk, S. R., & Karver, M. (2003). Prediction of treatment outcome from relationship variables in child and adolescent therapy: A meta-analytic review. *Journal of Consulting and Clinical Psychology, 71,* 452–464.

Silverman, W. K., & Ollendick, T. H. (2005). Evidence-based assessment of anxiety and its disorders in children and adolescents. *Journal of Clinical Child and Adolescent Psychology, 34,* 380–411.

Standards for Educational and Psychological Testing (1999). Washington, DC: American Psychological Association.

Steele, R. G., Nesbitt-Daly, J. S., Daniel, R. C., & Forehand, R. (2005). Factor structure of the Parenting Scale in a low-income African American sample. *Journal of Child and Family Studies, 14,* 535–549.

Task Force on Promotion and Dissemination of Psychological Procedures (1995). Training in and dissemination of empirically-validated psychological treatments: Report and recommendations. *Clinical Psychologist, 48,* 3–23.

Treatment for Adolescents with Depression Study (TADS) Team (2004). Fluoxetine, cognitive-behavioral therapy, and their combination for adolescents with depression: Treatment for adolescents with depression study (TADS) randomized controlled trial. *Journal of the American Medical Association, 292,* 807–820.

VanAcker, R., Yell, M. L., Bradley, R., & Drasgow, E. (2004). Experimental research designs in the study of children and youth with emotional and behavioral disorders. In R. B. Rutherford, M. M. Quinn, & S. R. Mathur (Eds.), *Handbook of Research in Emotional and Behavioral Disorders* (pp. 546–566). New York: Guilford Press.

Weber, K. P., Killu, K., Derby, K. M., & Barretto, A. (2005). The status of functional behavior assessment (FBA): Adherence to standard practice in FBA methodology. *Psychology in the Schools, 42,* 737–744.

Weersing, V. R., Weisz, J. R., & Donenberg, G. R. (2002). Development of the Therapy Procedures Checklist: A therapist-report measure of technique use in child and adolescent treatment. *Journal of Clinical Child and Adolescent Psychology, 31,* 168–180.

Weisz, J. R. (2004). *Psychotherapy for Children and Adolescents: Evidence-Based Treatments and Case Examples.* Cambridge: Cambridge University Press.

Weisz, J. R., & Addis, M. E. (2006). The research-practice tango and other choreographic challenges: Using and testing evidence-based psychotherapies in clinical care settings. In C. D. Goodheart, A. E. Kazdin, & R. J. Sternberg (Eds.), *Evidence-Based Psychotherapy: Where Practice and Research Meet* (pp. 179–206). Washington, DC: American Psychological Association.

Weisz, J. R., Suwanlert, S., Chaiyasit, W., Weiss, B., Walter, B., & Anderson, W. (1988). Thai and American perspectives on over- and undercontrolled child behavior problems: Exploring the threshold model among parents, teachers, and psychologists. *Journal of Consulting and Clinical Psychology, 56,* 601–609.

Wood, J. M., Nezworski, M. T., Lilienfeld, S. O., & Garb, H. N. (2003). *What's Wrong with the Rorschach?: Science Confronts the Controversial Inkblot Test.* San Francisco: Jossey-Bass.

Yeh, M., & Weisz, J. R. (2001). Why are we here at the clinic? Parent-child (dis)agreement on referral problems at outpatient treatment entry. *Journal of Consulting and Clinical Psychology, 69,* 1018–1025.

Youngstrom, E. A., Findling, R. L., Youngstrom, J. K., & Calabrese, J. R. (2005). Toward an evidence-based assessment of pediatric bipolar disorder. *Journal of Clinical Child and Adolescent Psychology, 34,* 433–448.

31

Graduate Training in Evidence-Based Practice in Psychology[1]

THAD R. LEFFINGWELL and FRANK L. COLLINS, JR.

Following the lead of most other health-care professions, endorsement of evidence-based practice in psychology (EBPP) became the official policy of the American Psychological Association in 2005 (APA Presidential Task Force on Evidence-Based Practice, 2006). This policy represents a culmination of two movements, one inside and one outside professional psychology, that converged to form this policy. Specifically, evidence-based practice in medicine is quickly becoming the norm and is a staple in most medical education programs. Likewise, within psychology, Division 12 of the American Psychological Association has worked hard to increase awareness of the efficacy of psychological treatments by recognizing empirically supported treatments (Task Force on Promotion and Dissemination of Psychological Procedures, 1995). These two movements, with their common ideals, goals, and motives, converged in psychology with the formation of a special task force on EBPP organized by then-president Ron Levant and, ultimately, the policy statement adopted in 2005.

The new policy statement is likely to have a strong influence on the professional practice of psychology in the future. For this reason, it is also likely to influence the training of professional psychologists. Psychologists in training need to attain the skills necessary to effectively perform EBPP to function maximally in the health-care system of the future. This chapter

---

[1] Portions of this chapter provide a synopsis of ideas outlined in Collins et al. (2007), Teaching evidence-based practice: Implications for Psychology. *Journal of Clinical Psychology*, 63, 657–670. Used with permission of the authors.

THAD R. LEFFINGWELL • Oklahoma State University and **FRANK L. COLLINS, JR.** • University of North Texas

describes some of the challenges EBPP presents for training and discusses some strategies for meeting these challenges. While graduate training in psychology includes academic training in a graduate program, a clinical internship, and often postdoctoral training, this chapter focuses primarily upon the academic graduate training program aspects of the total training experience.

DEFINITIONS OF EVIDENCE-BASED PRACTICE

To understand the implications of EBPP for training, one must first understand the components of EBPP. Several definitions of evidence-based practice exist. Sackett and colleagues (1996) devised the first widely used definition of evidence-based practice:

> Evidence based medicine is the conscientious, explicit, and judicious use of current best evidence in making decisions about the care of individual patients. The practice of evidence based medicine means integrating individual clinical expertise with the best available external clinical evidence from systematic research. (1996, p. 71)

The Institute of Medicine (IOM; 2001) adapted and expanded upon this definition in an influential report: "Evidence based practice is the integration of the best research evidence with clinical expertise and patient values" (p. 147). More recently, the American Psychological Association issued the landmark policy statement using a similar definition of EBP: "Evidence-based practice in psychology (EBPP) is the integration of the best available research with clinical expertise in the context of patient characteristics, culture and preferences" (APA Presidential Task Force on Evidence-Based Practice, 2006, p. 273).

Like the Sackett and IOM definitions before it, the APA definition of EBPP emphasizes the *integration* of research with clinical expertise and patient values. Importantly, the definition highlights EBPP as a *process* or *way of being* rather than as an *object* or an *outcome*. Unfortunately, the term "evidence-based practice" is already being confused with preexisting concepts like *empirically supported treatment*. In professional discussions with peers, it is not uncommon for the term "evidence-based practice" (as a *thing*, not a *process*) to be used interchangeably with "empirically supported treatment." We caution against this confounding of concepts. EBPP must be reserved for describing a process of integrating research evidence into practice, a *process* for which knowledge of empirically supported treatments is a critical resource. Empirically supported treatments (or, if one must, evidence-based treatments) refer to specific treatment approaches for which substantial valid and reliable empirical research evidence exists (Chambless & Hollon, 1998; Kendall, 1998). This distinction of definitions is critically important to the progress of the field embracing EBPP as well as to this chapter, as the definition of EBPP requires that we discuss how to train psychologists in the component competencies for EBPP and the *process* of *integration*, not simply in how to identify and use empirically supported treatments.

COMPETENCIES IN PSYCHOLOGY TRAINING

The EBPP movement has also coincided with a developing focus on professional competencies. Competencies have been conceptualized in a developmental framework that mirrors phases of training, including preparation for graduate education, predoctoral competencies, and postdoctoral competencies. For example, core competencies for practice have been identified (Collins et al., 2004; Kaslow et al., 2004) that include training in the scientific foundations of psychology (Bieschke et al., 2004), psychological interventions (Spruill et al., 2004), supervision (Falender et al., 2004), psychological assessment (Krishnamurthy et al., 2004), cultural and individual diversity (Daniel et al., 2004), consultation and interdisciplinary relationships (Arredondo et al., 2004), ethical, legal, and professional issues (de las Fuentes et al., 2005), and professional development (Elman et al., 2005).

The Association of Directors of Psychology Training Clinics (ADPTC) has developed a set of practicum competencies designed to identify those competencies that should be acquired prior to internship (Hatcher & Lassiter, 2005). An important aspect of these competencies is the identification of levels of expertise that are tied to specific competencies. Specifically, using the levels of expertise developed by Dreyfus and Dreyfus (1986) and Benner (1984), behavioral competencies can be identified as lying along a continuum from novice to expert. Training of psychologists should be guided by these competency definitions, and minimal levels of competence should be expected.

For example, it is thought that competencies that involve cognitive skills such as problem-solving ability, critical thinking, organized reasoning, intellectual curiosity, and flexibility should be at the "novice" level prior to beginning practicum. By "novice" we mean that these skills should reflect limited knowledge and understanding. However, by the time the trainee is "ready" to benefit from a clinical internship, he or she should show specific competencies that can be rated as "advanced" to "intermediate" in areas such as the ability to formulate and conceptualize cases, to integrate assessment data from different courses for diagnostic purposes, and to perform other cognitive skills. An individual with advanced to intermediate skills will be able to generalize to new situations (intermediate) and to develop long-term goals or plans of which he or she is consciously aware (advanced).

These competencies are clearly critical for the development of psychologists who can provide assessment and intervention services consistent with an EBPP model. These identified competencies are consistent with the necessity of integrating the best available research evidence with clinical expertise and patient values and are critical for training students in EBPP.

The greatest challenge in the area of clinical competencies is the lack of agreement as to how best to assess clinical competence. Roberts and colleagues (2005) have suggested that professional psychology needs to adopt both a culture of competence and a culture of assessment. As noted in this chapter, the culture of competence seems to be moving forward. There is general agreement as to the competencies needed for professional practice; however, the methods for assessing these competencies (and the need for systematic, consistent assessment) may be lagging. Specifically, assessment of competence involves both summative and formative assessment components. Summative assessment occurs at some endpoint in training or at some critical milestone. Thus, assessments such as comprehensive examinations and/or oral defense of the dissertation project, at the end of internship or prior to licensure, are typically summative and reflect some minimal demonstration of competency attainment. Formative assessment is ongoing and focuses on helping the trainee develop competencies by teaching him or her about the areas that need additional improvement. Both types of assessment are needed, however; trainees (and perhaps at times trainers) often do not differentiate between these types of assessment, which may result in confusion and misuse of assessment methods.

Clinical expertise, a core component of the APA's definition of EBPP, requires competence in each of these areas. As progress continues both conceptually and empirically toward defining and evaluating the critical competencies for professional psychology, progress will be made toward the ideal of EBPP.

EMPIRICAL STATUS OF CURRENT TRAINING

Given the recent release of the APA policy statement on EBPP, literature examining the current empirical status of training approaches in EBPP is nonexistent. However, some evidence exists regarding the prevalence and effectiveness of training in empirically supported treatments. In 1993, David Barlow, then-president of Division 12 of the American Psychological Association, commissioned a task force to enhance the visibility of the efficacy of psychological treatments (Task Force on Promotion and Dissemination of Psychological Procedures, 1995). Although the task force had a number of goals, two primary goals included (1) the generation of a list of known efficacious treatments for specific disorders (first called empirically validated treatments, later empirically supported treatments or ESTs) and (2) surveying training programs to evaluate the prevalence of graduate training in ESTs. The task force released a preliminary list of ESTs in 1995 (Chambless et al., 1996; Task Force on Promotion and Dissemination of Psychological Procedures, 1995), and updated lists were published in 1996 (Chambless et al., 1996) and 1998 (Chambless et al., 1998).

In addition to generating lists of empirically supported treatments, the Chambless Task Force also surveyed academic and internship training programs to evaluate the availability of training in ESTs. Their preliminary findings were discouraging, with the average academic program offering training in fewer than half of the known efficacious treatments and most internship programs offering no training in ESTs (Task Force on Promotion and Dissemination of Psychological Procedures, 1995). In a recently released follow-up report, little had changed in the years since the initial survey (Woody et al., 2005). Clearly, when looking at a relatively narrowly defined definition of simply offering training in ESTs (rather than the broader definition requiring integration of evidence, like that supporting ESTs), current training programs are falling short of the mark.

Other investigators have pursued other important questions related to training in ESTs. For example, a significant body of literature exists examining the efficacy of training for enhancing the competence of trainees to perform a treatment of choice. While on the whole this literature is encouraging and suggests that training does make a difference and can improve practitioner performance and outcomes, it also cautions that training may not be easy and that simple, brief workshops are likely inadequate for improving trainee performance (Miller et al., 2004; Sholomskas et al., 2005). Others have examined whether the introduction of ESTs via staff training in real-world clinics impacts staff performance or clinical outcomes. These studies suggest that both staff performance and clinical outcomes improve with training in ESTs (Cukrowicz et al., 2005).

SOURCES OF RESEARCH EVIDENCE

Certainly, one set of skills in learning the process of EBPP involves obtaining, evaluating, and implementing the best available research evidence. In medicine, Sackett and others (2000) recommend the use of rigorous secondary source materials by the practicing physician due to the overwhelming volume of primary source material. We would make a similar recommendation for the practicing psychologist seeking to implement EBPP. Evidence available in the literature grows exponentially in number over time and generally becomes more complex and sophisticated in regard to sampling, design, measurement, and analysis strategies as science progresses and the evidence base matures. To further complicate matters, the nature of scientific evidence is such that what once may have been known may have been superseded or replaced by new evidence, requiring all practitioners of EBPP to remain abreast of new developments in the research. The abundance of evidence and the dynamic nature of evidence are such that relying upon primary sources is simply not feasible (Sackett et al., 2000) and other means of obtaining and utilizing evidence are necessary (referred to as "evidence management" by McCabe, 2004). Members of the practice community often lack the time and resources (e.g., access to database searches or full-text copies of literature) to make personal primary-source searches for evidence practical or even possible. Fortunately, a growing number of resources are available that provide credible reviews and summaries of the most current evidence available, which are much more useful to practitioners.

Commissioned Reviews or Institute Reports

Given the importance of evidence-based practice to inform policy, governments may at times commission summaries of evidence to guide prudent use of our limited health-care resources. One example of this type of report from the field of psychotherapy is the reports by Roth and Fonagy (1996, 2004) commissioned by the National Health Service of the English Department of Health. Although not a government-issued report, the Division 12 Task Force list of empirically supported treatments described earlier represents another example.

Clinical Practice Guidelines and Consensus Statements

Another useful set of evidence summaries includes clinical practice guidelines or consensus statements. Occasionally, professional organizations or governments will issue practice guidelines or consensus statements including recommendations for best practices (this is especially the case for exceedingly common and costly problems). Such guidelines are based upon thorough and rigorous reviews of available research evidence, making them a useful source for credible summaries of current evidence. A leading force for clinical practice guidelines in the United States is the Agency for Healthcare Research and Quality [AHRQ; formerly the Agency for Health Care Policy and Research (AHCPR); www.ahrq.gov]. The AHRQ commissions the development of new practice guidelines and provides a mechanism for easy access to clinical practice guidelines, including both those commissioned by them and those produced by other professional bodies (www.guidelines.gov). Beginning in 1997, AHRQ launched an initiative to become a "science partner" with public and private organizations in order to improve the quality of health care by synthesizing the evidence and facilitating the translation of evidence-based research findings. The product of this effort is a number of "evidence reports" summarizing the current state of evidence regarding treatments for many common health reports.

Clinical practice guidelines can be initiated and produced by a variety of sources including governments (both federal and state) and professional organizations (like the American Psychiatric Association). Two examples of state-government–initiated evidence summaries include clinical practice guidelines prepared by the Michigan Quality Improvement Consortium (www.mqic.org) and evidence-based practices reports released by the Iowa Consortium for Substance Abuse Research and Evaluation (http://iconsortium.subst-abuse.uiowa.edu). A number of clinical practice guidelines already exist for psychological disorders and other behavioral problems. The National Guideline Clearinghouse lists 169 clinical practice guidelines for "mental disorders."

Some of the controversy surrounding EBPP includes concerns about a prescriptive approach that privileges some treatments while prohibiting others. Certainly, practice guidelines contribute to those fears because of a sense of such guidelines' imposing a particular choice and prohibiting other choices. However, we favor the recommendation of the American Psychological Association (2002b) stating that guidelines are aspirational rather than mandatory and should be used primarily to educate and inform practice. Further, we note that the APA recommendations (2002a) for treatment guidelines specifically recommend that such guidelines "… take into account research and relevant clinical consensus on other relevant patient characteristics" (Criterion 6.5, p. 1056). If all clinical practice guidelines followed this recommendation, it would be of tremendous service to practitioners attempting to employ EBPP, including integrating best research evidence with patient characteristics and values.

Cochrane Reviews

Since 1993, the Cochrane Collaboration has produced and distributed dozens of reviews of randomized controlled trials of treatments for health problems (www.cochrane.org). Although the collaboration's primary focus is on medical health care, the Cochrane Library (www.thecochranelibrary.com) also includes a number of reviews on the prevention and treatment of psychological and behavioral problems like drug and alcohol dependence and schizophrenia (pharmacological and psychosocial). As EBPP gains momentum, we anticipate a significant expansion of psychology-related reviews in the Cochrane Library.

Textbooks

A number of textbooks are also available, and many combine brief reviews of evidence with practical guidelines for the implementation of specific treatments. Notable examples relevant to psychological disorders include this text, as well as Barlow (2001) and Kazdin and Weiss (2003). Sackett and colleagues (2000) suggest caution in using textbooks as a *sole* source of evidence summaries because they may be biased editorially and become out-of-date quickly, as the status of the evidence is always changing. In general, we would caution against placing much trust in textbooks that offer little connection to research evidence or evidence-rich textbooks more than a few years old as authoritative guides for practice.

IMPLICATIONS OF EBPP FOR TRAINING FUTURE PSYCHOLOGISTS

One effective method in teaching science is to address common myths. Given the number of myths regarding EBPP, we recommend that education in EBPP focus on these common misconceptions as early in the curriculum as possible.

> *Myth 1. Teaching EBPP can be accomplished by training students in the use of empirically supported treatments (ESTs).* Although inclusion of empirically supported treatments is required for APA accreditation, and training in the most frequently used ESTs is certainly recommended (Chambless & Ollendick, 2001), such training alone is insufficient for EBPP. In addition to a requirement for integration of best research evidence with clinical expertise and patient values, teaching EBPP requires an explicit focus on competencies for lifelong learning

and professional development. A hallmark of EBPP is learning to critically appraise *current* evidence and *integrate* that evidence within existing practice competencies. Thus, successful training in EBPP cannot be understood merely in terms of the number of ESTs mastered, as learning to provide new treatments will be necessary throughout one's career. Students need to develop competencies for identifying and learning new treatments as evidence evolves and for integrating that knowledge with clinical expertise and patient values.

Myth 2. EBPP focuses solely on knowledge gained from randomized clinical trials (RCTs). Such is not the case. The emphasis in training in EBPP requires that students learn to identify the best evidence available. Practice then depends upon its integration with clinical expertise and patient values. The best choice for the patient sometimes depends on aspects unique to the clinical presentation rather than findings from RCTs. While it is noted that randomized clinical trials provide the highest level of scientific evidence for certain questions, e.g., the efficacy of the treatment (McCabe, 2004), other methods might provide the best evidence for a specific clinical decision. Students should be trained to appreciate the importance of randomized clinical trials but to appraise evidence obtained from other research methods as well and to understand how various methods contribute to our understanding of clinical phenomena. Examples of how this is done will be provided in the following section of this chapter.

Myth 3. EBPP requires only process learning, with a focus on "just-in-time" knowledge. Despite a focus on the critical appraisal process in training, and the realization that "just-in-time" knowledge is important in many clinical situations, EBPP also demands mastery of a core knowledge base. Clinicians must have broad knowledge of the science of behavior, the relationships between behavior and health, and mechanisms of behavior change. Education and training must include a special focus on biological, cognitive, affective, and cultural factors affecting health and health-care delivery, as well as issues of diversity. This knowledge, which is foundational for all APA-accredited professional psychology programs, is essential to interpret clinical observations, to evaluate whether research results are appropriate to the current clinical situation, and to integrate research findings with clinical expertise and patient values.

Myth 4. The extant scientific literature lacks clinical utility. Barlow and colleagues (1999) noted myths related to comorbidity and generalizability that affect practitioners' views of the utility of extant scientific literature. Their cogent analysis of the argument "my patients are different" is supported by data on the robustness of clinical research and the reality that there are often more similarities than differences in clinically significant variables. Further, recent evidence suggests that most clients in "real-world" settings who meet criteria for a diagnosis that has been included in one or more RCTs would have met inclusion criteria for that study (Stirman et al., 2003). Furthermore, when real-world patients fail to meet inclusion criteria, the most common reason is insufficient severity or duration of symptoms, and not comorbidity or other complicating factors. Trainees need to have this information integrated into their education programs to ensure that they are able to generalize beyond the research evidence.

Myth 5. EBPP is "cookbook" health care that ignores clinical experience and clinical intuition. By definition, this is not accurate. Clinical experience is an integral component of clinical expertise, which, in turn, is an integral component of EBPP. However, there is an emphasis on understanding the limitations of clinical experience just as there is an emphasis on understanding limitations of research findings. One could argue that since there are multiple components of EBPP (research evidence, clinical expertise, and patient values), one or more of these components might not be relevant for a specific case. However, EBPP is explicitly defined by the integration of all three components—a process for which there exists no cookbook. In addition, EBPP places as much of an emphasis on using knowledge from clinical experience to inform the scientific process as science informing practice. In this model, rather than science and practice being the endpoints of a continuum, they are intertwined in double-helix fashion, each providing a significant source of data, and each informing the other, much like the scientist-practitioner model in psychology education and training (Belar & Perry, 1992).

Myth 6. Clinical expertise = clinical experience. Clinical expertise and clinical experience are not equivalent. Although supervised clinical experience is required to develop clinical expertise, and ongoing clinical experience can serve to enhance it, clinical expertise is a far more complicated construct. It requires not only knowledge of current research, but skills in building therapeutic alliances, assessing and treating individual patients, monitoring patient progress, and clinical decision making. There is a robust literature on judgment and decision making that clinicians must learn to apply in their everyday work that requires a much higher-order intellectual process (involving both cognition and affect) than the attainment of experience alone. The focus of supervised clinical training must be on this process, and not just on "seeing cases" or following supervisor instructions.

TEACHING EBPP: CORE COMPONENTS

Teaching EBPP requires helping trainees develop skills in "data mining," including how to access various secondary sources and to critically appraise the information obtained.

For some faculty, the heavy reliance on secondary sources may require attitude change, since many faculty members have been trained to eschew secondary sources and to rely only on primary sources in synthesizing a literature. Although an analysis of primary sources remains critical to scholarly research, the explosion in knowledge combined with the time demands on the practitioner makes it impractical to conduct a review of the primary literature when information is needed immediately in the clinical situation. Moreover, if faculty members do not teach how to evaluate and utilize secondary resources, they have clearly failed to recognize this rapidly developing domain of scholarly research. Meta-analytic studies are increasingly more common, and there are now entire journals to support the dissemination of clinically relevant scientific knowledge (e.g., *Annual Review of Clinical Psychology, Clinical Psychology Review, Evidence-Based Medicine, Evidence-Based Nursing, Evidence-Based Mental Health*).

Other efforts have focused upon increasing standardization in reports of published randomized controlled trials (CONSORT Statement; Moher et al., 2001) and nonrandomized design studies (TREND Statement; Des Jarlais et al., 2004). Such efforts will improve the interpretability, generalizability, and comparisons of primary sources. To facilitate the accumulation of knowledge, some leading psychology journals have already adopted guidelines on reporting randomized trials, joining nearly all medical journals. For example, in August 2003, *Health Psychology* adopted the CONSORT guidelines for its authors (Stone, 2003).

A core component in the teaching of EBPP is ensuring that trainees have expertise in using resources such as the Cochrane Library, the Agency for Health Care Research and Quality's evidence reviews, and the National Guideline Clearinghouse as well as discipline-specific reviews. Of equal importance to developing skills in accessing information is systematic training in how to evaluate the quality of evidence available, for which there are a variety of systems of evaluation. Trainees also need to be aware of what practice guidelines might exist and the strength of the evidence supporting each recommendation. When recommendations are based on opinion, how those opinions were gathered must be evaluated as well. Articles on how to access, evaluate, and interpret the scientific literature in specific areas have been more common in medicine than in the psychology literature; this is an area in need of significantly more attention in psychology.

EBPP depends upon informatics—a core competency recommended for all health professions by the Institute of Medicine's Health Professions Education Summit (Institute of Medicine, 2002). Sometimes informatics is mistakenly viewed as interacting with computers to obtain knowledge, but such behavior is not equivalent to the application of informatics to patient care as described above. It is noteworthy that the IOM has already identified a number of priority areas for the development of a national information infrastructure for health-care quality improvement efforts (Institute of Medicine, 2003). Psychology trainees need to be aware of these efforts.

Teaching EBPP requires that faculty model the integration of science and practice.

Trainees need to witness firsthand their supervisors' appreciation of levels of evidence and understanding of how such evidence is integrated into clinical decision making. Supervisors can facilitate student learning by "thinking aloud" during clinical decision making rather than expecting trainees to accept the supervisor's judgment as evidence itself. Some teaching of EBPP can be done in the classroom, and some can be done by nonclinicians. However, given what we know about processes of professional socialization, there must be role models for the appraisal and integration of evidence with clinical expertise and patient values so that scientific evidence is seen as a central, not separate, component of clinical practice.

> *Teaching EBPP requires the development of evaluation methods that assess trainee ability to obtain, appraise, and apply facts to an individual patient situation.*

The use of standardized patients is very common in medicine, but not so in other disciplines. In general, more attention needs to be paid to performance-based assessment in psychology so that competence in evidence-based practice can be adequately assessed at all career stages. The IOM Health Professions Education Summit (Institute of Medicine, 2002) has recommended formal oversight groups to promote a more integrated approach to competency assurance across education, training, and credentialing processes in each profession.

Trainees also need systematic training in accurate self-assessment so that they can learn how to self-correct and to most appropriately engage in the lifelong learning required in all health professions (Belar et al., 2001). A commitment to self-assessment can be facilitated by faculty modeling self-assessment of their own teaching and practice.

> *Teaching EBPP requires a shift in supervisor role away from that as primary source of information.*

Berg (2000) points out that oftentimes the primary source of clinical advice is expert opinions. Thus, the trainee asks his or her supervisor a specific question and is typically provided a specific answer. However, if the same question is asked of a group of experts, these experts are likely to provide a range of answers rather than an answer based on the best available evidence. According to Berg (2000), supervisors (experts) would better serve their trainees if, rather than providing answers to clinical questions, they would teach students how to find the best evidence to answer the question. This requires a shift in where evidence is sought and in how a trainee evaluates evidence provided. As noted previously, reviews of randomized controlled trials (such as the Cochrane Reviews), meta-analyses, and other integrative reviews are often more helpful than classic textbooks or individual research studies (Sackett et al., 2000). It is also noteworthy that this approach to clinical teaching may be discomforting to some trainees, who would prefer to rely exclusively on the authority of the supervisor. As in any clinical training, students need to learn to tolerate more ambiguity than is sometimes comfortable for them.

> *Teaching EBPP requires program administrative support.*

Given the challenges to obtain external funding and to increase clinical income, teaching does not always obtain the administrative support required for teaching EBPP. The teaching of EBPP needs to be valued by the program, not just by individual faculty, as curriculum changes will be required that will need both financial and attitudinal support. In addition, evidence needs to be gathered on the outcomes of these educational interventions, so that results can be integrated with educational practice to facilitate evidence-based education and training.

TEACHING EBPP: ONE PROGRAM'S EXAMPLE

Obviously, there is no single or right way to teach EBPP, and we anticipate that ideas and strategies will continue to evolve over the coming decades. This section describes, for purposes of an example, the efforts of one program to integrate the teaching of EBPP into its curriculum.

Over the last several years, EBPP has "infused" much of the Oklahoma State University's Clinical Psychology Program. The program has been empirically oriented for a number of years with an emphasis on cognitive-behavioral therapy approaches, but only recently have emerging ideas from evidence-based medicine (and the recent APA policy regarding EBPP) provided a useful framework and language for infusing and integrating EBPP across the curriculum. Specifically, EBPP has influenced training in two areas—courses and clinical supervision. Examples of integration in each are described below.

EBPP and Courses

EBPP has become substantially integrated into at least two core courses in the clinical psychology curriculum, *PSYC 6083 Principles of Behavior Therapy* and *PSYC 5193 Ethics and Professional Development.* These two courses are taken early in the curriculum and provide students with different perspectives on EBPP.

PSYC 6083 Principles of Behavior Therapy

Integrating EBPP into a course in behavior therapy may appear logical given behavior therapy's long history of commitment to empirical methods as a source of knowledge and accountability. EBPP is an ever-present theme in this course, but the focus is more upon developing skills and competencies in evaluating research evidence than on the other two important components of EBPP—which are addressed elsewhere in the curriculum.

Students are provided an intensive opportunity to develop skills in evaluating research evidence through a major course project. For this project, teams of two or three students, in concert with the instructor, develop a 2.5-hour workshop on an empirically supported treatment for their peers. The collection of workshops is called the *Behavior Therapy Seminar Series* (Leffingwell, 2006). Each workshop is modeled after a beginner-level clinical workshop such as those found at national and regional professional conferences; it is meant to be an introduction to a treatment. The workshop includes three components: (1) a *theoretical and technical overview* in which the theoretical foundation, relevant scientific basis, and techniques typically included in the treatment are described; (2) an *empirical overview* in which the relevant efficacy and effectiveness data in the literature are summarized, including the strengths and weaknesses of the available literature; and (3) a few *clinical vignettes* in which students act out a few scenes depicting important or unique therapeutic skills or interventions included in the treatment. Students also develop a number of supporting documents for the workshops, including (1) a *treatment fact sheet* that summarizes the nature of the treatment and research evidence in a style appropriate for consumers and (2) a *quick-scan table* that summarizes the relative strengths and weaknesses of available published studies of the treatment. Creating the quick-scan summary and preparing the empirical overview portion of the workshop provide students with an intensive opportunity to review and scrutinize the literature regarding their treatment of choice. More details about this class project are available elsewhere (Leffingwell, 2006).

The *Behavior Therapy Seminar Series* is offered live only for student peers enrolled in the course. However, the workshops are digitally video-taped and archived on CD for use by other students and faculty in the program's training clinic who may be interested in the treatments included. In this way, the important role for psychologists as not only consumers of evidence but as disseminators is emphasized and modeled. Recently, both state and national organizations have expressed interest in the archived models as potentially useful for the broader professional community, perhaps as a source of continuing education.

PSYC 5193 Ethics and Professional Development

A major thrust of this course is commitment to the scientific bases of practice as an important ethical and professional issue. In this course, students are exposed to the definition and model of EBPP based upon Sackett et al. (1996) and the variety of secondary-source summaries of the literature. Students practice using these sources through a course project that requires them to develop a portfolio of EBPP based upon a client they are currently treating, have recently treated, or have observed in treatment as part of their clinical practica experience. For this project, students are asked to (anonymously) describe the client's presenting problem and associated information (including comorbid diagnoses and demographic variables). Students also provide a case conceptualization, treatment plan, and outcome data if available. Finally, students are asked to conduct a review of the scientific evidence for treatments specific to the client's presenting problem and provide an analysis of the fit of the evidence-based recommendations they uncover compared to the actual treatment plans and course of treatment for the specific case. Particular attention is paid to the methods used to review the treatment literature. To some extent, the methods used are more important to the evaluation of the student's professional development than the result of the review itself, although both are project components. The student is then required to discuss how the review of the evidence is linked to clinical expertise and patient values, with an emphasis on the integration of these three components. This analysis encourages students to consider how to integrate clinical judgment and patient values and preferences with the available scientific evidence in order to justify a treatment plan.

Other Courses

As mentioned previously, the concepts and language of EBPP are emerging as useful tools to create consistency across the clinical psychology curriculum. Instructors for other courses, including *Introduction to Clinical Methods*, *Systems of Psychotherapy*, *Child Psychopathology and Treatment*, and *Personality and Cognitive Assessment*, have expressed plans to incorporate EBPP language and models more explicitly into their courses and to create learning experiences for developing the competencies necessary for future EBPP-oriented practitioners and clinical scientists.

EBPP and Clinical Practica

Clinical practica are perhaps the ideal setting for providing teaching and training opportunities in the full spectrum of EBPP competencies. Our program, like most, includes both in-house practica supervised by core program faculty and external off-campus practica supervised by community partners and adjunct faculty. While we expect EBPP to be infused throughout all practica experiences, this section focuses upon our use of EBPP for in-house practica.

Our in-house practica structure includes both individual supervision of trainees with clinical caseloads and weekly team meetings with both didactic and group supervision components. The teams are vertically oriented, with each team including students at various stages of the training program. Students may be engaged in in-house practica in the department training clinic or in off-campus practica at various settings. The program typically has four active teams with six to nine students on each team. The EBPP model is influencing supervision on all teams, but some detail can be provided for how the model influences supervision for teams supervised by the authors.

Individual Supervision

Not all clients present with problems for which there is an abundance of evidence-based treatments available. Clients sometimes present with problems related to personal growth, adjustment issues, and general problems-in-living for which evidence is not well documented. In fact, this has been identified as the biggest obstacle to generalizing research findings to clinical samples (Stirman et al., 2003). Barlow (2004) has recently advocated for discriminating between *psychotherapy* (a relatively broad approach that may be appropriate for the problems described above) and *psychological treatment* (specific approaches with known efficacy for specific and reliably identifiable problems). For cases in which a psychological treatment model may be appropriate (e.g., primary Axis I disorders for which treatments may exist), supervisors in our program have moved away from instructing students what to do and handing them a manual, and have moved toward helping students craft the clinical question, probe the literature (beginning with secondary sources) for evidence, and then address how this information is integrated with clinical expertise and patient values.

Group Supervision

In addition to providing individual supervision that focuses on EBPP, one night a week, clients are seen by the clinic team where the focus is on group supervision with the "team" of trainees (and the supervisor) providing EBPP. After staffing an intake, the team divides up tasks and different trainees are sent out to research existing literature as well as to take an evaluative look at available treatment manuals and assessment approaches that might be of use in providing care for particular clients. Thus, this group or team approach allows for advanced students to play important roles that may be unique from others provided by trainees with less experience.

Practicum Team Meetings

Practicum team meetings are also part of the clinical training experience and typically described to students as the place where "science and practice come together." The explicit goal is to use scientific skills and resources to address real-life clinical questions. Activities include formal presentations of active cases and didactic discussions of clinically relevant topics of students' choosing. Team meetings are often situations where the integration of clinical judgment/expertise and patient values/preferences with research evidence is modeled and thus is a critical component to supervised clinical experience. In fact, team didactics often focus upon relevant themes including clinical judgment and decision making (both strengths and weaknesses) and patient values in practice (e.g., cultural diversity, spirituality). Participation in the team is conceptualized as an opportunity to "fill in the blanks" between the classroom and practice and to encourage and model an integration of the various didactic and experiential components of training.

THE FUTURE OF TRAINING IN EBPP

EBPP is the contemporary evolved state of a revolution in clinical practice that began both outside psychology (evidence-based medicine) and within psychology (empirically supported treatments). The operationalization of

EBPP provided by the APA policy statement (2006) is still very new, and the impacts upon training for the future generations of psychologists is unknown. In this chapter, we have highlighted important issues in the current status of our field in regards to evidence-based practice, speculated about some of the implications, and shared an example of how EBPP has influenced our training model. EBPP holds the promise of bridging the long-lamented divide between scientists and practitioners, thereby more closely approximating the ideals created by the developers of the Boulder model of scientist-practitioner training (Raimy, 1950). In our view, such a development would be welcome, indeed, and would serve the future of our profession well.

REFERENCES

American Psychological Association (2002a). Criteria for evaluating treatment guidelines. *American Psychologist, 57,* 1052–1059.

American Psychological Association (2002b). Criteria for practice guideline development and evaluation. *American Psychologist, 57,* 1048–1051.

APA Presidential Task Force on Evidence-Based Practice (2006). Evidence-based practice in psychology. *American Psychologist, 61,* 271–285.

Arredondo, P., Shealy, C., Neale, M., & Winfrey, L. L. (2004). Consultation and interprofessional collaboration: Modeling for the future. *Journal of Clinical Psychology, 60,* 787–800.

Barlow, D. H. (2001). *Clinical Handbook of Psychological Disorders: A Step-by-Step Treatment Manual,* 3rd ed. New York: Guilford Press.

Barlow, D. H. (2004). Psychological treatments. *American Psychologist, 59,* 869–879.

Barlow, D. H., Levitt, J. T., & Bufka, L. F. (1999). The dissemination of empirically supported treatments: A view to the future. *Behaviour Research & Therapy, 37,* 147–162.

Belar, C. D., Brown, R. A., Hersch, L. E., Hornyak, L. M., Rozensky, R. H., Sheridan, E. P., et al. (2001). Self-assessment in clinical health psychology: A model for ethical expansion of practice. *Professional Psychology: Research & Practice, 32,* 135–141.

Belar, C. D., & Perry, N. W. (1992). National conference on scientist-practitioner education and training for the professional practice of psychology. *American Psychologist, 47,* 71–75.

Berg, A. O. (2000). Dimensions of evidence. In J. P. Geyman, R. A. Deyo, & S. D. Ramsey (Eds.), *Evidence-Based Clinical Practice: Concepts and Approaches* (pp. 21–27). Boston: Butterworth Heinemann.

Bieschke, K. J., Fouad, N. A., Collins, F. L., Jr., & Halonen, J. S. (2004). The scientifically-minded psychologist: Science as a core competency. *Journal of Clinical Psychology, 60,* 713–723.

Chambless, D. L., Baker, M. J., Baucom, D. H., Beutler, L. E., Calhoun, K. S., Crits-Christoph, P., et al. (1998). Update on empirically validated therapies, II. *The Clinical Psychologist, 51,* 3–16.

Chambless, D. L., & Hollon, S. D. (1998). Defining empirically supported therapies. *Journal of Consulting & Clinical Psychology, 66,* 7–18.

Chambless, D. L., & Ollendick, T. H. (2001). Empirically supported psychological interventions: Controversies and evidence. *Annual Review of Psychology, 52,* 685–716.

Chambless, D. L., Sanderson, W. C., Shoham, V., Bennett Johnson, S., Pope, K. S., Crits-Christoph, P., et al. (1996). An update on empirically validated therapies. *The Clinical Psychologist, 49,* 5–18.

Collins, F. L., Jr., Kaslow, N. J., & Illfelder-Kaye, J. (2004). Introduction to the Special Issue. *Journal of Clinical Psychology, 60,* 695–697.

Cukrowicz, K. C., White, B. A., Reitzel, L. R., Burns, A. B., Driscoll, K. A., Kemper, T. S., et al. (2005). Improved treatment outcome associated with the shift to empirically supported treatments in a graduate training clinic. *Professional Psychology: Research and Practice, 36,* 330–337.

Daniel, J. H., Roysircar, G., Abeles, N., & Boyd, C. (2004). Individual and cultural-diversity competency: Focus on the therapist. *Journal of Clinical Psychology, 60,* 755–770.

de las Fuentes, C., Willmuth, M. E., & Yarrow, C. (2005). Competency training in ethics education and practice. *Professional Psychology: Research and Practice, 36,* 362–366.

Des Jarlais, D. C., Lyles, C., & Crepaz, N. (2004). Improving the reporting quality of nonrandomized evaluations of behavioral and public health interventions: The TREND statement. *American Journal of Public Health, 94,* 361–366.

Elman, N. S., Illfelder-Kaye, J., & Robiner, W. N. (2005). Professional development: Training for professionalism as a foundation for competent practice in psychology. *Professional Psychology: Research and Practice, 36,* 367–375.

Falender, C. A., Cornish, J. A. E., Goodyear, R., Hatcher, R., Kaslow, N. J., Leventhal, G., et al. (2004). Defining competencies in psychology supervision: A consensus statement. *Journal of Clinical Psychology, 60,* 771–785.

Institute of Medicine (2001). *Crossing the Quality Chasm: A New Health System for the 21st Century.* Washington, DC: National Academy Press.

Institute of Medicine (2002). *Health Professions Education: A Bridge to Quality.* Washington, DC: National Academy Press.

Institute of Medicine (2003). *Priority Areas for National Action: Transforming Health Care Quality.* Washington, DC: National Academy Press.

Kaslow, N. J., Borden, K. A., Collins, F. L., Jr., Forrest, L., Illfelder-Kaye, J., Nelson, P. D., et al. (2004). Competencies conference: Future directions in education and credentialing in professional psychology. *Journal of Clinical Psychology, 60,* 699–712.

Kazdin, A. E., & Weisz, J. R. (Eds.) (2003). *Evidence-Based Psychotherapies for Children and Adolescents.* New York: Guilford Press.

Kendall, P. C. (1998). Empirically supported psychological therapies. *Journal of Consulting and Clinical Psychology, 66,* 3–6.

Krishnamurthy, R., VandeCreek, L., Kaslow, N. J., Tazeau, Y. N., Miville, M. L., Kerns, R., et al. (2004). Achieving competency in psychological assessment: Directions for education and training. *Journal of Clinical Psychology, 60,* 725–739.

Leffingwell, T. R. (2006). The behavior therapy seminar series: A method for teaching evidence-based practice. *The Behavior Therapist, 29,* 77–80.

McCabe, O. L. (2004). Crossing the quality chasm in behavioral health care: The role of evidence-based practice. *Professional Psychology: Research & Practice, 35,* 571.

Miller, W. R., Yahne, C. E., Moyers, T. B., Martinez, J., & Pirritano, M. (2004). A randomized trial of methods to help clinicians learn motivational interviewing. *Journal of Consulting and Clinical Psychology, 72,* 1050–1062.

Moher, D., Schulz, K. F., & Altman, D. (2001). The CONSORT statement: Revised recommendations for improving the quality of reports of parallel-group randomized trials. *JAMA, 285,* 1987–1991.

Raimy, V. (Ed.) (1950). *Training in Clinical Psychology.* New York: Prentice-Hall.

Roberts, M. C., Borden, K. A., Christiansen, M. D., & Lopez, S. J. (2005). Fostering a culture shift: Assessment of competence in the education and careers of professional psychologists. *Professional Psychology: Research and Practice, 36,* 355–361.

Roth, A., & Fonagy, P. (1996). *What Works for Whom? A Critical Review of Psychotherapy Research.* New York: Guilford Press.

Roth, A., & Fonagy, P. (2004). *What Works for Whom? A Critical Review of Psychotherapy Research,* 2nd ed. New York: Guilford Press.

Sackett, D. L., Rosenberg, W. M., Gray, J. A., Haynes, R. B., & Richardson, W. S. (1996). Evidence based medicine: What it is and what it isn't. *British Medical Journal, 312,* 71–72.

Sackett, D. L., Straus, S. E., Richardson, W. S., Rosenberg, W. M., & Haynes, R. B. (2000). *Evidence Based Medicine: How to Practice and Teach EBM,* 2nd ed. London: Churchill Livingstone.

Sholomskas, D. E., Syracuse-Siewert, G., Rounsaville, B. J., Ball, S. A., Nuro, K. F., & Carroll, K. M. (2005). We don't train in vain: A dissemination trial of three strategies of training clinicians in cognitive-behavioral therapy. *Journal of Consulting & Clinical Psychology, 73,* 106–115.

Spruill, J., Rozensky, R. H., Stigall, T. T., Vasquez, M., Bingham, R. P., & De Vaney Olvey, C. (2004). Becoming a competent clinician: Basic competencies in intervention. *Journal of Clinical Psychology, 60,* 741–754.

Stirman, S. W., DeRubeis, R. J., Crits-Christoph, P., & Brody, P. E. (2003). Are samples in randomized controlled trials of psychotherapy representative of community outpatients? A new methodology and initial findings. *Journal of Consulting and Clinical Psychology, 71,* 963–972.

Stone, A. A. (2003). Editorial: Modification to "Instructions for Authors." *Health Psychology, 22,* 331.

Task Force on Promotion and Dissemination of Psychological Procedures (1995). Training in and dissemination of empirically validated psychological procedures: Report and recommendations. *The Clinical Psychologist, 48,* 3–23.

Woody, S. R., Weisz, J. R., & McLean, C. (2005). Empirically supported treatments: 10 years later. *The Clinical Psychologist, 58,* 5–11.

32

Emerging Issues in the Continuing Evolution of Evidence-Based Practice

T. DAVID ELKIN, MICHAEL C. ROBERTS, and RIC G. STEELE

As we noted in the opening chapters of this handbook, "evidence-based practice in psychology" (EBPP; American Psychological Association, 2006) is an evolving concept with a multitude of influences both within and outside the profession. Because it is evolving in response to many disparate influences (e.g., professional organizations, managed care, consumer advocates, researchers, and clinicians), no single entity "owns" the concept, and likewise, there is no single arbiter deciding what can be considered "evidence-based." Rather, as new methodologies and new findings emerge and as market and professional forces continue to exert their influences, assimilation *and* accommodation must keep the EBPP movement in equilibrium: assimilation of new evidence-based therapies into clinical practice, and accommodation of the conceptualization of EBPP to account for the new findings and methodologies.

In many respects, the current conceptualization of EBPP (APA, 2005) represents a more specific recast of the earlier "what works, for whom, and under what circumstances" discussions that occurred within the larger mental health community (e.g., Armstrong et al., 1992; Paul, 1967; Roth et al., 1996; Saxe et al., 1988). The questions of "what works, for whom, and under what circumstances" (and the attempts at answers), as well as the characterization of EBPP as a three-legged stool (i.e., "integration of the best available research with clinical expertise in the context of patient characteristics, culture, and preferences"; APA, 2005, p. 1), also provide a road map for the further development of professional psychology

T. DAVID ELKIN • University of Mississippi Medical Center, **MICHAEL C. ROBERTS, and RIC G. STEELE** • University of Kansas

and the tools that it uses. We see the current volume as one step in this development, specifically with regard to children, adolescents, and families.

WHAT WORKS?

Or rather, what *can* work? As the preceding chapters in this handbook have illustrated, much has been done in terms of investigating the efficacy and effectiveness of interventions for a wide range of disorders and conditions affecting children and adolescents. Of course, the treatment literature for some conditions (e.g., anxiety and elimination disorders) is farther along than it is for others (e.g., eating disorders). Likewise, some treatment approaches have been investigated more rigorously than others, allowing for firmer conclusions about the confidence that we (the editors) feel can be placed in the approaches. Clearly, much more work is needed in terms of investigating treatments for specific conditions as well as a more diverse array of clinical approaches. Nevertheless, for almost any disorder that a child or adolescent might present with, there is at least some empirical evidence on which a clinician can base treatment decisions (Hunsley & Lee, 2007).

This point necessitates some further commentary. As described earlier in this volume, some see EBPP and its reliance on empirical evidence as intrusions into a field that is essentially philosophical in nature and so should remain open to individual influences. These commentators assert their points in strong terms. Recognizing the value of a diversity of approaches to knowing, we would argue that if psychology is to remain a science, it must continue to base its decisions on empirical means of evaluating its claims (Melchert, 2007). In contrast to metaphysical matters, in which belief systems are not subject to "proof" or "evidence" external to the individual, we view psychotherapy outcomes within the domain of *provable matters* (see Lilienfeld, 2005). That is, even if we have not asked all of the right questions to date, whether an intervention is effective within a given population falls within the category of things that are "knowable" through empirical means. The same is true of many other issues touching upon the practice of psychology (e.g., the degree to which a therapist builds a relationship with a client, the degree to which the client feels understood by the therapist).

FOR WHOM?

The work that is reported in the chapters of this volume details tremendous efforts that are yielding tremendous fruits. However, to reverse the poet's metaphor: *Though much is taken, much abides* . We know an extraordinary amount about how to treat many disorders in children and adolescents, but there is, of course, much to learn. Among the most important questions for professional psychology to address is "For whom are these treatments most effective?" This question lies as the basis of one of the "legs" of the EBPP stool (i.e., "... in the context of patient characteristics, culture, and preferences") and has begun to be addressed by a number of clinical researchers.

Most frequently (but not frequently enough), this question has been asked in terms of ethnic or racial diversity: "What is the extent to which current evidence-based therapies can be applied to diverse populations?" As noted by Kotchick and Grover (Chapter 27), the majority of empirical research into the effectiveness of therapeutic approaches and techniques has been conducted within samples that lack significant cultural or ethnic diversity. Kotchick and Grover go on to suggest that this circumstance leaves the clinician with difficult choices: Does the clinician *assume* that a treatment validated primarily within European-American samples is likely to be equally effective for a client who is Latino/a? Or does the clinician *assume* that the approach is not likely to be effective and choose an alternate treatment approach that has yet to be empirically validated in any sample?

We would argue that either assumption does a disservice to the community. Specifically, that ignoring potential differences and responses to therapy across cultural groups is no more or less unethical than delivery of a treatment with no known efficacy. Given the evidence presented in many of the preceding chapters for the effectiveness of a number of treatments across cultural groups, we recommend the application of therapies with the best empirical support, delivered with cultural sensitivity. That is, delivered with enough flexibility and sensitivity to the individual clients' world-views and current circumstances to impart the "effective ingredients" of the therapy in a manner that can be understood and applied in the cultural milieu of the client (see Kendall & Beidas, 2007; Kotchick & Grover, Chapter 27). As will be discussed below, this assumes a high degree of general clinical competence as well as cultural competence on the part of the clinician working with diverse samples.

This recommendation in no way invalidates what we see as a significant need for additional research to examine cultural variables in relation to treatment response. However, rather than examining whether *Treatment X* is—or is not—effective within a particular culture, we recommend evaluation of theory-based reasons for differences in treatment response across cultural groups. Given the extreme diversity within both ethnic minority *and* majority cultural groups across a number of dimensions (e.g., socioeconomic, spiritual, political, etc.), a broader examination of what variables predict treatment adherence, acceptability, and response is imperative.

Equally important to the "for whom" question (but less frequently examined) are questions regarding the role of *client preferences* in treatment selection. This variable has been much more clearly articulated in the APA statement on EBPP (2005) than it has been empirically investigated. However, some studies already attest to the importance of treatment acceptability (or preference) on treatment selection. For example, Nelson et al. (2006) conducted focus groups among providers of child and adolescent mental health services at two community mental health centers. Results indicated that, among other client characteristics, therapists routinely consider client preference when choosing treatment approaches. Nevertheless, while some research exists on treatment acceptability, much more research into the construct is necessary if client preference is to be considered when designing, evaluating, disseminating, and choosing therapies.

One aspect of client preference is *consumer satisfaction*, which has enjoyed some popularity in the treatment outcomes literature and serves as a model for further investigation of client preference (Nelson & Steele, 2006; Roberts & Steele, 2005). A variety of different measures and approaches to measuring satisfaction has been employed (see Steele, Mize Nelson, & Nelson, Chapter 3). These instruments vary by length, reporter (child vs. adult), and focus. Cohen, McLaren, and Lim (Chapter 16) note the importance of dimensions such as environment, treatment acceptability, length of treatment, and cost and ease of implementation as important aspects of consumer satisfaction to consider. A commonality across most existing measures of satisfaction, however, is the retrospective nature of the measures. While this provides important information regarding how useful or effective the clients felt that a given therapy was, Nelson and Steele (2006) suggest that *prospective* evaluation of client preferences would be valuable in terms of designing and evaluating new therapies and translating such therapies into clinical practice.

UNDER WHAT CIRCUMSTANCES?

The final aspect of our question, "… under what circumstances?" is quite broad. Indeed, it may not be possible to adequately contain the myriad variables that affect, to one degree or another, the efficacy or effectiveness of treatment. However, two issues have recently come to the forefront of discussion in professional psychology, both bearing on the circumstances under which a particular intervention is likely to be effective.

First is the issue of training standards and clinical competence (viz., "integration of the best available research *with clinical expertise*…"; APA, 2005, p. 1). Regardless of the degree to which an intervention has demonstrated clinical effectiveness, the degree to which it is effective with a particular client depends on (i.e., is moderated by) the expertise of the clinician delivering it. At some level, one would hope that graduation from an accredited and reputable professional psychology training program and completion of an internship would, in and of itself, indicate a basic entry-level competence to practice psychology. Similarly, one would also hope that licensure at the state level would automatically indicate competence. However, as noted by the APA Task Force on the Assessment of Competence in Professional Psychology (2007), there is considerable latitude in what is considered competence within professional psychology and what can reasonably be expected of professionals at various levels across the professional lifespan.

Recent conferences, work groups, and task forces have begun the process of delineating core competencies that should be expected of trainees and assessed by training programs (see Kaslow, 2004; APA Task Force, 2007). As a result, consensus is beginning to emerge regarding the core and "foundational" competencies of professional psychology (APA, 2007; Kaslow, 2004). However, although the Committee on Accreditation has revised its guidelines to require training programs to demonstrate that they assess competencies (Committee on Accreditation, 2005), consensus has not yet been reached regarding when or how best to assess professional competencies.

Complicating the issue of expertise as it relates to the APA statement on EBPP is the fact that demonstration of core or foundational competencies does not translate directly into competency to administer a particular intervention. As noted above, EBPP will continue to evolve throughout the course of a professional's career, and it is certain that new therapies and approaches will develop well after a professional's formal training. Indeed, Nelson and colleagues' (2006) sample of community mental health providers noted a lack of time to learn emerging therapies as a hindrance from using newer evidence-based treatments. In partial answer to this problem, Roberts and colleagues (2005) have called for a shift toward ongoing professional assessment of competencies across the professional lifespan. Such a shift might include the assessment of the degree to which clinicians are staying abreast of the clinical treatment literature and seeking meaningful continuing education to maintain state-of-the-science standards of care. As noted by Leffingwell and Collins, Jr. (Chapter 31), a focus on the importance of life-long learning and regular self-assessment of clinical competencies (e.g., Belar et al., 2001) is essential for the continued growth and development of the professional.

Also making up the set of circumstances that affect treatment effectiveness is the relationship that the therapist creates with the client. Although few empirical studies of the impact of relational capacity or relational competence (e.g., therapeutic alliance) have been presented in the literature, we are encouraged by the few studies reviewed by Shirk and McMakin (Chapter 26). Of particular importance will be investigations further identifying the client and therapist variables that contribute to the relationship developed during therapy and subsequent studies evaluating the impact of such variables on treatment outcome.

CONCLUSIONS: WHERE DO WE GO FROM HERE?

And this is where the science of psychology must go. We need research not only on what types of EBPPs work, but also on how we train psychologists to deliver them. We need research on how effective these treatment modalities are, with clinician competence evaluated alongside patient values. We have a better idea of what treatments work than ever before, but we have only some emerging ideas of ways to measure who should deliver these treatments (i.e., competence) and how they are received by different populations (e.g., across heterogeneous preferences, values, cultures). Scientific foundations are necessary to all three components of the three-legged stool of EBPP. It is essential that, in addition, empirical research moves into these areas as well. And these investigations should look to and incorporate the expertise of independent practitioners, because these individuals have the experience and ability to devise interventions that can be delivered in the community.

Ultimately, the question comes down to this: How do we provide the best care for all human beings and yet respect human nature? Ethically, this is a consideration of beneficence and autonomy. But the real goal with EBPP is not to find the perfect manualized treatment for every shade of psychopathology, though this might be helpful. Rather, the true goal is to take known treatments and interventions and apply them in such a way that most people who receive them will benefit: in short, to have beneficence and autonomy together—which is, by the way, the goal of ethical behavior.

REFERENCES

American Psychological Association (2005). *Policy statement on evidence-based practice in psychology.* Accessed on January 6, 2007, from http://www.apa.org/practice/ebpstatement.pdf.

American Psychological Association Presidential Task Force on Evidence-Based Practice (2006). Evidence-based practice in psychology. *American Psychologist, 61,* 271–285.

American Psychological Association Task Force on the Assessment of Competence in Professional Psychology (2007, November). *Task Force on the Assessment of Competence in Professional Psychology: Executive summary.* Washington, DC: American Psychological Association.

Armstrong, M. I., Huz, S., & Evans, M. E. (1992). What works for whom: The design and evaluation of children's mental health services. *Social Work Research and Abstracts, 28,* 35–41.

Belar, C. D., Brown, R. A., Hersch, L. E., Hornyak, L. M., Rozensky, R. H., Sheridan, E. P., et al. (2001). Self-assessment in clinical health psychology: A model for ethical expansion of practice. *Professional Psychology: Research and Practice, 32,* 135–141.

Committee on Accreditation (2005). *Guidelines and Principles for Accreditation of Programs in Professional Psychology.* Washington, DC: American Psychological Association.

Hunsley, J., & Lee, C. M. (2007). Research-informed benchmarks for psychological treatments: Efficacy studies, effectiveness studies, and beyond. *Professional Psychology: Research and Practice, 38,* 21–33.

Kaslow, N. J. (2004). Competencies in professional psychology. *American Psychologist, 59,* 774–781.

Kendall, P. C., & Beidas, R. S. (2007). Smoothing the trail for dissemination of evidence-based practices for youth: Flexibility within fidelity. *Professional Psychology: Research and Practice, 38,* 13–20.

Lilienfeld, S. O. (2005). The 10 commandments of helping students distinguish science from pseudoscience in psychology. *The APS Observer, 18,* 39–40, 49–51.

Melchert, T. P. (2007). Strengthening the scientific foundations of professional psychology: Time for the next steps. *Professional Psychology: Research and Practice, 38,* 34–43.

Nelson, T. D., & Steele, R. G. (2006). Beyond efficacy and effectiveness: A multifaceted approach to treatment evaluation. *Professional Psychology: Research and Practice, 37,* 389–397.

Nelson, T. D., Steele, R. G., & Mize, J. (2006). Practitioner attitudes toward evidence-based practice: Themes and challenges. *Administration and Policy in Mental Health and Mental Health Services Research, 33 ,* 398–409.

Paul, G. L. (1967). Outcome research in psychotherapy. *Journal of Consulting Psychology, 31,* 109–118.

Roberts, M. C., Borden, K. A., Christiansen, M. D., & Lopez, S. J. (2005). Fostering a culture shift: Assessment of competence in the education and careers of professional psychologists. *Professional Psychology: Research and Practice, 36,* 355–361.

Roberts, M. C., & Steele, R. G. (2005). Program evaluation approaches to service delivery in child and family mental health. In R. G. Steele & M. C. Roberts (Eds.), *Handbook of Mental Health Services for Children, Adolescents, and Families* (pp. 351–369). New York: Kluwer Academic/Plenum Publishers.

Roth, A., Fonagy, P., Parry, G., Target, M., & Woods, R. (1996). *What Works for Whom? A Critical Review of Psychotherapy Research.* New York: Guilford Press.

Saxe, L., Cross, T., & Silverman, N. (1988). Children's mental health: The gap between what we know and what we do. *American Psychologist, 43,* 800–807.

Index